1001 Questions

An Interventional Cardiology Board Review

1001 Questions

An Interventional Cardiology Board Review

EDITORS

Debabrata Mukherjee, MD

Professor and Vice-Chairman of Medicine
Chief, Division of Cardiovascular Medicine
Department of Internal Medicine
Texas Tech University Health Sciences Center
Paul L. Foster School of Medicine
El Paso, Texas

Leslie Cho, MD

Director, Women's Cardiovascular Center
Section Head, Preventive Cardiology and Rehabilitation
Robert and Suzanne Tomsich Department of Cardiovascular Medicine
Cleveland Clinic
Cleveland, Ohio

David J. Moliterno, MD

Jack M. Gill Chair and Professor of Medicine
Department of Internal Medicine
Gill Heart Institute
University of Kentucky
Lexington, Kentucky

Julie P. Hoffmann

Publications Production Manager
Gill Heart Institute
University of Kentucky
Lexington, Kentucky

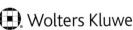

Wolters Kluwer | Lippincott Williams & Wilkins
Health

Philadelphia · Baltimore · New York · London
Buenos Aires · Hong Kong · Sydney · Tokyo

Acquisitions Editor: Frances R. DeStefano
Product Manager: Leanne Vandetty
Production Manager: Bridgett Dougherty
Senior Manufacturing Manager: Benjamin Rivera
Marketing Manager: Kimberly Schonberger
Design Coordinator: Stephen Druding
Production Service: SPi Global

Library of Congress Cataloging-in-Publication Data

1001 questions : an interventional cardiology board review / editors, Debabrata Mukherjee, Leslie Cho, David J. Moliterno.
     p. ; cm.
   One thousand one questions : an interventional cardiology board review
   One thousand and one questions : an interventional cardiology board review
   Rev. ed. of: 900 questions / editors, Debabrata Mukherjee ... [et al.]. c2007.
   Includes bibliographical references and index.
   ISBN 978-1-4511-1299-3 (pbk. : alk. paper) 1. Heart—Diseases—Treatment—Examinations, questions, etc. 2. Cardiovascular system—Diseases—Treatment—Examinations, questions, etc. I. Mukherjee, Debabrata. II. Cho, Leslie. III. Moliterno, David J. IV. 900 questions. V. Title: One thousand one questions : an interventional cardiology board review. VI. Title: One thousand and one questions : an interventional cardiology board review.
   [DNLM: 1. Cardiovascular Diseases—diagnosis—Examination Questions. 2. Cardiovascular Diseases—therapy—Examination Questions. WG 18.2]
   RC683.8.N564 2012
   616.1'20076—dc23
                                                                    2011025554

"To interventional fellows everywhere for their hard work and dedication to patient care; to my parents for their infinite patience, love, and understanding and who continue to be my source of inspiration; and to Suchandra, for her love and support."

—DEBABRATA MUKHERJEE

"To the interventional fellows at Cleveland Clinic past, present, and future for their dedication and hard work with gratitude."

—LESLIE CHO

"To my friends, colleagues, and fellows at the University of Kentucky who strive to find answers to the increasingly challenging questions being asked of us all in contemporary medical practice."

—DAVID J. MOLITERNO

Insightful questions have been used throughout the ages as a metric to assess one's knowledge, but when coupled with carefully delivered answers, they can become a powerful teaching tool. This book of questions and annotated answers covering the field of interventional cardiology is meant to serve as a helpful resource for individuals preparing for the interventional cardiovascular medicine board examination as well as for clinicians who wish to perform an in-depth self-assessment on individual topics or the full spectrum. The book has many key features, which we believe will make the reader successful in passing the boards and improving clinical practice.

Of foremost importance, the areas covered are relevant not only to the day-to-day practice of interventional cardiology but have also been patterned in scope and content to the actual board examination. The book begins with several chapters dedicated to the anatomy and physiology associated with interventional cardiology and the pathobiology of atherosclerosis and inflammation. This corresponds to the 15% of the board examination targeting material in basic science. The subsequent chapters focus on the essential interventional pharmacotherapy of antiplatelets, anticoagulants, and other commonly used medications in the catheterization laboratory and outpatient setting for patients with atherosclerosis. These chapters correspond to the next 15% of the boards centering on pharmacology. A similar-sized 15% of the board examination is directed toward imaging, and the book includes specific chapters on radiation safety, catheterization laboratory equipment and technique, contrast agents, and intravascular ultrasound. The two largest areas of the examination, each covering 25% of the content, include case selection–management and procedural techniques. The review book dedicates 28 chapters to comprehensively cover these areas. Finally, we have included chapters for the miscellaneous remaining areas covered by the board examination, including peripheral vascular disease, cerebrovascular and structural heart interventions, ethics, statistics, and epidemiology, as well as a chapter directed at improving test-taking skills.

Also essential to the quality and appropriateness of the questions and annotated answers is the expertise of the chapter authors. We are fortunate to have assembled the "who's who of academic interventional cardiology." The contributing authors from leading medical centers around the world have over 6,000 articles cited in PubMed. We are greatly indebted to these authors who are recognized both for their interventional expertise and for their teaching skills. In the end, the true value of this textbook is not only the relevance of the questions, the outstanding quality of the authors, but also the value of the annotated answers. The text includes 1110 questions and 411 figures and tables. The corresponding answers have been appropriately detailed to provide relevant facts and information as well as up-to-date journal citations.

The practice of interventional cardiology is exciting, rewarding, and a privilege each of us enjoys. Likewise, it has been our privilege to work with the superb contributors, our colleagues in interventional cardiology, as well as the editorial team at the University of Kentucky and Lippincott Williams & Wilkins. It is our personal hope that you will enjoy this book and that it will be a valuable resource to you in passing the board examination and providing the highest quality care possible to your patients.

Debabrata Mukherjee, MD
Leslie Cho, MD
David J. Moliterno, MD

Carlos L. Alviar, MD

Chief Resident, Internal Medicine
St. Luke's - Roosevelt Hospital Center
Columbia University College of Physicians and Surgeons
New York, New York

Dominick J. Angiolillo, MD, PhD

Associate Professor of Medicine
Director, Cardiovascular Research
University of Florida College of Medicine
Jacksonville, Florida

Robert J. Applegate, MD

Professor of Internal Medicine
The Heart Center at Wake Forest Baptist Medical Center
Wake Forest University
Winston-Salem, North Carolina

Joseph Babb, MD

Professor of Medicine
Cardiovascular Sciences
East Carolina University Brody School of Medicine
Greenville, North Carolina

Thomas M. Bashore, MD

Professor of Medicine
Clinical Chief, Division of Cardiology
Duke University Medical Center
Durham, North Carolina

David C. Booth, MD

Endowed Professor of Medicine
University of Kentucky
Chief of Cardiology
Lexington VA Medical Center
Lexington, Kentucky

Sorin J. Brener, MD

Professor of Medicine
Weill Cornell Medical College
Director, Cardiac Catheterization Laboratory
New York Methodist Hospital
Brooklyn, New York

Ivan P. Casserly, MD

Associate Professor of Medicine
University of Colorado Hospital
Aurora, Colorado

Leslie Cho, MD

Section Head, Preventive Cardiology and Rehabilitation
Robert and Suzanne Tomsich Department of Cardiovascular
    Medicine
Cleveland Clinic Foundation
Cleveland, Ohio

Antonio Colombo, MD

Interventional Cardiology Unit
San Raffaele Scientific Institute
EMO-GVM Centro Cuore Columbus
Milan, Italy

Harold L. Dauerman, MD

Professor of Medicine
Director, Cardiovascular Catheterization Laboratories
University of Vermont
Fletcher Allen Health Care, Cardiac Unit
Burlington, Vermont

Steven R. Daugherty, PhD

Department of Psychology
Rush Medical College
Chicago, Illinois

Gregory J. Dehmer, MD

Professor of Medicine
Texas A & M Health Science Center College of Medicine
Director, Cardiology Division
Scott & White Healthcare
College Station and Temple, Texas

José G. Díez, MD

Medical Director Cardiovascular Program
CHRISTUS St. Catherine Hospital
Professional Staff Interventional Cardiology
St. Luke's Episcopal Hospital/Texas Heart Institute
Houston, Texas

Steven P. Dunn, PharmD

Pharmacy Clinical Coordinator, Cardiology
Department of Pharmacy Services
University of Virginia Health System
Charlottesville, Virginia

Mark J. Eisenberg, MD, MPH

Professor of Medicine
Jewish General Hospital
McGill University
Montreal, Quebec, Canada

Amy L. Elsass, MD

Solaris Heart and Vascular
Marietta, Georgia

David P. Faxon, MD

Senior Lecturer
Harvard Medical School
Vice Chair of Medicine for Strategic Planning
Brigham and Women's Hospital
Boston, Massachusetts

Joel A. Garcia, MD

Assistant Professor of Medicine
University of Colorado Hospital
Director, Cardiac Catheterization Laboratories
Denver Health Medical Center
Denver, Colorado

Thomas Gehrig, MD

Assistant Professor of Medicine
Division of Cardiovascular Medicine
Duke University Medical Center
Durham, North Carolina

Bernard Gersh, MD, ChB, DPhil

Professor of Medicine
Mayo Clinic College of Medicine
Consultant in Cardiovascular Diseases
Mayo Clinic
Rochester, Minnesota

John C. Gurley, MD, MBA

Professor of Medicine
Division of Cardiovascular Medicine
Director, Interventional Cardiology
University of Kentucky
Lexington, Kentucky

Robert A. Harrington, MD

Professor of Medicine
Division of Cardiology
Director, Duke Clinical Research Institute
Durham, North Carolina

Stephen A. Hart, MD

Resident, Pediatrics
Children's Hospital of Pittsburgh
University of Pittsburgh Medical Center
Pittsburgh, Pennsylvania

Howard C. Herrmann, MD

Professor of Medicine
Cardiovascular Division, Department of Medicine
Director, Cardiac Catheterization Laboratories
University of Pennsylvania School of Medicine
Philadelphia, Pennsylvania

L. David Hillis, MD

Professor and Chairman
Department of Internal Medicine
University of Texas Health Science Center
San Antonio, Texas

Alice K. Jacobs, MD

Professor of Medicine
Boston University School of Medicine
Director, Cardiac Catheterization Laboratories
Boston Medical Center
Boston, Massachusetts

Hani Jneid, MD

Assistant Professor of Medicine
Baylor College of Medicine
Assistant Director of Interventional Cardiology
Michael E. DeBakey VA Medical Center
Houston, Texas

Arun Kalyanasundaram, MD, MPH

Interventional Cardiology Fellow
Robert and Suzanne Tomsich Department of Cardiovascular
  Medicine
Cleveland Clinic Foundation
Cleveland, Ohio

David E. Kandzari, MD

Director, Interventional Cardiology and Interventional
  Cardiology Research
Piedmont Heart Institute
Atlanta, Georgia

Samir Kapadia, MD

Professor of Medicine
Director, Sones Cardiac Catheterization Laboratories
Robert and Suzanne Tomsich Department of Cardiovascular
  Medicine
Cleveland Clinic Foundation
Cleveland, Ohio

Dimitri Karmpaliotis, MD

Interventional Cardiology
Piedmont Heart Institute
Atlanta, Georgia

Prashant Kaul, MD

Assistant Professor of Medicine
UNC Center for Heart & Vascular Care
Division of Cardiology
University of North Carolina
Chapel Hill, North Carolina

Morton J. Kern, MD

Professor of Medicine
Chief of Cardiology, Long Beach VA Hospital
Associate Chief of Cardiology
University California Irvine School of Medicine
Orange, California

Richard A. Krasuski, MD

Director of Adult Congenital Heart Disease Services
Robert and Suzanne Tomsich Department of Cardiovascular
   Medicine
Cleveland Clinic Foundation
Cleveland, Ohio

Richard A. Lange, MD

Professor and Executive Vice-Chairman
Department of Internal Medicine
University of Texas Health Science Center
San Antonio, Texas

Azeem Latib, MD

Interventional Cardiology Unit
San Raffaele Scientific Institute
EMO-GVM Centro Cuore Columbus
Milan, Italy

Evan Lau, MD

Interventional Cardiology Fellow
Robert and Suzanne Tomsich Department of Cardiovascular
   Medicine
Cleveland Clinic Foundation
Cleveland, OH

Ferdinand Leya, MD

Director of Interventional Cardiology
Cardiology Department
Loyola University, Chicago
Maywood, Illinois

Tracy E. Macaulay, PharmD

Assistant Professor
College of Pharmacy
Clinical Pharmacy Specialist, Cardiology
University of Kentucky
Lexington, Kentucky

Andrew O. Maree, MD

Associate Professor of Medicine
Boston University School of Medicine
Boston Medical Center
Boston, Massachusetts

Bernhard Meier, MD

Professor and Chairman of Cardiology
Department of Cardiology
Swiss Cardiovascular Center Bern
University Hospital
Bern, Switzerland

Timothy A. Mixon, MD

Associate Professor of Medicine
Department of Medicine
Texas A & M Health Science Center College of Medicine
Scott & White Healthcare
College Station and Temple, Texas

David J. Moliterno, MD

Jack M. Gill Chair and Professor of Medicine
Department of Internal Medicine
Gill Heart Institute
University of Kentucky
Lexington, Kentucky

Pedro R. Moreno, MD

Associate Professor of Medicine
Director, Translational Research
Interventional Cardiology
Mount Sinai School of Medicine
New York, New York

Debabrata Mukherjee, MD

Professor and Vice-Chairman of Medicine
Chief, Division of Cardiovascular Medicine
Texas Tech University Health Sciences Center
Paul L. Foster School of Medicine
El Paso, Texas

Brahmajee K. Nallamothu, MD, MPH

Associate Professor of Internal Medicine
Interventional Cardiology
University of Michigan Cardiovascular Center
Ann Arbor, Michigan

Craig R. Narins, MD

Associate Professor of Medicine
Cardiology Division
University of Rochester Medical Center
Rochester, New York

Zoran S. Nedlijkovic, MD

Assistant Professor of Medicine
Boston University School of Medicine
Director, Interventional Cardiology Fellowship Program
Boston Medical Center
Boston, Massachusetts

Stephane Noble, MD

Division of Cardiology
University Hospital
Geneva, Switzerland

Igor F. Palacios, MD

Associate Professor of Medicine
Harvard Medical School
Director, Knight Catheterization Laboratory
Massachusetts General Hospital
Boston, Massachusetts

Karen S. Pieper, MS

Associate Director, Clinical Trial Statistics
Duke Clinical Research Institute
Durham, North Carolina

Thomas Pilgrim, MD

Department of Cardiology
Swiss Cardiovascular Center Bern
Bern University Hospital
Bern, Switzerland

Sunil V. Rao, MD

Associate Professor of Medicine
Duke University Medical Center
Director, Cardiac Catheterization Laboratories
Durham VA Medical Center
Durham, NC

Michael C. Reed, MD

Interventional Cardiology
International Heart Institute of Montana Foundation
St. Patrick's Hospital
Missoula, MT 59802

Eric Reyes, MS

Clinical Trial Statistics
Duke Clinical Research Institute
Durham, North Carolina

Marco Roffi, MD

Associate Professor
Director, Interventional Cardiology Unit
Division of Cardiology
University Hospital
Geneva, Switzerland

Raul A. Schwartzman, MD

Staff Physician
New York Methodist Hospital
Brooklyn, New York

Avi Shimony, MD

Department of Cardiology
Jewish General Hospital
McGill University
Montreal, Quebec, Canada

Mehdi H. Shishehbor, DO, MPH

Staff, Interventional Cardiology and Vascular Medicine
Associate Program Director, Interventional Cardiology
Robert and Suzanne Tomsich Department of Cardiovascular
    Medicine
Cleveland Clinic Foundation
Cleveland, Ohio

Paul Sorajja, MD

Associate Professor of Medicine
Mayo Clinic College of Medicine
Mayo Clinic
Rochester, Minnesota

James E. Tcheng, MD

Professor of Medicine
Professor of Community and Family Medicine
Duke University Medical Center
Durham, North Carolina

E. Murat Tuzcu, MD

Professor of Medicine
Vice-Chairman, Cardiovascular Medicine
Cleveland Clinic Foundation
Cleveland, Ohio

Christopher R. Walters, MD

Assistant Professor of Medicine
Duke Cardiology of Lumberton
Southeastern Regional Medical Center
Lumberton, North Carolina

Peter Wenaweser, MD

Associate Professor of Cardiology
Director, Invasive Cardiology
Swiss Cardiovascular Center
University Hospital Bern
Bern, Switzerland

Stephan Windecker, MD

Professor and Chief of Cardiology
Director of Structural Invasive Cardiology
Swiss Cardiovascular Center Bern
Bern University Hospital
Bern, Switzerland

Brion M. Winston, MD, MPH

Regional Health Doctors
Rapid City Regional Hospital
Rapid City, South Dakota

Khaled M. Ziada, MD

Gill Foundation Professor of Interventional Cardiology
Director, Cardiac Catheterization Laboratories
Gill Heart Institute
University of Kentucky
Lexington, Kentucky

CONTENTS

AAA	abdominal aortic aneurysm
ABI	ankle-brachial index
ABIM	American Board of Internal Medicine
ACAS	Asymptomatic Carotid Atherosclerosis Study
ACC	American College of Cardiology
ACCF	American College of Cardiology Foundation
ACE	angiotensin-converting enzyme
ACEI	angiotensin-converting enzyme inhibitor
ACGME	Accredited Council for Graduate Medical Education
ACLS	Advanced Cardiac Life Support
ACP	American College of Physicians
ACS	acute coronary syndrome
ACT	Acetylcysteine for Contrast-Induced Nephropathy Trial
ACT	activated clotting time
ACUITY	Acute Catheterization and Urgent Intervention Triage strategy
AD	advance directive
ADP	adenosine diphosphate
AHA	American Heart Association
AIVR	accelerated idioventricular rhythm
ALARA	As Low As Reasonably Achievable
ALI	acute limb ischemia
AMI	acute myocardial infarction
ANA	antinuclear antibody
Apo E	apolipoprotein E
aPTT	activated partial thromboplastin time
APV	average peak velocity
ARC	Academic Research Consortium
ARFD	acute renal failure requiring dialysis
AS	aortic stenosis
ASA	acetylsalicylic acid
ASD	atrial septal defect
ATP III	Adult Treatment Panel III
AV	atrioventricular

AVM	arterial-venous malformation
AVR	aortic valve replacement
AYMYDA	atorvastatin for reduction of myocardial damage during angioplasty
BARI	Bypass vs. Angioplasty Revascularization Investigation
BE	balloon-expandable
BMI	body mass index
BMS	bare-metal stent
BNP	Brain natriuretic peptide
BP	blood pressure
BSA	body surface area
BVS	bioresorbable vascular scaffold
CABG	coronary artery bypass graft
CAD	coronary artery disease
cAMP	cyclic adenosine monophosphate
CAS	Carotid artery stenting
CBC	complete blood count
CCA	common carotid artery
CCD	charge-coupled device
CCS	Canadian Cardiovascular Society
CCU	coronary care unit
CEA	carotid endarterectomy
CFR	coronary flow reserve
CHD	coronary heart disease
CHF	congestive heart failure
CI	confidence interval
CKD	chronic kidney disease
CK-MB	creatine kinase-MB
CME	continuing medical education
CMR	Cardiovascular magnetic resonance
CNS	central nervous system
CO	cardiac output
COPD	chronic obstructive pulmonary disease
COX	cyclooxygenase
CPO	Cardiac power output
CREDO	clopidogrel for the reduction of events during observation

CREST	Carotid Revascularization Endarterectomy vs. Stenting Trial
CRP	C-reactive protein
CSA	cross-sectional area
CT	computed tomography
CTA	computed tomography angiography
CTFC	corrected TIMI Frame count
CTO	chronic total occlusion
CVA	cerebrovascular accident
CVD	comorbid cardiovascular disease
2D	two-dimensional
D2B	door-to-balloon
DAP	dose area product
DAT	dual antiplatelet therapy
DCA	directional coronary atherectomy
DES	drug-eluting stent
DM	diabetes mellitus
DNA	deoxyribonucleic acid
DNR	do not resuscitate
DREAM	Dutch Endovascular Aneurysm Management
DSA	digital subtraction angiography
DVT	deep vein thrombosis
EAST	Emory Angioplasty vs. Surgery Trial
ECA	external carotid artery
ECG	electrocardiogram
ECST	European Carotid Surgery Trial
ED	emergency department
EDRF	endothelial-derived relaxing factor
EEM	external elastic media
EEOC	Equal Employment Opportunity Commission
EES	everolimus-eluting stent
EF	ejection fraction
EKG	electrocardiogram
EMERALD	enhanced myocardial efficacy and recovery by aspiration of liberated debris
EMS	Emergency medical services
EP	electrophysiologic
EPC	endothelial progenitor cell
EPD	emboli protection device
ER	emergency room
ERBAC	excimer laser, rotational atherectomy, and balloon angioplasty comparison
ESSENCE	efficacy and safety of subcutaneous enoxaparin in non–q-wave coronary events

EVAR	endovascular aneurysm repair
FDA	Food and Drug Administration
FFR	fractional flow reserve
FIRE	FilterWire EX Randomized Evaluation
FMD	fibromuscular dysplasia
GERD	Gastroesophageal reflux disease
GFR	glomerular filtration rate
GIK	glucose–insulin–potassium
GP	glycoprotein
GPI	glycoprotein IIb/IIIa inhibitor
GRACE	Global Registry of Acute Coronary Events
HCM	hypertrophic cardiomyopathy
HDL	high density lipoprotein
HF	heart failure
HIT	heparin-induced thrombocytopenia
HMG-CoA	hydroxymethyl glutaryl coenzyme A
HORIZONS-AMI	Harmonizing Outcomes with Revascularization and Stents in Acute Myocardial Infarction
HPS	The Heart Protection Study
HR	hazard ratio
HR	heart rate
HS	hockey stick
HTN	hypertension
IABP	intraaortic balloon pump
IC	intermittent claudication
ICA	internal carotid artery
ICAM	intercellular cell adhesion molecule
ICD	Implantable cardioverter defibrillator
ICE	intracardiac echo
IC NTG	intracoronary nitroglycerin
ICU	intensive care unit
IgE	immunoglobulin E
IL	interleukin
IMA	inferior mesenteric artery
IMA	internal mammary artery
IPA	Inhibition of platelet aggregation
IRB	Institutional Review Board
ITT	intention-to-treat
IV	intravenous
IVC	inferior vena cava
IVUS	intravascular ultrasound
KERMA	kinetic energy released to matter
LA	left atrium
LAD	left anterior descending

LAD	leukocyte adhesion deficiency
LAO	left anterior oblique
LBBB	left bundle-branch block
LCB	left coronary bypass
LCX	left circumflex
LDH	lactate dehydrogenase
LDL	low-density lipoprotein
LDL-C	low-density lipoprotein cholesterol
LIMA	left internal mammary artery
LM	left main
LMCA	left main coronary artery
LMT	left main trunk
LSVC	left-sided vena cava
LTA	light transmittance aggregometry
LV	Left ventricular
LVEDP	left ventricular end dialostic pressure
LVEF	left ventricular ejection fraction
LVH	left ventricular hypertrophy
LVOT	left ventricular outflow tract
MA	malignant arrhythmias
MACE	major adverse cardiac events
MAP	mean arterial pressure
MBG	myocardial blush grade
MCA	middle cerebral artery
MCE	myocardial contrast echocardiography
MDR	multidrug resistance
MERLIN	Middlesbrough Early Revascularization to Limit Infarction
MI	myocardial infarction
MLA	minimum lumen area
MLD	minimal lumen diameter
MONA	morphine, oxygen, nitroglycerin, and aspirin
MP	multipurpose
MPA	maximal platelet aggregation
MR	mitral regurgitation
MRA	magnetic resonance angiography
MS	mitral stenosis
MVD	multivessel disease
MVP	mitral valve leaflet prolapse
NASCET	North American Symptomatic Carotid Endarterectomy Trial
NCEP	National Cholesterol Education Program
Nin-IRA	non–infarct-related artery
NNT	number needed to treat

NO	nitric oxide
NPH	neutral protamine Hagedorn
NSAID	nonsteroidal anti-inflammatory drug
NSTEMI	non–ST-segment elevation myocardial infarction
NSVT	non sustained ventricular tachycardia
NTG	nitroglycerine
NTR	no-torque right
NYHA	New York Heart Association
OCT	optical coherence tomography
OM	obtuse marginal
OR	odds ratio
PA	plasminogen-activator
PA	pulmonary arterial
PA	pulmonary artery
PAD	peripheral arterial disease
PAF	paroxysmal atrial fibrillation
PAI-1	plasminogen activator inhibitor-1
PAR-1	protease-activator receptor-1
PAV	percent atheroma volume
PB	plaque burden
PBMA	poly n-butyl methacrylate
PCI	percutaneous coronary intervention
PCL	poly(ε-caprolactone)
PCW	pulmonary capillary wedge
PCWP	pulmonary capillary wedge pressure
PD	pharmacodynamic
PDA	patent ductus arteriosus
PDA	posterior descending artery
PE	pulmonary embolism
PES	paclitaxel-eluting stent
PEVA	polyethylene-co-vinyl acetate
PFO	patent foramen ovale
PFT	pulmonary function test
PGA	poly(glycolic acid)
PK	pharmacokinetics
PKC	protein kinase C
PLC	phospholipase C
PLE	protein-losing enteropathy
PLLA	poly-L-lactic acid
PPI	proton pump inhibitor
PT	prothrombin time
PTA	percutaneous transluminal angioplasty
PTCA	percutaneous transluminal coronary angioplasty

PTSMA	Percutaneous Transluminal Septal Myocardial Ablation
PV	peripheral vascular
PV	pulmonary vein
QCA	quantitative coronary angiography
RA	right atrial
RAGE	receptor for advanced glycation end products
RAO	right anterior oblique
RAS	renin-angiostensin system
RBC	red blood cell
RCA	right coronary artery
RCB	right coronary bypass
rCRF	relative CRF
RCT	randomized clinical trial
RD	reference diameter
RI	ramus intermedius
RIMA	right internal mammary artery
RN	registered nurse
RP	retroperitoneal
RPH	retroperitoneal hematoma
RV	right ventricular
RVSP	right ventricular systolic pressure
SA	stable angina
SAFER	Saphenous Vein Graft Angioplasty Free of Emboli Randomized
SBP	systolic blood pressure
SCAI	Society of Coronary Angiography and Interventions
sCD40L	soluble CD40 ligand
SCI	Spinal cord ischemia
SD	sudden death
SE	self-expanding
SES	sirolimus-eluting stent
SFA	superficial femoral artery
SI	silent ischemia
SMA	superior mesenteric artery
SOB	shortness of breath
SS	spot stenting
STEMI	ST-elevation myocardial infarction
STR ST	resolution
SVC	superior vena cava

SVG	Saphenous vein graft
SYC	syncope
TAA	thoracic aortic aneurysm
TAPAS	Thrombus Aspiration During Percutaneous Coronary Intervention in Acute Myocardial Infarction Study
TAV	total atheroma volume
TAVI	transcatheter aortic valve replacement
TCFA	thin cap fibroatheromas
TEE	transesophageal echocardiogram
TFC	TIMI frame count
TFPI	tissue factor pathway inhibitor
TG	triglycerides
ThCFA	thick-cap fibroatheroma
TIA	transient ischemic attack
TIMI	thrombolysis in myocardial infarction
TLR	target lesion revascularization
TMP	TIMI myocardial perfusion
TMPG	TIMI myocardial perfusion grade
TNF	tumor necrosis factor
Tnl	troponin l
TnT	troponin T
TOF	Tetralogy of Fallot
TOPAS	Thrombolysis or peripheral arterial surgery trial
TOSCA	Total Occlusion Study of Canada
tPA	tissue plasminogen activator
TS	traditional stenting
TVR	target vessel revascularization
UA	unstable angina
UFH	unfractionated heparin
VASP	vasodilator-stimulated phosphoprotein
VCAM	vascular cell adhesion molecule
VF	ventricular fibrillation
VH	virtual histology
VKOR	vitamin K epoxide reductase
VL	voda left
VLDL	very low-density lipoprotein
VSD	ventricular septal defect
VSR	ventricular septal rupture
ZES	zotarolimus-eluting stent

1001 Questions

An Interventional
Cardiology Board Review

1

Vascular Biology

Pedro R. Moreno and Carlos L. Alviar

1.1 A 64-year-old female with diabetes, hypertension, and an active smoking history undergoes cardiac catheterization and stent implantation in a 90% obstructive lesion found in her left anterior descending (LAD) artery. In addition to the stented lesion, she is found to have an additional nonobstructive lesion in her proximal right coronary artery (RCA). You are suspecting that the nonobstructive lesion has a large necrotic lipid core, as shown in Figure Q1-1. The following statements are true regarding this plaque containing a lipid core, EXCEPT:

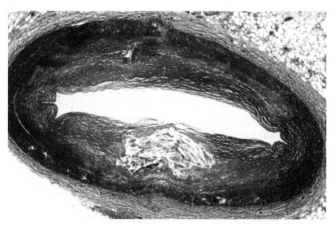

Figure Q1-1 (see color insert)

(A) It is composed of cholesterol crystals and collagen
(B) The predominant cell is the smooth muscle cell
(C) It is reflected a green structure on polarized microscopy using the Picosirius red stain
(D) It may be suitable for imaging using percutaneous techniques

1.2 You are evaluating a 59-year-old male patient with a history of diabetes, hypertension, peripheral vascular disease, hypercholesterolemia, and coronary artery disease. He has previously undergone coronary artery bypass grafting, drug-eluting stent implantation twice, and bilateral below the knee amputation. His laboratory results showed an elevated hs-CRP. Which of the following statements is FALSE regarding the pathophysiology of the atheroma of this patient?

(A) Given this advanced atherosclerosis burden, this patient has a defective resolution of inflammation
(B) The complex atherosclerotic plaques in this patient are rich in neovascularization, which is promoted by inflammation
(C) Macrophages are the main source of metalloproteinases in the plaque
(D) Plaque stabilization is characterized by defective efferocytosis

1.3 Which of the following best describes the coronary substrate that leads to the clinical presentation of this patient?

A 49-year-old male who is an active smoker is rushed into the catheterization laboratory after presenting to the emergency department with a 20 minutes history of excruciating, pressure-like substernal chest pain radiated to his left arm and associated with nausea and diaphoresis, which occurred while rapidly climbing upstairs. The initial coronary angiogram is shown in Figure Q1-3. A successful thrombectomy was performed.

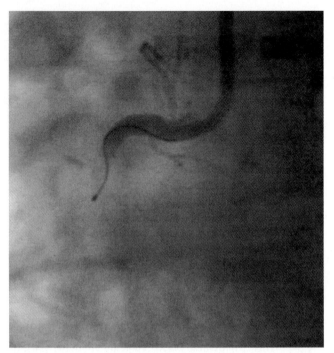

Figure Q1-3

(A) A ruptured atherosclerotic plaque with increased collagen content
(B) A ruptured atherosclerotic plaque with decreased lipid content
(C) A ruptured atherosclerotic plaque with increased proteoglycan content
(D) A ruptured atherosclerotic plaque with increased matrix metalloproteinase expression

1.4 In the patient mentioned in Question 1.3, the atherosclerotic plaque responsible for his clinical event would be characterized by the following, EXCEPT:

(A) A thrombotic thin-cap fibroatheroma characterized by cap thickness < 65 μm, macrophages, and large lipid core
(B) A ruptured plaque with extravasation of RBC's within the lipid core
(C) A plaque with multiple ruptures and extensive collagen production leading to severe stenosis (healed plaque)
(D) A plaque with increased vasa-vasorum neovascularization

1.5 You are called by the senior pathology resident at your institution, who is doing an autopsy on a 61-year-old male who died from an acute coronary syndrome. The resident reports to you evidence of intramyocardial microembolization while examining the specimens. Intravascular ultrasound of the patient performed by yourself 1 month before his death revealed a nonobstructive plaque in the proximal LAD as demonstrated

in the angiogram (Fig. Q1-5). The following statements about microemboli from epicardial vessels are true, EXCEPT:

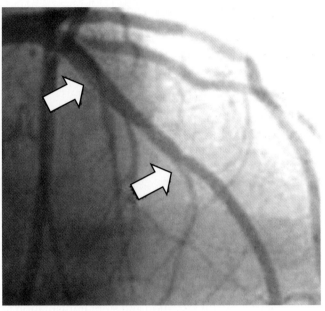

Figure Q1-5

(A) Microemboli and occluded intramyocardial vessels are most common in the RCA
(B) Microemboli contains predominately cholesterol crystals
(C) Mean stenoses of the culprit lesions is similar in those with emboli and in those without emboli
(D) Intramyocardial microemboli is more common in plaque rupture than in erosion

1.6 A 75-year-old female patient is undergoing elective cardiac catheterization for a positive stress test. As shown in Figure Q1-6, the coronary angiogram reveals a 30% lesion (left panel) in her proximal LAD artery and a 90% lesion (right panel) in her proximal RCA. Based on evidence, which of the following statements is FALSE?

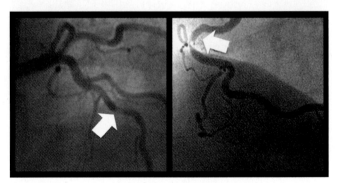

Figure Q1-6

(A) Nonobstructive lesions, like the one found in the LAD of this patient, are the most frequent cause of acute myocardial infarction (MI)

(B) A nonobstructive lesion, such as the one shown in the LAD of this angiogram, has low potential of evolving into complete occlusion silently

(C) The individual risk for plaque progression to complete occlusion is higher in nonobstructive lesions

(D) Vulnerable plaques are located predominately in the proximal segments of the coronary arteries

1.7 You are called by the emergency department to see a 38-year-old female patient who was admitted with substernal chest pain, radiating to the jaw, associated with dyspnea and vomiting. She denies smoking. All other known cardiovascular risk factors are negative. Her initial troponin is 5.4 ng/ml, and her electrocardiogram (ECG) is shown in Figure Q1-7. All of the following statements regarding plaques precipitating this problem are true, EXCEPT:

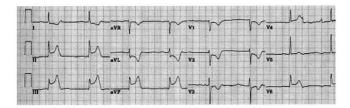

(A) It is highly possible that this patient has a ruptured atherosclerotic plaque, as these are the most common lesions responsible for coronary thrombosis in premenopausal females

(B) The most likely histologic lesion related to this patient's presentation is plaque erosion, as eroded plaques associated with thrombosis are more frequently seen in nonsmoker females

(C) Plaques with calcium nodules can precipitate coronary thrombosis in 5% of cases

(D) If this patient were to have a rupture atherosclerotic plaque, a histologic evaluation of this lesions would reveal increased macrophage content

1.8 A 72-year-old patient develops sudden onset excruciating substernal chest pain associated with severe shortness of breath. He is rapidly taken to the cardiac catheterization laboratory, where a drug-eluting stent implantation is successfully performed, as shown in Figure Q1-8.

Based on previous evidence, you consider the most likely histopathologic event leading to this patient's clinical presentation is plaque rupture. All of the following statements are true, EXCEPT:

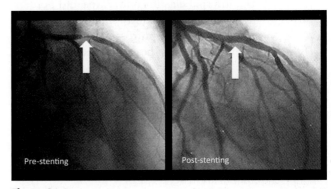

Figure Q1-8

(A) Plaque rupture may occur simultaneously in two different arteries

(B) Plaque healing after rupture is mediated by smooth muscle cell production of collagen type III

(C) Smooth muscle cells are responsible for weakening the fibrous cap

(D) T lymphocytes increase proteolytic activity and decrease collagen synthesis

1.9 A 67-year-old male sustained a witnessed cardiac arrest after complaining of sudden onset severe chest pain. He undergoes a total of 40 minutes of CPR and advanced life support without surviving the event. The family requests an autopsy; it reveals multiple nonobstructive plaques with different stages of complexity, including thrombotic occlusions (Fig. Q1-9) as well as previously healed plaques and thrombi formation. The relationship of thrombus healing to plaque morphology in sudden coronary death is characterized by the following, EXCEPT:

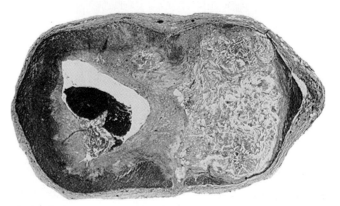

Figure Q1-9

(A) When analyzed by histology, the majority are early (<1 day) thrombus

(B) Macrophages are increased in ruptured plaques with thrombus when compared to eroded plaques with thrombus

(C) The internal elastic lamina area and percent stenosis are significantly smaller in erosions compared with ruptures

(D) Thrombus length is not associated with healing

1.10 A 67-year-old male is referred to you for evaluation after a positive stress test. His laboratory evaluation included an elevated low-density lipoprotein level, low levels of high-density lipoprotein (HDL) and elevated C-reactive protein (CRP) levels. Regarding CRP, all of the following statements are true, EXCEPT:

(A) CRP is an acute phase reactant that binds to phosphocholine in dying cells or bacteria

(B) CRP is produced in the liver as a proinflammatory response to IL-4

(C) CRP has been found within the plaque at the lipid core

(D) CRP has intrinsic atherogenic properties stimulating foam cell formation

1.11 A cardiac catheterization performed in a 58-year-old demonstrates nonobstructive lesions in the proximal part of the RCA. You confirm these findings with quantitative coronary angiography (QCA) and intravascular ultrasound (Fig. Q1-11) and suspect that these lesions could represent thin cap fibroatheromas (TCFA). All of the following statements about TCFA are true, EXCEPT:

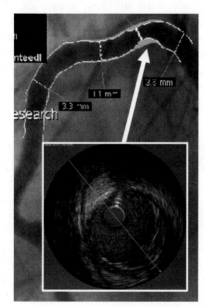

Figure Q1-11

(A) The nonthrombosed lesion that most resembles the acute plaque rupture is the TCFA

(B) TCFA is characterized by a necrotic core with an overlying fibrous cap measuring < 65 μm, containing rare smooth muscle cells but numerous macrophages

(C) TCFAs are most frequently observed in patients dying with acute MI and least common in plaque erosion

(D) TCFAs have a greater degree of calcification than other advanced plaques

1.12 You are evaluating a 64-year-old with a history of multiple MIs, who is visiting your office for the first time. You notice that the patient has high levels of inflammatory markers including hs-CRP and leukocytosis. All of the following statements about inflammation are true, EXCEPT:

(A) Inflammation is associated with TCFA

(B) Randomized trials have shown no benefit for steroids in unstable angina

(C) Leukocytosis is an independent predictor for future events

(D) The beneficial effects of aspirin in primary prevention are independent of degree of inflammation, measured as plasma hs-CRP levels

1.13 A 69-year-old male patient with history of hypertension, uncontrolled diabetes, and smoking undergoes cardiac catheterization and intravascular ultrasound imaging that reveal numerous atherosclerotic plaques with positive remodeling as seen in Figure Q1-13. All of the following statements are true, EXCEPT:

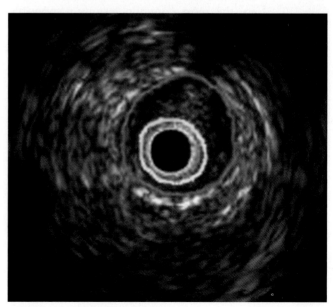

Figure Q1-13 (see color insert)

(A) Remodeling preserves the lumen and protects from heart attacks
(B) Positive remodeling is most frequently seen in unstable syndromes
(C) Positive remodeled plaques have more macrophages
(D) Plaques can grow up to 40% area stenosis without obstructing the lumen

1.14 In the patient from Question 1.13, you are concerned that most of the nonobstructive lesions observed during his coronary angiogram are vulnerable plaques. Which of the following statements is FALSE regarding vulnerable plaques?

(A) The main source of neovessels is vasa vasorum
(B) Are mostly lipid-rich, with increased macrophage infiltration
(C) Exhibit positive remodeling
(D) Can be identified by angioscopy, showing a white-colored surface

1.15 The cardiac catheterization laboratory at your institution is part of a multicenter prospective study that evaluates the use of optical coherence tomography (OCT) in coronary plaque characterization. One of your patients, a 61-year-old female, is enrolled in the study. During the OCT pullback, you observed a dense layer of tissue covering an atherosclerotic lesion as showed in Figure Q1-15. This plaque can be classified as:

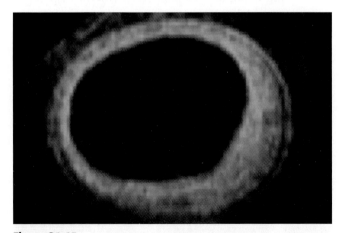

Figure Q1-15

(A) Plaque rupture
(B) Thin cap fibroatheroma
(C) Thick cap fibroatheroma
(D) Plaque erosion

1.16 The angiogram of a 49-year-old male with atypical chest pain is presented in Figure Q1-16. After 100 µg of intracoronary nitroglycerin, the angiogram dramatically improves. The following statements are true, EXCEPT:

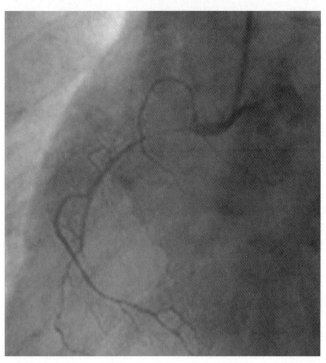

Figure Q1-16

(A) The improvement is related to increased endothelial-dependent relaxation
(B) The improvement is related to increased endothelial-independent relaxation
(C) This patient will benefit from long-acting calcium channel blockers
(D) Coronary stenting is associated with repeat spasm in nonstented areas

1.17 Regarding the patient presented in Question 1.16, which of the following statements best describes the role of nitric oxide (NO) in the vascular tissue?

(A) Blocks endothelial-dependent vasodilation
(B) Activates thrombin
(C) Induces smooth muscle cell proliferation
(D) Activates cGMP

1.18 A 58-year-old male patient with a history of smoking and early coronary artery disease in both parents is undergoing a diagnostic cardiac catheterization. Optical coherence tomography is performed and demonstrates areas of high-intensity signal with stripe pattern shadow suggestive of macrophage infiltration (Fig. Q1-18). This increased macrophage activity in vulnerable plaques can lead to:

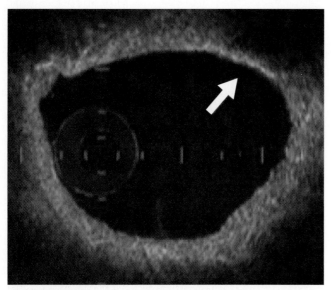

Figure Q1-18

(A) Expression of matrix metalloproteinases

(B) Antiapoptotic cell survival

(C) Production of nitric oxide

(D) Expression of antithrombin III

1.19 You are doing rounds evaluating patients after cardiac catheterization. One of your patients, a 65-year-old female, with advanced diabetes and history of multiple coronary events, CABG, and stent implantation asks you to explain why she has had multiple cardiovascular complications. Which one of the following is true about diabetic atherosclerosis?

(A) Associated with decreased atherosclerotic burden

(B) Characterized by decreased plaque macrophage infiltration

(C) Associated with lower levels of hs-CRP

(D) Associated with upregulation of macrophage receptor for advanced end-glycation (RAGE) products

1.20 An autopsy performed in a 75-year-old-male who died from an acute coronary syndrome reveals atherosclerotic plaques with increased inflammatory components as shown in the immunohistochemistry image in Figure Q1-20. The following statements about inflammation are true, EXCEPT:

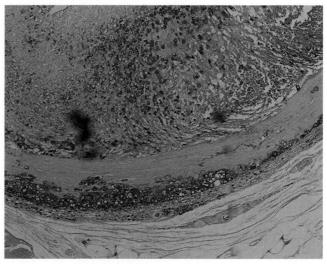

Figure Q1-20 (see color insert)

(A) T cells are less frequently found when compared to macrophages

(B) Plaque inflammation is associated with increased neovascularization

(C) Cell-adhesion molecules (VCAM, ICAM) are mostly expressed in the endothelium and less expressed in plaque neovessels

(D) Is reduced after lipid-lowering therapy

1.21 Intravascular ultrasound imaging performed in a 62-year-old diabetic female patient reveals positive remodeling in several vascular segments as shown in Figure Q1-21. Which of the following is not an independent predictor of positive remodeling?

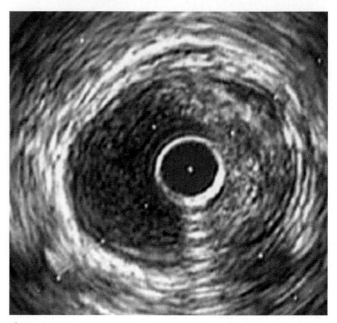

Figure Q1-21

(A) Inflammation
(B) Calcification
(C) Medial atrophy
(D) Cigarette smoking

1.22 A 72-year-old male patient is brought to the cardiac catheterization laboratory for an ST-elevation MI. During the procedure the patient has a cardiac arrest secondary to ventricular fibrillation. The patient undergoes 40 minutes of advanced cardiac life support but does not survive. The autopsy of this patient reveals a nonocclusive atherosclerotic plaque with superimposed thrombus completely occluding the proximal segment of the LAD artery. Notably, you observe areas of positive glycophorin A-antibody staining and Mallory's stain for iron suggestive of intraplaque hemorrhage. Which of the following statements is FALSE regarding intraplaque hemorrhage?

(A) Is associated with increased neovascularization
(B) Is associated with symptomatic carotid disease
(C) Red blood cell extravasation stimulates lipid core expansion
(D) Downregulates macrophage CD-163 receptor
(E) Increases the production of reactive oxygen species

1.23 In the aforementioned case (Question 1.22), tissue immunostaining reveals areas with dense neovascularization (Fig. Q1-23). Which of the following statements is FALSE regarding plaque neovascularization?

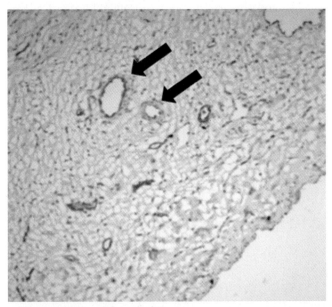

Figure Q1-23 (see color insert)

(A) Is increased in ruptured plaques
(B) Is associated with inflammation
(C) Hypoxic Factor 1 alpha triggers plaque angiogenesis
(D) The vast majority of neovessels communicate with the vessel lumen to nurture the base of the plaque

1.24 A 71-year-old female diabetic patient undergoes bare-metal stent implantation in a 78% lesion in her mid-RCA after a positive nuclear stress test. The patient undergoes a follow-up coronary angiogram with OCT imaging as part of a clinical trial, in which he was enrolled at the time of the stenting. OCT reveals neointimal coverage over the implanted stent struts as shown in Figure Q1-24. Which of the following statements is FALSE regarding smooth muscle cell proliferation after stent deployment?

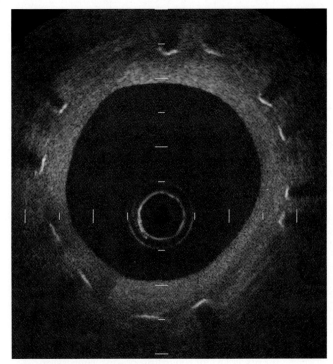

Figure Q1-24 (see color insert)

(A) Is increased in diabetic lesions after bare-metal stenting
(B) Is characterized by increased production of collagen I
(C) Is associated with inflammation
(D) Is reduced after complete endothelialization
(E) Is associated with increased cell apoptosis

1.25 A 64-year-old male patient with history of hypertension, hypercholesterolemia, and previous cigarette smoking presents to the emergency room with chest pain in the mid-chest radiating to his back and left shoulder. An ECG taken upon arrival is displayed in Figure Q1-25. His pain starts to improve after two sublingual nitroglycerin tablets. His initial troponin-I level is 3.5 ng/ml. He is taken to the cardiac care unit at your institution for medical management. Which of the following statements is FALSE regarding coronary thrombosis in unstable angina and NSTEMI?

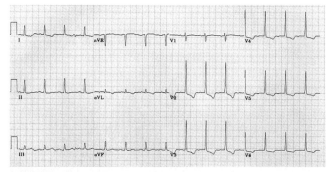

Figure Q1-25

    (A) Is more frequently mediated by plaque rupture rather than erosion

    (B) Can induce distal emboli, predominately composed by cholesterol crystals and necrotic debris

    (C) Thrombolysis reduces embolization and facilitates intervention

    (D) Is associated with increased circulating tissue factor particles and cell apoptosis

1.26 You are evaluating a 65-year-old female patient with family history of coronary artery disease who has been referred to you for a coronary CT-angiogram that revealed extensive coronary atherosclerosis in the RCA (Fig. Q1-26). The patient is asymptomatic and obsessively asks about disease regression. Which of the following statements is FALSE regarding plaque regression?

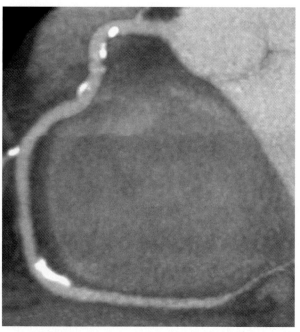

Figure Q1-26

    (A) Follows an eccentric pattern, reducing plaque volume before improving the lumen

    (B) Can be obtained by aggressive lipid-lowering therapy

    (C) Improves the lumen and therefore reduces coronary events

    (D) Is associated with reverse lipid transport from the plaque to the liver

1.27 A 78-year-old female patient is admitted to the medical service with a 6-hour history of weakness and paresthesias in the left upper and lower extremities. On physical exam, besides her motor and sensory deficits in the left limbs, she also presents right mouth droop and a right carotid bruit. You order a carotid ultrasound that shows an 80% atherosclerotic plaque in the right internal carotid artery (Fig. Q1-27), so you call for a neurosurgery consult. Studies of carotid endarterectomy have shown all of the following, EXCEPT:

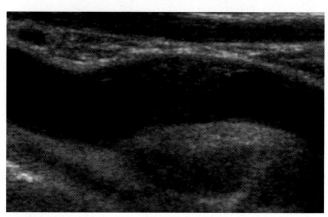

Figure Q1-27

(A) Thrombotic plaques are more frequently observed in patients with stroke as compared to transient ischemic attack

(B) Asymptomatic patients can have thrombotic carotid plaques in up to 27% of individuals

(C) Hypertension and low HDL-cholesterol are associated with vulnerable and thrombotic carotid plaques

(D) Low HDL cholesterol does not correlate with macrophage infiltration

1.28 A 67-year-old male patient, active smoker and with history of dyslipidemia, obesity, and hypertension undergoes a coronary CT-angiogram, as recommended by his primary care physician. The report of the test reveals extensive coronary calcification and a high coronary calcium score (Fig. Q1-28). The following statements about coronary calcification are true, EXCEPT:

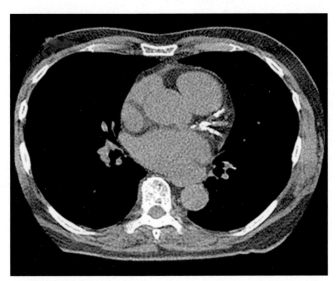

Figure Q1-28

(A) Coronary calcification is a predictor for future coronary events

(B) Coronary calcification typically reflects advanced disease by histologic criteria

(C) Plaque erosion is more frequently seen in smokers

(D) Chronic stable angina lesions may be healed ruptured plaques

(E) Plaque rupture more frequently occurs at the center of the fibrous cap

1.29 A 52-year-old diabetic female with history of two episodes of pulmonary thromboembolism and several third trimester miscarriages is referred to you for follow-up after being discharged for an NSTEMI. Given her high incidence of thrombotic events, you decide to perform a workup for hypercoagulable state. In regards to vascular thrombosis, all of the following statements are true, EXCEPT:

(A) Her coronary thrombus is predominately platelet-rich

(B) Her DVT and PE are mostly fibrin-rich

(C) Her natural anticoagulants to be evaluated include protein-C, protein S, and TFPI

(D) Her plasminogen-activator inhibitor-1 (PAI-1) level will be low

1.30 While talking to the pathologist who has performed the autopsy on a 70-year-old male who experienced sudden cardiac death, he describes to you that the immunostaining analysis of the specimens revealed abundant matrix metalloproteinases as observed in the following image (Fig. Q1-30). The role of these matrix metalloproteinases is relevant for the following, EXCEPT:

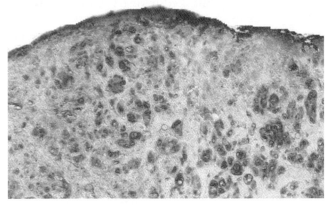

Figure Q1-30 (see color insert)

(A) Positive remodeling, by digesting the internal elastic lamina

(B) Plaque angiogenesis, by mediating tunnelization of neovessels

(C) Plaque rupture, by digesting the collagen of the fibrous cap

(D) Myocardial salvage, preventing expansion and remodeling

1.31 In further evaluation of the specimen from the patient in Question Q1-30, the pathologist also describes significant amounts of monocyte-derived macrophages infiltrating the atheroma (Fig. Q1-31). The role of these monocyte-derived macrophages in atherosclerosis can be described by the following, EXCEPT:

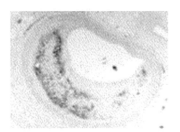

Figure Q1-31

(A) Removal of oxidized LDL by the scavenger receptor CD-36

(B) Transfer of free cholesterol to HDL by the ABC1 and ABCG transporters

(C) Removal of apoptotic bodies from the plaque

(D) Antithrombogenic effects during apoptosis by the expression of protein C

1.32 A 49-year-old male patient with history of smoking, morbid obesity, and marked hyperlipidemia is brought to the emergency department after complaining of sudden onset shortness of breath. Upon arrival, the patient is hypotensive with jugular venous distention and bilateral crackles. The ECG shows an acute anterior MI, and the patient is rushed into the cardiac catheterization laboratory but died during PCI on autopsy An acute thrombus of the proximal LAD is observed (Fig. Q1-32). Given this patient's clinical presentation, you suspect a vulnerable plaque leading to this presentation. The following statements are true, EXCEPT:

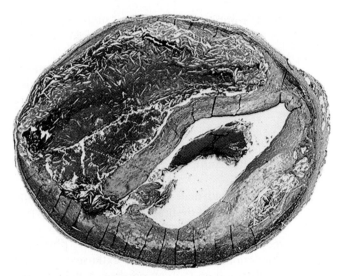

Figure Q1-32 (see color insert)

(A) The fibrous cap is composed of collagen and smooth muscle cells

(B) The shoulders of the plaque are in contact with the internal elastic lamina

(C) Plaque burden can be quantified by intravascular ultrasound

(D) Plaque neovessels are responsible for intraplaque hemorrhage

1.1 **Answer B.** A necrotic core characterizes plaque rupture with an overlying thin-ruptured cap infiltrated by macrophages and lymphocytes. There are few or no smooth muscle cells within the cap. With polarized microscopy, collagen fibers will be bright yellow or orange and the thinner fibers will be green. The lipid core is suitable for imaging using radiofrequency analysis of intravascular ultrasound (virtual histology) or near infrared spectroscopy. More recently, intracoronary OCT, a technique that measures backscattered light, or optical echoes, derived from an infrared light source directed at the arterial wall, has been proposed as a high-resolution analogue of intravascular ultrasound. (*Arterioscler Thromb Vasc Biol* 2010;30:1282-1292.)

1.2 **Answer D.** Plaque stabilization is characterized by *effective*, not defective, efferocytosis, which relates to the ability of macrophages to remove apoptotic bodies from the core of atherosclerotic plaques. (*Nat Rev Immunol* 2010;10:36-46.) All other statements are true.

1.3 **Answer D.** Ruptured plaques are characterized by decreased collagen content, increased lipid content, and increased metalloproteinase expression (*Arterioscler Thromb Vasc Biol* 2010;30:1282-1292).

1.4 **Answer D.** Healed plaques with increased vasavasorum neovascularization are characteristic of stable angina patients and typically do not present with acute MI. (*Heart* 1999;82:265-268.)

1.5 **Answer D.** Microemboli and microvascular obstruction are common in patients dying of acute coronary thrombosis, most frequently seen in RCA. Microemboli are composed of cholesterol crystal embolization. Plaque erosion is more likely to cause emboli. These emboli and microvessel obstruction have a prominent clinical role since microemboli leads to myonecrosis. (*J Am Coll Cardiol* 2009;54:2167-2173.)

1.6 **Answer C.** The individual risk for plaque progression to complete occlusion is lower in nonobstructive lesions (<5%) when compared to obstructive lesions (24%). (*J Am Coll Cardiol* 1993;22:1141-1154.) Most MIs are caused by nonobstructive lesions and plaque rupture or erosion with superimposed thrombosis.

1.7 **Answer B.** Eroded plaques are more frequently seen in smoker females. (*Thromb Haemost* 1999;82(suppl 1):1-3.) All other statements are true.

1.8 **Answer C.** Smooth muscle cells are responsible for strengthening, not weakening, of the fibrous cap. All other statements are correct.

1.9 **Answer A.** Approximately two-thirds of coronary thrombi in sudden coronary deaths are late (>1 day). Late stage is characterized in phases of lytic (1 to 3 days), infiltrating (4 to 7 days), or healing (>7 days). All other statements are correct. (*J Am Coll Cardiol* 201012;55:122-132.)

1.10 **Answer B.** CRP is produced in the liver as a pro-inflammatory response to IL-6, and not to IL-4.

1.11 **Answer D.** TCFAs have a lesser degree of calcification than other advanced plaques. (*J Am Coll Cardiol* 2006;47(8 suppl):C13-C18.) Other statements are correct.

1.12 **Answer D.** The beneficial effects of aspirin in primary prevention are closely related to CRP levels. (*N Engl J Med* 1997;336:973-979.) In patients with the lowest quintile of CRP, ASA does not prevent cardiovascular events (13% reduction when compared to placebo; $P = NS$). However, in patients with the highest quintile of CRP, aspirin prevents cardiovascular events (53% reduction when compared to placebo; $p < 0.0001$).

1.13 **Answer A.** Remodeling preserves the lumen but does not protect from heart attacks. It is actually more frequent in plaques from patients with acute coronary events. (*Circulation* 2000;101:598-603.)

1.14 **Answer D.** On angioscopy, vulnerable plaques are associated with a glistening yellow color. Stable plaques are white. (*Am Heart J* 1995;130:195-203.)

1.15 **Answer C.** A plaque with a dense layer of tissue covering the lipid core is considered a thick cap fibroatheroma.

1.16 **Answer A.** Nitroglycerin acts directly on the smooth muscle cell of the tunica media, classically known as endothelial-independent relaxation. Coronary stenting is associated with repeat spasm in nonstented areas and is not indicated.

1.17 **Answer D.** The mechanism of action of nitric oxide is related to the activation of cGMP.

1.18 **Answer A.** Increased macrophage activity in vulnerable plaques can lead to expression of matrix metalloproteinases.

1.19 **Answer D.** Diabetes atherosclerosis is characterized by increased atherosclerotic burden, increased, higher levels of CRP plaque macrophage infiltration and upregulation of RAGE. (*Atherosclerosis* 2006;185:70-77.)

1.20 **Answer C.** Cell-adhesion molecule expression is two to three times higher in plaque neovessels than in the luminal endothelium. (*J Clin Invest* 1993;92:945-951.) All other statements are correct.

1.21 **Answer D.** The independent predictors of positive remodeling include inflammation, calcification, and medial atrophy. (*Circulation* 2002;105:297-303.) Cigarette smoking is associated with plaque erosion but not positive remodeling.

1.22 **Answer D.** Intraplaque hemorrhage upregulates macrophage CD-63 receptor, increasing inflammation and foam cell formation. (*Atherosclerosis* 2002;163:199-201.) All other statements are correct.

1.23 **Answer D.** The majority of neovessels are derived from adventitial vasa-vasorum. Only the minority originate or communicate from the lumen. (*Hum Pathol* 1995;26:450-456.)

1.24 **Answer B.** Smooth muscle cell proliferation after stent deployment is characterized by

increased production of Collagen III, not collagen I. All other statements are correct.

1.25 **Answer C.** Coronary thrombosis in unstable angina and NSTEMI is mediated by platelet-rich thrombus (*J Am Coll Cardiol* 2005;46:937-954.) Thrombolysis activates platelets and may be harmful in ACS and should not be used. Other statements are correct.

1.26 **Answer C.** Plaque regression follows an eccentric pattern, improving initially the plaque burden associated with positive remodeling. Most importantly, plaque regression is associated with a significant reduction of new plaque formation thereby preventing plaque rupture, and reducing acute coronary events and not necessarily related to improved lumen. (*J Am Coll Cardiol* 2005;46:937-954.)

1.27 **Answer D.** Low HDL cholesterol is an independent predictor for macrophage infiltration in carotid endarterectomy studies in humans. In addition, asymptomatic patients can have thrombotic carotid plaques up to 27% of the cases. (*Atherosclerosis* 2010;208:572-580.)

1.28 **Answer E.** Plaque rupture more frequently occurs at the shoulders, not the center of the fibrous cap. (*Lancet* 1989;2:941-944.) Other statements are correct.

1.29 **Answer D.** Plasminogen-activator inhibitor-1 is increased in diabetic plaques not lowered. (*Cardiovasc Diabetol* 2009;8:48.) All other statements are true.

1.30 **Answer D.** Metalloproteinases do not salve myocardium. On the contrary, MMPs are associated with expansion and remodeling of the ventricle after MI. (*Circulation* 2002;105:753-758.) Other statements are correct.

1.31 **Answer D.** Macrophages are associated with thrombogenic effects during apoptosis by the expression of tissue factor. Other statements are correct.

1.32 **Answer B.** The shoulders of the plaque are in contact with the lumen, not with the internal elastic lamina. Other statements are true.

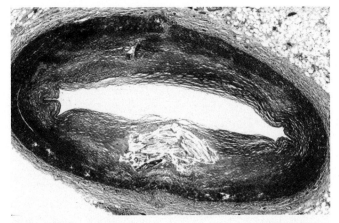

Figure Q1-1

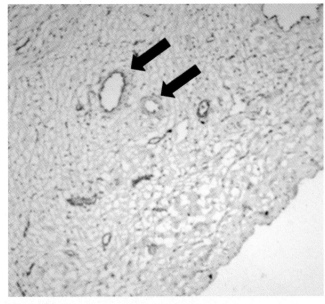

Figure Q1-23

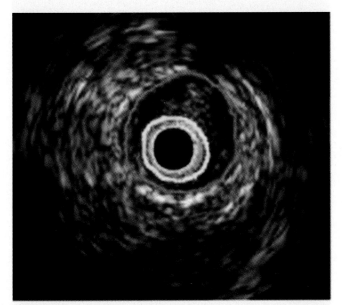

Figure Q1-13

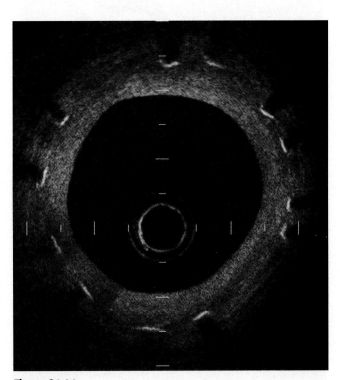

Figure Q1-24

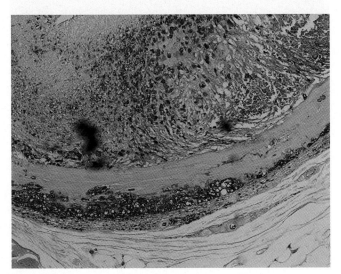

Figure Q1-20

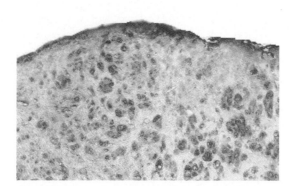

Figure Q1-30

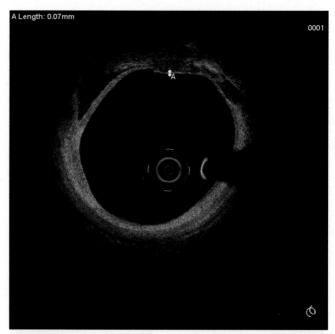

Figure Q12-24

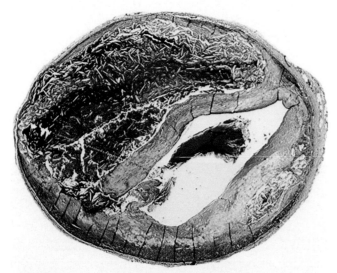

Figure Q1-32

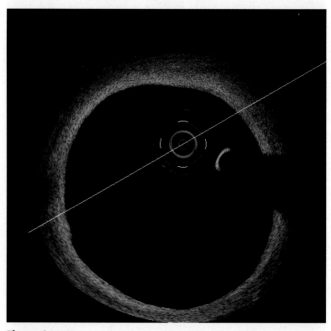

Figure Q12-25

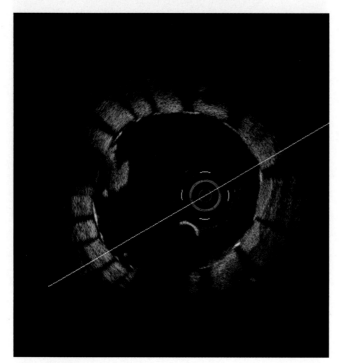

Figure Q12-22

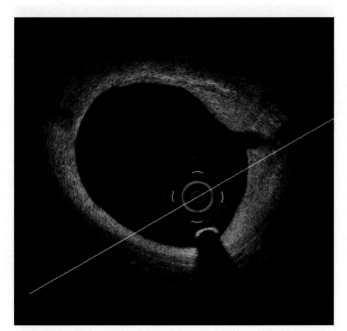

Figure Q12-26

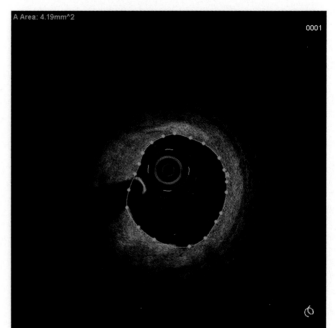

Figure Q12-28

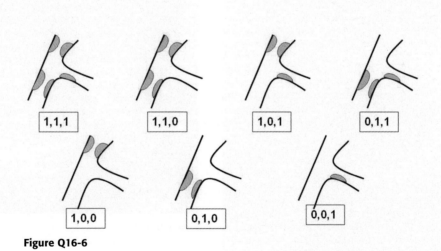

Figure Q16-6

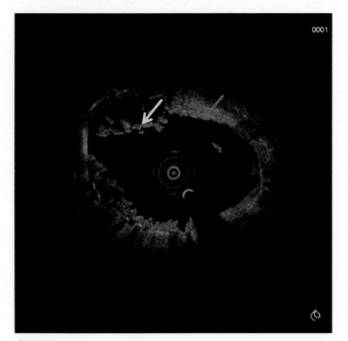

Figure Q21-23

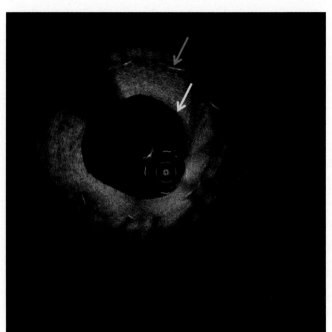

Figure Q21-25

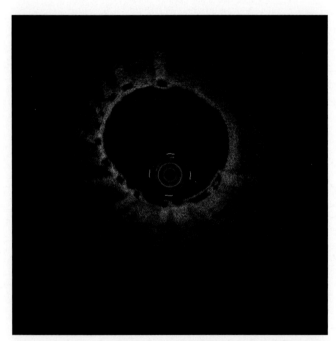

Figure A21-30. Example of 6 month follow-up OCT image of a BVS stent showing complete coverage of the stent struts.

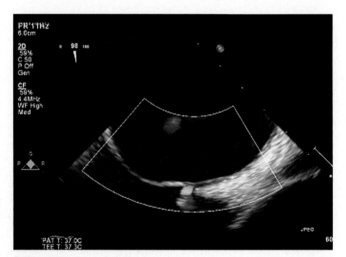

Figure Q24-3

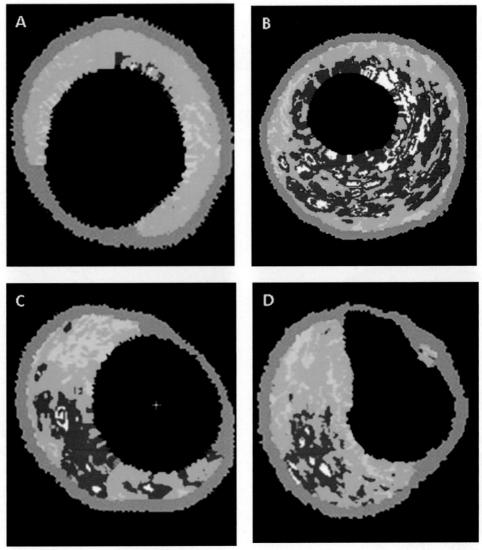

Figure Q27-16

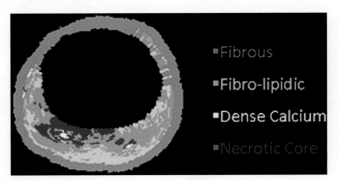

- Fibrous
- Fibro-lipidic
- Dense Calcium
- Necrotic Core

Figure A27-3

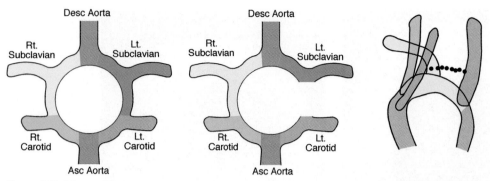

Figure A29-16

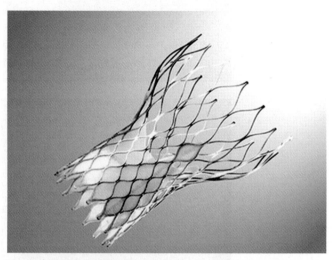

Figure Q31-24. Medtronic percutaneous aortic CoreValve.

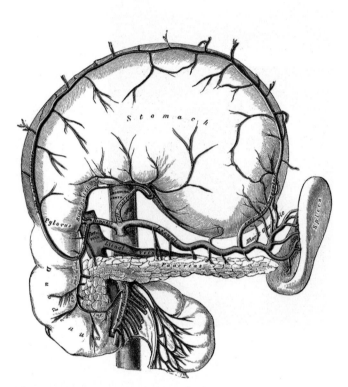

Figure A29-18

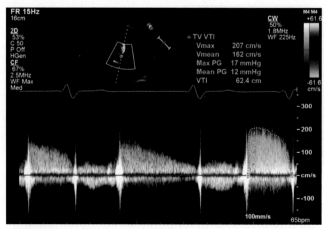

Figure Q31-7. A representative echo Doppler tracing through a prosthetic tricuspid valve replacement with mean gradient of 12 mm Hg.

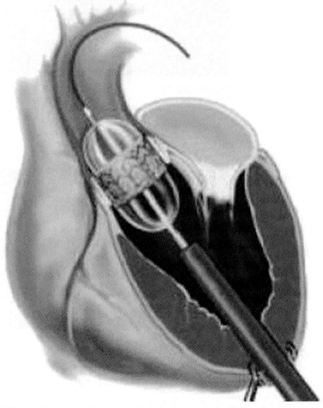

Figure A31-24. Cartoon depicting transapical placement of a percutaneous SAPIEN aortic valve.

2 Anatomy and Physiology

Richard A. Lange and L. David Hillis

QUESTIONS

2.1 An 80-year-old man is referred for coronary angiography for evaluation of retrosternal pain at rest. Pressure recordings from the coronary catheter tip during its engagement in the coronary ostium and withdrawal (see arrow, Fig. Q2-1) into the aorta indicate:

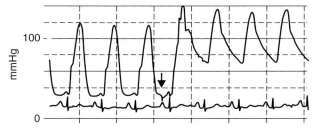

Figure Q2-1

(A) Collateral coronary flow
(B) Severe aortic stenosis
(C) Anomalous origin of a coronary artery
(D) Obstruction of antegrade coronary flow by the catheter

2.2 Which of the following projections allows the operator to visualize a proximal left circumflex (LCX) stenosis optimally?

(A) 30-degree right anterior oblique (RAO)
(B) 30-degree RAO, 30-degree cranial
(C) 60-degree left anterior oblique (LAO), 30-degree cranial
(D) 30-degree RAO, 30-degree caudal

2.3 A 45-year-old man with a bicuspid aortic valve is found to have a left dominant coronary circulation at cardiac catheterization. What is the incidence of this?

(A) 90%
(B) 50%
(C) 30%
(D) 10%

2.4 A 55-year-old man undergoes coronary angiography for evaluation of nonexertional chest pain. The left lateral view of the left anterior descending (LAD) artery obtained during diastole (panel A) and systole (panel B) is displayed in Figure Q2-4. He has:

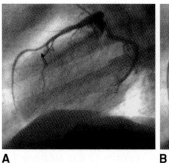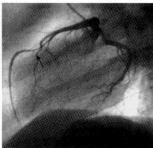

A   B
Figure Q2-4. (Image reproduced from Bauters C, Chmait A, Tricot O, et al. Coronary thrombosis and myocardial bridging. *Circulation* **2002;105;130, with permission.)**

(A) An eccentric atherosclerotic stenosis
(B) Myocardial bridging
(C) Prinzmetal's angina
(D) Coronary dissection

2.5 In order to obtain a "spider view" to visualize the left main (LM) coronary artery as well as the proximal LAD and LCX arteries optimally, the image intensifier should be positioned:

(A) 50 degrees LAO, 20 degrees caudal
(B) 30 degrees RAO, 30 degrees caudal
(C) 50 degrees LAO, 35 degrees cranial
(D) 15 degrees RAO, 30 degrees cranial

2.6 In a 30-year-old survivor of sudden cardiac death, left ventriculography in the 30-degree RAO projection shows a "button" projecting from the aortic root (Fig. Q2-6). This suggests the patient has:

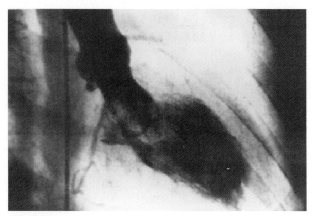

Figure Q2-6

(A) Occlusion of the proximal right coronary artery (RCA)
(B) Anomalous origin of the LCX artery
(C) Pseudoaneurysm of the proximal ascending aorta
(D) Coronary ectasia from Kawasaki's disease

2.7 In routine clinical practice, the severity of coronary stenosis is estimated from visual inspection of the coronary angiogram. Compared with quantitative coronary angiography, such a visual estimation of coronary stenoses usually:

(A) Provides similar results
(B) Underestimates the severity of the stenosis by 35%
(C) Underestimates the severity of the stenosis by 20%
(D) Overestimates the severity of the stenosis by 20%

2.8 Impaired vasodilator reserve is first noted when the coronary luminal diameter narrowing (e.g., stenosis) is:

(A) 50%
(B) 60%
(C) 75%
(D) 90%

2.9 What is a Kugel's artery?

(A) Anomalous origin of the LAD coronary artery from the pulmonary artery
(B) Coronary arteriovenous fistula
(C) Conus artery branch
(D) Right-to-right collateral (from proximal to distal RCA through the atrioventricular [AV] node branch)

2.10 A 55-year-old woman with exertional chest pain and an abnormal myocardial perfusion scan has a coronary angiogram that demonstrates a 50% stenosis of the mid RCA. This corresponds to a cross-sectional area narrowing of:

(A) 50%
(B) 60%
(C) 75%
(D) 90%

2.11 Catheterization reveals a 70% stenosis in the proximal LCX artery. All the following would indicate that this is a hemodynamically significant coronary stenosis, EXCEPT:

(A) A fractional flow reserve (FFR) of 0.80
(B) An impaired pattern of phasic coronary flow distal to the stenosis, with a diastolic to systolic ratio < 1.5
(C) Impaired coronary hyperemic flow (less than two times basal values)
(D) A translesional pressure gradient > 30 mm Hg

2.12 In what percentage of individuals does the LCX coronary artery provide the blood flow to the sinoatrial node?

(A) 10%
(B) 40%
(C) 60%
(D) 90%

2.13 All the following are endothelial-derived vasodilators, EXCEPT:

(A) Nitric oxide (NO)
(B) Thromboxane
(C) Prostacyclin
(D) Prostaglandin I_2

2.14 Which of the following is true of the coronary venous system?

(A) Veins and venules are innervated by sympathetic nerves

(B) Venous volume increases with sympathetic stimulation

(C) Veins dilate in response to local metabolic factors

(D) Veins are constricted in the basal state

2.15 All the following are true regarding coronary vascular resistance, EXCEPT:

(A) Left ventricular (LV) hypertrophy can impair microcirculatory (R3) resistance

(B) In the absence of stenosis, R1 (epicardial vessel) resistance is trivial

(C) The R2 (prearteriolar) vessels are responsible for most of the total coronary resistance

(D) The R3 (arteriolar and intramyocardial) vessels are regulated neurogenically and locally

2.16 Under normal physiologic conditions, endothelial cell surface proteins prevent thrombosis of arteries and veins. One of the endothelial cell surface proteins responsible for these anticoagulant properties is:

(A) Thrombomodulin

(B) von Willebrand factor

(C) Tissue factor

(D) Plasminogen activator inhibitor

2.17 Before placement of a catheter in the coronary sinus, a venogram is performed (Fig. Q2-17). What does the arrow denote?

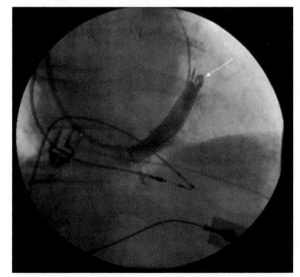

Figure Q2-17. (Habib A, Lachman N, Christensen KN, et al., The anatomy of the coronary sinus venous system for the cardiac electrophysiologist *Europace* 2009;11:15–21, by permission of Oxford University Press.)

(A) A prominent Vieussens valve is visualized

(B) The proximal coronary sinus has a thrombotic occlusion

(C) The middle cardiac vein is seen coursing superiorly after emptying into the coronary sinus

(D) A persistent left superior vena cava is visualized

2.18 The CORRECT formula for determining myocardial oxygen consumption (MVO_2) from the coronary arterial or venous flow (Q), arterial oxygen content (AoO_2), and coronary sinus oxygen content (CSO_2) is:

(A) $MVO_2 = Q/(AoO_2 - CSO_2)$

(B) $MVO_2 = (AoO_2 - CSO_2)/Q$

(C) $MVO_2 = Q \times (AoO_2 - CSO_2)$

(D) Cannot calculate with the data provided

2.19 The "abbreviated" form of the Gorlin formula (so-called Hakki equation: valve area (cm^2) = flow (L/min)/$\sqrt{}$peak-to-peak pressure gradient) is often used to estimate valve area in patients with valvular stenosis referred for catheterization. It may be inaccurate in which of the following circumstances?

(A) Valve area < 1.0 cm^2

(B) High cardiac output

(C) Low transvalvular gradient

(D) Bradycardia (heart rate < 60 bpm) or tachycardia (heart rate > 100 bpm)

2.20 In which of the following circumstances may the use of an LV–Ao pullback pressure recording to assess aortic valve area yield inaccurate results?

(A) Low (<35 mm Hg) transvalvular gradient

(B) Atrial fibrillation

(C) Immediately after left ventriculography

(D) All the above

2.21 Endothelial dysfunction can be identified by:

(A) Inability to vasodilate in response to intracoronary nitroprusside

(B) Vasoconstrictor response to intracoronary acetylcholine

(C) Intravascular ultrasound (IVUS) imaging

(D) Reduced coronary sinus blood levels of endothelial-derived relaxing factor (EDRF) and NO

2.22 Coronary venous oxygen saturation is typically:

(A) 30%

(B) 50%

(C) 65%

(D) 80%

2.23 Each of the following is true of coronary blood flow, EXCEPT:

(A) Most coronary flow occurs during ventricular diastole

(B) There is compression of intramyocardial vessels during systole

(C) Compression of microvessels during systole is more prominent in the subendocardial than the subepicardial layer

(D) The subepicardium is more susceptible to hypoperfusion than the subendocardium

2.24 Which of the following coronary artery anomalies does NOT often course between the aorta and pulmonary artery?

(A) Anomalous origin of the LCX artery from the right cusp

(B) Anomalous origin of the LAD artery from the right cusp

(C) Anomalous origin of the RCA from the left cusp

(D) Anomalous origin of the LM from the right cusp

2.25 Which of the following is NOT true of coronary flow reserve (CFR)?

(A) It is computed as hyperemic flow velocity divided by basal mean flow velocity

(B) It can be used to assess the physiologic significance of stenoses in epicardial coronary vessels

(C) Normal CFR is 2.5 to 5

(D) Maximal hyperemia is attained with intracoronary injections of adenosine, papaverine, or acetylcholine

2.26 Which is true of the capillary vessels?

(A) They consist of a single layer of endothelial cells

(B) They lack the ability to change their diameter actively because they have no smooth muscle cells

(C) They have the largest cross-sectional and surface area of the vessels in the vasculature

(D) All the above

2.27 Coronary blood flow velocity is:

(A) Proportional to cross-sectional area of the artery

(B) Proportional to vascular resistance

(C) Proportional to blood flow

(D) All the above

2.28 Which of the following induces coronary arterial vasodilatation?

(A) Angiotensin II

(B) Vasopressin

(C) Alpha-1 adrenergic receptor stimulation

(D) Beta-2 adrenergic receptor stimulation

2.29 Coronary angiography in a 50-year-old man with an acute inferior MI demonstrates a mid-right coronary arterial stenosis, with penetration of contrast material to the distal arterial segment but without perfusion. This would be characterized as:

(A) Thrombolysis in myocardial infarction (TIMI) 0 flow

(B) TIMI 1 flow

(C) TIMI 2 flow

(D) TIMI 3 flow

2.30 In a normal subject at rest, coronary blood flow is what percentage of cardiac output?

(A) 40%

(B) 20%

(C) 10%

(D) 5%

2.31 Which is true of the vasa vasorum?

(A) Intimal lesion formation is associated with a decrease in vasa vasorum density

(B) Regression of atherosclerosis with medical therapy (e.g., statins) is associated with proliferation of the vasa vasorum

(C) Hypoperfusion of the vasa vasorum may lead to atherosclerotic changes in the intima

(D) Unlike the coronaries, blood flow in the vasa vasorum is not regulated by endothelial-derived vasoactive agents

2.32 A 45-year-old woman developed acute-onset, severe substernal chest pain and anterior ST elevation on her electrocardiogram following an intense argument with her son (Fig. Q2-32A). Arteriography demonstrated no significant coronary stenoses, and her left ventriculogram is shown in Figure Q2-32B,C. She most likely has:

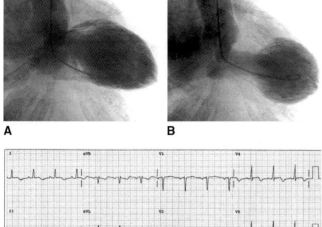

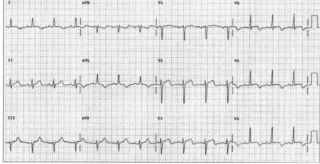

C

Figure Q2-32. (Reproduced from Witzke C, Lowe HC, Waldman H, et al. Images in cardiovascular medicine: transient left ventricular apical ballooning. *Circulation* 2003;108:2014, with permission.)

(A) Prinzmetal's angina
(B) Myopericarditis
(C) Dilated cardiomyopathy
(D) Takotsubo cardiomyopathy

2.33 A 70-year-old woman presents with an acute inferior MI. Following primary PCI of an occluded RCA, coronary angiography shows persistent staining of the inferior myocardium, with the blush persisting at the time of the next coronary injection (Fig. Q2-33). Using the TIMI myocardial perfusion grade (TMPG) system, you would classify this as:

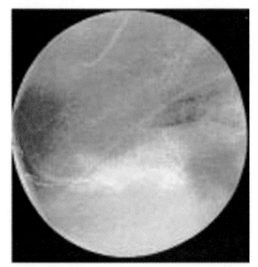

Figure Q2-33. (Image reproduced from Gibson CM, Schömig A. Coronary and myocardial angiography: angiographic assessment of both epicardial and myocardial perfusion. *Circulation* 2004;109;3096–3105, with permission.)

(A) TMPG 0
(B) TMPG 1
(C) TMPG 2
(D) TMPG 3

2.34 A 71-year-old male smoker presents with chest pain. Coronary angiography reveals a normal left coronary artery and severe stenoses in the proximal and mid RCA (Fig. Q2-34A). Immediately following successful stenting of the RCA (Fig. Q2-34B), the patient developed severe chest pain and marked anterior ST segment elevation (Fig. Q2-34C). The most likely cause is:

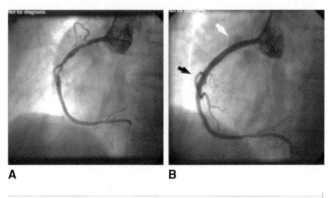

A   B

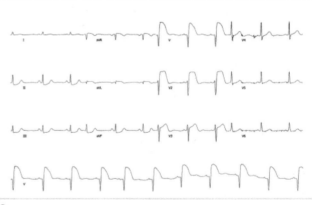

C

Figure Q2-34. (Image reproduced from Eichhöfer J, Curzen N. Unexpected profound transient anterior ST elevation after occlusion of the conus branch of the right coronary artery during angioplasty. *Circulation* 2005;111;e113–e114, with permission.)

(A) Microvascular obstruction
(B) Occlusion of sinoatrial branch of the RCA
(C) Occlusion of right ventricular branch of the RCA
(D) Occlusion of the conus branch of the RCA

2.35 A 60-year-old man with previous coronary artery bypass surgery for LM disease undergoes coronary angiography for the evaluation of angina with minimal exertion (Fig. Q2-35), which demonstrates occlusion of the LM and a patent RCA. The LAD, LCX, and ramus intermedius arteries are perfused via collaterals (solid black arrow), the source (open arrow) of which is:

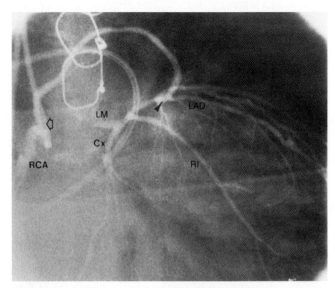

Figure Q2-35. (Image reproduced from O'Leary EL, Garza L, Williams M, et al. Vieussens' Ring. *Circulation* 1998;98;487–488, with permission.)

(A) Kugel's artery
(B) Aorta-coronary fistula
(C) Anomalous origin of the LAD from the pulmonary artery (Bland-Garland-White syndrome)
(D) Vieussens' ring

2.1 **Answer D.** The pressure recording shows "ventricularization," in which diastolic pressure is reduced but systolic pressure is preserved. Normally, the catheter tip pressure and the peripheral arterial pressure are similar. If an ostial coronary stenosis is present, engagement of the catheter may obstruct antegrade blood flow and cause ventricularization of the catheter pressure waveform (*Am Heart J* 1989;118:1160–1166).

2.2 **Answer D.** In the 30-degree RAO projection, one is looking down the AV plane, in which the LCX artery resides. Because the proximal portion of the vessel is foreshortened in this view, caudal angulation must be employed to unforeshorten it. With the other angles listed, the proximal LCX is foreshortened or overlapped by other vessels.

2.3 **Answer C.** In the general population, only 10% of individuals are left dominant (e.g., the posterior descending artery arises from the distal LCX artery), but 30% of subjects with a bicuspid valve are left dominant (*Am J Cardiol* 1978;42:57–59).

2.4 **Answer B.** Not infrequently, the LAD will course beneath a muscle bundle on the epicardial surface of the heart, resulting in its compression during ventricular systole; this is known as myocardial bridging. It is usually an incidental finding of no consequence, but rarely it has been associated with myocardial ischemia (Bauters et al., *Circulation* 2002;105;130).

2.5 **Answer A.** The LAO caudal view projects the LAD upward from the LM in the appearance of a spider and permits improved visualization of the LM and the bifurcation.

2.6 **Answer B.** The most common coronary anomaly is origin of the LCX artery from the right sinus of Valsalva. This can often be visualized during left ventriculography (30-degree RAO projection) as a "dot" or "button" projecting from the aortic root as the LCX courses posterior to the aorta (*Circulation* 1974;50:768–773, *Ann Thorac Surg* 1997;63:377–381).

2.7 **Answer D.** Visual estimation of coronary stenoses is subject to substantial operator variability and a systematic form of "stenosis inflation," in which the operator's estimate of diameter stenosis is approximately 20% greater than that measured by quantitative coronary angiography (*Circulation* 1990;82:2231–2234). Therefore, a stenosis that measures 50% by quantitative angiography is typically called 70% by visual estimation.

2.8 **Answer A.** A 50% reduction in luminal diameter (hence, a 75% reduction in cross-sectional area) is "hemodynamically significant," in that it impairs CFR (i.e., the three- to fourfold augmentation in coronary flow in response to increased myocardial oxygen demands). The ability to increase flow during vasodilator stimulus is first impaired when luminal diameter is reduced 50% and abolished when it is reduced >70% (*N Engl J Med* 1994;330:1782–1788).

2.9 **Answer D.** A Kugel's artery passes from either the proximal right or left coronary artery along the anterior margin of the atrial septum to anastomose with the AV nodal branch of the distal RCA to provide blood supply to the posterior circulation (Fig. A2-9). (*Tex Heart Inst* 2004;31:267–270; *Am Heart J* 1950;40:260–270.)

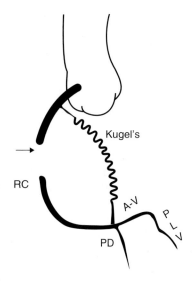

Figure A2-9

2.10 **Answer C.** A 50% stenosis represents a 75% narrowing in cross-sectional area (Fig. A2-10).

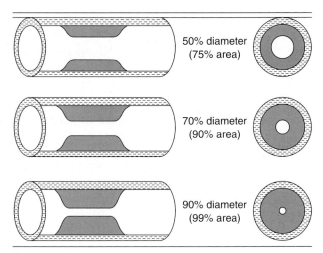

50% diameter
(75% area)

70% diameter
(90% area)

90% diameter
(99% area)

Figure A2-10

2.11   **Answer A.** An FFR > 0.75 is associated with the absence of exercise-induced myocardial ischemia and a low incidence of clinical events (*J Am Coll Cardiol* 1998;31:841-847; *Circulation* 1995;92:39-46).

2.12   **Answer B.** The sinus node artery originates from the LCX artery in 40% of individuals and from the proximal RCA in 60%, regardless of whether the patient is right or left dominant.

2.13   **Answer B.** Nitric oxide, prostacyclin, and prostaglandin I_2 are vasodilators that are produced by endothelial cells. Thromboxane is a potent vasoconstrictor that is released from platelet secretory granules in response to platelet activation.

2.14   **Answer A.** Like arterioles, veins and venules are innervated by sympathetic nerves, with increased sympathetic tone resulting in venoconstriction and a decrease in venous volume. Unlike arteries, the venous system is not regulated by local metabolic factors and has little basal tone. Therefore, veins are generally in a dilated state.

2.15   **Answer C.** In the absence of stenoses, the R3 vessels (arteriolar and intramyocardial) are responsible for 40% to 50% of total coronary resistance, the R2 vessels (prearteriolar) are responsible for 25% to 35%, and the R1 (epicardial) vessels contribute little to coronary resistance.

2.16   **Answer A.** Under normal physiologic conditions, antithrombotic properties dominate in the vasculature as a result of endothelial cell surface expression of thrombomodulin, heparin sulfate proteoglycans, plasminogen activators,

and eicosanoids. When the integrity of the blood vessel wall is compromised, exposure of blood constituents to von Willebrand factor, tissue factor, and plasminogen activator inhibitor in the subendothelium leads to a prothrombotic state.

2.17   **Answer A.** The valve of Vieussens lies at the junction of the great cardiac vein and the coronary sinus. Its position is marked by the vein of Marshall, which can be seen coursing superiorly after emptying into the coronary sinus. In this particular patient, the valve of Vieussens is preventing reflux of contrast material from the coronary sinus into the great cardiac vein.

2.18   **Answer C.** According to the Fick principle, the uptake of a substance (e.g., oxygen or MVO_2) is the product of flow (Q) and the arteriovenous concentration difference of the substance ($AoO_2 - CSO_2$). Therefore, $MVO_2 = Q \times (AoO_2 - CSO_2)$.

2.19   **Answer D.** At extremes of heart rate (<60 bpm or >100 bpm), the Hakki equation should not be used to estimate valve area, as it may be inaccurate (*Kardiologiia* 1991;31:40-44).

2.20   **Answer D.** Assessment of the transvalvular aortic gradient with nonsimultaneous measurement of LV and aortic pressures may be inaccurate when the transvalvular gradient is low, the systolic pressure is fluctuating (e.g., with atrial fibrillation), or contrast material administered during left ventriculography causes depression of ventricular systolic function and systemic vasodilatation (*Am Heart J* 1992;123:948-953).

2.21   **Answer B.** Nitroprusside is an endothelium-independent vasodilator, whereas acetylcholine is an endothelium-dependent vasodilator. Nitroprusside induces vasodilation by acting directly on the vascular smooth muscle. Acetylcholine causes vasodilation if the endothelium is intact and vasoconstriction if the endothelium is absent or dysfunctional. IVUS provides images of the arterial wall (i.e., intima, media, and adventitia), but it does not provide an assessment of endothelial function. Endothelial dysfunction results in reduced local concentrations of EDRF and NO; however, they have a very short half-life, so that changes in their concentrations cannot be detected in coronary sinus blood.

2.22   **Answer A.** At rest, transmyocardial oxygen extraction is nearly maximal, with typical coronary venous oxygen saturations of 25% to 35%.

2.23 **Answer D.** Most coronary flow occurs during diastole, because compression of intramyocardial vessels occurs during systole. Compression of microvessels during systole is more prominent in the subendocardium than the subepicardium, and the subendocardial layer is more susceptible to hypoperfusion because ventricular diastolic pressure opposes the driving pressure for flow.

2.24 **Answer A.** The most common coronary anomaly is origin of the LCX artery from the right proximal RCA or sinus of Valsalva (top panel), from which it courses posterior to the aorta (Fig.A2-24). With an anomalous RCA (or LAD), the vessel may course anterior to the pulmonary artery (middle panel) or between the aortic root and the pulmonary artery (bottom panel), which is associated with sudden cardiac death.

Anomalous left circumflex

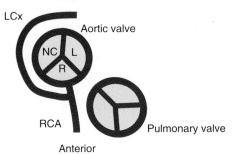

Anomalous right coronary

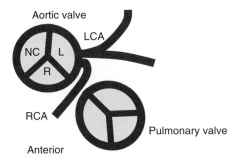

Anomalous right coronary (anterior course)

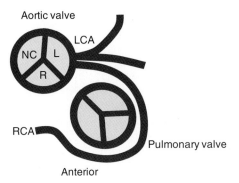

Figure A2-24

2.25 **Answer D.** CFR is the hyperemic flow (or velocity) divided by the basal flow (or velocity); it normally ranges from 2.5 to 5. A reduction in CFR occurs with a hemodynamically significant stenosis (>50% luminal diameter narrowing). Maximal hyperemia is attained with intracoronary injections of dipyridamole, adenosine, or papaverine (not acetylcholine). Intracoronary acetylcholine causes vasodilation if the endothelium is normal and vasoconstriction if the endothelium is absent or dysfunctional.

2.26 **Answer D.** Capillaries are the smallest vessels in the vasculature with the largest cross-sectional and surface area. The capillary wall consists of a single layer of endothelial cells, thereby allowing the capillaries to act as the exchange vessels of the cardiovascular system. Because they contain no smooth muscle cells, they lack the ability to change their diameters in response to stimuli.

2.27 **Answer C.** Velocity (V) is proportional to blood flow (Q) and inversely proportional to the cross-sectional area (A) of the artery and vascular resistance (R). This can be expressed as: $V=Q/A$. Since flow (Q) is proportional to the pressure gradient (ΔP) and inversely proportional to resistance ($Q = \Delta P/R$), then velocity $(V) = \Delta P/(A \times R)$. Thus, blood flow velocity (V) increases when flow (Q) increases and decreases if the cross-sectional area of the artery (A) or vascular resistance increases.

2.28 **Answer D.** Stimulation of vascular beta-2 adrenergic receptors causes vasodilatation, whereas stimulation of alpha-1 adrenergic receptors causes vasoconstriction. Since beta-2 receptors are more sensitive to epinephrine, moderately elevated levels of circulating epinephrine typically cause vasodilatation, whereas higher levels cause alpha-1 receptor–mediated vasoconstriction. Angiotensin II and vasopressin are potent vasoconstrictors.

2.29 **Answer B.** As initially defined by the TIMI investigators (*N Engl J Med* 1985;312:932–936), TIMI 0 flow represents no perfusion; TIMI 1 flow represents penetration of contrast material without perfusion (e.g., contrast material is visualized beyond the area of obstruction but fails to opacify the entire distal coronary bed); TIMI 2 flow represents impaired (slowed) antegrade perfusion (contrast material is visualized in the coronary artery distal to the obstruction, but it arrives there and then dissipates slowly); and TIMI 3 flow represents normal perfusion.

2.30 **Answer D.** Coronary blood flow is approximately 250 mL/min, which represents 4% to 5% of cardiac output.

2.31 **Answer C.** Hypoperfusion of the vasa vasorum may lead to atherosclerotic changes in the intima. A direct relationship between the severity of atherosclerosis and the density of vasa vasorum is noted. Regression of atherosclerosis with medical therapy (e.g., statins) is associated with a decrease in the density of the vasa vasorum. Blood flow in the vasa vasorum is regulated by endothelial-derived vasoactive agents (i.e., adenosine and endothelin-1).

2.32 **Answer D.** Takotsubo cardiomyopathy is characterized by systolic apical ballooning of the ventricle with preservation of basal contraction. Excessive amounts of epinephrine (endogenous or exogenous) are thought to cause it. The ventricular regional wall motion abnormalities do not follow any particular coronary anatomic pattern and probably are not a result of transient coronary arterial occlusion. The acute onset of severe chest pain following emotional stress and the pattern of ventricular involvement are not characteristic of myopericarditis.

2.33 **Answer B.** In the TMPG system, TMPG 0 represents minimal or no myocardial blush; with TMPG 1, contrast material stains the myocardium, and the stain persists on the subsequent injection; in TMPG 2, contrast material reaches the distal vessel lumen but dissipates slowly; and in TMPG 3, normal vessel perfusion is noted (*Circulation* 2004;109;3096–3105).

2.34 **Answer C.** The post-PCI angiogram shows occlusion of the conus branch of the RCA, whereas the right ventricular branch is patent. Anterior ST segment elevation due to occlusion of a right ventricular RCA branch has been reported previously and is thought to be a mirror image of right ventricular ischemia. Occlusion of the sinoatrial branch of the RCA may cause dysrhythmias but not anterior ST segment elevation, and microvascular obstruction of the RCA would typically cause inferior, rather than anterior, ST segment alterations.

2.35 **Answer D.** The patient has a large (3.3-mm) conus branch off the RCA that passes upward and over the right ventricular outflow tract to provide collateral flow to the LAD and subsequently the other vessels of the left coronary artery system. This type of collateral system is known as Vieussens' ring.

3

Radiation Safety, Equipment, and Basic Concepts

John C. Gurley and David J. Moliterno

QUESTIONS

3.1 In an attempt to decrease vascular complications, contemporary catheterization laboratory practice has increased utilization of radial artery access. In the RIVAL (Radial vs. Femoral Access for Coronary Intervention) trial, 7,021 patients were randomized to radial vs. femoral artery access, and the 30-day composite occurrence of death, myocardial infarction (MI), stroke, and bleeding was similar between the two groups. In addition to a lower frequency of vascular complications in the radial artery access group, another finding in RIVAL was that fluoroscopy time was:

(A) Similar according to access site
(B) Shorter with radial artery access
(C) Longer with radial artery access
(D) Not assessed in this trial

3.2 The arteriogram shown in Figure Q3-2 was obtained with digital subtraction technique, which eliminates background structures and enhances the visibility of contrast-filled vessels. Which of the following statements about digital subtraction angiography and radiation is TRUE?

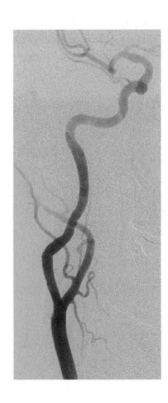

Figure Q3-2

(A) Compared to cardiac "cine" acquisitions, each frame of a subtraction study delivers a much larger dose of radiation to the patient
(B) A principal advantage of digital subtraction technique is that each frame delivers a reduced dose of radiation to the patient
(C) Digital subtraction is a form of postprocessing that does not influence patient dose
(D) Subtraction technique can enhance low-quality images obtained with very low x-ray exposure settings

3.3 Which of the following statements regarding fluoroscopy in the modern cardiac catheterization laboratory is TRUE?

(A) The x-ray exposure for fluoroscopy is much lower than the exposure for diagnostic cineangiography

(B) Most reports of radiation skin injury due to fluoroscopy occurred before 1996 and were linked to improperly calibrated, analog imaging equipment

(C) The federal government limits the maximum allowable fluoroscopic exposure rate to 10 R per minute, a rate that is below the known threshold for skin burns

(D) Modern catheterization laboratories have reduced the potential for x-ray exposure to patients and operators

3.4 The interventional cardiologist shown in Figure Q3-4 wishes to minimize his own radiation exposure during a procedure that will require imaging in a lateral projection. Which of the following statements is TRUE?

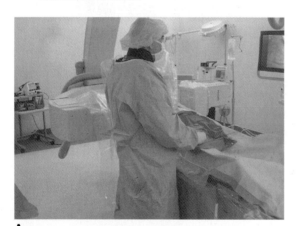

A

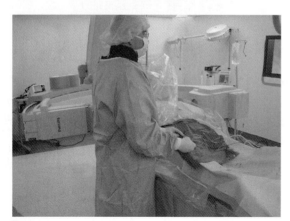

B

Figure Q3-4

(A) Panel B is preferred because the principal source of scatter radiation is positioned farthest from the operator

(B) Panel A is preferred because the x-ray beam is directed away from the operator

(C) There is no difference as long as the distances between the x-ray tube, patient, and image receptor are held constant

(D) There is no difference because the x-ray beam penetrates the same thickness of tissue

3.5 The images in Figure Q3-5 were obtained from the same patient, with the same radiographic equipment. Panel A has a grainy appearance, whereas Panel B is smoother and sharper. Which of the statements best explains the difference?

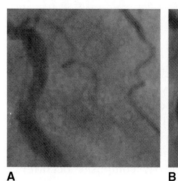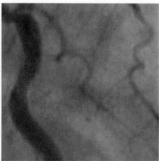

A **B**

Figure Q3-5

(A) Panel A was acquired with an excessively high milliampere (mA) setting

(B) Panel B has been electronically processed with an edge enhancement filter

(C) The speckled appearance of Panel A could have been improved by decreasing the pulse width

(D) Panel B is visually superior because it was made with a larger dose of x-rays

(E) Panel A indicates that the charge-coupled device (CCD) camera is out of focus and should be recalibrated by the service technician

3.6 The three plots in Figure Q3-6 depict the energy spectra of x-rays produced by a typical cardiac fluoroscopy unit. In each case, the dashed line represents a change that has been made to the settings. Which of the following statements is TRUE?

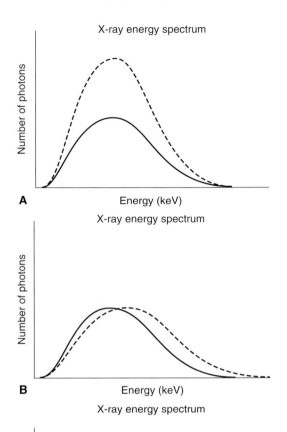

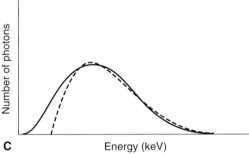

Figure Q3-6

(A) The dashed line in A indicates that kVp has been increased
(B) The dashed line in B indicates that mA has been increased
(C) The dashed line in B indicates that the pulse width has been increased
(D) The dashed line in C indicates that the beam has been hardened by placing copper or aluminum filters over the output port of the x-ray tube

3.7 Which of the following statements about tube filament current (mA) is CORRECT?

(A) Doubling the mA will decrease the patient dose rate by 50%
(B) Doubling the mA will increase the patient dose rate by 50%

(C) Doubling the mA will double the patient dose rate
(D) Doubling the mA will quadruple the patient dose rate

3.8 Patients are increasingly exposed to radiation given the proclivity toward diagnostic and therapeutic imaging procedures. If a patient is to receive 10 mSv of radiation during a routine cardiac catheterization and PCI procedure, what is the equivalent number of chest radiographs this exposure would represent and how long would it take for such an exposure to occur from natural background radiation?

(A) 50, 1 year
(B) 500, 3 years
(C) 50, 10 years
(D) 500, 30 years

3.9 Figure Q3-9 illustrates the use of collimation during coronary arteriography. Which of the following statements about collimation is FALSE?

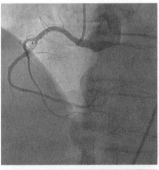

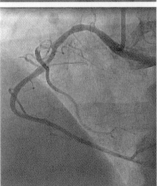

Figure Q3-9

(A) Collimation reduces the skin entrance dose
(B) Collimation reduces x-ray exposure everywhere in the room
(C) Collimation improves image quality
(D) As a means of reducing x-ray exposure, collimation is superior to selecting a smaller field of view (higher magnification) that just encompasses the area of interest

3.10 In Figure Q3-10, a dotted line has been superimposed on the plot of photon energies produced by a typical cardiac fluoroscopy unit. Which of the following statements about this dotted line is TRUE?

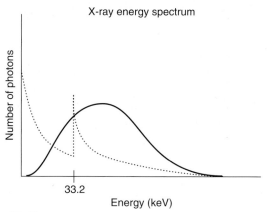

Figure Q3-10

(A) The spike in the dotted line depicts Compton scatter, which peaks at 33.2 keV

(B) The dotted line illustrates how copper beam filters reduce skin dose by eliminating x-rays with energies above 33.2 keV

(C) The spike in the dotted line depicts characteristic x-rays originating from the K shell of the tungsten atom

(D) The spike in the dotted line depicts the bremsstrahlung effect

(E) The dotted line depicts the absorption spectrum of iodine, with an absorption peak at 33.2 keV

3.11 Time, distance, and shielding are the three variables that determine exposure to scatter radiation during catheterization procedures. Which of the following statements about shielding is FALSE?

(A) Lead aprons typically provide the equivalent of 0.5-mm lead thickness and block >90% of scatter radiation

(B) Lead eyeglasses reduce radiation exposure to the lens by approximately 35%

(C) Operators who find leaded glasses uncomfortable can utilize a transparent, movable shield to provide good protection

(D) A transparent, movable shield should be placed between the operator and the face of the image intensifier or flat-panel detector

(E) Assistants can reduce their exposure to scatter radiation by standing behind the primary operator

3.12 Which of the following statements is TRUE about the function of the grid?

(A) The grid reduces the radiation dose received by the patient

(B) The grid improves image quality

(C) The grid is applied to the surface of the x-ray tube

(D) The grid should be removed when imaging larger patients

3.13 Which of the following statements about occupational exposure to x-rays in the cardiac catheterization laboratory is FALSE?

(A) The lifetime risk of developing cancer in the United States is approximately 20%

(B) A career in interventional cardiology can be expected to measurably increase the risk of developing cancer

(C) A reasonable annual dose limit for an interventional cardiologist is 50 mSv

(D) Background radiation delivers an equivalent dose of approximately 3 to 4 mSv per year

(E) Cataract is a major occupational hazard for interventional cardiologists

3.14 Modern cardiac fluoroscopy systems display values for air kinetic energy released to matter (KERMA) and dose area product (DAP). Interventional cardiologists should understand what these values mean. Which of the following statements is TRUE?

(A) Air KERMA estimates the skin dose and can be used to predict the risk of radiation skin injury

(B) DAP is a valuable measure of total x-ray exposure because it cannot be manipulated by collimation or any other operator-controlled variable

(C) Air KERMA is a measure of scatter radiation in the air surrounding the image receptor (intensifier or flat detector)

(D) Air KERMA and DAP are instantaneous values that should never be used to infer the skin dose or the total absorbed dose

3.15 The operator in Figure Q3-15 has selected the right radial approach to coronary arteriography for an obese patient with a very large abdominal pannus. Which of the following statements about this situation is FALSE?

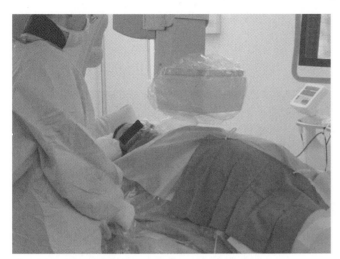

Figure Q3-15

(A) He should obtain eye protection and a radiation shield and stand back as far as possible because the x-ray exposure levels needed to penetrate this heavy patient will increase exponentially with patient thickness

(B) He has lowered the table as far as possible; this will minimize the risk of radiation skin injury

(C) He should expect low-quality images

(D) He should utilize a large field of view (low magnification) and minimize panning

(E) It is unethical to perform the procedure on an extremely obese patient in whom large doses of x-ray will be needed to generate low-quality images

(F) He should add "skin burns" to the consent document

3.16 To minimize radiation exposure to the patient, the operator, and the catheterization laboratory staff, the invasive cardiologist should be familiar with variants of arterial anatomy. Which of the following variants of the aortic arch vessels is the most common?

(A) Right common carotid originating from the innominate

(B) Right common carotid originating from the arch

(C) Common origin of the left carotid and the innominate

(D) Common origin of the right carotid and the innominate

3.17 The operator controls several factors that significantly influence radiation exposure and image quality. Among these are table height, tube position, and image detector position. In

Figure Q3-17, the image detector (*arrow*) is positioned well above the patient's chest. Which of the following statements is TRUE?

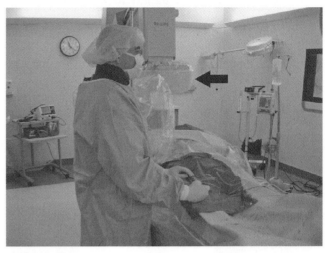

Figure Q3-17

(A) The operator has placed an air gap between the patient and the image detector to reduce his dose of scatter radiation

(B) The operator has placed an air gap between the patient and the image detector to improve image quality

(C) The operator should lower the detector to the patient's chest in order to reduce the skin entrance dose

(D) The operator should lower the table as much as possible to minimize the skin entrance dose

3.18 Which of the following statements about radiation safety terminology is TRUE?

(A) ALARA is the adjusted lifetime average of radiation accumulated

(B) The unit of measure for the quantity of radiation absorbed is the roentgen (R)

(C) The unit of measure for radiation exposure is the sievert (Sv)

(D) The unit of measure for the quantity of radiation absorbed is the gray (Gy)

3.19 A 23-year-old woman has developed pulmonary edema during her second trimester of pregnancy. Echocardiography demonstrates critical rheumatic mitral stenosis, and the patient is now referred for balloon valvotomy. Which of the following statements is TRUE regarding radiation exposure during pregnancy?

(A) Pregnancy is an absolute contraindication to cardiac fluoroscopy

(B) The procedure can be performed safely as long as proper shielding is applied to the abdomen and pelvis

(C) The radiation hazard to the fetus is very small, and shielding is not necessary

(D) The most likely adverse effect is intrauterine growth retardation because rapidly growing tissues are extremely sensitive to small doses of ionizing radiation

3.20 Which of the following statements about the device shown in Figure Q3-20 is TRUE?

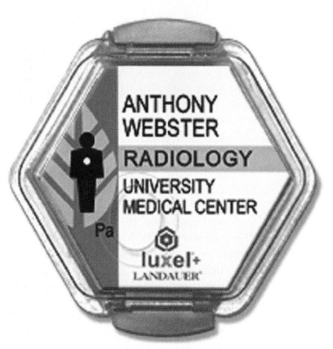

Figure Q3-20

(A) If a single film badge is worn, it should be placed under the apron at waist level

(B) If a single film badge is worn, it should be placed on the outside of the apron at waist level

(C) If a single film badge is worn, it should be placed on the outside of the thyroid collar on the side closest to the source of scatter radiation

(D) Acceptable readings indicate that the operator is using safe radiologic practices

(E) This device protects the operator against cumulative doses of radiation that are above the threshold for stochastic effects

3.21 Figure Q3-21 depicts coronary arteriograms obtained from two different patients, utilizing the same radiographic equipment. In Panel A, the arteries are well opacified with excellent contrast between contrast-filled vessels and background structures. In Panel B, the arteries are not as dark, and they do not stand out as well against the background. Which of the following statements best explains the difference?

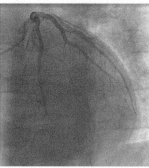
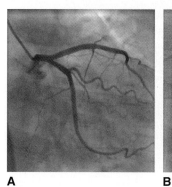

A   B

Figure Q3-21

(A) The operator injected less contrast agent in Panel B, so fewer iodine atoms are available to absorb x-rays

(B) A higher mA setting was used in Panel B

(C) A shorter pulse width was used in Panel A

(D) A higher peak kilovoltage (kVp) setting was used in Panel B

3.22 Figure Q3-22 depicts a flat-detector catheterization laboratory. Which of the following statements about this technology is FALSE?

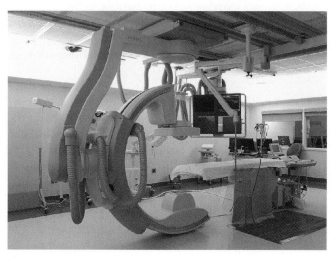

Figure Q3-22

(A) Flat-panel detectors and image intensifiers are similar in that they both require a fluorescent phosphor to convert x-rays into visible light

(B) Flat-panel systems typically deliver 30% to 50% less x-ray exposure than image intensifier–based systems

(C) Flat-panel systems use a conventional x-ray tube

(D) Flat-panel detectors are solid-state devices, whereas image intensifiers use a large vacuum tube

(E) Flat-panel detectors require a high-speed CCD video camera

3.23 Which of the following patients would you be most concerned for potentially developing a malignancy from radiation exposure?

(A) A 78-year-old female undergoing CT of the head and neck and then undergoing carotid angiography with ad hoc angioplasty and bilateral stent placement

(B) A 17-year-old male undergoing CT of the chest and abdomen/pelvis following a motor vehicle accident

(C) A 52-year-old male with recurrent sinus infections requiring repeat head CT

(D) A 49-year-old female undergoing a barium enema for a suspected colonic mass

3.24 Figure Q3-24 is a schematic diagram of a simple x-ray tube, along with a plot of the energy it produces. Which of the following statements is TRUE?

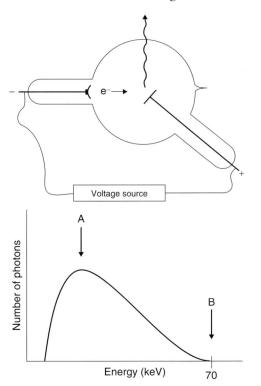

Figure Q3-24

(A) Arrow *A* marks the kVp of the x-ray tube

(B) The x-rays were made with a peak filament current of 70 mA

(C) Arrow *B* indicates the power rating of the tube

(D) Up to 70,000 V was applied to this tube

3.25 Which of the following statements is TRUE regarding safe operation of x-ray equipment by the physician during cardiac catheterization?

(A) Selecting 15 frames per second instead of 30 frames per second will cut the dose rate exactly in half

(B) An interventional cardiologist who constantly switches "fluoro" on and off every time he glances at his hands is not reducing x-ray exposure as expected; this is due to a power surge at start-up

(C) Virtual collimators do not reduce x-ray doses as effectively as standard lead collimators

(D) Each person in the room is responsible for his or her own radiation safety

3.26 The patient in Figure Q3-26 complained to his family physician about an uncomfortable "rash" on his right lower back that appeared 3 weeks after he was hospitalized for chest pain. Which of the following statements is TRUE?

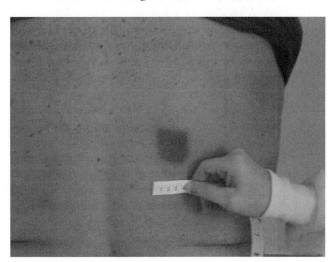

Figure Q3-26

(A) The photograph illustrates a deterministic effect of radiation

(B) This type of injury is very unpredictable

(C) The delayed appearance makes radiation skin injury unlikely

(D) The photograph illustrates a stochastic effect of radiation

3.27 A 56-year-old man has been referred to you for a second attempt at catheter-based repair of a chronic, total circumflex artery occlusion. He had not seen a physician until 1 week ago, when he presented with heart failure and angina. During the past week, he underwent diagnostic coronary arteriography, an unsuccessful percutaneous coronary intervention, and successful implantation of a biventricular defibrillator. The transfer records note hyperglycemia and obesity (weight 329 lb). You realize that two of the three procedures performed during the past week probably involved prolonged fluoroscopy, so radiation skin injury is a very real possibility. Before beginning another procedure, which of the following should you do?

(A) Examine the back of the chest for signs of hair loss (epilation)
(B) Examine the back of the chest for signs of telangiectasia
(C) Examine the back of the chest for signs of dermal atrophy or necrosis
(D) Examine the back of the chest for signs of moist desquamation
(E) None of the above

3.28 Figure Q3-28 is a radiograph of a line-pair phantom that can be used by radiation physicists and service technicians to measure high-contrast spatial resolution. Which of the following statements about calibration and maintenance is FALSE?

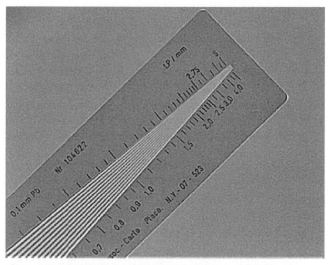

Figure Q3-28

(A) A physicist should measure radiation levels and image quality parameters on a regularly scheduled basis
(B) Image quality and dose measurements are still necessary for modern flat-detector systems
(C) The physicist and service technician should strive for the best possible image quality
(D) Image quality can be improved by simply increasing the dose

ANSWERS AND EXPLANATIONS

3.1 **Answer C.** The RIVAL trial was the first large-scale study assessing the impact of access site on coronary angiography and interventional outcome. Patients were enrolled from 32 countries. No difference was found in the 30-day composite of ischemic and bleeding events (3.7% in the radial group vs. 4.0% in the femoral group), but vascular complications were less frequent in the radial artery access group (1.4% vs. 3.7%). The occurrence of crossover in access site (7.6% vs. 2.0%) and fluoroscopy time (9.3 vs. 8.0 minutes) was greater ($p < 0.0001$) in the radial artery group (*Lancet* 2011;377:1409–1420).

3.2 **Answer A.** In digital subtraction angiography, a non–contrast-filled (mask) image is subtracted from a contrast-filled (live) image. Constant densities, such as bone, are neutralized, leaving only the contrast column. The pattern created by random noise is different on the mask and live images, so subtraction accentuates the noise inherent in low-dose images. To suppress noise, each frame of a subtraction study requires a substantially larger dose of radiation than is needed for a cardiac cine frame. A typical subtraction study can deliver more than 10 times the dose per frame to the patient. Scatter exposure to the operator and room staff is increased commensurately. Subtraction studies are usually acquired at low frame rates of 1 to 6 per second, but this only partially mitigates the higher dose per frame. Subtraction cannot create image detail that was not present in the original image.

3.3 **Answer A.** In recent years, the scope and complexity of interventional procedures have expanded greatly. Although it is true that refinements to imaging systems have reduced x-ray exposure rates, the greater duration of therapeutic procedures has actually *increased* the potential for radiation exposure to patients and operators.

The x-ray exposure rates for fluoroscopy are typically 15 to 20 times lower than those used for diagnostic ("cine" mode) acquisitions. Nevertheless, during interventional procedures, most x-ray exposure to patients and operators comes from fluoroscopy. Procedures that utilize only fluoroscopy are capable of delivering skin doses sufficient to cause severe burns.

The recognition that diagnostic x-ray systems can cause skin injury to patients is a relatively recent phenomenon. The first U.S. Food and Drug Administration (FDA) advisory was published in 1994 and the first reports of radiation skin necrosis due to fluoroscopy did not appear in the medical literature until 1996 (www.fda. gov/cdrh/fluor.html. 2006; *Radiographics* 1996; 16:1195–1199). Even modern, properly calibrated systems are capable of causing radiation skin injury. The risk is greatest with prolonged or repeated procedures, heavy patients, and when body parts are positioned close to the x-ray tube.

The FDA limits the maximum exposure rate for diagnostic fluoroscopy, but this does not guarantee patient safety. Body parts that are positioned close to the x-ray tube (such as the arm in a lateral projection) can receive much more than the calibrated 10 R per minute limit. Prolonged exposures can further increase the risk of injury.

3.4 **Answer A.** Scatter radiation is the main source of exposure to the operator, to laboratory staff, and to patient body parts outside the x-ray beam. Most scatter to the operator originates from the beam entry point, where incoming x-rays strike the table and body surface. In Panel B, the source of scatter is farther from the operator, so exposure is reduced as predicted by the inverse square law. In addition, the patient's body is positioned as a shield between the source of scatter and the operator. By choosing Panel B, this operator can estimate a 10-fold reduction in personal exposure.

The primary beam is collimated, by law, to the size of the image receptor. Therefore, the operator in these illustrations would not be exposed to the primary beam.

3.5 **Answer D.** The background granularity of the image on the left is known as "quantum mottle." It is due to random variation in the distribution of x-ray photons striking the image detector, and it is most apparent when very few photons are available to generate an image. The images obtained through night-vision goggles are grainy for the same reason—few light photons. X-rays and visible light are both forms of electromagnetic radiation, with energy carried in discrete packets or quanta.

Quantum mottle is a form of noise that degrades the detectability of vessel edges and low contrast structures. Increasing the tube filament current (mA) or the pulse width would generate more x-ray photons and thereby suppress quantum mottle. Small amounts of x-ray are used during fluoroscopy, whereas larger amounts of x-ray are used to produce archive quality images such as the one on the right.

Quantum mottle does not indicate a lack of focus or any other problem with the equipment. In fact, the ability to appreciate quantum mottle should reassure the operator that the fluoroscopic dose settings are appropriately low.

The image on the left was obtained with "low-dose" fluoroscopy, whereas that on the right was obtained in the "cine" acquisition mode. The difference in x-ray dose to the patient and operator was approximately 40-fold.

3.6 **Answer D.** An increase in filament current (mA) increases the number of photons produced without altering the distribution of photon energies, as depicted in Panel A. An increase in kVp shifts the energy spectrum toward the right, increasing the proportion of high-energy photons (Panel B). Because high-energy photons are more likely to penetrate the patient, they are less likely to be absorbed and therefore less likely to deposit their energy into tissues. Low-energy photons are absorbed by the skin at the beam entry point; they deposit all their energy into tissues and do not contribute to an image. Obviously, the higher energy photons are desirable for imaging, but only to a point. High-energy photons are poorly absorbed by iodine, so they produce low-contrast arteriograms. Copper and aluminum filters are routinely utilized to absorb the low-energy x-rays that would contribute to skin dose but not to image production. The effect is illustrated in Panel C.

3.7 **Answer C.** Tube filament current (mA) is directly proportional to the number of x-ray photons being produced. Doubling the mA will double the patient's skin entry dose and it will also double the amount of scatter radiation for operators and room staff.

3.8 **Answer B.** Exposure to radiation is a progressively worrisome issue as more and more tests are becoming available and patients are being exposed at younger ages. Cardiac computed tomography (cardiac CTA) studies are becoming more popular, though fortunately with newer scanners and algorithms, the dose of radiation is decreasing to the 5- to 10-mSv range, whereas earlier in this technology development, it was much higher. A chest radiograph has an effective

dose of 0.02 mSv in comparison, and the natural background radiation in the United States is in the range of 2 to 4 mSv per year.

3.9 **Answer A.** Collimators are lead shutters that restrict the size and shape of the x-ray beam as it leaves the tube. The amount of radiation exiting the tube is directly proportional to the area of the beam.

The uncollimated beam used to create the image on the left exposes tissues outside the area of interest to useless radiation. This creates scatter radiation that unnecessarily exposes the operator, patient, and room staff. Scatter that reaches the detector fogs the desirable portion of the image, reducing contrast and overall image quality.

The exposed area of the collimated image on the right is less than half of the uncollimated image. This means that exposure for everyone in the room is less than half of what it would be without collimation.

Although collimation reduces the area of skin exposed, it does not reduce the dose absorbed by skin cells within the irradiated area. In some cases, tight collimation can actually increase the skin dose (this happens if the collimator blades fall within the sampling area for automatic brightness compensation).

3.10 **Answer E.** The black line represents the energy *emission* spectrum of an x-ray tube. The dotted line represents the x-ray *absorption* spectrum of iodine. A sudden jump in absorption occurs when the photon energy is just above the binding energy of the K-shell electron of the iodine atom. The process is known as *photoelectric absorption*. Iodine is a good agent for contrast angiography because it is relatively nontoxic and has a K-shell binding energy of 33.2 keV, which is close to the peak of the output spectrum of medical x-ray machines. Barium has a K edge of 37.4 keV, so it would make a good contrast agent if it were not toxic.

X-rays are produced when electrons emitted from the cathode are accelerated into a tungsten target. When a high-speed electron approaches a dense, positively charged tungsten nucleus, it is deflected and slowed, and its kinetic energy is released in the form of an x-ray photon. These photons are called *bremsstrahlung* or *braking x-rays*. Almost all the x-rays produced by a medical x-ray machine are bremsstrahlung rays.

A few of the high-speed electrons that interact with the target cause the ejection of orbital electrons from shells close to the tungsten nucleus. When an electron from a higher shell drops down to fill the void, the difference in binding energy between the two shells is released in the form of an x-ray photon. These x-rays always have the same wavelength, which is *characteristic* of the target metal and the specific shells involved. The production of bremsstrahlung and characteristic x-rays is illustrated in Figure A3-10.

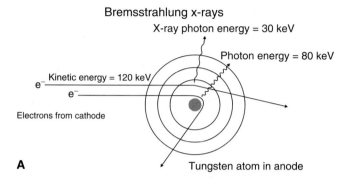

Bremsstrahlung x-rays

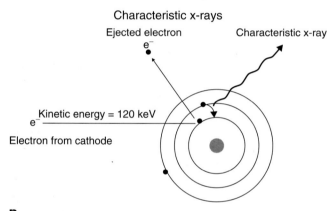

Characteristic x-rays

B

Figure A3-10

It is apparent that many of the x-rays produced by a fluoroscopy unit have energies that are either too low to penetrate the patient or too high to be absorbed by iodine. Copper filters screen out the low-energy photons that would contribute to skin dose but have no imaging value. An ideal x-ray beam for angiography would contain photons in the range between 30 and 70 keV.

Compton scattering occurs when the incoming x-ray photon energies are much greater than the electron binding energies in body tissues. The incoming photon transfers enough energy to completely eject an electron from its atom; it then continues as a lower energy x-ray in a different direction (to conserve momentum of the system). Most of the scatter radiation in a catheterization laboratory comes from Compton interactions.

3.11 **Answer C.** A movable acrylic shield should be part of every catheterization laboratory. Because most scatter radiation originates from the area where the x-ray beam first strikes the patient's chest wall, the shield should be positioned between the beam entry port and the operator's face. It is important to remember that scatter radiation comes from the patient, not from the image detector. A well-positioned acrylic shield will reduce exposure to the operator's eyes, chest, and thyroid by 90%. An assistant who stands in the "shadow" of the primary operator can reduce his or her exposure by two methods. First, the increased distance alone can reduce exposure by 90% compared to the primary operator (inverse square law). Second, scatter rays must penetrate the body of the operator plus two layers of lead worn by the operator. This can be expected to attenuate the scatter beam by >99%.

3.12 **Answer B.** The antiscatter grid is a plate-like device that attaches to the face of the image intensifier or flat detector. It functions like the slats of a Venetian blind, allowing straight-line rays from the x-ray tube to pass through while blocking tangentially directed scatter rays. The grid improves image quality by reducing the fogging effect of scatter, but it does so at the expense of increased patient doses. The grid can more than double the entrance doses received by the patient. Because small children and very thin adults produce little scatter, removing the grid can reduce patient exposure without compromising image quality. This might be important in cases in which the operator wishes to minimize radiation exposure to sensitive areas such as the breast.

3.13 **Answer E.** The lifetime risk of cancer in the United States is approximately 20%. The cumulative occupational dose acquired during a busy interventional career can be projected to increase that risk by 3% to 4%. Although no amount of radiation can be considered safe, the generally accepted annual dose limit is 50 mSv. To place this amount in perspective, average background radiation delivers 3 to 4 mSv per year.

Cataract formation is a deterministic effect of x-ray exposure that depends on a threshold dose and dose rate. Early fluoroscopists who looked directly into the x-ray beam received large doses of radiation in a short period, and they did develop cataracts. With modern equipment, the risk of developing a cataract is probably very low. Even so, eye protection is a reasonable precaution.

3.14 **Answer A.** The transfer of x-ray energy to tissues is estimated with an air-filled ionization chamber placed within the beam, inside the x-ray tube housing. The KERMA is then calculated for a point that approximates the location of the skin surface when the heart is at the isocenter. The cumulative air KERMA displayed on the monitor, in units of gray, can be a very good substitute for skin dose, which is difficult to measure directly. This assumes a typical table height and a single projection. Air KERMA will overestimate the skin dose when multiple projections are utilized because the dose spreads over several different entry ports. It will underestimate the skin dose and the risk of injury whenever body parts are placed close to the x-ray tube.

DAP is the air KERMA multiplied by the beam cross-sectional area. The cumulative DAP is a good measure of the total amount of radiation absorbed by the patient. It is also a good indicator of total room exposure. Collimation reduces beam area, DAP, total patient dose, and room exposure.

3.15 **Answer B.** Shielding and distance are highly effective methods of reducing operator exposure. Because the intensity of scatter radiation is inversely proportional to the square of the distance from the source, one step backward can reduce exposure 10-fold.

To produce an image, x-rays must penetrate the patient and enter the detector. Because absorption increases exponentially with increasing tissue thickness, obese patients require far greater input levels of radiation.

In obese patients, the generator control computer will automatically increase the kVp in an attempt to maintain image brightness, and this will reduce image contrast. It may also increase the pulse width, which can blur moving vessels. These effects, along with increased scatter, will markedly degrade the image quality. This operator should select a large field of view and avoid panning if possible. This will minimize the skin entry dose, keep kVp to a minimum, maximize image contrast, and minimize motion blur.

The operator cannot deny this patient a necessary procedure, but he must be responsible for balancing the risks and benefits. For most patients, the potential for radiation skin injury is so low that a discussion of risk is not necessary. However, for interventional procedures in extremely obese patients, the operator should probably discuss the possibility of skin injury.

Lowering the table as much as possible would place the skin entry in the most concentrated portion of the x-ray beam. This would markedly increase the skin dose and the risk of skin injury.

Figure A3-15 illustrates what happens when the table is lowered as much as possible. A smaller area of skin is exposed to more intense radiation.

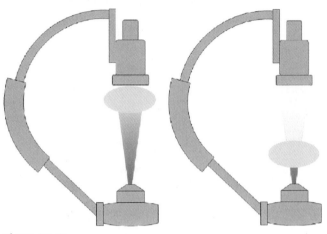

Figure A3-15

3.16 **Answer C.** "Normal" aortic arch anatomy includes the right carotid artery originating from the innominate (bifurcation of the innominate into the subclavian and carotid arteries) with the left carotid and left subclavian originating separately and directly from the aorta. The most frequent variant is a common origin of the innominate and left carotid artery. This erroneously is referred to as a "bovine arch." Technically cattle have a single brachiocephalic trunk from which all arch vessels originate.

3.17 **Answer C.** The table height and detector position are key determinants of x-ray exposure, and both are under the operator's control. The x-ray beam diverges and becomes less intense as it leaves the tube, just like a beam of light diverges and becomes less intense as it leaves a flashlight.

Raising the detector, as shown in the photograph, forces the generator control computer to increase x-ray output to compensate for lost image brightness. This markedly increases the patient skin dose, as well as the scatter dose absorbed by everyone in the room. The computer also increases the kVp, which diminishes image contrast. The detector should always be placed as close to the patient as possible.

Lowering the table will place the patient's skin in the most concentrated portion of the x-ray beam, increasing skin dose rates. This is why some medical x-ray tubes have spacers to keep body parts away from the intense beam. Spacers must never be removed.

Figure A3-17 depicts how an x-ray beam diverges and becomes less intense with distance from the source. The left panel is a photograph of a typical image intensifier–based cardiac system. The right panel is a schematic diagram showing how the beam at point A is less likely to cause skin injury than the same beam at point B.

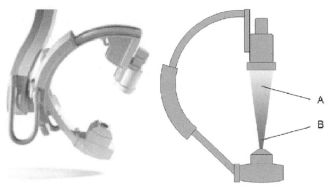

Figure A3-17

3.18 **Answer D.** It is useful to think of radiation in three dimensions: intensity of exposure, absorption, and biologic effect. An analogy is the transfer of heat energy that occurs when one briefly passes a hand through a candle flame. The brief exposure to intense heat transfers very little energy, which is insufficient to injure tissue. Prolonged exposure to warm air on a summer day can cause heat stroke, a profound whole-body effect.

The unit used to measure the *intensity* of x-ray exposure is the roentgen (R). Simplistically, this value tells you whether you are dealing with a candle flame or with warm air. The intensity of radiation diminishes with the square of the distance from the source (inverse square law). This is why distance is an excellent way to minimize operator exposure. If you know that you are dealing with a candle flame, it is best not to put your hand too close. Unfortunately, operators cannot see or feel x-rays. This is why cardiac fluoroscopy systems have instrumentation that displays the intensity of radiation.

The concentration of radiation at a given location can be determined by exposing some material to x-rays, then measuring the KERMA. Catheterization laboratory x-ray machines use air as material. They count ionizations in a chamber with a known volume of material (air) and then calculate air KERMA.

Absorbed dose refers to the concentration of energy transferred to tissue, and the unit of measure for *absorption* is the gray (Gy). In cardiac fluoroscopy, this is an important measure of the potential risk of skin injury.

The sievert (Sv) is a measure of the whole-body biologic effect of one or more absorbed doses. This value can be used to estimate the long-term risk of cancer in an operator.

ALARA is an acronym for as low as reasonably achievable. It is the guiding principle for everyone who uses x-rays.

3.19 **Answer C.** Pregnancy is not a contraindication to necessary cardiac catheterization procedures. External shielding is useless because the fetus is not exposed to the primary beam, only to scatter radiation originating from the mother's chest, and most of this scatter is absorbed by the abdominal viscera. The very small doses of radiation reaching the pelvis would not be expected to cause cell damage (a deterministic effect) leading to intrauterine growth retardation. However, even the smallest dose of ionizing radiation could increase the future risk of malignancy in an unpredictable manner. Fetuses and newborns are known to be at least an order of magnitude more susceptible to radiation-induced malignancy than adults, so the risk is not entirely theoretical. (*Med Phys* 2001;28:1543–1545, Committee on the Biological Effects of Ionizing Radiation. *National research council: health effects of exposure to low levels of ionizing radiation*, 1990).

The operator should discuss the very small cancer risk with the patient and utilize the smallest amount of radiation needed to conduct the procedure safely. The operator should limit the beam to the chest and utilize fluoroscopy instead of cine mode acquisition whenever possible.

3.20 **Answer C.** This is a film badge type of dosimeter that records the accumulated dose of scatter radiation over a period of time. Ideally, two badges should be worn, one on the thyroid collar and one under the apron at waist level. If a single badge is used, it should be placed on the outside of the thyroid collar on the side closest to the source of scatter radiation. Acceptable readings do not indicate safe practice. An operator who performs a limited number of procedures can expose his patient and his room staff to unnecessary radiation while recording low badge readings. There is no threshold for stochastic effects, including genetic defects and cancer. A badge will not protect anyone. The best protection is a good understanding of radiation safety.

3.21 **Answer D.** The difference in image quality stems from the greater thickness and density of tissue that must be penetrated in Panel B. The image in Panel A was obtained from an average-sized patient, in a shallow RAO projection, with the lung as the background. The image in Panel B was obtained from a large patient, in a cranial projection, with the spine as the background.

When steep projections are used in large patients, the generator control system automatically increases the kVp, often to >90 kVp, in an attempt to maintain image brightness. This produces more energetic photons that are able to penetrate tissues better. Unfortunately, many of these photons are too energetic to be absorbed by the iodine, which has a K-edge absorption peak at 33.2 keV.

It does appear that the iodine concentration is too low in Panel B, but the same contrast medium was used and both arteries were well injected. The problem is not the concentration of iodine, but rather that iodine is transparent to high-energy photons. The washed-out image is characteristic of a high kVp.

3.22 **Answers B and E.** Flat-panel detectors and image intensifiers utilize phosphors that convert x-ray photons into faint scintillations of visible light. Early fluoroscopists looked directly at the phosphor in darkened rooms, but this delivered high radiation doses to the eyes and caused cataracts. Image intensifiers brighten the image with a large photomultiplier tube, to the point where it can be captured with a video camera and displayed on a television monitor. With flat detectors, the input phosphors are bonded directly to photodiode arrays that convert the visible light into digital signals.

Both systems use a conventional x-ray tube and similar x-ray exposure levels. Because flat detectors are solid-state devices, they tend to be smaller and lighter, and their performance is more stable over time. Flat-panel catheterization systems are rapidly replacing image intensifier–based systems.

3.23 **Answer B.** All radiation exposure potentially adds to the lifetime risk of developing a malignancy, and this risk is cumulative according to effective doses of exposure and time at risk. As such, younger patients are of particular concern

when receiving radiation-exposing diagnostic studies. In this series of patients, it is known that a head CT has the lowest typical effective dose (2 to 3 mSv), whereas CT scans of the abdomen/pelvis produce an effective dose several times higher (8 to 10 mSv). While patient A may have a slightly higher total effective dose than patient B, given patient B is markedly younger, this is the patient at greatest lifetime risk.

3.24 **Answer D.** This type of x-ray tube was used in the late 1890s by Roentgen and other pioneers to produce amazingly high-quality radiographs. Electrons from the cathode are accelerated by a high voltage until they collide with the metal anode. The maximum voltage across the tube determines the maximum energy of the x-ray photons produced. In this example, the 70,000 V peak (70 kVp) produces x-rays with energies up to 70 keV.

Modern cardiovascular tubes utilize the same principle, with a few refinements to increase the output of x-rays. The cathode consists of a white-hot filament that boils off the large quantities of electrons needed to make large amounts of x-rays. The anode consists of a rotating tungsten disk that absorbs and dissipates heat much better than a stationary target, which would quickly melt if used for cardiac angiography.

X-ray production is very inefficient. Only approximately 1% of the electrical energy delivered to the tube is converted into x-rays; the remaining 99% is converted to heat that must be dissipated. For years, heat dissipation was a major technical challenge for cardiovascular x-ray tubes. The problem has largely been solved by liquid cooling systems that work like automobile radiators.

3.25 **Answer A.** Most cardiac systems now operate at 15 frames per second. Thirty frames per second are sometimes used for pediatric patients with high heart rates and for ventricular wall motion studies.

Limiting the beam on time is one of the most effective methods of reducing radiation exposure. The operator should *never* make x-rays unless he is looking directly at the monitor and prepared to work. Live fluoroscopy should never be used when an operator is manipulating equipment under direct vision, and it should never be used when contemplating the next move. "Last image hold" and "fluoro replay" features provide the same information without unnecessary radiation.

Virtual collimators are software-generated lines on the last recorded image. They allow the operator to position the collimators without stepping on the "fluoro" pedal. They are an excellent way to minimize radiation exposure.

The physician in charge is responsible for the radiation safety of everyone in the room. The operating physician must be knowledgeable enough to recognize and correct unsafe practices.

3.26 **Answer A.** Stochastic effects pertain to deoxyribonucleic acid (DNA) injury that may increase the probability of genetic defects or cancer at some point in the future. Theoretically, even a single x-ray photon can induce DNA injury in a single cell that leads to fatal lymphoma 20 years later. A greater exposure and one of a longer duration will increase the probability of a stochastic effect, but there is no safe threshold and the consequences are unpredictable. Cancer caused by a single x-ray photon is just as bad as cancer caused by millions of photons.

Deterministic effects pertain to cell injury that occurs shortly (hours to months) after a threshold dose of radiation is exceeded. Skin injury is the most common deterministic effect of diagnostic x-ray exposure. Because skin cells divide continuously, they are susceptible to injury from large doses of radiation that can occur at the beam entrance port. The injury becomes apparent weeks to months after exposure, when cells lost by normal desquamation are no longer replaced. Because of the delay, patients and physicians may not even suspect the cause.

The photograph illustrates radiation skin injury from fluoroscopy used during a percutaneous coronary intervention. The size and location indicate that the operator worked in the left anterior oblique (LAO) projection and utilized square collimators. This type of injury can progress for months, sometimes leading to deep, nonhealing ulcers that require grafting. It is important to know that deterministic effects are predictable and therefore preventable.

3.27 **Answer E.** Because of his obesity, this patient will receive substantially increased skin entry doses during cardiac fluoroscopy. The recent exposures will lower the threshold for skin injury with the next procedure. Diabetes may further increase the susceptibility to skin injury. In addition to discussing the risks and benefits, and considering the alternatives to another fluoroscopic procedure, this operator should examine the patient carefully for signs of radiation skin injury.

All the answers list deterministic effects of radiation. However, hair loss does not appear until 3 weeks after the exposure, and the latent period is even longer for desquamation (4 weeks), dermal atrophy or necrosis (3 months), and telangiectasia formation (1 year). Erythema can develop within hours to days.

3.28 **Answer C.** The objective of cardiac fluoroscopy is not to make the best possible image, but rather to strike a balance between image quality and dose. A good image contains some degree of noise. To achieve this objective, a regularly scheduled testing program is necessary for all fluoroscopy systems. Older image intensifier systems are especially susceptible to loss of contrast that can be partially compensated by increasing the input dose.

4 Inflammation and Arterial Injury

Harold L. Dauerman

QUESTIONS

4.1 A 54-year-old man presents to your office 2 weeks after sirolimus-eluting stent (SES) placement with diffuse hives and pruritus. There is no wheezing, and his blood pressure is stable. The patient is on chronic aspirin therapy and was started on an ACE inhibitor, statin, and clopidogrel during his recent hospitalization. The patient shows you a journal article given to him by a physician who is a family friend. He asks if the problem reported in the article (Fig. Q4-1) is the cause of his "rash." You review the article and advise him to:

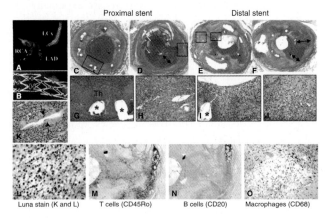

Figure Q4-1. (Reproduced from Virmani R, Guagliumi G, Farb A, et al. Localized hypersensitivity and late coronary thrombosis secondary to a sirolimus-eluting stent: should we be cautious? *Circulation* 2004;109:701–705.)

(A) Discontinue clopidogrel
(B) Discontinue aspirin
(C) Start antihistamines and steroids
(D) Stop statin and ACE inhibitor; consider changing from clopidogrel to prasugrel; start antihistamines and possibly oral steroids

4.2 A 43-year-old woman presents for elective cardiac catheterization and asks that you use ticagrelor as opposed to clopidogrel if stenting is required. Data that support the patient's request include which of the following?

(A) Ticagrelor suppresses postpercutaneous coronary intervention (PCI) inflammation to a greater degree than clopidogrel
(B) Ticagrelor decreases cardiovascular events compared to clopidogrel in patients with acute coronary syndromes
(C) Ticagrelor is a more potent inhibitor of the glycoprotein IIb/IIIa receptor than clopidogrel
(D) Ticagrelor decreases ischemic cardiovascular events compared to clopidogrel in patients with stable coronary syndromes undergoing PCI

4.3 A 65-year-old woman comes to your office after seeing a television report about stents, and she is concerned that her drug-eluting stent (DES) is a "ticking time bomb in my chest." She wants proof that DES are at the same risk as bare-metal stents (BMS) for late stent thrombosis. She has done some research on the Internet and shows

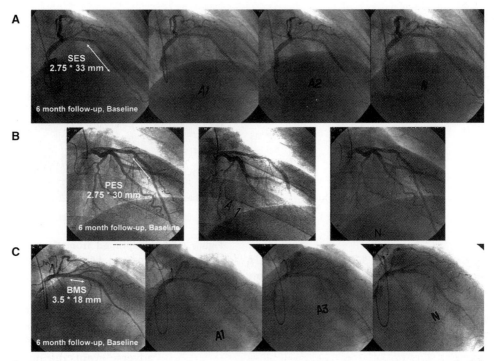

Figure Q4-3. (Reprinted from Pendyala LK, Yin X, Li J, et al. The first-generation drug-eluting stents and coronary endothelial dysfunction. *JACC Cardiovasc Interv* 2009;2:1169–1177, with permission from Elsevier.)

you a figure (Fig. Q4-3) that depicts the impact of intracoronary acetylcholine (A) and nitroglycerin (N) administered 6 months after BMS and DES (SES, sirolimus-eluting stent; PES, paclitaxel-eluting stent) implantation. Your interpretation of this experiment is:

(A) BMS and DES have a similar acute vasodilatory response to acetylcholine consistent with a similar chronic risk of inflammation and stent thrombosis

(B) First-generation DES (sirolimus and paclitaxel) demonstrate an enhanced risk of chronic endothelial dysfunction compared to BMS, consistent with the patient's concerns about chronically enhanced inflammation and thrombotic risk with DES

(C) First-generation DES (sirolimus and paclitaxel) have similar risk of chronic endothelial

dysfunction, and thus there is no increased risk of inflammation and thrombosis with DES

(D) First-generation DES (sirolimus and paclitaxel) cause more chronic endothelial dysfunction, but this dysfunction is only at the proximal edges of the stent and should not cause any increased inflammation or thrombotic risk in the distal vasculature

4.4 The same 65-year-old woman as in the previous question is now more concerned than ever about her lifetime risk of stent thrombosis. She has looked up her stent type and found it to be a second-generation (zotarolimus-eluting) stent. You show her Figure Q4-4 and explain this experiment as follows:

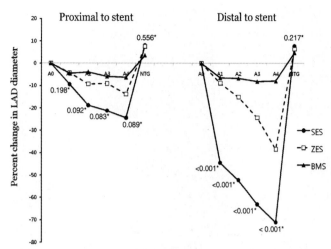

Figure Q4-4. (Reprinted from Kim JW, Seo HS, Park JH, et al. A prospective, randomized, 6-month comparison of the coronary vasomotor response associated with a zotarolimus- versus a sirolimus-eluting stent: differential recovery of coronary endothelial dysfunction. *J Am Coll Cardiol* 2009;53:1653–1659, with permission from Elsevier.)

(A) Risks of acute, late, and very late stent thrombosis are the same with sirolimus- vs. zotarolimus-eluting stents
(B) Zotarolimus-eluting stents cause more chronic endothelial dysfunction than SES
(C) BMS cause the most chronic endothelial dysfunction and thus have the highest likelihood of chronic inflammation and thrombosis
(D) While zotarolimus-eluting stents cause more chronic inflammation than BMS, the chronic endothelial dysfunction and thus inflammatory response is better than SES, and this may translate into a lower risk of late thrombosis

4.5 An 82-year-old man received two everolimus-eluting stents (EES) in the left anterior descending coronary artery and had relief of angina. Would this patient's risk of chronic inflammation and stent thrombosis be less with either a bioabsorbable stent or bioabsorbable polymer as shown in Figure Q4-5?

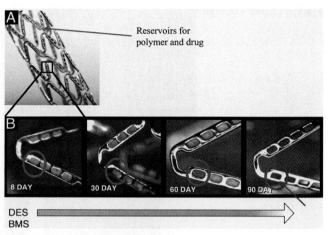

Figure Q4-5. (Reprinted from Garg S, Serruys PW. Coronary stents: looking forward. *J Am Coll Cardiol* 2010;56:S43–S78, with permission from Elsevier.)

(A) Compared to a permanent polymer DES, bioabsorbable polymer DES in the LEADERS trial demonstrated a decreased risk of adverse events during follow-up
(B) Bioabsorbable polymers on DES do not decrease ischemic events, but late events are prevented with a fully bioabsorbable stent
(C) A fully bioabsorbable stent may eliminate risk of chronic inflammation but has not been tested in a large enough clinical trial to determine its role in preventing late stent thrombosis
(D) Permanent polymers do not cause chronic inflammation or increased risk of stent thrombosis

4.6 You are deciding between eptifibatide vs. bivalirudin for PCI of an LAD lesion in a patient with an acute coronary syndrome. The TIMI 30-PROTECT trial data suggest that you should choose a platelet IIb/IIIa inhibitor over bivalirudin if the goal is to reduce:

(A) The risk of bleeding complications after the PCI
(B) The duration of asymptomatic ischemia on Holter monitoring after the PCI
(C) The inflammation measured as a rise in interleukin-6, C-reactive protein (CRP), and soluble CD40 ligand after the PCI
(D) The risk of ischemic events after the PCI

4.7 After coronary stenting, which of the following cell types would NOT be part of the initial injury response?

(A) Platelets
(B) Lymphocytes and macrophages
(C) Alpha-actin–positive smooth muscle cells
(D) Neutrophils

4.8 How does arterial injury caused by angioplasty differ from injury due to DES placement?

(A) Negative remodeling may be a major factor in DES-related healing
(B) DES abolishes the early phases of platelet activation and inflammatory cytokine increases
(C) Polymer coating of the stent limits migration of smooth muscle cells
(D) Both neointimal hyperplasia and negative remodeling play major roles in the long-term healing response to balloon angioplasty

4.9 All of the following may contribute to arterial injury and inflammation, EXCEPT:

(A) Stent coating with selected polymers/drugs
(B) Increased stent strut thickness and specific geometric factors
(C) Stent deployment with struts in contact with damaged media or lipid core
(D) Stent deployment with struts in contact with fibrous plaque

4.10 Considering the photomicrographs in Figure Q4-10, the panel (A) is a histopathologic section from a rabbit artery stented with polymer and a high dose of paclitaxel. Panel (B) is from an artery stented with polymer alone. How did this high dose of paclitaxel influence the healing response?

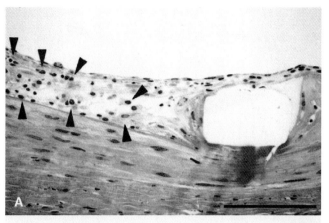

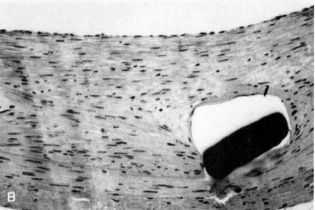

Figure Q4-10. (Reproduced from Farb A, Heller PF, Shroff S, et al. Pathological analysis of local delivery of paclitaxel via a polymer-coated stent. *Circulation* 2001;104:473–479.)

(A) Decreased intimal hyperplasia in the paclitaxel polymer–coated stent
(B) Increased inflammatory reaction in the polymer-only stent
(C) Decreased intimal hyperplasia in the polymer-only stent
(D) Persistent fibrin deposition in the polymer-only stent

4.11 Figure Q4-11 shows a histopathologic analysis 1 day after implantation of a coronary artery stent. What does the asterisk (*) demonstrate?

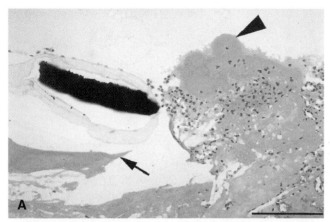

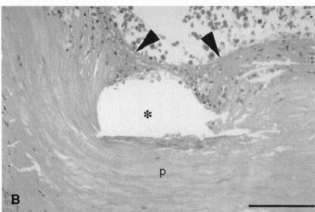

Figure Q4-11.   (Reproduced from Farb A, Sangiorgi G, Carter AJ, et al. Pathology of acute and chronic coronary stenting in humans. *Circulation* 1999;99:44–52.)

(A) Platelet-rich thrombus
(B) Lipid-rich vulnerable plaque
(C) Site of stent strut
(D) Fibrous plaque

4.12 Late stent thrombosis after DES placement has been associated with which of the following?

(A) Warfarin anticoagulation in addition to dual antiplatelet therapy
(B) A localized, hypersensitivity (eosinophilic, giant cell) reaction to the polymer
(C) Implantation of DES in the setting of ST-segment elevation myocardial infarction
(D) Geographic miss during DES implantation

4.13 A patient develops acute chest pain and ECG changes within 1 minute of stent implantation. What type of arterial injury is shown just distal to the stent (Fig. Q4-13)?

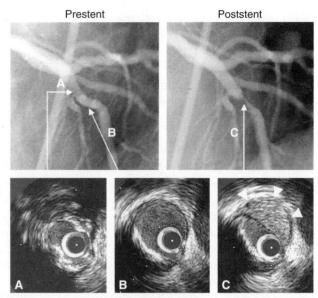

Figure Q4-13.   (Reproduced from Maehara A, Mintz GS, Bui AB, et al. Incidence, morphology, angiographic findings, and outcomes of intramural hematomas after percutaneous coronary interventions. *Circulation* 2002;105:2037–2042.)

(A) Acute intramural hematoma
(B) Intraprocedural stent thrombosis
(C) Spontaneous rupture of distal lipid-rich plaque
(D) Acute platelet-rich thrombus due to stent-mediated hypersensitivity

4.14 Arterial injury due to stent placement induces a systemic inflammatory response. Figure Q4-14 shows the systemic rise of which inflammatory marker after stenting?

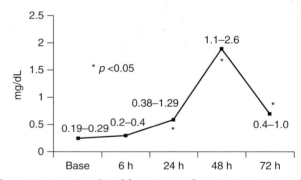

Figure Q4-14.   (Reprinted from Gaspardone A, Crea F, Versaci F, et al. Predictive value of C-reactive protein after successful coronary-artery stenting in patients with stable angina. *Am J Cardiol* 1998;82:515–518, with permission from Elsevier.)

(A) Serum amyloid A
(B) CRP
(C) Soluble CD40 ligand
(D) IL-6

4.15 A 73-year-old retired physician with stable angina discusses risk and benefit of PCI prior to his procedure. He is concerned about the risk of stent thrombosis and wants the stent that will "heal the best." He shows you Figure Q4-15 and asks which stent you plan to use:

(C) Use a bare-metal stent if rapid and complete healing is the goal
(D) Use a second-generation DES (ZES or EES) as healing and inflammation are the same as with BMS

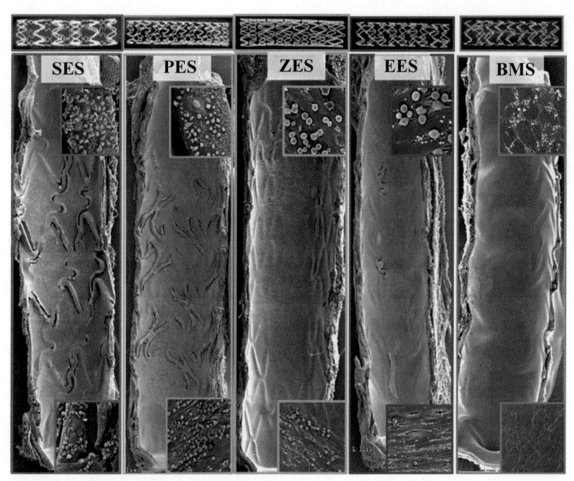

Figure Q4-15. (Reprinted from Joner M, Nakazawa G, Finn AV. Endothelial cell recovery between comparator polymer-based drug-eluting stents. *J Am Coll Cardiol* 2008;52:333–342, with permission from Elsevier.)

(A) Use the SES stent as it has the most years of experience as a DES
(B) Use the PES stent as overall risk of late adverse events is superior with this DES type

4.16 Optical coherence tomography is performed on a patient 12 months after DES implantation. Figure Q4-16 shows what phenomenon and what potential mechanisms are a reasonable explanation of this occurrence?

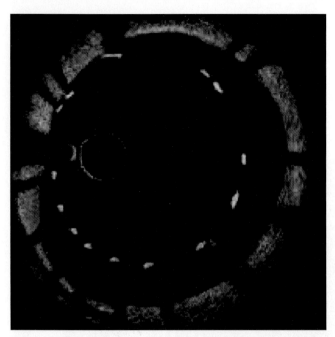

Figure Q4-16. (Reprinted from Garg S, Serruys PW. Coronary stents: current status. *J Am Coll Cardiol* 2010;56:S1–S42, with permission from Elsevier.)

(A) Persistent intramural hematoma caused by extensive coronary dissection

(B) A predominantly eosinophilic inflammatory response that is associated with increased risk of incomplete stent apposition

(C) Spontaneous dissection postprocedure that is associated with overexpansion or stent diameter in great excess to the reference vessel diameter

(D) Pseudoaneurysm associated with inappropriate extent of anticoagulation during the procedure

4.17 Activated macrophages, recruited after arterial injury, secrete which systemic mediators of inflammation?

(A) CRP
(B) Soluble CD40 ligand
(C) IL-1 and IL-6
(D) P selectin

4.18 A 56-year-old woman with anterior ischemia on stress testing is found to have a long segment of LAD disease. The lesion length is 23 mm. You have the option of using one 28-mm DES or two 15-mm DES. Figure Q4-18 is from a porcine model and shows the consequences of your choice and is best interpreted as follows:

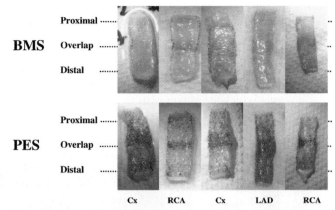

Figure Q4-18. (Reprinted from Chen JP, Hou D, Pendyala L, et al. Drug-eluting stent thrombosis: The Kounis hypersensitivity-associated acute coronary syndrome revisited. *JACC Cardiovasc Interv* 2009;2:583–593, with permission from Elsevier.)

(A) A single long DES has an enhanced inflammatory response compared to two shorter DESs

(B) Overlap of DES may cause an enhanced inflammatory response at the overlap sites

(C) Drug-elution patterns are similar at overlap sites as compared to nonoverlap sites

(D) You should use a BMS to avoid increased risk of stent thrombosis due to overlapping DESs

4.19 Arterial injury leads to a cascade of platelet activation followed by local and systemic inflammation. Figure Q4-19 demonstrates vasoconstriction occurring after exercise in a patient who received an SES more than 6 months prior to the stress test. Which answer is INCORRECT?

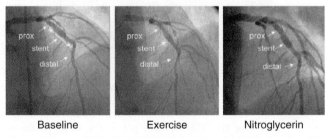

Figure Q4-19. (Reprinted from Togni M, Windecker S, Cocchia R, et al. Sirolimus-eluting stents associated with paradoxic coronary vasoconstriction. *J Am Coll Cardiol* 2005;46:231–236.)

(A) The patient might also have abnormal flow-independent dilation of the brachial artery

(B) The patient might also have abnormal flow-mediated dilation of the brachial artery

(C) DES lead to delay in endothelial regeneration after injury

(D) Chronic endothelial dysfunction suggests durable polymers lead to chronic inflammation

4.20 Figure Q4-20 demonstrates a similar extent of DES- and BMS-induced systemic inflammation after PCI. If inflammation after arterial injury is important in developing restenosis, what best explains the 50% to 80% reduction in restenosis with DES vs. BMS?

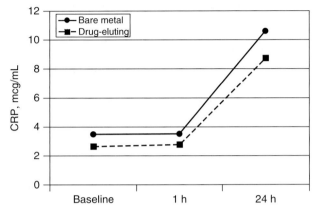

Figure Q4-20. (Reprinted from Gogo PB, Schneider DJ, Watkins MW, et al. Systemic inflammation after drug-eluting stent placement. *J Thromb Thrombolysis* **2005;19:87–92, with permission from Springer.)**

(A) DES decrease initial and chronic platelet activation compared to BMS

(B) DES decrease the early systemic inflammatory response to stenting compared to BMS

(C) DES decrease systemic inflammation occurring between 24 hours and 9 months after stenting

(D) DES decreases the local, but not systemic, impact of stenting on inflammation

4.21 An enhanced systemic inflammatory response may occur after PCI for cardiogenic shock. This inflammatory response may lead to:

(A) Up-regulation of nitric oxide synthase leading to vasodilation and hypotension

(B) Severe vasoconstriction thus resulting in a decreased cardiac output

(C) A down-regulation of nitric oxide synthase leading to pulmonary edema

(D) Up-regulation of natriuretic peptides leading to hypotension via excessive diuresis

4.22 All of the following drugs have been shown to have a potential favorable impact on the acute inflammatory response after PCI, EXCEPT:

(A) Atorvastatin

(B) Clopidogrel

(C) Abciximab

(D) Beta-blockers

4.23 In the IMPRESS randomized trial, prednisone or placebo was given for 45 days after BMS implantation with a reduction in 6-month cardiovascular event rates (Fig. Q4-23). What was the key entry requirement to be randomized in this trial?

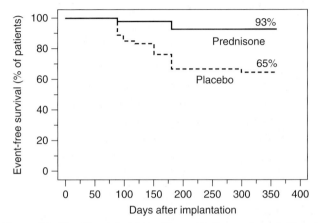

Figure Q4-23. (Reprinted from Versaci F, Gaspardone A, Tomai F, et al. Immunosuppressive therapy for the prevention of restenosis after coronary artery stent implantation (IMPRESS study). *J Am Coll Cardiol* **2002;40:1935–1942, with permission from Elsevier.)**

(A) Elevated preprocedural levels of soluble CD40 after stent placement

(B) High risk for restenosis based upon presence of diabetes mellitus

(C) Elevated preprocedural levels of CRP

(D) A persistently elevated CRP level 72 hours after stent placement

4.24 Which patients undergoing PCI may benefit the most from preprocedural clopidogrel administration?

(A) Patients at lower risk for inflammation as defined by a CRP < 1.0

(B) Patients with a heightened inflammatory status as defined by an elevated CRP prior to the PCI

(C) Patients undergoing PCI for stable angina, but not acute coronary syndromes

(D) Patients with a heightened inflammatory status as defined by soluble CD40 ligand

4.25 Eptifibatide and tirofiban have been shown to clearly have which effects after PCI?

(A) Decrease intimal hyperplasia via a direct effect on macrophage accumulation

(B) Decrease intimal hyperplasia via inhibition of smooth muscle cell hyperplasia

(C) Decrease the rise of CRP and IL-6 in the first 24 hours after PCI compared to heparin alone

(D) Decrease platelet aggregation and the incidence of periprocedural myonecrosis

ANSWERS AND EXPLANATIONS

4.1 Answer D. The figure incidentally shows a case of intense eosinophilic reaction to a DES associated with late stent thrombosis. The patient is correct that DES can elicit a chronic inflammatory response even after the drug has fully eluted. This reaction is generally localized and hypothesized to be associated with increased risk of very late stent thrombosis. In this patient's case, a systemic allergic response is much more likely to be drug mediated and careful alteration of medications is warranted. A chronic systemic reaction to the permanent components of the stent (nickel, polymer) is extremely rare but is a potential explanation for symptoms if medication changes do not relieve the hypersensitivity reaction (*Circulation* 2004;109:701–705).

4.2 Answer B. Ticagrelor is a more potent platelet $P2Y_{12}$ receptor antagonist than clopidogrel. In the PLATO trial, cardiovascular events were decreased with ticagrelor as compared to clopidogrel among patients with acute coronary syndromes—a trial of ticagrelor in stable, elective catheterization patients has not yet been reported. While more potent inhibition of $P2Y_{12}$ receptor–mediated platelet activation could plausibly impact platelet–monocyte interactions and post-PCI inflammation, a positive impact on arterial injury mediated inflammation has not yet been demonstrated (*N Engl J Med* 2009;361:1045–1057).

4.3 Answer B. The figure demonstrates significantly more proximal and distal vasoconstriction with PES and SES vs. BMS among patients tested with ascending doses (A1, A2) of intracoronary acetylcholine 6 months after stent implantation. Non–endothelium-dependent vasodilation (N = nitrates) is similar among all three groups. It should be appreciated that any drug should have fully eluted 6 months after DES implantation, so this chronic endothelial dysfunction likely represents a chronic inflammatory response to permanent polymer. This pathophysiologic finding has not been clearly linked to increased risk of clinical late stent thrombosis (*JACC Cardiovasc Interv* 2009;2:1169–1177).

4.4 Answer D. Vasoreactivity is abnormal for both SES (sirolimus) and ZES (zotarolimus) 6 months after stent implantation compared to BMS. But the relative vasoconstriction is much more intense proximally and distally with the first-generation SES. This suggests more intense endothelial dysfunction due to chronic inflammation with the SES vs. ZES stent. Of note, the BASKET-PROVE trial compared SES vs. second-generation EES and did not show a difference in death, infarction, or stent thrombosis despite a possible difference in inflammatory responses based on generation of DES.

4.5 Answer C. The concept of reducing chronic DES inflammation and possible enhanced risk of very late stent thrombosis has led to development of DES with bioabsorbable polymers (e.g., Nevo stent, as shown in the figure) and fully bioabsorbable DES platforms. To date, trials have not demonstrated a difference in late stent thrombosis rates with these emerging DES concepts (*EuroIntervention* 2010;6:233–239).

4.6 Answer B. All stenting elicits a rapid systemic inflammatory response including a rise of cytokines (IL-6 and CRP). Glycoprotein IIb/IIIa inhibitors have been shown to blunt the rise of CRP after coronary intervention in the EPIC trial. The TIMI 30-PROTECT trail randomized ACS patients to bivalirudin or eptifibatide with stenting and found no difference in peak levels of cytokines, suggesting no difference in acute inflammatory modulation with these pharmacologies. There was also no difference in ischemic events in this trial. On the other hand, bleeding events were less with bivalirudin and Holter monitor–measured ischemia was less with eptifibatide (*J Am Coll Cardiol* 2006;47:2364–2373; *Circulation* 2001;104:163–167).

4.7 Answer C. Coronary stenting is a model for arterial injury, and the healing response proceeds in phases. Phase I is de-endothelialization followed by deposition of platelets and fibrin. Via platelet activation and cytokine increases, acute inflammatory cells are then recruited in the first few days after stenting. Phase 2 involves release of growth factors from platelets and leukocytes driving proliferation and migration of smooth muscle cells and chronic inflammatory cells. Phase 3 (weeks to months after injury) is characterized by migration of alpha-actin–positive smooth muscle cells into the neointima, extracellular matrix deposition, and re-endothelialization of the stent (*J Am Coll Cardiol* 2000;35:157–163; *Arterioscler Thromb Vasc Biol* 2002;22:1769–1776).

4.8 **Answer D.** All forms of arterial injury lead to platelet activation, inflammation, and smooth muscle cell–mediated chronic healing. Paclitaxel and sirolimus decrease the amount of neointimal hyperplasia compared to bare-metal stenting, but the underlying polymer has no favorable effect on the healing process. All stents in general abolish two adverse components of the healing response: an acute decrease in vessel diameter (recoil) and a chronic decrease in the external elastic membrane dimension (negative remodeling). Incomplete stent apposition may rarely occur as part of the healing process after stenting. This is related to positive remodeling during the healing process and does not contribute to restenosis after bare-metal or drug-eluting stenting (*Circulation* 1997;96:475–483; *Circulation* 2003;107:2660–2663).

4.9 **Answer D.** The inflammatory response to stent-mediated arterial injury determines adverse healing responses. Among the factors that may increase inflammation and restenosis are (a) certain polymers/drugs, (b) stent strut thickness and geometric factors, and (c) medial injury or lipid core penetration by stent struts. Deployment of stents in fibrous plaque without causing medial damage reduces the inflammatory response to stenting (*Circulation* 2002;106:2649–2651; *J Am Coll Cardiol* 2003;41:1283–1288).

4.10 **Answer A.** Paclitaxel successfully reduced the thickness of intimal hyperplasia in the top picture, as compared to polymer alone. At this high dose of paclitaxel, though, the inflammatory response is augmented (*arrowheads*) as compared to polymer alone. Adverse events related possibly to chronic inflammation and delayed healing due to high-dose paclitaxel were seen with the QuaDS QP-2 stent. Similar adverse clinical events were not seen using the different polymer/paclitaxel dosing regimen of the TAXUS-IV trial (*Circulation* 2001;104:473–479; *N Engl J Med* 2004;350:221–231).

4.11 **Answer C.** Both panels show the acute response to arterial injury. In the top panel (A), platelet-rich thrombus (*arrowhead*) is seen. Numerous acute inflammatory cells are also present within the thrombus; focal fibrous cap disruption is also demonstrated (*arrow*). In Panel B, an asterisk shows the site of the stent strut with associated fibrin-rich thrombus (*arrowheads*). Fibrous plaque (*p*) is present below the strut.

4.12 **Answer B.** The major cause of DES thrombosis is early cessation of dual antiplatelet therapy. But case reports demonstrate rare hypersensitivity reactions after implantation of SES that may be associated with stent thrombosis. While other causes of hypersensitivity reactions may occur (i.e., clopidogrel or aspirin allergies), an eosinophilic reaction can occur at the site of the stent strut and be associated with fatal stent thrombosis. This could be due to either drug or polymer, but early drug elution suggests that an allergic reaction to the permanent polymer may have been implicated in some cases of late stent thrombosis (*JAMA* 2005;293:2126–2130).

4.13 **Answer A.** Arterial injury can manifest itself angiographically immediately after stent deployment. Causes of acute vessel closure in the stent era include intraprocedural stent thrombosis, extensive dissection, or intramural hematoma formation (*Circulation* 2004;109:2732–2736). Intramural hematoma complicates approximately 7% of PCI procedures, and the angiogram may show stenosis, dissection, or even a normal appearance. By intravascular ultrasound, intramural hematomas are crescent shaped, homogenous, hyperechoic areas with an entry site from dissection into the media.

4.14 **Answer B.** The most extensively studied systemic marker of inflammation is CRP; the magnitude of pre- and post-PCI levels of CRP has been associated with adverse events after stenting. The systemic rise in CRP after injury is fairly slow, with no rise appreciated until at least 24 hours after PCI. The slow systemic rise of CRP after stenting is most consistent with production of CRP primarily in the liver and a downstream role of this cytokine in the response to injury.

4.15 **Answer C.** The figure shows a scanning electron micrograph comparing various DES and BMS at 28 days after implantation in a rabbit iliac model. There are significant differences in inflammation and healing among the different stents with healing grades being greatest in BMS, then second-generation DES, and worst with first-generation DES. As the patient requested the stent with the best healing, BMS would win in this animal model. But, for clinical performance in humans, EES and SES provide similar outcomes in the BASKET PROVE trial, and both stents demonstrate improved efficacy compared to BMS (*J Am Coll Cardiol* 2008;52:333-342).

4.16 Answer B. Late acquired incomplete stent apposition is more common after DES than BMS (and not related to underdeployment of stents at time of implantation). While the exact mechanism is unknown, the clinical consequences of incomplete apposition may be an increased risk of stent thrombosis. Potential mechanisms of increased risk of incomplete apposition after DES include inflammation, delayed healing, underlying soft plaque, and a chronic eosinophilic response to DES implantation.

4.17 Answer C. CRP is an acute-phase reactant produced by the liver. IL-6 is the main hepatic stimulus for CRP production and is produced by macrophages. CRP in turn stimulates further production of inflammatory cytokines such as IL-1, IL-6, and TNF-alpha by macrophages. P selectin is stored in the alpha granules of platelets. CD40 ligand, a transmembrane protein, was originally identified on CD4+ T cells, and recently found on activated platelets. Both membrane-bound and soluble forms of this ligand may interact with CD40, which is expressed on vascular cells, resulting in a variety of inflammatory responses (*Circulation* 1999;100:614-620; *Am Heart J* 2003;145:563-566).

4.18 Answer B. While lesion length and multiple DES may be predictors of DES stent thrombosis, the clinical results of overlapping DES are not entirely clear. Overlapping DES, though, is clearly associated with variable drug elution and an enhanced chronic inflammatory response at the overlap sites as shown in this porcine PES histology. Since BMS do not elute drugs, there is no increased inflammatory response at BMS overlap sites, but intimal hyperplasia is abundant. Use of a single longer DES obviates both the altered drug elution and increased inflammation associated with overlapping multiple DES.

4.19 Answer A. Flow-mediated dilation of the brachial artery reflects systemic endothelial dysfunction while flow-independent dilation reflects smooth muscle function. Patients have abnormal endothelial function early after PCI, but it is somewhat surprising that abnormal endothelial function can be seen >6 months after DES placement. As sirolimus is no longer present on the stent at that time, the etiology of this longer term endothelial dysfunction is most likely related to durable polymer (*J Am Coll Cardiol* 2005;46:231-236; *Am J Cardiol* 2004;94:1420-1423; *Eur Heart J* 2006;27:166-170).

4.20 Answer D. While prior literature has suggested that the post-PCI rise of cytokines is predictive of restenosis, this has not been confirmed in the DES era. In fact, it appears that systemic cytokine rise after PCI is marked and similar for both DES and BMS. No difference in platelet activation has been shown for various stent types. Given the markedly lower restenosis rates for DES, it is likely local drug delivery works via local suppression of inflammation and smooth muscle cell migration despite a similar systemic inflammatory response (*J Thromb Thrombolysis* 2005;19:87-92; *Am Heart J* 2005;150:344-350).

4.21 Answer A. Cardiogenic shock has traditionally been thought of as massive myonecrosis leading to reduced cardiac output and compensatory vasoconstriction. In the SHOCK trial, though, systemic vascular resistance was not markedly elevated in most cardiogenic shock patients. Newer evidence suggests that shock induces a systemic inflammatory response leading to nitric oxide synthase overproduction. This leads to inappropriate vasodilation and may play an important role in the refractory hypotension associated with cardiogenic shock (*Circulation* 2003;107:2998-3002; *Eur Heart J* 2003;24:1287-1295).

4.22 Answer D. Atorvastatin, clopidogrel, and abciximab may blunt the inflammatory response after PCI as one mechanism of their beneficial impact on PCI. Abciximab blunted the rise of CRP and IL-6 after PCI in a subset of patients in the EPIC trial. Clopidogrel may attenuate the increased risk associated with PCI among patients with high CRP levels. Similarly, statin therapy prior to PCI seems to have the most benefit among patients with the highest level of pre-PCI inflammation. While none of these systemic medications clearly impact long-term healing (stent restenosis), local applications of statin drugs may be promising given their potential effects on inflammation and smooth muscle cell migration (*Am J Cardiol*

2001;88:672–674; *Circulation* 2003;107:1750–1756; *Circulation* 2003;107:1123–1128; *Am J Cardiol* 2002;90:786–789).

4.23   **Answer D.** The IMPRESS (Immunosuppressive Therapy for the Prevention of Restenosis after Coronary Artery Stent Implantation) trial hypothesized that patients with persistent inflammation after PCI would benefit from anti-inflammatory therapy. Eighty-three patients undergoing successful bare-metal stenting with CRP levels >0.5 mg/dL measured 72 hours after the procedure were randomized to receive oral prednisone or placebo for 45 days. As shown above, this trial supports the importance of inflammation after bare-metal stenting by demonstrating decreased events in the prednisone group. As 93% event-free survival can also be seen with drug-eluting stenting without prednisone, it is not clear whether adjunctive oral steroids would be beneficial in the current era (*J Am Coll Cardiol* 2002;40:1935–1942).

4.24   **Answer B.** In addition to inhibiting platelet aggregation, clopidogrel may have an impact on inflammation after PCI. One mechanism of clopidogrel benefit on inflammation may be via decreased expression of P selectin after clopidogrel administration. P selectin may play a key role in activation of tumor necrosis factor-alpha as well as other cytokines. Thus, treatment with clopidogrel prior to PCI may be especially beneficial among patients with heightened inflammatory status as defined by CRP.

4.25   **Answer D.** Glycoprotein IIb/IIIa inhibitors decrease platelet aggregation and periprocedural myonecrosis. While the EPIC trial suggests that abciximab decreased the rise of CRP and IL-6 after PCI as compared to heparin alone, there are little data to suggest that eptifibatide or tirofiban significantly suppress the inflammatory response to PCI. It is possible that the inferiority of tirofiban compared to abciximab in the TARGET trial may relate to both inadequate tirofiban dosing and lack of tirofiban anti-inflammatory effects. None of the glycoprotein IIb/IIIa inhibitors have been clearly shown to prevent intimal hyperplasia and in-stent restenosis (*N Engl J Med* 2001;344:1888–1894; *Am J Cardiol* 2003;91:334–336).

5

Antiplatelet, Antithrombotic, and Thrombolytic Agents

David J. Moliterno and Tracy E. Macaulay

QUESTIONS

5.1 An 81-year-old African American male has just undergone successful percutaneous coronary intervention (PCI) and had placement of a femoral arteriotomy closure suture using a Perclose device. Unfortunately, soon thereafter he has several episodes of emesis followed by severe groin pain. He now has an enlarging hematoma. You appropriately choose to give intravenous protamine since unfractionated heparin had been given during the case. At the same time, local pressure is applied to the hematoma. Which of the following statements best describes protamine?

(A) It is a weak anticoagulant
(B) Patients allergic to fish may have an anaphylactoid reaction to protamine
(C) Doses >50 mg should be avoided
(D) Patients regularly taking neutral protamine Hagedorn (NPH) insulin should not receive protamine
(E) All of the above

5.2 Which of the following best describes the reason prasugrel provides more potent and consistent platelet aggregation inhibition as compared with clopidogrel?

(A) It is absorbed over a broader gastric pH range and is therefore less affected by proton pump inhibitors
(B) The active metabolite is formed by a single oxidative step
(C) The effect of foods, such as grapefruit juice, is lesser on prasugrel
(D) All of the above

5.3 The TRITON-TIMI 38 (Trial to Assess Improvement in Therapeutic Outcomes by Optimizing Platelet Inhibition With Prasugrel-Thrombolysis In Myocardial Infarction 38) trial compared prasugrel with clopidogrel among patients with an acute coronary syndrome (ACS) and intending to undergo PCI. At >1-year follow-up, how did the occurrence of ischemic events (cardiovascular death, myocardial infarction [MI], and stroke) and major non–coronary artery bypass graft (CABG) bleeding events compare with prasugrel vs. clopidogrel?

(A) Decreased, decreased
(B) Decreased, no change
(C) Decreased, increased
(D) Increased, no change

5.4 In the GUSTO-I (Global Utilization of Streptokinase and Tissue plasminogen activator for Occluded Arteries) trial, ischemic events and bleeding events were correlated with the activated partial thromboplastin time (aPTT) 12 hours after heparin therapy was initiated. The investigators described an optimal therapeutic range for aPTT where the risk of death and moderate or severe bleeding was lowest. This range, from point A to point B (Fig. Q5-4A,B), was found to be:

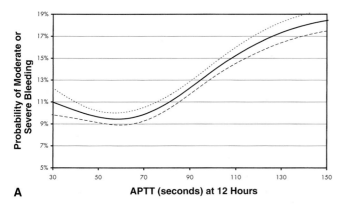

A

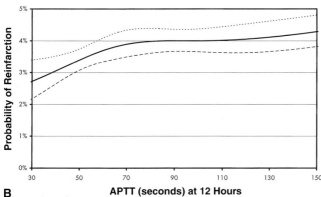

B

Figure Q5-4

(A) 40 to 60 seconds
(B) 50 to 70 seconds
(C) 70 to 90 seconds
(D) 90 seconds

5.5 Which of the following is NOT an absolute contraindication for thrombolytic therapy for treatment of ST-segment elevation MI?

(A) Active menses
(B) Hemorrhagic stroke >1 year earlier
(C) Suspected aortic dissection
(D) Intracranial arteriovenous malformation
(E) Recent, severe head trauma

5.6 Which of the following describes thrombocytopenia associated with abciximab?

(A) Thrombocytopenia can be quickly predicted with a simple laboratory test before abciximab administration
(B) Although infrequent, severe thrombocytopenia can often be detected within 2 to 4 hours of drug administration
(C) The occurrence of thrombocytopenia is roughly 10-fold higher among patients receiving repeat dosing of abciximab within a 2-week interval
(D) The nadir platelet count usually occurs 4 to 6 days after receiving abciximab

5.7 Unfractionated heparin affects several factors in the coagulation cascade. What is the effect of heparin on levels of tissue factor pathway inhibitor (TFPI)?

(A) Increased
(B) Decreased
(C) Unchanged

5.8 A 61-year-old Caucasian female was found to have a positive stress test result on preoperative evaluation. She underwent successful implantation of a paclitaxel-eluting stent into the left anterior descending coronary artery. Approximately 6 weeks later, you are contacted by the patient's orthopedic surgeon who wishes to proceed with a planned knee surgery. Your recommendations are:

(A) Proceed with planned surgery, but discontinue clopidogrel at least 5 days in advance
(B) Admit the patient to hospital, discontinue clopidogrel, and begin intravenous eptifibatide
(C) Discontinue clopidogrel, and after 2 days, admit the patient to hospital for fondaparinux injections
(D) Postpone surgery for 11 months

5.9 You are asked to see a 42-year-old man who is hospitalized for a deep vein thrombosis (DVT). No risks for DVT are apparent in the history and physical examination. What is the most commonly present hypercoagulable state in westernized countries?

(A) Protein C deficiency
(B) Protein S deficiency
(C) Factor V Leiden mutation
(D) Lupus anticoagulant
(E) Antiphospholipid antibody syndrome

5.10 Which of the following characteristics accurately describes bivalirudin?

(A) 20 amino acids: 25-minute half-life; <25% removal with dialysis
(B) 65 amino acids: 75-minute half-life; immunogenic
(C) Arginine derivative: 50-minute half-life; hepatic clearance
(D) 20 amino acids: 25-minute half-life; hepatic clearance
(E) 65 amino acids: 75-minute half-life; leech derivative

5.11 As compared with second- and third-generation fibrinolytic agents, which of the following statements regarding streptokinase is FALSE?

(A) Streptokinase is less fibrin specific
(B) Streptokinase is an indirect activator of plasminogen
(C) Streptokinase is the most fibrinogenolytic (depletes fibrinogen) of the agents
(D) Streptokinase has the shortest half-life

5.12 You are asked to see a 59-year-old African American woman who is referred for preoperative assessment. She is planning to have a breast mass removed. Her past medical history is remarkable for successful placement of a stent in her LCX approximately 8 years ago. Five years ago she had aortic valve replacement using a St. Jude mechanical prosthesis. As part of her evaluation, a treadmill nuclear stress test was performed. This revealed a large anterolateral reversible defect at a moderate workload. Her protime-international normalization ratio (INR) is 2.9. Which of the following plans should be implemented for her to undergo coronary angiography?

(A) Admit the patient to hospital, discontinue warfarin, and begin bivalirudin
(B) Discontinue warfarin 3 to 4 days before outpatient catheterization and measure the protime-INR on the day of planned catheterization
(C) Continue warfarin and use a 5 French diagnostic coronary artery catheter
(D) Administer fresh frozen plasma on the day of planned catheterization
(E) Admit the patient to hospital, discontinue warfarin, and begin enoxaparin

5.13 Which of the following factors associated with coagulation is NOT released from activated platelets?

(A) Fibrinogen
(B) Tissue plasminogen activator (tPA)
(C) Adenosine diphosphate (ADP)
(D) Plasminogen activator inhibitor-1 (PAI-1)
(E) Soluble CD40 ligand (sCD40L)

5.14 Which of the following factors at presentation LEAST strongly predicts 30-day mortality following ST-elevation myocardial infarction (STEMI)?

(A) Age
(B) MI location
(C) History of hypertension
(D) Killip class
(E) Heart rate on presentation

5.15 You receive a call from a physician in the emergency room who recently heard about a new medication called ticagrelor and wonders how this drug is administered, as well as its antiplatelet affect and mechanism. Which of the following best describes the administration and activity of ticagrelor?

(A) Oral, irreversible, direct-acting $P2Y_{12}$ receptor antagonist
(B) Oral, reversible, direct-acting $P2Y_{12}$ receptor antagonist
(C) Oral, reversible, indirect-acting $P2Y_{12}$ receptor antagonist
(D) Intravenous, irreversible, indirect-acting $P2Y_{12}$ receptor antagonist

5.16 In the Platelet Inhibition and Patient Outcomes (PLATO) trial testing ticagrelor as compared with clopidogrel among patients with an ACS, how did ticagrelor affect the rates of mortality and non-CABG major bleeding?

(A) Decreased mortality, decreased non-CABG bleeding
(B) Decreased mortality, increased non-CABG bleeding
(C) Unchanged mortality, increased non-CABG bleeding
(D) Unchanged mortality, unchanged non-CABG bleeding
(E) Unchanged mortality, decreased non-CABG bleeding

5.17 Platelet aggregability is increased by numerous factors (thrombin, epinephrine, ADP) including hypertriglyceridemia. Elevation of which of the following lipoproteins is associated with reduced platelet aggregability?

(A) High-density lipoprotein (HDL)
(B) Low-density lipoprotein (LDL)
(C) Very low-density lipoprotein (VLDL)
(D) Lipoprotein(a)
(E) Apolipoprotein E (apo E)

5.18 Which of the following is NOT an action of thrombin?

(A) Converts fibrinogen to fibrin
(B) Activates factors V and XII
(C) Causes normal endothelium to vasoconstrict
(D) Stimulates platelet aggregation

5.19 You recently started working in a rural hospital that has started a primary angioplasty program. One of the catheterization laboratory nurses begins asking questions about the measurement of activated clotting time (ACT). Which of the following is FALSE regarding the ACT test?

(A) An agent, such as kaolin or diatomaceous earth, stimulates the intrinsic pathway of coagulation

(B) Currently available measures of the ACT have been developed to assess anticoagulation produced by unfractionated heparin

(C) The ACT is similar for arterial and venous blood samples

(D) The ACT is unaffected by most coagulation factor deficiencies such as hemophilia

5.20 Which of the following antithrombotic drugs used during PCI has the shortest half-life?

(A) Unfractionated heparin

(B) Low-molecular-weight heparin

(C) Lepirudin

(D) Bivalirudin

(E) Argatroban

5.21 Which of the following practices in interventional cardiology has reduced the occurrence of bleeding associated with PCI?

(A) Using weight-based heparin dosing

(B) Decreasing arterial sheath size

(C) Removing sheaths on the same day of the procedure

(D) Avoiding the use of heparin postprocedure

(E) All of the above

5.22 As the ACT increases among patients receiving heparin with a glycoprotein IIb/IIIa inhibitor, the occurrence of ischemic events:

(A) Gradually increases

(B) Gradually decreases

(C) Remains largely unchanged

5.23 Which factor is UNIMPORTANT in assessing whether patients being treated with enoxaparin have adequate anticoagulation during percutaneous coronary revascularization?

(A) Timing of the last enoxaparin dose

(B) The current ACT

(C) The dose of enoxaparin being given

(D) The number of subcutaneous doses of enoxaparin received

(E) The estimated creatinine clearance

5.24 Which of the following drugs is NOT known to be associated with antibody formation?

(A) Unfractionated heparin

(B) Low-molecular-weight heparin

(C) Argatroban

(D) Lepirudin

(E) Abciximab

5.25 Which of the following statements accurately describes heparin-induced thrombocytopenia (HIT)?

(A) The diagnosis of HIT is a clinical one and should be suspected when the platelet count is below 150,000 per mm³ or has decreased 50% from baseline

(B) The likelihood of HIT substantially increases for patients receiving heparin for ≥ 4 days

(C) Antibodies related to HIT remain present for about 3 to 4 months

(D) All of the above

5.26 Advantages that low-molecular-weight heparins have over unfractionated heparins include all of the following, EXCEPT:

(A) Bind less to plasma proteins, thereby producing a more consistent effect

(B) Have better subcutaneous absorption

(C) Do not require anticoagulant monitoring

(D) Can be used safely in patients with heparin–PF4 antibodies or HIT

(E) Have a several-fold longer half-life

5.27 Meta-analysis of clinical trials testing enoxaparin vs. unfractionated heparin for the medical treatment of unstable angina has shown enoxaparin to lower the composite relative risk of death or MI at 6 weeks by:

(A) 0%

(B) 5% to 10%

(C) 10% to 15%

(D) 15% to 20%

5.28 Your junior partner refers his mother to you for elective PCI. She is a 62-year-old with hypertension and hypercholesterolemia. She has never used tobacco products. When talking with you, she relates that she is terrified about the procedural risk of major bleeding. You explain that major bleeding, as defined by the thrombolysis in myocardial infarction (TIMI) study criteria, occurs at which of the following rates in prospective PCI trials?

(A) 1% to 2%

(B) 3% to 5%

(C) 6% to 8%

(D) >10%

5.29 Reasonable measures to decrease bleeding complications among patients receiving IIb/IIIa inhibitors include all EXCEPT:

(A) Targeting lower ACT values by using a lower bolus dose of heparin
(B) Using smaller arterial access sheaths
(C) Giving clopidogrel after the coronary intervention procedure is completed
(D) Removing vascular access sheaths on the same day as the procedure

5.30 Which of the following drugs should have its dose adjusted in renal insufficiency?

(A) Argatroban
(B) Tirofiban
(C) Abciximab
(D) None of the above

5.31 Pharmacotherapies known to reduce the occurrence of death or MI among patients with non–ST-segment elevation myocardial infarction (NSTEMI) include all of the following, EXCEPT:

(A) Aspirin
(B) Clopidogrel
(C) Unfractionated heparin
(D) Low-molecular-weight heparin
(E) Fibrinolytic agents

5.32 PCI trials testing IIb/IIIa inhibitors have used a 30-day composite end point of death, MI, and urgent target vessel revascularization (TVR). What percentage of this composite end point is accounted for by a periprocedural rise in creatine kinase-MB (CK-MB)?

(A) 20%
(B) 40%
(C) 60%
(D) 80%

5.33 For which of the following does abciximab have a class III indication?

(A) Left main coronary artery stenting
(B) As medical therapy among patients with ACS
(C) Angioplasty in patients older than 90 years
(D) Percutaneous coronary revascularization among patients with recent stroke

5.34 The time required for maximal clinical benefit of a 300-mg loading dose of clopidogrel in a post hoc analysis of the CREDO (Clopidogrel for the Reduction of Events During Observation) trial was found to be:

(A) 2 hours
(B) 6 hours

(C) 24 hours
(D) 96 hours

5.35 Which anticoagulant is represented in Figure Q5-35?

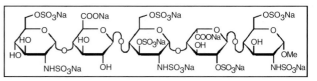

Figure Q5-35

(A) Unfractionated heparin
(B) Enoxaparin
(C) Fondaparinux
(D) Bivalirudin
(E) Eptifibatide

5.36 A 73-year-old Caucasian woman weighing 62 kg undergoes an uneventful percutaneous coronary revascularization procedure by you. Because she had an ACS and evidence of residual thrombus in the culprit lesion, procedural abciximab and bivalirudin were utilized. Following the procedure, the patient is found to be hypotensive and tachycardiac, and a retroperitoneal hemorrhage is diagnosed. Which of the following measures would be the next step in her treatment to reverse the effects of abciximab?

(A) Transfuse random donor platelets
(B) Administer intravenous protamine
(C) Request fresh frozen plasma from the blood bank
(D) Intravenous bolus of cryoprecipitate

5.37 Several small randomized studies have suggested the benefit of triple-antiplatelet therapy by adding cilostazol to aspirin and clopidogrel for patient undergoing drug-eluting stent placement. Recently, the CILON-T (influence of CILostazol-based triple antiplatelet therapy ON ischemic complication after drug-eluting stenT implantation) investigators randomized nearly 1,000 patients receiving a drug-eluting stent to aspirin and clopidogrel or a combination of aspirin, clopidogrel, and cilostazol. While the P2Y$_{12}$ reactivity units were lower among patients receiving triple-antiplatelet therapy, there was no difference in the 6-month rate of a composite of cardiovascular death, MI, ischemic stroke, and target lesion revascularization. Which of the following describes the cellular mechanism of cilostazol?

(A) It directly binds the protease-activator receptor (PAR-1)
(B) It is an ADP (P2Y$_{12}$) receptor agonist
(C) It inhibits cellular phosphodiesterase III
(D) It blocks the collagen (glycoprotein VI) platelet receptor

5.38 A 72-year-old retired lawyer presents with an NSTEMI, and at angiography a severe right coronary artery stenosis with a large thrombus is found. You plan to use a IIb/IIIa inhibitor, though the patient comments he has heard a lot of negative information about those drugs. Which of the following statements is FALSE concerning IIb/IIIa inhibitors?

(A) Bleeding is infrequent although it usually occurs in hollow organs (gastrointestinal, genitourinary, and vascular)

(B) Severe thrombocytopenia occurs in approximately 1% of patients

(C) Thrombocytopenia is more frequent with abciximab, especially with early repeat administration

(D) TIMI major bleeding is increased by approximately 1% when using a IIb/IIIa inhibitor, and this is predominately due to an increase in intracranial hemorrhage

5.1 **Answer E.** Protamine is currently synthesized by way of biotechnology but was originally produced from fish products. Patients with a strong fish allergy or those who take NPH insulin should not receive protamine due to the increased risk of histamine-mediated reaction. Theoretically, protamine in higher doses can act as an anticoagulant.

5.2 **Answer B.** Both prasugrel and clopidogrel require hepatic cytochromes for oxidation to their corresponding active drug metabolite. Whereas prasugrel requires only a single oxidative step involving CYP2c19, clopidogrel requires two oxidative steps.

5.3 **Answer C.** At approximately 15-month follow-up, the composite ischemic end point decreased from 12.1% to 9.9% with prasugrel ($p < 0.001$). In contrast, the major bleeding rate increased from 1.8% to 2.4% with prasugrel, $p = 0.03$ (*NEJM* 2007;357:2001–2015).

5.4 **Answer B.** Granger et al. found 50 to 70 seconds to be this optimal therapeutic range, which fortunately minimized both ischemic and bleeding events. Before this study, a number of investigators and clinicians used a therapeutic range of 60 to 85 seconds. Since this manuscript, most subsequent studies and clinicians have chosen 50 to 70 seconds. In the GUSTO-II trial, a 20% increase in the dose of heparin resulted in a 5- to 10-second higher aPTT as compared with results from the GUSTO-I trial. This increase in aPTT was associated with a doubling in the rate of intracranial hemorrhage among patients treated with thrombolytic therapy (*Circulation* 1996;93:870–878).

5.5 **Answer A.** The absolute contraindications for thrombolytic therapy are solely centered on life-threatening bleeding such as intracranial hemorrhage. Any history of previous hemorrhagic stroke is an absolute contraindication. Active internal bleeding is considered a contraindication except for menses.

5.6 **Answer B.** Thrombocytopenia associated with abciximab (*Semin Thromb Hemost* 2004;30:569–577) occurs very quickly, and therefore it is recommended that a platelet count be performed 2 hours after drug administration. There is no quick laboratory test to predict thrombocytopenia caused by abciximab. The occurrence of severe thrombocytopenia (platelet count < 20 × 10⁹/l) among patients receiving abciximab is approximately 2%, and this occurrence is roughly doubled (not 10-fold) among patients who receive repeat administration of abciximab within 2 weeks. Severe thrombocytopenia secondary to abciximab administration should prompt immediate drug discontinuation and future avoidance.

5.7 **Answer A.** Unfractionated heparin affects coagulation factors in the intrinsic, extrinsic, and common pathways of coagulation. The extrinsic pathway, including tissue factor and factor VII, is affected by unfractionated heparin since it increases levels of TFPI.

5.8 **Answer D.** The need for surgery in the early weeks to months following drug-eluting stent placement is a vexing problem. No large-scale prospective data are available. It is well recognized that premature discontinuation of adequate antiplatelet therapy markedly increases the risk for stent thrombosis. In one large-scale registry, it was found that premature antiplatelet therapy discontinuation was associated with a hazard ratio of 90 (95% CI, 30–270) for stent thrombosis (*JAMA* 2005;293:2126–2130). Current expert consensus suggests 12 months of dual antiplatelet therapy after DES, though some data suggest decreasing benefit beyond 6 months.

5.9 **Answer C.** Factor V Leiden mutation is present in roughly 6% of the population. Most thrombotic events from this deficiency are venous, although arterial thrombosis does infrequently occur.

5.10 **Answer A.** Bivalirudin is a short amino acid sequence with the shortest half-life among the intravenous direct thrombin inhibitors. It is poorly dialyzable. Answer B is a description for lepirudin, while Answer C best describes argatroban. Choices D and E do not accurately characterize any of the direct thrombin inhibitors.

5.11 **Answer D.** Streptokinase, a first-generation fibrinolytic agent, is least fibrin specific and also depletes fibrinogen levels the greatest. As such, patients have a longer time of coagulation abnormality and hence do not require early heparin administration. Separately, streptokinase has an intermediate half-life (20 minutes) as compared with tPA, which has the shortest half-life (5 minutes).

5.12 **Answer B.** The patient's stent placement was done many years before so there is no particular concern for stent thrombosis. Perioperative unfractionated heparin therapy is recommended for patients in whom the risk of bleeding with oral anticoagulation is high and the risk of thromboembolism without anticoagulation is also high (mechanical valve in the mitral position, Bjork-Shiley valve, recent [i.e., <1 year] thrombosis or embolus, or three or more of the following risk factors: atrial fibrillation, previous embolus at any time, hypercoagulable condition, mechanical prosthesis, and LVEF < 30%). For patients between these two extremes, physicians must assess the risk and benefit of reduced anticoagulation vs. perioperative heparin therapy. Since the patient's INR is 2.9, it is reasonable to simply discontinue the warfarin and measure the protime-INR on the third or fourth morning. If the patient's INR still remains >1.5, using a particularly small arterial sheath and/or possibly an arteriotomy closure device could be considered.

5.13 **Answer B.** Many factors associated with coagulation, inflammation, or cell repair and growth are released from platelets. Most factors either accelerate coagulation (ADP, fibrinogen) or promote inflammation (sCD40L). Platelets do not contain tPA but rather release PAI-1 (the natural inhibitor of tPA) when activated.

5.14 **Answer C.** All these factors are independent predictors of 30-day mortality. A history of hypertension, however, represents <1% of predictive models for mortality. MI location and heart rate are each roughly 10 times more powerful predictors than hypertension. In fact, most of the predictive factors for 30-day mortality can be assessed by the ambulance driver or triage nurse before the patient's arrival at the hospital.

5.15 **Answer B.** Ticagrelor is the first orally available P2Y$_{12}$ receptor antagonist that reversibly affects the receptor.

5.16 **Answer B.** PLATO randomized 18,624 patients with an ACS at 12 months. Ticagrelor significantly reduced the primary end point of death from vascular causes, MI, or stroke. Impressively, death from vascular causes was significantly reduced (HR 0.79; 95% CI, 0.69–0.91). While overall bleeding was not increased, the rate of non–CABG-related major bleeding was increased from 3.8% to 4.5% (HR 1.19; 95% CI, 1.02–1.38) (*N Engl J Med* 2009;361:1045–1057).

5.17 **Answer A.** The elevation of most lipid and lipoprotein levels is associated with increased platelet aggregation. Triglyceride-rich lipids increase a number of procoagulant factors and increase blood viscosity. On the other hand, HDL reduces PAI-1, and high levels of HDL inhibit platelet aggregability (*Atherosclerosis* 1998;140:271–280).

5.18 **Answer C.** Among the primary activities of thrombin is causing the conversion of fibrinogen to fibrin. Thrombin does activate a number of other coagulation pathway factors including V, VIII, and XII as it autoamplifies its production. Normal endothelium, in response to thrombin, releases tPA and also vasodilates. Abnormal endothelium vasoconstricts (through endothelin) in response to thrombin. Another important activity of thrombin is that it is one of the most potent stimulators of platelet aggregation.

5.19 **Answer D.** The ACT initiates the intrinsic pathway of coagulation. The commercially available assays are almost exclusively designed for measuring therapeutic levels of unfractionated heparin. The assay is poorly sensitive to most factor Xa inhibitors and low-molecular-weight heparins. The ACT can measure the extent of anticoagulation from direct thrombin inhibitors, although it is less accurate than other assays. Clinically important coagulation factor deficiencies, such as with hemophilia, substantially prolong the ACT as well as other clotting time assays.

5.20 **Answer D.** At therapeutic doses, unfractionated heparin half-life ranges from 30 to 60 minutes, while half-life of LMWH is largely dependent on rate of creatinine clearance. Bivalirudin has the consistently shortest half-life of these drugs, and it is approximately 20 to 25 minutes. The other direct thrombin inhibitors have half-lives of approximately 60 minutes (*Am Heart J* 2003;146:S23–S30).

5.21   Answer E. The rate of major bleeding in randomized clinical trials and in practice has substantially decreased over the last decade from 2%–4% to <1%. Many changes in practice have resulted in this decrease in bleeding despite the use of multiple antiplatelets and anticoagulants (aspirin, clopidogrel, IIb/IIIa inhibitors, and potent antithrombins).

5.22   Answer C. As compared with heparin alone, when increasing ACT is associated with a decreasing ischemic event rate, the rate of ischemic events among patients receiving heparin with a glycoprotein IIb/IIIa inhibitor is largely unchanged from an ACT in the range of approximately 200 to 400 seconds. For this reason, there is no need to attain an ACT higher than approximately 200 seconds when using a IIb/IIIa inhibitor.

5.23   Answer B. Several factors are important when deciding if a patient remains adequately anticoagulated from enoxaparin. These include the amount of enoxaparin given and the number of hours since this last dose. Likewise, patients who have received only one subcutaneous dose of enoxaparin will be therapeutic for a shorter interval than patients who have reached steady state following several subcutaneous doses. It is also important whether the patient has received intravenous or subcutaneous enoxaparin. The ACT is an unreliable measure of the extent of anticoagulation provided by enoxaparin. Since the primary excretion for low-molecular-weight heparins is renal, the creatinine clearance can have an important influence on the extent and duration of anticoagulant effect.

5.24   Answer C. Both unfractionated heparins and fractionated or low-molecular-weight heparins, by interacting with PF4, can lead to antibody formation. Abciximab, having a protein-antibody structure, can act as an antigen and cause antibody formation. Hirudin and lepirudin are polypeptides and may lead to relevant antibody formation, whereas argatroban is a synthetic arginine derivative and has not been found to cause antibody formation.

5.25   Answer D. The suspicion and diagnosis of HIT should be made near solely on clinical grounds. Laboratory-based assays for HIT can be diagnostic, but should be confirmatory. While unfractionated heparin is much more likely than low-molecular-weight heparin to cause HIT, all heparins can cause and exacerbate HIT. Fondaparinux has not been associated with HIT. The mechanism of HIT is antibody generation in response to a heparin–platelet factor complex. This antibody formation usually takes exposure to several days of heparin to occur, and the antibody remains present for several months.

5.26   Answer D. Low-molecular-weight heparins provide several advantages over unfractionated heparin since they bind less to the endothelium, plasma proteins, and macrophages, thereby providing a more consistent effect. They are also better absorbed subcutaneously and have a longer half-life. Although low-molecular-weight heparins are less likely to cause formation of heparin-induced platelet antibodies than unfractionated heparin, both agents are unsafe once antibodies are formed, and a direct thrombin inhibitor should be used instead.

5.27   Answer D. A meta-analysis combining data from ESSENCE (Efficacy and Safety of Subcutaneous Enoxaparin in Non–Q-wave Coronary Events) and TIMI-11B showed that the 43-day incidence of death or nonfatal MI was reduced by 17% (*N Engl J Med* 1997;337:447–452; *Circulation* 1999;100:1593–1601).

5.28   Answer A. The TIMI major bleeding definition has been used for many years in thrombolytic therapy trials as well as in percutaneous revascularization trials. For several reasons, including the fact that TIMI major bleeding has occurred in only approximately 1% of patients in recent PCI trials, more clinically relevant bleeding definitions have been defined and used in several studies such as REPLACE-2. The REPLACE-2 major bleeding definition, as compared with the TIMI major bleeding definition, includes transfusion of ≥2 units of packed red blood cell, observed blood loss with >3 g/dL Hgb blood loss, and retroperitoneal hemorrhage (*JAMA* 2003;289:853–863).

5.29   Answer C. The primary measures by which vascular bleeding events have decreased in the setting of IIb/IIIa inhibitor use center around using lower bolus doses of heparin and removing the arterial access sheaths the same day as the procedure (as opposed to leaving them overnight).

Clopidogrel should be given preprocedure when possible.

5.30   Answer B. Abciximab is largely cleared by the reticuloendothelial system and not by the kidney. Therefore, the dose does not need to be adjusted for renal insufficiency. This is in contrast to the small-molecule IIb/IIIa inhibitors such as tirofiban. Likewise, argatroban is hepatically metabolized.

5.31   Answer E. Placebo-controlled trials have shown many antiplatelet and antithrombin therapies to reduce death or MI among patients with NSTEMI. Several studies, including TIMI-IIIB, showed patients with NSTEMI-ACS receiving fibrinolytic therapy to have a worse outcome—primarily a higher rate of MI (*Circulation* 1999;100:1593–1601).

5.32   Answer D. Periprocedural MI accounts for nearly 90% of the 30-day composite of ischemic end points. In current practice, in-hospital death and urgent TVR each occur in fewer than 1% of patients undergoing nonemergent PCI.

5.33   Answer B. While there are a number of reasons not to use abciximab, using it as medical therapy alone among patients with ACS is a class III indication. This distinction is given because of the results of GUSTO-IV trial (*Lancet* 2001;357:1915–1924), which showed no benefit but rather a nonsignificant increase in adverse events among patients receiving abciximab alone (without PCI) for ACS.

5.34   Answer C. While no prospective large-scale study has been completed to discern the exact time interval required to receive maximal benefit from a clopidogrel loading dose, a post hoc analysis from the CREDO trial observed the maximal separation of the adverse event curves

between the group of patients pretreated with placebo and those receiving a 300-mg loading dose to occur maximally at 24 hours. No statistically significant difference was seen in the clinical outcome until after 15 hours. At this time point, a 59% reduction in the ischemic event rate was noted relative to placebo (*J Am Coll Cardiol* 2006;47:939–943).

5.35   Answer C. The diagram shows a 5-sugar unit entity, namely, a pentasaccharide (fondaparinux).

5.36   Answer A. Abciximab, being a monoclonal antibody, avidly binds to platelet receptors. Protamine would be a useful treatment to reverse the effects of heparin; however, it will have no effect on abciximab. Administering cryoprecipitate or plasma products will be of little to no value because of the mechanism of abciximab binding. Rather, transfusion of platelets will provide additional IIb/IIIa receptors to facilitate appropriate coagulation. In addition, abciximab can migrate among platelets, and the transfused platelets will aid in decreasing the number of abciximab molecules on the originally affected platelets, thereby allowing their earlier recovery. Bivalirudin has a very short half-life and effect should be gone rapidly.

5.37   Answer C. Cilostazol is a quinolinone derivative that inhibits cellular phosphodiesterase. While this cellular mechanism can reduce the activity of the P2Y$_{12}$ receptor, it does not directly block this receptor. Likewise, it does not affect the thrombin (PAR-1) receptor.

5.38   Answer D. Although TIMI major bleeding is increased by approximately 1%, this is not due to an increase in intracranial hemorrhage. Intracranial hemorrhage occurs in 0.1% of patients undergoing PCI, and this is not particularly increased with the use of IIb/IIIa inhibitors.

6

Pharmacogenomics and Drug Monitoring

Dominick J. Angiolillo

QUESTIONS

6.1 Which of the following BEST describes the pharmacogenetics of cardiovascular drugs?

(A) Discipline evaluating the impact of specific gene variants on the variability in patient response to a given drug

(B) Discipline evaluating the impact of an individual gene on cardiovascular outcomes

(C) Discipline evaluating the impact of several genes on cardiovascular outcomes, irrespective of pharmacologic treatment

(D) None of the above

6.2 Which of the following mechanisms leads to inhibition of platelet function following treatment with $P2Y_{12}$ receptor inhibitors, such as clopidogrel?

(A) Reduction of cyclic adenosine monophosphate (cAMP) levels

(B) Increased phosphorylation status of vasodilator-stimulated phosphoprotein (VASP-P)

(C) Inhibition of phospholipase C (PLC)

(D) Inhibition of adenylyl cyclase

(E) Inhibition of protein kinase C (PKC)

6.3 Proton pump inhibitors (PPIs) such as omeprazole have shown to reduce the pharmacokinetic and pharmacodynamic effects of clopidogrel by modulating the effects of which of the following?

(A) Glycoprotein (GP) IIb/IIIa receptor expression

(B) Cytochrome P450 (CYP) 2C19 enzymatic activity

(C) Cytochrome P450 (CYP) 3A4 enzymatic activity

(D) Intestinal P-glycoprotein transport activity

6.4 The Food and Drug Administration has issued a genetic-related boxed warning for clopidogrel. This boxed warning derives from studies showing that clopidogrel at recommended doses forms less of its metabolite and has a smaller effect on platelet function in patients who are CYP2C19 "poor metabolizers." Also, "poor metabolizers" with acute coronary syndrome or undergoing percutaneous coronary intervention treated with clopidogrel at recommended doses exhibit higher cardiovascular event rates than do patients with normal CYP2C19 function. Which of the following represents a CYP2C19 genotype identifying a clopidogrel "poor metabolizer"?

(A) wt/wt (wt: wild type)

(B) wt/*2

(C) wt/*17

(D) *2/*17

(E) *2/*2

6.5 Which of the following guideline recommendations has been given for platelet function testing in clopidogrel-treated patients?

(A) Class I—Level of Evidence B

(B) Class IIa—Level of Evidence B

(C) Class IIb—Level of Evidence B

(D) Class IIa—Level of Evidence C

6.6 Platelet function testing comparing prasugrel with clopidogrel has shown which of the following?

(A) Prasugrel 60-mg loading dose to be associated with more potent platelet inhibition compared with a 300-mg clopidogrel loading dose, but not a 600-mg clopidogrel loading dose

(B) Prasugrel 60-mg loading dose and 10-mg maintenance dose to be associated with more potent platelet inhibition compared with clopidogrel, irrespective of loading (300 to 600 mg) or maintenance (75 to 150 mg) dose used

(C) Prasugrel 60-mg loading dose to be associated with more potent platelet inhibition compared with clopidogrel 600-mg loading dose, but with slower effects

(D) Prasugrel 60-mg loading dose to be associated with more potent platelet inhibition compared with clopidogrel 600-mg loading dose, but similar effects when transitioning to maintenance therapy

6.7 A patient undergoes platelet function testing using LTA (light transmittance aggregometry) with 20 μmol/L ADP stimulation before and 24 hours after a loading dose of clopidogrel. Pre and post maximal platelet aggregation values are 80% and 40%, respectively. The inhibition of platelet aggregation (IPA) of this patient is:

(A) 30%

(B) 40%

(C) 50%

(D) 60%

6.8 A patient comes to your clinic and informs you that he participated in a research study in which he was found to be "aspirin resistant." The patient had a drug-eluting stent implanted in his mid RCA 8 months ago and is currently asymptomatic on treatment with aspirin (81 mg/day), clopidogrel (75 mg/day), and atorvastatin (40 mg/day). What do you believe should be the most appropriate therapeutic approach in this patient?

(A) Given the history of aspirin resistance, the patient should have the dose of aspirin increased to overcome resistance

(B) Given the history of aspirin resistance, the patient should maintain clopidogrel and stop aspirin at 1 year post-PCI

(C) Given the history of aspirin resistance, the patient may also be clopidogrel resistant and should be tested for this

(D) Although the patient has shown aspirin resistance, no changes in his medical management should be made at the current time; ensure that the patient is compliant to his medication

6.9 Which of the following has been shown to be the most important determinant of inadequate clopidogrel-induced antiplatelet effects?

(A) Genetic polymorphisms of the P2Y$_{12}$ receptor

(B) Interaction with atorvastatin

(C) Up-regulation of nonpurinergic signaling pathways

(D) Noncompliance and underdosing

(E) Accelerated platelet turnover

6.10 True statements about aspirin include all of the following, EXCEPT:

(A) The antiplatelet effects of aspirin can be diminished with concomitant nonsteroidal anti-inflammatory drug use

(B) Aspirin exerts its antiplatelet effects through inhibition of the platelet thrombin receptor (PAR) for the life span of the platelet

(C) Aspirin is a relatively weak inhibitor of platelet aggregation in vitro

(D) When chewed or solubilized, the full antiplatelet effects of aspirin can be achieved in approximately 15 minutes

(E) Aspirin exerts its antiplatelet effects through irreversible blockade of the COX-1 enzyme

6.11 Which of the following platelet function tests assessing antiplatelet drug response has been mostly associated with adverse outcomes and considered the gold standard assay?

(A) VerifyNow Assay

(B) PFA-100

(C) P-selectin assessed by whole blood cytometry

(D) Light transmittance aggregometry

(E) GP IIb/IIIa activation assessed by whole blood cytometry

6.12 Polymorphisms of which of the following genotypes can modulate intestinal absorption of several cardiovascular drugs?

(A) ABCB1 (also known as multidrug resistance–associated protein [MDR]-1)

(B) Cytochrome P450 enzymes

(C) *PlA* polymorphisms

(D) Vitamin K epoxide reductase (*VKOR*)

6.13 Antithrombotic agents with linear pharmacokinetics (PK) have a more predictable pharmacodynamic (PD) response. Which of the following antithrombotic agents has the BEST PK/PD response profile?

(A) Unfractionated heparin
(B) Low-molecular-weight heparin
(C) Bivalirudin
(D) Warfarin

6.14 Which of the following statements is CORRECT with regards to heparin dosing and ACT monitoring in patients undergoing PCI who do not receive GP IIb/IIIa inhibitors?

(A) Unfractionated heparin should be given during coronary angioplasty to achieve an ACT of 250 to 300 seconds with the HemoTec device and 300 to 350 seconds with the Hemochron device
(B) A weight-adjusted bolus heparin (70 to 100 IU/kg) can be used to avoid excess anticoagulation

(C) If the target values for ACT are not achieved after a bolus of heparin, additional heparin boluses (2,000 to 5,000 IU) can be given
(D) All of the above

6.15 Which of the following statements is CORRECT with regards to heparin dosing and ACT monitoring in patients undergoing PCI receiving GP IIb/IIIa inhibitors?

(A) The unfractionated heparin bolus should be 50 to 70 IU/kg in order to achieve a target ACT of 200 seconds
(B) The unfractionated heparin bolus should be 70 to 100 IU/kg in order to achieve a target ACT of 300 seconds
(C) A fixed (non–weight-based) bolus of 5,000 IU should be given without monitoring of ACT
(D) None of the above

6.1   **Answer A.** Pharmacogenetics is a field that tries to identify specific gene variants that are able to explain the variability among patients' responses to a given drug. This variability may explain the efficacy of a specific drug in a given patient as well as its adverse side effects. Polymorphisms affecting genes that encode disposition, metabolism, transporters, or targets of the drug can all potentially modify an individual's response to one therapy and thus explain its efficacy and safety profiles (*Am Coll Cardiol* 2009;54:1041–1057). Cardiovascular disease is complex and multifactorial; therefore, multiple genes, including many that are as yet unidentified, are likely to be involved in cardiovascular risk. However, the influence of only 1 polymorphism of a candidate gene is likely to be weak, and certainly much weaker than that of clinical risk factors. Several large-scale studies have demonstrated only a minor role of many different polymorphisms in development and prognosis of cardiovascular events.

Figure A6-1 is an example of pharmacogenetics of clopidogrel effects. Different targets can be identified that may modulate clopidogrel effects. Clopidogrel is a prodrug that, after intestinal absorption, is metabolized in the liver by cytochrome (P450 CYP) system to generate an active metabolite. The active metabolite then irreversibly inhibits the platelet $P2Y_{12}$ receptor, which in turn blocks platelet activation and subsequent aggregation ultimately mediated by the GP IIb/IIIa receptor. Genetic polymorphisms of targets in this metabolic pathway (intestines, liver, platelet membrane) may all potentially influence clopidogrel-induced antiplatelet effects.

6.2   **Answer B.** The active metabolite of clopidogrel inhibits the ADP $P2Y_{12}$ receptor. The downstream effects of this are an increase in cAMP levels and VASP-P. This overall inhibits platelet activation and thus aggregation processes. Activation of ADP $P2Y_{12}$ receptor signaling inhibits adenylyl cyclase, which reduces cAMP levels and thus the status of VASP-P. PLC and PKC are part of the $P2Y_1$ receptor signaling pathway (Fig. A6-2) (*J Am Coll Cardiol* 2007;49:1505–1516).

Pharmacogenetics of Cardiovascular Antithrombotic Therapy

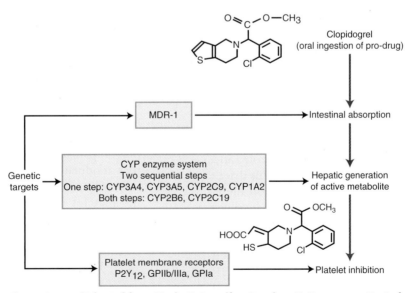

Figure A6-1. (Adapted from Marin F, González-Conejero R, Capranzano P, et al. Pharmacogenetics in cardiovascular antithrombotic therapy. *J AM Coll Cardiol* 2009; 54:1041–1057.)

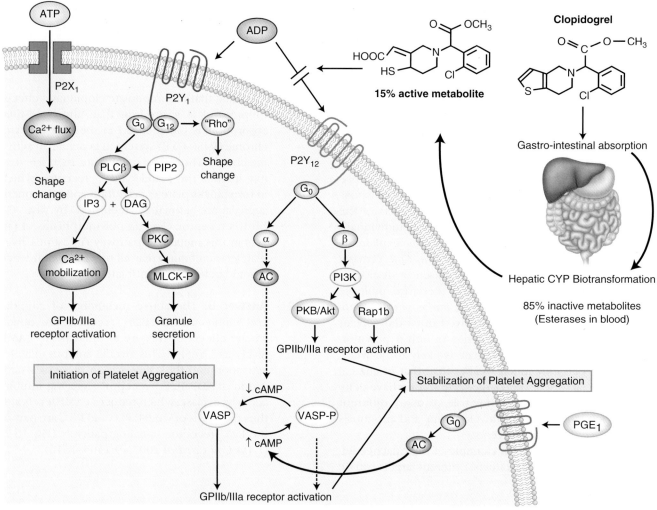

Figure A6-2. (Adapted from Angiolillo DJ, Fernandez-Ortiz A, Bernardo E, et al. Variability in individual responsiveness to clopidogrel: clinical implications, management, and future perspectives. *J Am coll Cardiol* 2007;49:1505–1516.)

6.3 **Answer B.** Several factors have been associated with reduced pharmacokinetic (PK) and pharmacodynamic (PD) response profiles to clopidogrel. Among these, a drug interaction between PPIs, in particular omeprazole, and clopidogrel has been demonstrated. This drug–drug interaction is due to the common metabolic pathway of these agents, which involves the cytochrome P450 (CYP) 2C19 enzyme (*Clin Pharmacol Ther* 2011;89:65-74). This drug interaction is also reflected in a boxed warning issued by the FDA. The CYP2C19 isoenzyme is of particular importance since it is involved in both oxidation steps required for clopidogrel prodrug to generate its active metabolite. Therefore, intrinsic (e.g., genetic polymorphisms) or extrinsic (e.g., drugs) factors modulating the activity of this enzyme may affect active metabolite levels and thus the platelet inhibitory effects of clopidogrel. Other drugs may interfere with different targets involved in clopidogrel metabolism (Fig. A6-3) (*J Am Coll Cardiol* 2011;57: 1251-1263).

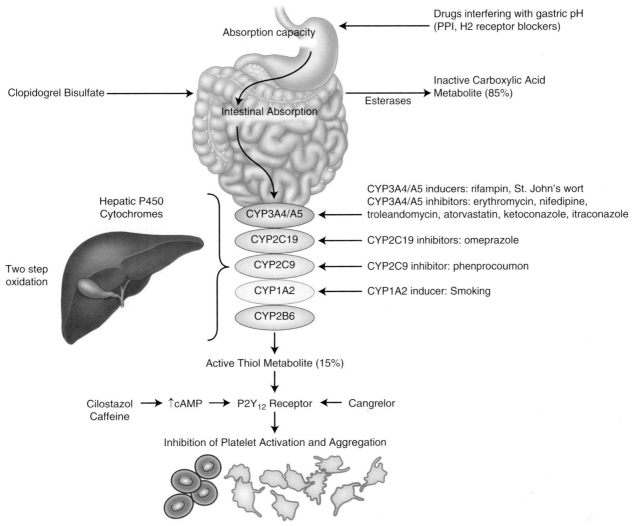

Figure A6-3. (Adapted from Bates ER, Lau WC, Angiolillo DJ. Clopidogrel–drug interactions. *J Am Coll Cardiol* **2011;57:1251–1263.)**

6.4 **Answer E.** The genes that encode the CYP enzymes are polymorphic, with certain alleles demonstrated to confer reduced enzymatic function, thereby interfering with production of the drug metabolites. These reduced-function alleles, particularly in CYP2C19, have been shown to affect the PK and PD responses to clopidogrel. Moreover, in the setting of treatment with clopidogrel, patients carrying reduced-function CYP2C19 alleles compared with noncarriers have substantially higher rates of major adverse cardiovascular events, including stent thrombosis (*N Engl J Med* 2009;360:354–362). The boxed warning issued by the FDA is for poor metabolizers only. Poor metabolizer status is defined by the presence of 2 reduced-function alleles. The most common reduced-function allele is *2 and the most common poor metabolizer status is *2/*2, which has a prevalence of approximately 3% among Caucasians, 5% in African Americans,

and up to 15% in Asians. Other reduced-function alleles are shown in the table below. An increased function allele has also been identified (*17). The wild-type (wt) allele is indicated as *1. The table below indicates the classification of CYP2C19 metabolic status.

a. Ultrarapid: *1/*17, *17/*17
b. Extensive: *1/*1
c. Intermediate: *1/*2-*8, *17/*2-*8
d. Poor: *2-*8/*2-*8

6.5 **Answer C.** The recent 2011 ACCF/AHA Focused Update of the Guidelines for the Management of Patients With Unstable Angina/Non-ST-Elevation Myocardial Infarction (Wright RS, Anderson JL, Adams CD, et al. 2011 ACCF/AHA Focused Update of the Guidelines for the Management of Patients With Unstable Angina/Non-ST-Elevation Myocardial Infarction, *J AM Coll Cardiol* 2011;57: 1920-1959) provides new recommendations for platelet function and genetic testing. Both new recommendations are Class IIb but differ in level of evidence. Guidelines state the following: (1) Platelet function testing to determine platelet inhibitory response in patients with UA/NSTEMI (or, after ACS and PCI) on thienopyridine therapy may be considered if results of testing may alter management (*Level of Evidence: B*); (2) Genotyping for a CYP2C19 loss of function variant in patients with UA/NSTEMI (or, after ACS and with PCI) on clopidogrel therapy might be considered if results of testing may alter management (*Level of Evidence: C*).

6.6   Answer B. Pharmacodynamic studies in which various platelet function tests have been used have shown a 60-mg loading dose of prasugrel to be more potent than clopidogrel loading, even when used at high doses (≥600 mg). More potent antiplatelet effects are achieved more rapidly and are sustained in the maintenance phase using a 10-mg maintenance dose of prasugrel compared with clopidogrel irrespective of maintenance dosing (75 to 150 mg) (*Circulation* 2007;116:2923–2932).

6.7   Answer C. Apply the following formula:

$$IPA = \frac{(MPA_{Pre} - MPA_{Post}) \times 100\%}{MPA_{Pre}}$$

$$50\% = \frac{(80\% - 40\%) \times 100\%}{80\%}$$

6.8   Answer D. Although some small studies have shown that increasing the dose of aspirin may overcome aspirin resistance, most studies have not. In fact, increasing the dose of aspirin does not further inhibit the COX-1 enzyme. Recent studies have shown that the most important cause of aspirin resistance is noncompliance to medication. Therefore, compliance to antiplatelet therapy should be evaluated in patients shown to be resistant in a platelet function test. Importantly, there are no studies showing that increasing the dose of aspirin in these patients or switching treatment is clinically beneficial. Increasing the dose of aspirin is known to increase the risk of bleeding, in particular in patients concomitantly treated with clopidogrel. Although some functional studies have shown that patients with aspirin resistance may also be clopidogrel resistant, there is no indication to test for this in routine clinical practice. At the current time, the patient should maintain without modifications his dual antiplatelet dose

regimen. The patient should maintain aspirin indefinitely and clopidogrel up to 1 year (*Am J Cardiol* 2009;103:27A–34A).

6.9   Answer D. Numerous factors account for inadequate clopidogrel-induced antiplatelet effects. These include genetic, cellular, and clinical factors. However, noncompliance and underdosing seem to play the most important role. Dose-finding studies supporting currently recommended dosages of clopidogrel were designed to achieve a degree of platelet inhibition similar to 250 mg/b.i.d. of ticlopidine. Importantly, these studies did not take into consideration the prothrombotic milieu of high-risk subjects, such as those with acute coronary syndromes or undergoing percutaneous coronary interventions. Numerous platelet function studies have shown that when increasing the loading and maintenance dose of clopidogrel enhanced antiplatelet effects are achieved (*Am J Cardiol* 2009;103:27A–34A).

6.10   Answer B. Concomitant use of NSAID such as ibuprofen, indomethacin, and naproxen can prevent aspirin from acetylating the platelet COX-1 enzyme. COX-1 inhibition (and not PAR inhibition) is the mechanism through which aspirin exerts its effects and blocks platelet's ability to synthesize thromboxane A2. While it is a weak inhibitor of platelet aggregation in vitro, it does decrease the incidence of peri-PCI thrombotic events by up to 75%. Chewing approximately 162 to 325 mg of aspirin allows for the achievement of its full effects within approximately 15 minutes (*N Engl J Med* 2005;353:2373–2383).

6.11   Answer D. The vast majority of data available in the scientific literature associating antiplatelet drug resistance with clinical outcomes has utilized LTA (light transmittance aggregometry), which despite its numerous pitfalls is still considered the gold standard assay for platelet function. Although point-of-care assays (VerifyNow and PFA-100) and platelet membrane receptors (assessed by flow cytometry) have also been implied in determining adverse clinical outcomes, the degree of evidence is less robust compared to LTA (*Am J Cardiol* 2009;103(3 suppl):27A–34A).

6.12   Answer A. A key protein involved in thienopyridine absorption is the efflux pump P-glycoprotein, which is encoded by *ABCB1* (also known as *MDR1*, located on chromosome 7). P-glycoprotein is an ATP-dependent efflux pump that transports various molecules across extracellular and intracellular membranes. It is expressed, among other places, on intestinal epithelial cells, where increased expression or function can affect bioavailability of drugs that are substrates. Studies have shown that following clopidogrel administration individuals with genetic variants in *ABCB1* (specifically those who are TT homozygotes for the 3435C→T variant) have reduced concentrations of the active drug metabolite and increased rates of adverse clinical outcomes (*Lancet* 2010;376:1312–1319). Polymorphisms of cytochrome P450 enzymes have been implied in modulating clopidogrel response through its hepatic metabolism. Controversial data exist on the modulating role of *Pl^A* polymorphisms on antiplatelet agents, which encode for the platelet glycoprotein IIb/IIIa receptor. *VKOR* polymorphisms are involved in modulating warfarin effects (Fig. A6-12) (*J Am Coll Cardiol* 2009;54:1041–1057).

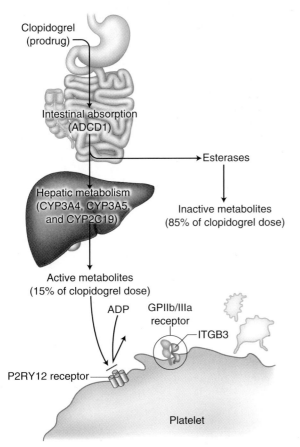

Figure A6-12. **(Adapted from Simon T, Verstuyft C, Mary-Krause M, et al. Genetic determinants of response to clopidogrel and cardiovascular events. *N Engl J Med* 2009;360:363–375.)**

6.13 **Answer C.** Unfractionated heparin, low-molecular-weight heparin, bivalirudin, and warfarin are all anticoagulant agents. Pharmacokinetic studies have shown that bivalirudin has a linear dose–plasma concentration relationship (*Circulation* 1993;87:1622). This translates into more predictable anticoagulant effects as assessed in pharmacodynamic studies. The effects of unfractionated heparin, low-molecular-weight heparin, and warfarin are influenced by multiple factors, which ultimately lead to broad variability in intersubject anticoagulant effects.

6.14 **Answer D.** In patients undergoing PCI who do not receive GP IIb/IIIa inhibitors, guidelines (*Circulation* 2006;113:e166–e286) recommend that (a) unfractionated heparin should be given during coronary angioplasty to achieve an ACT of 250 to 300 seconds with the HemoTec device and 300 to 350 seconds with the Hemochron device; (b) a weight-adjusted bolus heparin (70 to 100 IU/kg) can be used to avoid excess anticoagulation; and (c) if the target values for ACT are not achieved after a bolus of heparin, additional heparin boluses (2,000 to 5,000 IU) can be given (*Circulation* 2001;103:961–968). No large randomized study has established the optimal dose of heparin or target ACT, especially in the contemporary device and drug era. Many interventionalists begin with a 50-U/kg bolus of heparin (Fig. A6-14).

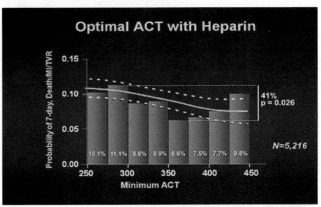

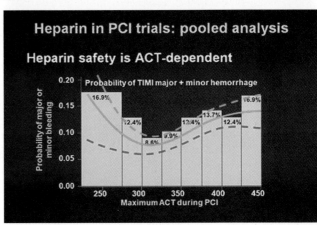

Figure A6-14. **(Reproduced from Chew DP, Bhatt DL, Lincoff AM, et al. Defining the Optimal Activated Clotting Time During Percutaneous Coronary Intervention: aggregate Results From 6 Randomized, Controlled Trials. *Circulation* 2001;103:961–968, with permission.)**

6.15 **Answer A.** In patients undergoing PCI receiving GP IIb/IIIa inhibitors, guidelines recommend (*Circulation* 2006;113:e166–e286) that the unfractionated heparin bolus should be 50 to 70 IU/kg in order to achieve a target ACT of 200 seconds irrespective of device that is being used to measure ACT. Higher doses of unfractionated heparin (70 to 100 IU/kg) have been associated with increased risk of bleeding and should be reserved for patients undergoing PCI without the use of GP IIb/IIIa inhibitors. A fixed (non–weight-based) bolus of 5,000 IU, without ACT monitoring, is subject to broad variability in ACT levels (*Circulation* 2001;103:961–968). Often times an ACT of >200 seconds can be achieved with a low dose (50 U/kg) of heparin (Fig.A6-15).

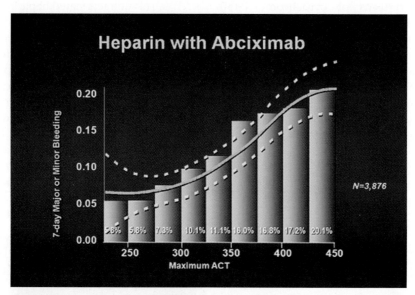

Figure A6-15. (Reproduced from Chew DP, Bhatt DL, Lincoff AM, et al. Defining the Optimal Activated Clotting Time During Percutaneous Coronary Intervention: aggregate Results From 6 Randomized, Controlled Trials. *Circulation* 2001;103:961–968, with permission.)

7 Antiarrhythmics, Sedatives, and Lipid-lowering Agents

Steven P. Dunn and David J. Moliterno

QUESTIONS

7.1 A 68-year-old Caucasian male with a history of hypertension, diabetes, and hyperlipidemia presents 6 hours after the onset of substernal chest pressure with an ECG significant for ST elevation in leads V4 to V6. He is seen in the emergency department and then taken to the catheterization suite for coronary angiography and possible percutaneous coronary intervention. After injecting the left coronary artery, the nurse notifies you of a rapid heart rate (Fig. Q7-1). The aortic pressure is noted to be 65/30 mm Hg and the patient does not respond to questions. What is the best treatment?

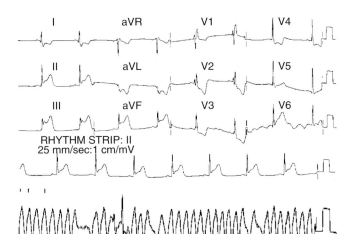

Figure Q7-1

(A) Immediate lidocaine 100 mg IV bolus
(B) Electrical cardioversion
(C) Rapid atrial pacing

(D) Give metoprolol 5 mg IV push
(E) Load with IV amiodarone 300 mg

7.2 Which of the following is the most appropriate description of amiodarone dosing for stable ventricular tachycardia (assume long-term continuation)?

(A) 150-mg IV bolus, followed by a 200-mg daily maintenance dose
(B) 300-mg IV bolus, followed by a 1-mg/min IV infusion for 6 hours, followed by a 0.5-mg/min IV infusion for 18 hours, followed by an oral loading dose for 5 to 7 days
(C) A 1-mg/min IV infusion for 6 hours, followed by a 0.5-mg/min IV infusion for 18 hours
(D) 400-mg oral maintenance dose

7.3 Which of the following methods of administration for amiodarone is most likely to cause hypotension?

(A) Amiodarone oral loading dose
(B) Amiodarone continuous intravenous infusion
(C) Amiodarone maintenance dose
(D) Amiodarone intravenous bolus

7.4 Accumulating evidence has demonstrated that the development of new atherosclerotic lesions, as opposed to the treatment of restenosis or previously intervened upon lesions, is a leading cause for recurrent coronary artery disease and symptoms. As such, it is crucial following percutaneous coronary interventions to aggressively treat lipid abnormalities. Assuming you are treating a patient naïve to medical therapy undergoing initial percutaneous coronary intervention, which of the following lipid-lowering therapies would you prescribe to achieve the greatest risk reduction of both stable and unstable coronary artery lesions, irrespective of abnormalities on the patient's lipid panel?

(A) Atorvastatin
(B) Fenofibrate
(C) Niacin
(D) Omega-3 fatty acids
(E) Colesevelam

7.5 An 87-year-old woman undergoes left heart catheterization and diagnostic angiography following suspected unstable angina. The night prior to the procedure, she was anxious and had difficulty sleeping. She received 5 mg of zolpidem for sleep and 2 mg of lorazepam for anxiety. The morning of the catheterization, she received 25 mg of diphenhydramine orally. Near the time her femoral arterial sheath was placed, she complained of back pain and received two tablets of oxycodone/acetaminophen 5/325 since there was a PRN order. Prior to obtaining arterial access, conscious sedation procedures are initiated with 50 µg of intravenous fentanyl. Over the next several minutes, her oxygen saturation decreased to <80% and she was difficult to arouse. Her vital signs were stable except her respiratory rate was decreased. The next appropriate step would be to administer:

(A) Midazolam
(B) Atropine
(C) Flumazenil
(D) Naloxone
(E) Epinephrine

7.6 Atropine is used in the cardiac catheterization laboratory particularly among patients who are experiencing vasovagal bradycardia and/or hypotension. Which of the following statements is true for the use of atropine in the cardiac catheterization laboratory?

(A) It should be used in caution among patients with a history of diabetes
(B) It may cause anticholinergic side effects
(C) It should be used among patients who have a substantial decrease in heart rate
(D) It should be used in small doses (<0.4 mg) especially among patients with diabetes
(E) It should be given in large doses (>2 mg) among patients with a large body mass index (>30)
(F) All of the above

7.7 On your morning rounds, you plan to discharge a 62-year-old man who had been admitted several days prior with non–ST-elevation myocardial infarction. He underwent successful angioplasty and bare-metal stent placement to the proximal left anterior descending artery. You notice his fasting cholesterol profile reveals the total cholesterol to be 332, triglycerides (TG) 600, and high-density lipoprotein (HDL) 48. The low-density lipoprotein (LDL) is unable to be calculated. Which of the following lipid-lowering therapies would be appropriate for this patient?

(A) Simvastatin
(B) Niacin
(C) Gemfibrozil
(D) Simvastatin plus niacin
(E) Simvastatin plus fenofibrate

7.8 Assuming the same patient as in Question 7.7, which of the following lipid abnormalities matched with the appropriate drug is the most appropriate to target first, assuming limited financial means?

(A) Triglycerides → Niacin
(B) Total Cholesterol → Statin
(C) Triglycerides → Gemfibrozil
(D) HDL → Gemfibrozil

7.9 Assuming you are ready to discharge the patient in Question 7.7 home, the medical resident on your team presents the following as his medication regimen upon discharge: aspirin 325 mg daily, clopidogrel 75 mg daily, simvastatin 80 mg nightly, metoprolol 25 mg twice daily, gemfibrozil 600 mg twice daily, and lisinopril 5 mg daily. Which of the following combinations represents a clinically important drug–drug interaction that requires therapeutic modification?

(A) Clopidogrel–Simvastatin
(B) Simvastatin–Gemfibrozil
(C) Aspirin–Clopidogrel
(D) Aspirin–Lisinopril
(E) None of the above

7.10 A 75-year-old man with a past medical history of stroke, coronary artery disease, ischemic cardiomyopathy, hypertension, and chronic kidney disease with a creatinine clearance of 30 mL/min undergoes angioplasty and direct stent placement, which are successful. However, he develops atrial fibrillation overnight and further discussion with the patient reveals a history of palpitations over the past several months. Which antiarrhythmic medication(s) would be reasonable treatment options for this patient at this time?

(A) Sotalol
(B) Flecainide
(C) Mexiletine
(D) Dofetilide

7.11 A 62-year-old woman with renal insufficiency, atrial fibrillation, and a CHADS$_2$ score of 3 is being discharged after a hospitalization where she received a drug-eluting stent. Your resident informs you of the final medication regimen at discharge, which includes aspirin 325 mg daily, clopidogrel 75 mg daily, warfarin 5 mg daily, simvastatin 40 mg nightly, amiodarone 200 mg daily, digoxin 125 μg daily, and metoprolol 25 mg twice daily. Which of the following is a clinically significant drug–drug interaction, requiring either increased monitoring or therapeutic intervention?

(A) Amiodarone–Digoxin
(B) Amiodarone–Simvastatin
(C) Amiodarone–Warfarin
(D) All of the above

7.12 Assuming again the same patient above eventually progresses to end-stage renal disease requiring hemodialysis, which of the following antiarrhythmic medications would be most preferable?

(A) Sotalol
(B) Amiodarone
(C) Flecainide
(D) Mexiletine
(E) Dofetilide

7.13 Which of the following lipid-lowering therapies does not result in a drug–drug interaction when given with warfarin?

(A) Ezetimibe
(B) Cholestyramine
(C) Lovastatin
(D) Simvastatin

7.14 A 56-year-old man with a positive nuclear stress test and exertional angina is referred for coronary angiography and possible stent placement. The patient is prepped and local anesthesia is administered around the access site. At this time, which of the following medications is appropriate for inducing conscious sedation?

(A) Lidocaine 100 mg IV
(B) Midazolam 2 mg IV
(C) Diphenhydramine 50 mg IV

(D) Succinylcholine 100 mg IV
(E) None of the above

7.15 Which of the following patient parameters most closely describes characteristics of the level of sedation recommended for cardiac catheterization procedures?

(A) Purposeful response to commands
(B) Maintenance of pulmonary ventilation and oxygenation
(C) Maintenance of cardiovascular function
(D) All of the above
(E) None of the above

7.16 Assuming the patient above has an allergy to benzocaine, which of the following actions with local anesthesia initiation is appropriate?

(A) Abandon the procedure since cross-allergenicity is possible with all anesthetics
(B) Administer larger doses than usual of fentanyl in order to "make up" for the lack of a local anesthetic
(C) Proceed with administration of lidocaine, but choose a preservative-free solution without vasoconstrictor components
(D) None of the above

7.17 Which of the following local anesthetics is associated with the most adverse effects on the cardiovascular system?

(A) Lidocaine
(B) Ropivacaine
(C) Bupivacaine
(D) Benzocaine

7.18 An 82-year-old African American male with a history of coronary artery disease, hypertension, diabetes, and chronic kidney disease presents with an inferolateral STEMI and receives primary PCI to the RCA. Following the procedure, he remains bradycardic with a heart rate in the 40s and hypertensive with a systolic blood pressure of 140s to 150s. His serum creatinine at baseline is 2.3 but is found to be now 3.0 after obtaining labs post-PCI. The decision is made to try to increase his heart rate in an attempt to improve renal perfusion. He declines consent for a temporary pacing wire due to lack of desire for further invasive procedures so he must be paced using pharmacologic measures. Which of the following would be the least appropriate method for pharmacologic pacing at this time?

(A) Isoproterenol
(B) Dopamine
(C) Dobutamine
(D) None of the above

7.19 The patient's serum creatinine in the above question eventually returns to baseline and pharmacologic pacing is withdrawn several days following his acute myocardial infarction. He does not appear to require a permanent pacemaker (and would refuse if one was offered) but his heart rate remains in the 50s. Prior to discharge, the patient develops atrial fibrillation with a slow ventricular response on telemetry for which he feels light-headed and dizzy despite normal hemodynamics. This rhythm resolves spontaneously. Which of the following medications would be the optimal choice to maintain the patient in sinus rhythm, assuming such a strategy is used?

(A) Amiodarone
(B) Diltiazem
(C) Dofetilide
(D) Metoprolol

7.20 If dofetilide is chosen as the antiarrhythmic strategy, which of the following is true regarding the patient's disposition?

(A) The patient can go home the same day it is initiated
(B) The patient must receive a prescription from an attending cardiologist
(C) The patient must be hospitalized for the first 3 days of therapy with a prescription written upon discharge by an approved dofetilide prescriber
(D) The patient must be hospitalized for the first 3 days of therapy, but any licensed provider can write the prescription
(E) None of the above

ANSWERS AND EXPLANATIONS

7.1 **Answer B.** Figure Q7-1 shows a tracing of ventricular tachycardia that is associated with hypotension and reduced mental status (the patient does not respond to your question). In this scenario, the best treatment is direct current cardioversion to immediately restore sinus rhythm. Although amiodarone and lidocaine are Advanced Cardiovascular Life Support (ACLS) drugs of choice for hemodynamically stable VT, the goal in this patient is to rapidly convert the patient to a more stable rhythm (*Circulation* 2010;122:S250–S275). Metoprolol would be less desirable in a hypotensive patient.

7.2 **Answer B.** Amiodarone is a complex drug to administer, requiring a bolus followed by a prolonged loading period. Answers A and D are incorrect due to the lack of an appropriate total loading dose (usually 8 to 10 g for VT). Answer C is also incorrect due to the lack of an initial IV dose to attempt to terminate the rhythm and also due to lack of follow-up beyond the 24-hour infusion period. Therefore B is the most appropriate answer, assuming amiodarone is continued beyond the short-term period.

7.3 **Answer D.** Intravenous amiodarone contains a polysorbate compound that is known to cause hypotension upon rapid infusion. While all methods of amiodarone administration are associated with some effects on hemodynamic parameters, due to effects of the compound on beta and calcium channels, the intravenous bolus is most consistently the cause of hemodynamically significant hypotension (*Drugs* 1992;43:69–110). Additionally, aqueous amiodarone solutions are also now available, which may be associated with less hypotension during the bolus phase of administration (*Am J Cardiol* 2004;93:576–581).

7.4 **Answer A.** HMG-CoA reductase inhibitors ("statins") have been extensively shown to reduce the secondary development of both unstable and stable coronary artery disease. Indeed, intensive statin therapy has also remarkably shown regression in coronary artery plaque. While other therapies on this list may alter lipid parameters, none have demonstrated reduction

in events similar to statin drugs and are indicated in virtually all patients with known coronary artery disease.

7.5 **Answer D.** Pharmacologic reversal is indicated due to her decreased oxygen saturation and altered mental status. Midazolam would be inappropriate in this scenario as benzodiazepines can further induce respiratory dysfunction, an effect that can also be synergistic in combination with opiate analgesics. Atropine additionally has no indication in this scenario due to the stable hemodynamics. Flumazenil would potentially be indicated if the patient had received intravenous benzodiazepines for sedation, but from this scenario, only fentanyl had been given. The lorazepam from the previous evening is probably not significantly present in the body at this time. Epinephrine is also not indicated due to the stable hemodynamic profile. Naloxone would be the most appropriate choice to the immediate onset after the administration of intravenous opiate therapy.

Table A7-5. Reversal Agents for Conscious Sedation Procedures

	Dose	Peak Effect	Duration of Effect
Flumazenil (benzodiazepine antagonist)	0.2 mg initial Max (total): 1 mg	6–10 min	1–4 h
Naloxone (opioid antagonist)	0.4 mg initial Max (total): 2 mg	5–10 min	45 min–3 h

7.6 **Answer B.** Atropine is a very valuable drug in the cardiac catheterization laboratory and can quickly reverse the bradycardia and hypotension sometimes associated with infarction, ischemia, and inappropriate vagal tone. Diabetes is not a concern when administering atropine. Additionally, the relative degree of decrease in heart rate is not a significant factor when deciding whether or not to administer atropine, rather bradycardia with hemodynamic compromise should be the indication. Doses <0.4 mg should not be administered due to potential for a paradoxical bradycardic reaction. Finally, a patient's body weight does not influence the initial dose of atropine given. Atropine does, however, antagonize muscarinic receptors and exerts its therapeutic effect via anticholinergic mechanisms. Therefore, other anticholinergic effects may be present with the use of atropine but should dissipate within a few hours and not be considered significant barrier to its use.

7.7 **Answer E.** This patient has severe dyslipidemia that will require combination therapy to achieve optimal levels. Niacin seems reasonable, as it will potentially affect LDL, HDL, and TG but will not be enough by itself, and its primary target, HDL, is at goal. Statins are certainly indicated but will do little to achieve goal levels of TG. Gemfibrozil will not significantly change HDL and LDL levels. Therefore, E is the best answer.

7.8 **Answer C.** Per the ATP guidelines (*JAMA* 2001;285:2486-2497), TG of >500 mg/dL should be treated as the primary lipid abnormality to reduce the acute risk of pancreatitis. In reality, this can and should be paired with an affordable statin, although answer B is incorrect as total cholesterol is not the appropriate primary target with statin therapy. Answer A is incorrect as TG will not be significantly reduced with niacin alone. Answer D is incorrect since gemfibrozil will not significantly increase HDL.

7.9 **Answer B.** The combination of statin and fibrates may be utilized, but multiple reports exist describing the increased risk of muscle toxicities, including rhabdomyolysis, associated with the combination. Therefore, the choice of fibrate and the dose of statin make a clinically significant difference. Gemfibrozil inhibits certain proteins that uptake statins into the liver and therefore will increase levels of virtually all statin medications. Simvastatin may be utilized in combination, but it is recommended to be dosed no higher than 10 mg daily. Additionally, fenofibrate affects statin bioavailability to a lesser degree and may be more safely utilized with statin therapy. While some literature exists regarding statin medication interfering with the antiplatelet effect of clopidogrel, this has not been found to be clinically significant, making B incorrect. Aspirin and clopidogrel do increase the risk of bleeding but are therapeutically indicated in this patient due to the recent stent, which makes C incorrect. Aspirin has also been shown to interfere with the vasodilating effects of angiotensin-converting enzyme inhibitors (ACEI), but not enough data exist to suggest modification of therapy in this patient. Therefore, B is the correct answer.

7.10 **Answer D.** The decision to use an antiarrhythmic in a patient with extensive cardiovascular disease and altered metabolic function is complex. Sotalol could initially be considered but is not recommended for use in patients with heart failure. Mexiletine is not effective for atrial arrhythmias. Flecainide is also not recommended for patients with structural heart disease due to risk of proarrhythmia. As such, it is very reasonable to treat this patient with either amiodarone, which is entirely metabolized by the liver, or dofetilide, which is primarily eliminated by the kidney but can be adjusted for renal dysfunction. Both agents can be used successfully not only in acute atrial fibrillation but also as prophylactic agents to prevent recurrent atrial fibrillation. Additionally, both amiodarone and dofetilide are the only recommended antiarrhythmic drugs to be used chronically in patients with a history of heart failure.

7.11 **Answer D.** All of the above are significant drug–drug interactions, which require either increased monitoring or therapeutic intervention. Amiodarone inhibits P-glycoprotein, which partially metabolizes digoxin prior to absorption. Therefore, amiodarone initiation in a patient receiving digoxin will necessitate a dose reduction of digoxin. Amiodarone inhibits CYP3A4, a major metabolic pathway for simvastatin and warfarin. The maximum dose of simvastatin recommended with warfarin is 20 mg/day. Additionally, initiation of warfarin in a patient receiving amiodarone will require close monitoring, and it is recommended that an empiric 50% reduction in the dose of warfarin be performed.

7.12 **Answer B.** Sotalol and dofetilide are contraindicated in hemodialysis-dependent patients. Flecainide is not a preferable agent in patients with structural heart disease and mexiletine is not effective for atrial fibrillation. Therefore, B is the best answer. Amiodarone is metabolized by the liver and is not significantly affected by renal function.

7.13 **Answer A.** Many lipid-lowering therapies inhibit metabolism of warfarin (such as many statins) or, in the case of cholestyramine, absorption of warfarin, both of which can affect the resultant anticoagulant effect of warfarin. Ezetimibe is not known to affect either hepatic metabolism of warfarin or vitamin K production in the gut (*Clin Pharmacokinet* 2005;44:467-494).

Table A7-14. **Benzodiazepines in Conscious Sedation**

	Dose		Peak Effect	Duration of Effect	Metabolic Pathway	Active Metabolite	Protein Binding (%)
Midazolam	**Oral:** NA	**IV:** 0.5–2 mg Max: 5–10 mg	3–5 min	30–80 min	Oxidation	Yes	95
Diazepam	**Oral:** 5 mg	**IV:** 2–5 mg Max: 10 mg	**Oral:** 30 min **IV:** 8–10 min	2–4 h	Oxidation	Yes	80
Lorazepam	**Oral:** 4 mg	**IV:** 2 mg Max: 4 mg	**Oral:** 60–90 min **IV:** 15–20 min	6–8 h	Conjugation	No	85

7.14 **Answer B.** Short-acting, intravenous benzodiazepines are the method of choice to induce conscious/moderate sedation in patients undergoing catheterization. The table below (Table A7-14) illustrates potential benzodiazepine options in the catheterization lab. Intravenous lidocaine would have no effect on the level of sedation. Diphenhydramine is often administered to patients undergoing catheterization as a premedication to induce a baseline level of sedation, but this ideally should be done at least 30 minutes prior to the procedure. Succinylcholine is a neuromuscular blocker, that would be inappropriate to give for sedation, and would additionally result in a loss of respiratory function.

7.15 **Answer D.** Conscious (or moderate) sedation is the recommended level of sedation for cardiac catheterization procedures. This level of sedation is a drug-induced depression of consciousness that still allows for the patient to respond to commands and for maintenance of pulmonary and cardiovascular function. The patient's ability to respond to commands is particularly critical in the catheterization laboratory since patient symptoms can often be the first indicator of procedural success or complications.

7.16 **Answer C.** True local anesthetic allergies are uncommon. However, amine-containing anesthetics (benzocaine, prilocaine, or tetracaine) do contain a potentially immunogenic substitution. Amide-containing anesthetics (such as lidocaine) should not be cross-reactive in patients with "amine" allergies. In addition, preservative-free solutions of lidocaine can also be utilized. Patients also may have allergic reaction to sulfite compounds in vasoconstrictors, which can also be avoided in a patient with a local anesthetic allergy. While similar anesthesia may be obtained with intravenous opiates, this should be considered a less preferential pathway due to the potential for oversedation and respiratory dysfunction. Therefore, C is the best answer.

7.17 **Answer C.** Bupivacaine is widely regarded as the local anesthetic with the most potential for cardiotoxicity. Cardiotoxicity with local anesthetics typically results from the same nerve blocking mechanism extending to the myocardial conduction system, resulting in potential bradyarrhythmias. Additionally, anesthetics may promote ventricular arrhythmias via unidirectional block and reentry pathways. Lidocaine is typically considered the local anesthetic of choice due to its rapid onset, offset, and minimal potential for cardiotoxic effects.

7.18 **Answer B.** In general, all of the above medications are options for pharmacologic pacing due to the fact that all of these options stimulate β-1 receptors, which should result in an increase in both inotropic and chronotropic effects. However, dopamine is inappropriate in this situation given that the patient is already hypertensive at baseline. Dopamine stimulates dopaminergic, β-1, and α-1 receptors in a dose-dependent manner and is the most likely drug to further increase the patient's blood pressure. Isoproterenol and dobutamine would be better choices due to the lack of alpha-stimulating activity. Both isoproterenol and dobutamine stimulate β-1 and β-2 receptors, which may actually result in hypotension.

7.19 **Answer C.** A rhythm-control strategy may be reasonable in this patient, since they are symptomatic in atrial fibrillation despite a slow ventricular rate. Diltiazem and metoprolol would be primarily rate-control strategies, although they may have some benefit in maintaining the patient in sinus rhythm, particularly metoprolol. However, both would be contraindicated in this patient with bradycardia due to effects on AV and SA node conduction. Amiodarone would be an effective antiarrhythmic but also has effects on beta and calcium channels (and therefore heart rate), which would not be desirable. Since the patient's serum creatinine has returned to baseline, dofetilide would be an ideal choice as a pure potassium channel antagonist since it does not affect chronotropy in any significant way.

7.20   **Answer C.** As part of the restrictions for approval of dofetilide, the patient must be hospitalized for the first 3 days of therapy and a licensed dofetilide prescriber must write the prescription upon discharge. This does not, however, have to be a cardiologist but any prescriber must complete an online mandatory training course. Additionally, only a licensed pharmacy can fill the prescription. These measures were put into place in order to minimize the risk of potentially life-threatening QT-interval prolongation and drug-induced torsades de pointes.

8

Inotropes, Vasopressors, and Vasodilators

Tracy E. Macaulay and David J. Moliterno

QUESTIONS

8.1 A 68-year-old female patient presents to the emergency room complaining of chest pain, and her ECG reveals a new left bundle branch block (LBBB). Upon arrival to the cardiac catheterization laboratory, the patient's systolic blood pressure (SBP) is 85 mm Hg, heart rate is 115 bpm, cardiac index (CI) is 1.9 L/min, and pulmonary capillary wedge pressure (PCWP) is 19 mm Hg. An intra-aortic balloon pump (IABP) is placed; however, blood pressure and CI remain low. Which of the following is the drug of choice in this setting?

(A) Dopamine
(B) Vasopressin
(C) Epinephrine
(D) Norepinephrine

8.2 Which of the following scenarios would be most appropriate for initiation of milrinone 0.375 μg/kg/min in a patient undergoing a right heart catheterization?

(A) Mean pulmonary arterial pressure 22 mm Hg, mean arterial pressure (MAP) 55 mm Hg, cardiac index (CI) 4.0 L/min, systemic vascular resistance (SVR) 800 dynes × s/cm^5, pulmonary capillary wedge pressure (PCWP) 8 mm Hg, heart rate (HR) 110 bpm
(B) Mean pulmonary arterial pressure 22 mm Hg, MAP 70 mm Hg, CI 3.5 L/min, SVR 1,000 dynes × s/cm^5, PCWP 8 mm Hg, HR 90 bpm
(C) Mean pulmonary arterial pressure 38 mm Hg, MAP 70 mm Hg, CI 2.0 L/min, SVR 1,600 dynes × s/cm^5, PCWP 36 mm Hg, HR 110 bpm
(D) Mean pulmonary arterial pressure 38 mm Hg, MAP 55 mm Hg, CI 2.0 L/min, SVR 1,000 dynes × s/cm^5, PCWP 36 mm Hg, HR 105 bpm

8.3 A 74-year-old patient with ischemic cardiomyopathy (LVEF 20% to 30%) is undergoing elective PCI for progressive anginal symptoms. During the procedure, he begins to experience hypotension (MAP 55 mm Hg) and shortness of breath. Chest x-ray reveals pulmonary edema and the SVO$_2$ is 65%. Which of the following is the most appropriate pharmacotherapy?

(A) Nesiritide 0.01 μg/kg/min
(B) Dopamine 10 μg/kg/min
(C) Nitroprusside 15 μg/min
(D) Milrinone 0.5 μg/kg/min

8.4 No-reflow can be a significant problem, in patients with high thrombus load or undergoing vein graft PCI. Which one of the following agents has NOT offered therapeutic benefit?

(A) Hydralazine
(B) Sodium nitroprusside
(C) Adenosine
(D) Verapamil
(E) Nicardipine

8.5 You are using a radial approach to perform PCI on a proximal LAD lesion in a 61-year-old woman. Following performance of balloon angioplasty, slow flow remains, and the entire vessel appears constricted. Which of the following agents would NOT be appropriate to administer?

(A) Diltiazem
(B) Sodium nitroprusside
(C) Nitroglycerin
(D) Acetylcholine

8.6 A 24-year-old with juvenile rheumatoid arthritis presents to cardiology clinic with marked limitations in physical activity secondary to progressive shortness of breath. Thus far, workup has revealed a normal ECG and echocardiographic changes consistent with pulmonary arterial hypertension. For further diagnosis, you decide to perform a right heart catheterization and vasodilatory study. Which vasodilatory regimen would be appropriate?

(A) Nesiritide 2 μg/kg bolus every 10 minutes to a maximum of 16 μg/kg

(B) Nitroglycerin 50 to 100 μg/min as a continuous infusion

(C) Epoprostenol 2 ng/kg/min titrated every 5 minutes to a maximum of 10 mg/kg/min

(D) Verapamil 20 mg IV bolus, followed by 10 mg/h

8.7 Which of the following is an endothelium-dependent vasodilator?

(A) Adenosine

(B) Serotonin

(C) Nitric oxide

(D) Nitroglycerin

(E) Verapamil

8.8 Which of the following statements best describes the activity of norepinephrine?

(A) Norepinephrine, similar to epinephrine, primarily exerts its effect on the β_1 receptors resulting in potent cardiostimulatory effects

(B) Norepinephrine exhibits vasodilatory effects at low doses, inotropic effects at moderate doses, and vasoconstrictive effects at high doses

(C) Norepinephrine and phenylephrine are preferred over epinephrine in vasodilatory shock as they produce more vasoconstrictive than cardiostimulatory effects

(D) Norepinephrine is favored over vasopressin among patients with low pH and cardiopulmonary arrest

8.9 Which one of the following statements is most CORRECT about contrast media–induced anaphylactoid reactions and their treatment?

(A) Urticaria should be immediately treated with subcutaneous epinephrine

(B) Intravenous steroid injection is effective at ameliorating the acute hemodynamic effects of contrast-mediated anaphylactoid reactions

(C) Angioedema should be treated with 0.3 mL of 1:1,000 epinephrine given IV push

(D) Cardiogenic shock should be treated with a 10-μg intravenous bolus of epinephrine followed by continuous infusion of 1 to 4 μg/min as needed

(E) Significant anaphylactoid reactions to contrast media occur in 2% to 3% of all patients undergoing selective coronary angiography, and intravenous diphenhydramine is the initial treatment of choice.

8.10 The vascular endothelium produces a number of vasoactive molecules. Which of the following is NOT produced by the endothelium?

(A) Nitrous oxide

(B) Endothelin

(C) Thromboxane

(D) Prostacyclin

8.11 Methergine is used as the "gold standard" vasoactive agent for the diagnosis of coronary artery spasm. Which of following is most CORRECT about methergine?

(A) Methergine stimulates abnormal vascular endothelium to produce large amounts of endothelin, causing vasoconstriction

(B) Methergine causes coronary vasoconstriction by up-regulating thromboxane production in abnormal vascular endothelium

(C) Methergine is a serotonin receptor agonist that causes vasodilation in normal endothelium but vasoconstriction in unhealthy endothelium

(D) Methergine is a vasopressin agonist that directly activates the coronary vascular smooth muscle in patients prone to coronary artery spasm

8.12 While PCI was performed on a saphenous vein graft in a 74-year-old male, he developed "slow flow" that was treated with intracoronary nitroprusside (400 μg). Subsequently, the patient developed hypotension (MAP 52 mm Hg) and tachycardia (HR 96 bpm). Which of the following is the BEST agent to reverse hypotension in this patient?

(A) Dopamine

(B) Isoproterenol

(C) Epinephrine

(D) Phenylephrine

(E) Norepinephrine

8.13 Which of the following is TRUE regarding the advantages of vasopressin over dopamine in resuscitation following cardiac arrest?

(A) Vasopressin increases SVR, the chronotropic and inotropic state of the myocardium, whereas dopamine only increases SVR

(B) All vasopressin receptors cause intense vasoconstriction, thereby increasing SVR more potently than dopamine

(C) Reflex vasoconstriction, from vasopressin-induced bradycardia, increases the effect on SVR, making it a more potent vasoconstrictor than dopamine

(D) Vasopressin receptors in the brain mediate vasodilatation, and vasopressin receptors in the periphery mediate vasoconstriction, thereby preserving cerebral perfusion

8.14 Which of the following statements is TRUE regarding the angiographic no-reflow phenomenon in the setting of myocardial infarction?

(A) Adventitial endothelial cell edema is a leading contributor to no-reflow

(B) The presence of no-reflow alone poorly predicts mortality

(C) Direct stenting reduces the incidence of no-reflow

(D) Vasodilators like verapamil and sodium nitroprusside improve survival in patients with no-reflow

(E) Reactive oxygen species play a significant role in no-reflow

8.15 Protamine sulfate reverses nearly all the anticoagulant effect of unfractionated heparin and reverses roughly 60% of the effect of low-molecular-weight heparin. Adverse reactions to the administration of protamine can occur following several situations. These include all of the following EXCEPT:

(A) Previous administration of protamine

(B) Vasectomy

(C) Allergy to fish

(D) Use of amiodarone

(E) Use of NPH insulin

8.16 A 51-year-old female with history of hypertension, hyperlipidemia, and pulmonary arterial hypertension secondary to COPD presents with the onset of severe chest pain. Her ECG reveals new ST-segment depression. Her BP is 132/88 mm Hg and HR is 93 bpm. Which of the following should be administered cautiously in this patient?

(A) Metoprolol 12.5 mg po every 12 hours

(B) Nitroglycerin continuous infusion starting at 10 to 20 μg/min

(C) Aspirin 324 mg chewed or crushed and then swallowed

(D) Unfractionated heparin 60 units/kg bolus followed by 12 units/kg/h

(E) Enoxaparin 1 mg/kg SQ every 12 hours

8.17 A 61-year-old man is brought to the emergency department (ED) after a witnessed cardiac arrest. He had return of spontaneous rhythm following advanced cardiac life support including CPR and defibrillation. At the time of arrival, his blood pressure is 75/40 mm Hg, and his heart rate is 45 bpm. In the ED, he is started on dopamine at 15 μg/kg/min and placed on a mild therapeutic hypothermia protocol. The telemetry monitor shows an RBBB pattern with second degree AV-block. In the cardiac catheterization laboratory, an IABP is placed with 2:1 augmentation; the patient remains hypotensive with a SBP < 90 mm Hg. Which of the following will be most helpful?

(A) Switch dopamine to epinephrine

(B) Administer intravenous fluid boluses

(C) Change IABP 1:1 augmentation to provide better SBP support

(D) Add milrinone to increase his HR, CO, and BP

8.18 Nitric oxide (NO) has many physiologic effects on vascular endothelium and the underlying smooth muscle. Which of the following is NOT CORRECT about nitric oxide?

(A) NO inhibits neutrophil adhesion by decreasing production of neutrophils

(B) NO decreases cGMP in vascular smooth muscle cells

(C) NO causes inhibition of platelet aggregation

(D) NO inhibits adhesion molecule production by vascular endothelial cells

8.19 While performing PCI on a 65-year-old male with a history of hypertension and diabetes, the patient develops chest pain, and his BP steadily climbs to 195/107 mm Hg with an HR of 120 bpm. The patient then develops flash pulmonary edema. Which of the following treatments would be best for this acute situation?

(A) Nitroglycerin 5 μg/min continuous infusion

(B) Phentolamine 1 mg/h continuous infusion

(C) Diltiazem 5 mg/h continuous infusion

(D) Fenoldopam 0.1 to 1 μg/kg/min continuous infusion

(E) Labetalol 10 to 20 mg IV push every 5 to 10 minutes as needed

8.20 Which of the following statements best describes the use of sodium nitroprusside?

(A) Sodium nitroprusside has a long elimination half-life which precludes its use in acute settings

(B) Cyanide toxicity is only seen at very high doses with prolonged infusion

(C) It is particularly useful in patients with low-output, left-sided heart failure because of balanced arteriole and venous vasodilation

(D) It is the treatment of choice for patients with cardiorenal syndrome

ANSWERS AND EXPLANATIONS

8.1 **Answer D.** Based on the data given about this patient, she is exhibiting signs of cardiogenic shock (SBP < 90 mm Hg, CI < 2.2 L/min, PCWP > 12 mm Hg). According to the subgroup analysis from the SOAP II trial, patients with cardiogenic shock (n = 280) who were randomized to receive norepinephrine had decreased rates of death compared to those who were randomized to receive dopamine (p = 0.03). This may have been related to a decrease in arrhythmic events in patients treated with norepinephrine compared to dopamine. (N Engl J Med 2010;362:779-789).

8.2 **Answer C.** Milrinone is a phosphodiesterase inhibitor that induces positive inotropic effects via inhibition of the breakdown of cyclic AMP, which causes an intracellular shift of calcium ion to produce an increase in myocardial contractility. It also has a dose-dependent vasodilatory effect by inducing peripheral vascular muscle relaxation. This effect is not present with other inotropic agents (dobutamine, isoproterenol, or dopamine), making it the ideal choice in patients with low cardiac index and elevated systemic vascular resistance as well as pulmonary artery pressures.

8.3 **Answer B.** All are potential options for patients with left ventricular systolic dysfunction in certain clinical circumstances. Nitroprusside and nesiritide are vasodilators and therefore should be avoided for inpatients who are exhibiting signs of shock. Milrinone may increase this patient's SVO_2; however, given its peripheral vasodilatory properties, it may further lower the patient's blood pressure. In this case, dopamine, given at a dose that results in both inotropy and vasoconstriction, is the most appropriate choice.

8.4 **Answer A.** Useful medical therapies (i.e., intracoronary vasodilators) include verapamil, adenosine, diltiazem, papaverine, nicardipine, and sodium nitroprusside. There is a suggestion in the literature that "combination therapy" with adenosine and nitroprusside is better than adenosine alone. Infusion of vasodilators into the distal vascular bed, instead of through the guide catheter, using a pulse spray method (perfusion catheter) may also improve angiographic outcome. However, angiographic improvement does not clearly alter subsequent morbidity and mortality (J Am Coll Cardiol 2001;37:1335-1343; Cathet Cardiovasc Diagn 1998;45:360-356; J Invasive Cardiol 2002;14:299-302; Catheter Cardioavasc Interv 2006;68:671-676).

8.5 **Answer D.** This patient's response is suggestive of diffuse vasospasm. The treatment of choice for vasospasm is administration of a vasodilator, such as diltiazem, sodium nitroprusside, or nitroglycerin (Fig. A8-5). These agents are all preferred over acetylcholine, as they are endothelium-independent vasodilators, whereas acetylcholine is an endothelium-dependent vasodilator. In patients such as this one, with coronary artery disease, endothelial dysfunction is common rendering agents such as acetylcholine ineffective or may cause further vasoconstriction (N Engl J Med 1986;315:1046-1051).

Table A8-3.

Dopamine Dose	α	β_1	β_2	DA	VD	VC	INT
1–3 μg/kg/min	−	+	−	++++	+	−	++
3–10 μg/kg/min	−	++++	++	++++	+	−	++++
>10–20 μg/kg/min	+++	++++	+	−	−	+++	+++

Dopamine pharmacologic and clinical effects.
DA, dopamine receptor; VD, Vasodilation; VC, Vasoconstriction; INT, inotropic.

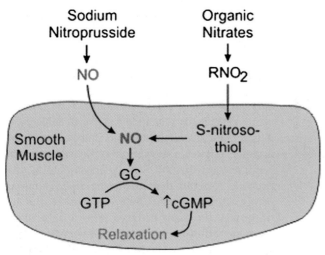

Figure A8-5

8.6 **Answer C.** Multiple agents have been used for acute vasodilatory challenges in patients undergoing evaluation of pulmonary arterial hypertension. In addition to epoprostenol intravenously, some studies have evaluated other prostacyclin analogs given intravenously as well as inhaled iloprost. Additionally, intravenous adenosine and inhaled nitric oxide have been used. All of these have a rapid onset and produce little rebound hypertension. Inhaled options offer the advantage of avoiding systemic effects (*Circulation* 2008;118:1195–1201).

8.7 **Answer B.** Nitric oxide is the *product* of the endothelium being stimulated by an endothelium-dependent vasodilator like acetylcholine or serotonin. Therefore, nitric oxide is an endothelium-independent vasodilator. Indeed, the nitrate-based, endothelium-independent vasodilators used in clinical practice, such as sodium nitroprusside and nitroglycerin, produce nitric oxide spontaneously or enzymatically that acts directly on vascular smooth muscle. A healthy endothelium is not needed for nitrates or the active molecule nitric oxide to cause vasodilation. Calcium channel blockers and adenosine have mechanisms of action that are also independent of the vascular endothelium.

8.8 **Answer C.** Norepinephrine is an important vasoactive medication with mixed effects on the α_1 and β_1 receptors across all doses. Due to the potent effects on the α_1, administration increases SVR, PAWP, MAP, and HR, but has a somewhat neutral effect on cardiac output. The usual starting dose is 2 μg/min and ranges up to 30 μg/min. Norepinephrine, often in combination with vasopressin, appears to be the drug of choice in septic

shock. In cardiogenic shock, recent studies have suggested that norepinephrine may decrease mortality compared to dopamine (*N Engl J Med* 2010;362:779–789). Norepinephrine and phenylephrine are preferred over epinephrine in vasodilatory shock as they produce more vasoconstrictive than cardiostimulatory effects due to predominantly α_1 effect.

8.9 **Answer D.** Anaphylactoid reactions secondary to contrast media occur in <0.5% of patients undergoing coronary angiography. Early treatment should include intravenous steroids; however, it will take several hours for steroids to have an effect. Therefore, if hypotension (vasodilatory shock) is evident, epinephrine should be administered in bolus doses of 10 μg every minute until MAP > 60 mm Hg. A 10-μg dose can be easily made by diluting 0.1 mL of 1:1,000 (1 mg/mL) epinephrine in 9.9 mL of 0.9% NS, resulting in a final concentration of 10 μg/mL. If continued epinephrine support is needed, then 1 to 4 μg/min continuous infusion may be given. For minor or moderate reactions, epinephrine can be administered subcutaneously with 0.3 mL of 1:1,000 solution (0.3 mg) every 15 minutes up to a total dose of 1 mg. Minor reactions such as isolated urticaria can be treated with diphenhydramine 25 to 50 mg given intravenously.

8.10 **Answer A.** Prostacyclin and thromboxane are products of cyclooxygenase and are produced by the vascular endothelium. Endothelin is a protein produced by the endothelium and is one of the most potent vasoconstrictors known. Nitric oxide is a free radical produced by the constitutive enzyme eNOS (endothelial nitric-oxide synthase) in normal endothelial cells in nonpathologic situations. There is also an inducible form of nitric oxide synthase—iNOS—that can be rapidly induced by a number of pathologic or inflammatory processes including ischemia-reperfusion injury and the sepsis syndrome. Nitric oxide is the putative endothelium-derived relaxing factor that is also a neurotransmitter in the brain, and one of the principal mediators of flow-dependent vasodilation. Nitrous oxide is an inhaled anesthetic and is not produced by the endothelium.

8.11 **Answer C.** Methergine is a synthetic analog of ergonovine, which causes serotonin receptor agonism resulting in effects on both the vascular endothelium and the vascular smooth muscle. When the vascular endothelium is healthy, methergine produces vasodilation via an endothelium-dependent (nitric oxide-mediated) mechanism that overpowers the direct vasoconstrictor effects on the vascular smooth muscle. However, if the endothelium in coronary artery segments is unhealthy, methergine stimulation does not result in increased amounts of endothelium-dependent vasodilators, and the direct vasoconstrictor action on the vascular smooth muscle is unopposed, thereby causing "spasm" in that coronary artery segment. Methergine has no effect on vasopressin receptors, thromboxane, or endothelin. Additionally, endothelin is a protein, not a small molecule, and it takes much more time for its production due to translation, transcription, and secretion of protein products from endothelial cells.

8.12 **Answer D.** Phenylephrine is a pure alpha agonist with no to minimal beta-adrenergic effects. Isoproterenol is incorrect as you would not want to lower heart rate in this clinical situation as it is likely secondary to vasodilation and will CORRECT in vasoconstriction.

8.13 **Answer D.** Vasopressin receptors in the brain are mediators of endothelium-dependent cerebral vasodilation. In the periphery, vasopressin receptors mediate vasoconstriction. This combination of peripheral vasoconstriction and cerebral vasodilation is an ideal hemodynamic combination for resuscitation, and vasopressin has been recommended as an alternative agent to dopamine by the Emergency Cardiac Care committee in Advanced Cardiac Life Support protocols. Dopamine, in the doses suggested by ACLS recommendations, increases SVR and the chronotropic state of the heart by stimulating α and β receptors.

8.14 **Answer E.** No-reflow is a complex pathophysiologic phenomenon that was first described in animal models of ischemia-reperfusion injury. As oxygen is reintroduced following anoxia, reactive oxygen species like superoxide anion, hydroxyl radical, and hydrogen peroxide cause free radical–mediated cell injury. Intimal, not adventitial endothelial cell edema, capillary plugging with neutrophils, platelet plugs, and eventually red cells all contribute to the no-reflow seen angiographically. In addition, microvascular vasospasm, atheroembolic debris, and endothelial dysfunction also participate in the no-reflow phenomenon. While there are several available treatments for no-reflow, none have

been shown to improve survival (*Am Heart J* 2003;145:42–46; *Catheter Cardiovasc Interv* 2004;61:484–491).

8.15 **Answer D.** With the exception of amiodarone, each of the factors listed are associated with an increased risk of reaction to protamine. Antibodies to medicinal protamine can develop following administration of protamine resulting in reactions with repeat exposure. These antibodies can also develop in 22% to 33% of patients undergoing vasectomy as nucleoprotamines are a normal component of human sperm cells. Protamine is derived from salmon testes, creating the potential for reaction in patients allergic to fish. The risk to have a severe allergic reaction to protamine among NPH (Neutral Protamine Hagedorn)-dependent diabetes is 27% compared to 0.5% in patients without NPH exposure. (*Urology* 1983;22:493–495; *Circulation* 1984;70:788–792).

8.16 **Answer B.** Before administration of nitroglycerin, this patient should be questioned about medical management of her pulmonary arterial hypertension. A common treatment in patients with pulmonary arterial hypertension is phosphodiesterase inhibitors, which have the potential to interact with nitrates. Nitrodilators stimulate cGMP production while cGMP degradation is inhibited by phosphodiesterase inhibitors. When combined, these two drug classes greatly potentiate cGMP levels, which can lead to hypotension and impaired coronary perfusion. All other therapies listed here would be appropriate for management of her acute coronary syndrome.

8.17 **Answer B.** This patient is having an inferior wall myocardial infarction possibly with right ventricular involvement. Switching from high-dose dopamine to epinephrine is unlikely to be beneficial. Increasing the rate of IABP will not affect SBP (but will increase the diastolic pressure). Milrinone could increase myocardial ischemia and worsen hypotension. The initial treatment for hypotension associated with inferior wall and right ventricular infarction is generous intravenous volume administration.

8.18 **Answer B.** Nitric oxide diffuses rapidly from endothelial cells into the surrounding vascular smooth muscle cells and increases production of cGMP that initiates a cascade of events leading to vascular smooth muscle relaxation. Nitric oxide is a potent inhibitor of platelet aggregation, in conjunction with endothelial-derived prostacyclin. Nitric oxide also inhibits adhesion of neutrophils by at least two mechanisms: nitric oxide production reduces expression of adhesion molecules in normal vascular endothelium, and it also has a direct effect on neutrophils preventing adhesion.

8.19 **Answer E.** Labetalol is a beta-blocker with α_2 vasodilatory properties. Along with esmolol, labetalol is considered the preferred treatment of hypertensive crisis in patients with cardiac ischemia. Nitroglycerin is an excellent adjunct therapy, especially in patients with evidence of pulmonary edema, although it is not the preferred first-line therapy as its utility is often limited by side effects. Phentolamine is useful in patients with catecholamine-induced hypertension, such as those with pheochromocytoma. Unlike dihydropyridine calcium channel blockers, diltiazem is more useful in patients needing control of heart rate as opposed to blood pressure. Fenoldopam is a selective dopamine-1 receptor agonist approved for the management of severe hypertension. It may be useful as an adjunct in this setting (for hypertension uncontrolled by labetalol and nitroglycerin), or as a first line in patients with acute renal injury.

8.20 **Answer C.** Sodium nitroprusside contains 44% cyanide by weight, which is released nonenzymatically from nitroprusside. Both cyanide and its renally eliminated metabolite, thiocyanate, can cause toxicity including respiratory failure, coma, delirium, psychosis, and hypothyroidism. Sodium nitroprusside has an immediate onset and a very short half-life that make it easily titratable. However, given the potential, it should be used at the lowest effective dose for the shortest duration possible, ideally <72 hours.

9 Guide Catheter Selection for Coronary Intervention

Timothy A. Mixon and Gregory J. Dehmer

9.1 You are performing coronary angiography from the femoral approach on a 56-year-old commercial airline pilot with atypical chest pain and a small inferior perfusion defect. After attempting to cannulate the left main with a JL 4 catheter, the coronary angiogram in Figure Q9-1 is obtained. The most likely diagnosis and a maneuver to obtain additional angiograms are:

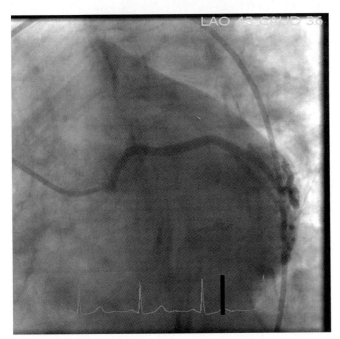

Figure Q9-1

(A) Anomalous origin of a coronary artery from the right sinus of Valsalva; change to a multipurpose (MP 1) catheter and look for the anomalous artery in the right cusp

(B) Separate coronary ostia; change to a JL 3.5

(C) Separate coronary ostia; change to a JL 4.5

(D) Anomalous origin of a coronary artery from the pulmonary artery, perform a pulmonary angiogram

(E) Stop the procedure and perform a CT coronary angiogram

9.2 A 78-year-old woman with a history of coronary artery bypass surgery and aortic valve replacement is referred for angiographic evaluation because of increasing and very limiting angina. Bypass grafts to the LAD and right coronary artery (RCA) are patent, but a vein graft to the left circumflex artery (LCX) is occluded. Angiography shows a stenosis within the distal LCX system for which percutaneous coronary intervention (PCI) has been requested (Figure Q9-2, although the distal stenosis is not seen in this view). The diagnostic angiograms were obtained using an MP 1 catheter. Expecting you will need strong support to treat the distal circumflex lesion, which of the following would be the best choice for a guide catheter?

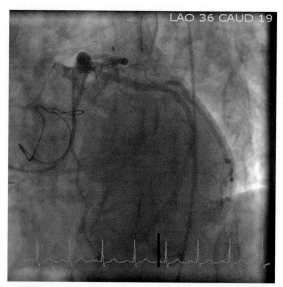

Figure Q9-2

    (A) JL 3.5
    (B) Q 4
    (C) AL 0.75
    (D) Voda left (VL) 4
    (E) Hockey stick (HS) catheter

9.3 Angiography is performed in a patient with a remote history of coronary artery bypass surgery, which included a vein graft to the RCA. After imaging the RCA with a JR 4 catheter, you seek the vein graft with the same catheter and obtain the image shown in Figure Q9-3. The angiogram obtained is felt to be inadequate. An alternative catheter choice for more selective images would be:

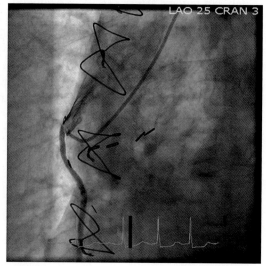

Figure Q9-3

    (A) AL 1
    (B) MP 1

    (C) No-torque right (NTR)
    (D) Hockey stick (HS)
    (E) Internal mammary artery (IMA)

9.4 You are asked to perform ad hoc PCI of a long stenosis in the LCX and marginal artery in a woman with an occluded bypass graft to the LCX. You note that the vessel is somewhat tortuous and mildly calcified (Fig. Q9-4). Diagnostic angiography was performed from the right radial artery. Which of the following is the most reasonable plan for guide catheter support during PCI?

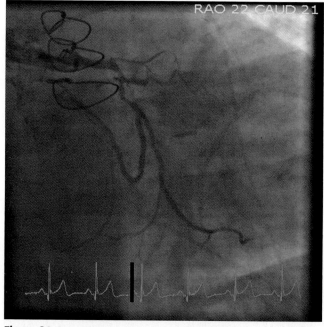

Figure Q9-4

    (A) Continue from the radial approach using a 6-F system with plans to enhance support using a 6-F GuideLiner or Proxis device, if necessary
    (B) This is unlikely to be successful from the radial approach due to the lesion length and tortuosity. Convert to a femoral approach
    (C) This can be done from the radial approach using a 6-F JL 4
    (D) Upsize to an 8-F system for enhanced support and proceed from the radial site
    (E) Continue from the radial approach but use a guide catheter with side holes and deep seat the catheter into the mid LCX

9.5 Which of the following is a concern that should be considered when selecting larger French size guide catheters over smaller diameter guide catheters?

(A) Increased potential for trauma at the ostium of the artery selected for intervention

(B) Larger arteriotomy site with increased risk of bleeding and delay to ambulation

(C) Increased contrast volume use

(D) Increased potential for embolization of atherosclerotic debris from the aortic wall

(E) All of the above

9.6 You are performing coronary angiography in a 52-year-old man with typical angina and a reversible lateral wall defect demonstrated on a stress myocardial perfusion study. There were no coronary stenoses seen in the vessels arising from the left main, and the RCA has minimal atherosclerotic narrowing. The angiogram in Figure Q9-6 is obtained. Since the lesion found matches the area of abnormal perfusion, you proceed with PCI. Which of the following would be a poor choice for a guide catheter in this case?

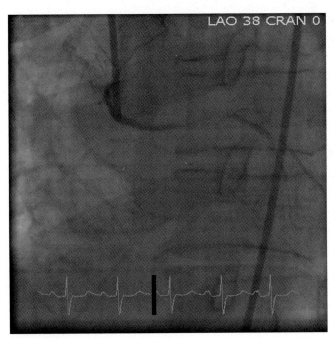

Figure Q9-6

(A) JR 4

(B) MP 1

(C) AR 1

(D) VL 4

(E) HS

9.7 You are asked to perform PCI on a calcified mid-LAD stenosis in a 76-year-old woman with exertional angina and an abnormal stress test. She is 5'4" tall and weighs 112 lb. A limited femoral angiogram shows a small femoral artery. You conclude that a 6-F sheath is the largest her

artery can safely accommodate. You plan to use a 6-F Q-curve guiding catheter. What is the largest rotablator burr that can be used with this guide catheter?

(A) 1.5-mm burr

(B) 1.75-mm burr

(C) 2.0-mm burr

(D) 2.15-mm burr

(E) 2.25-mm burr

9.8 A 55-year-old woman with diabetes and prior stenting of her RCA 6 years ago presents with exertional angina. Angiography reveals occlusion of her mid-RCA stent (type 4 in-stent restenosis), as shown in Figure Q9-8. In planning PCI, an appropriate guide catheter choice might include:

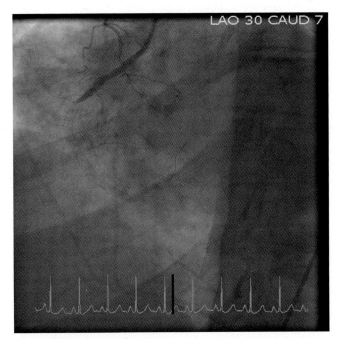

Figure Q9-8

(A) IM

(B) AL 1

(C) JR 4

(D) AR 1

(E) ART 1

9.9 You are performing coronary angiography before possible PCI in a 60-year-old man who presented late after an inferior myocardial infarction. He now has angina during his daily activities. He is 5'10" tall, has a normal build, and has no history of hypertension. You are planning access from the right radial artery since his Allen's test is normal. Acceptable guide catheter choices, should intervention be needed, include all of the following, EXCEPT:

(A) JL 3.5
(B) Jacky catheter
(C) Kimny catheter
(D) JR 3.5
(E) JR 4.5

9.10 You are asked to treat a bifurcation stenosis that consists of two, approximately equal-sized branches, with disease located at the ostium of each branch. You elect a strategy of simultaneous kissing stents. Which of the following is the smallest French guide catheter that would provide an adequate lumen size for your planned approach?

(A) 6-F guide catheter
(B) New generation large lumen 7-F guide catheter
(C) 8-F guide catheter
(D) 5-F guide catheter
(E) 8-F large lumen guide catheter

9.11 A 45-year-old construction worker presents with progressive angina for the past year. He has been reluctant to seek medical attention because of fear he will lose his job, but he can no longer perform his regular work duties because of angina. After failing a stress test, coronary angiography is performed showing an occluded mid LAD. One of your colleagues has unsuccessfully attempted to open the chronic total occlusion (CTO) via an antegrade approach, so the patient is referred to you to consider a retrograde approach through one of the septal collateral channels (Fig. Q9-11A-B). When considering guide catheter choice, you should consider all of the following, EXCEPT:

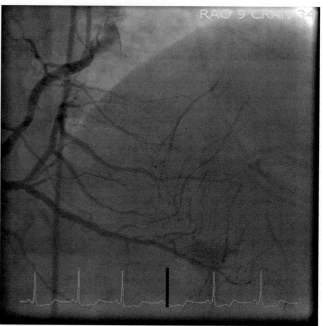

A

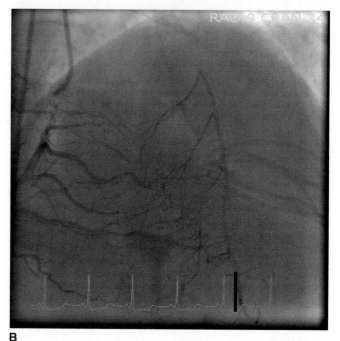

B

Figure Q9-11

(A) Shortening the guide catheter in anticipation of a long course for CTO wires and balloons due to the retrograde approach
(B) Use an 8-F guide catheter, for enhanced support
(C) Use a 6-F JL 5, to minimize vessel trauma
(D) Use an AL 1 with side holes, for enhanced support
(E) Use two 8-F guide catheters, to allow visualization of the occluded vessel from an antegrade and retrograde view

9.12 Treatment of a distal LAD stenosis through a long, tortuous left IMA bypass graft is most likely to be successful using the following guide catheter:

(A) Standard IMA guide catheter
(B) Newer, IMC guide catheter
(C) JR 4 guide catheter
(D) 90-cm IM guide catheter
(E) A left radial approach with a standard IM guide catheter

9.13 You initially have difficulty cannulating the left main artery in a woman who is 5'0" tall and weighs 245 lb. Your assessment of the JL 4 catheter shows the tip to consistently lie in the left cusp just inferior to the origin of the left main origin (Fig. Q9-13). Which of the following maneuvers is most likely to engage the left main?

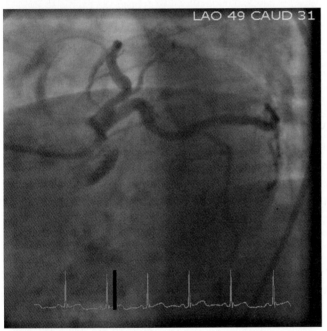

Figure Q9-13

(A) Change to a JL 5
(B) Have the patient take a deep breath and attempt to engage the left main again
(C) Change to an MP 1 catheter
(D) Change to an AL 2
(E) Change to a Voda 4 (VL 4)

9.14 A 56-year-old man with a history of prior bypass surgery presents with increasing exertional angina. During a stress test, he develops 2 mm of horizontal ST-segment depression in the anterior leads at a heart rate of 104 beats/min. Diagnostic angiography shows a severe stenosis in the body of the vein graft to the LAD. Which of the following guide catheters is least likely to cannulate the vein graft and provide adequate support for PCI?

(A) NTR
(B) JR 4
(C) HS
(D) Left coronary bypass (LCB), or left graft seeker
(E) AL 1

9.15 A 64-year-old man with a recent transient ischemic attack is found to have a 90% stenosis of his proximal right internal carotid artery. He has a prior history of surgery and radiation for a squamous cell carcinoma of the neck and is deemed to be high risk for carotid endarterectomy. He is referred to you for carotid stenting. His initial aortogram is shown in Figure Q9-15. Which of the following is the best guide catheter to cannulate the innominate artery?

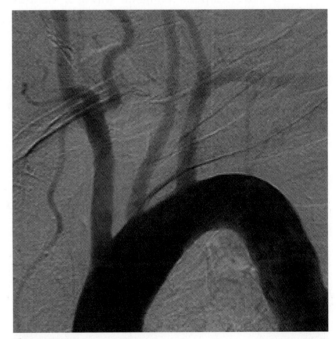

Figure Q9-15

(A) JR 4
(B) IM
(C) Simmons 1
(D) Vertebral catheter
(E) JB 1

9.16 You are asked to treat a heavily calcified mid-RCA stenosis. Considerations for proper guide catheter selection before rotational atherectomy include all of the following, EXCEPT:

(A) Adequate French size to accommodate the anticipated required burr
(B) Presence of side holes
(C) Coaxial positioning at the vessel ostium
(D) Deep seating potential to allow maximum support
(E) Adequate catheter tip stiffness to maintain position in the coronary ostium

9.17 A 60-year-old man with a history of a prior bypass operation 7 years ago presents with increasing angina and has an abnormal stress myocardial perfusion image showing inferior ischemia. Coronary and bypass graft angiography shows that the vein graft to the RCA is occluded as is the native RCA at its ostium. The LAD is occluded, but there is a patent LIMA graft to the mid LAD, which then provides several transseptal collaterals to the posterior descending artery (PDA). Medical therapy is not controlling his angina. Before attempting retrograde wiring of the RCA via the LAD septal collaterals (Fig. Q9-17A,B), you anticipate the need to have a shortened IM guide. Unfortunately, you have no 90-cm guides available in the lab because they are on back order, so you decide to shorten the guide catheter yourself. Which of the following statements is correct for safe and successful creation of a shortened guide catheter?

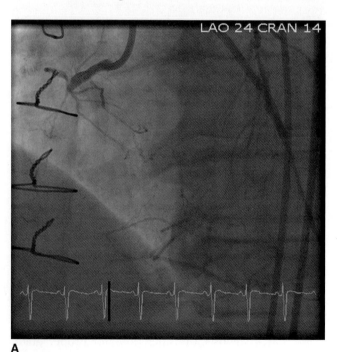

B
Figure Q9-17

(A) It is best to remove 10 to 15 cm of guiding catheter near the midshaft of the guide
(B) Remove the last 10 to 15 cm including the hub, and then connect to a Tuohy-Borst system
(C) To shorten a 7-F guide, you will need to use a piece of 7-F sheath to reconnect
(D) To shorten a 7-F guide, you will need to use a piece of 6-F sheath to reconnect
(E) Remove the proximal 12 cm of the guide catheter and reshape the tip using a heat gun

9.18 After diagnostic angiography with a 5-F system, you are asked to treat a focal stenosis in the mid LAD. Upon placement of a 7-F JL 4 guide catheter, you notice significant dampening of the pressure waveform (Fig. Q9-18). Which of the following is the best course of action?

A

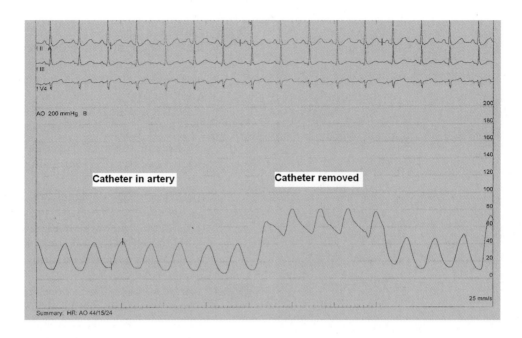

Figure Q9-18

(A) Manipulate the catheter in the left main in an attempt to improve the waveform

(B) Change to a catheter with side holes

(C) Perform intravascular ultrasound to better understand the geometry and presence of any disease in the left main

(D) Downsize to a 6-F guide catheter

(E) Proceed with the PCI, but disengage the guide once the wire is across the stenosis

9.19 You are asked to perform PCI on a stenosis in the distal RCA through a saphenous vein graft in a 67-year-old woman who presented with unstable angina and small increase in her troponin-I. Which of the following guide catheters is least likely to allow satisfactory completion of the procedure?

(A) Multipurpose A curve (MP A)

(B) Judkins right

(C) Right coronary bypass (RCB)

(D) Left coronary bypass (LCB)

(E) Amplatz left II or III curve

9.20 You are asked to perform PCI to correct a severe stenosis in a large third marginal branch of a fairly tortuous LCX. Which of the following catheters is least likely to provide adequate backup support?

(A) XB 3.5

(B) EBU 4

(C) AL 2

(D) JL 4

(E) VL 3.5

9.21 A 60-year-old woman presented with atypical angina. A dobutamine echocardiogram showed mild hypokinesis of the inferior wall. Coronary angiography showed no disease in the left coronary, but an anomalous RCA originating superior to the usual location and midway between the left coronary and the usual position of the RCA ostium. The operator performing the diagnostic study had considerable difficulty engaging the anomalous RCA, but the angiograms showed a severe stenosis in the mid-to-distal RCA. Which of the following types of guide catheters is least likely to successfully cannulate the RCA?

(A) Judkins right family

(B) Voda (XB, EBU)

(C) Judkins left family

(D) Amplatz left family

(E) Q-curve catheter

9.22 After diagnostic angiography, PCI is requested of a mid-RCA stenosis. The diagnostic operator had difficulty accessing the aorta from the femoral artery and subsequently "kinked" a 6-F JR 4 catheter while attempting to rotate it into the RCA ostium. Angiography of the iliac vessels reveals extremely tortuous, although widely patent, vessels (Fig. Q9-22). Which of the following options is least likely to result in a smooth and successful procedure?

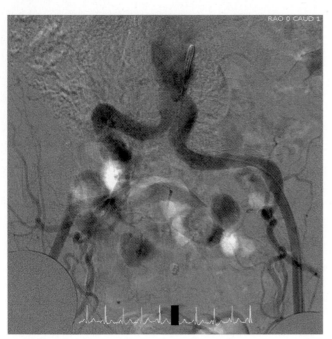

Figure Q9-22

(A) Convert to a radial artery approach
(B) Using an Amplatz wire, exchange the short diagnostic sheath for a 7-F, 45-cm sheath
(C) Upsize to a short, 8-F sheath and use an 8-F guide catheter
(D) Use a 6-F JR 4 guide catheter
(E) Use a long 8-F sheath and a 7-F JR 4 guide catheter

9.23 Upon placement of a 6-F guide catheter into the ostium of the coronary artery with a significant stenosis, the waveform in Figure Q9-23 is observed. The catheter is immediately removed from the ostium but the waveform remains the same. What is the most likely explanation for this waveform?

(A) Kinking of the guide catheter
(B) Excessively deep intubation into the coronary artery
(C) Unappreciated significant stenosis at the ostium
(D) Obstruction of the guide lumen or pressure tubing with air or thrombus
(E) This is a normal waveform

9.24 You are asked to assist a colleague who has been unable to pass an embolic protection device into a tortuous, proximal vein graft to a circumflex marginal artery (Fig. Q9-24). A 6-F JR 4 guide catheter was being used but the guide catheter repeatedly disengaged from the graft ostium when the protection device was advanced. In addition to upsizing to an 8-F guide catheter, which of the following strategies would you recommend?

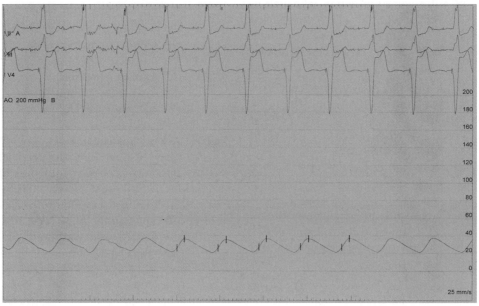

Figure Q9-23

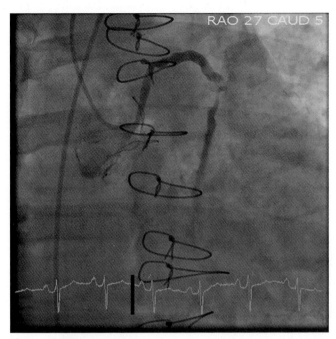

Figure Q9-24

(A) Change to an AL 1 guide

(B) A JR 4 guide in 8-F size will be adequate

(C) IM guide

(D) JL 5

(E) Any of the above is likely to be successful in an 8-F size

9.25 To achieve optimal support and coaxial alignment in treating an RCA with a "shepherd's crook" (upward takeoff) configuration, which of the following guide catheters would be best?

(A) AR 1

(B) JR 4

(C) AL 1

(D) HS

(E) NTR

9.1 **Answer B.** Separate ostia of the left coronary or a very short left main artery is one of the most common coronary anomalies and must be recognized by the operator. In this circumstance, it is often better to selectively cannulate and obtain separate angiograms of the left circumflex (LCX) and leukocyte adhesion deficiency (LAD) than to obtain inadequate angiograms of both vessels by a suboptimal catheter position. In this patient, a JL 4 catheter selectively entered the LCX. The most likely maneuver to selectively cannulate the LAD is to change to the next smaller Judkins curve size, in this case a JL 3.5 (Fig. A9-1A–C). Other maneuvers that may work are to withdraw the JL 4 slightly and apply clockwise rotation that will direct the tip anteriorly allowing cannulation of the LAD. A longer Judkins catheter (JL 4.5) would place the tip inferior to the LCX ostium. CT coronary angiography can be very helpful to define the course of anomalous coronary arteries in difficult cases, but there is no reason to abort the case at this point without trying other maneuvers. This patient was found to have no significant coronary narrowings.

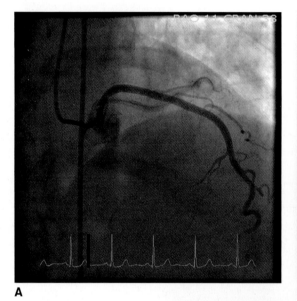

A

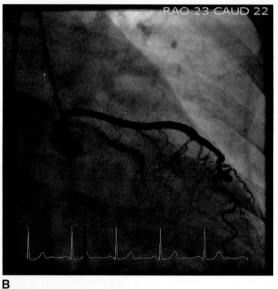

B

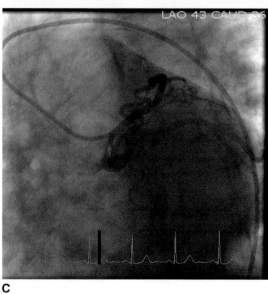

C

Figure A9-1

9.2 **Answer D.** Note that in Figures Q9-2 and A9-2A, the MP 1 catheter reflects off the aortic cusp and into the left main. The most robust backup support will come from a catheter that not only engages the left main but also makes contact with the opposite aortic wall. A Voda catheter with the proper curve size for the aorta is designed to accomplish this. While a VL 3.5 will typically function well in a patient with a normal-sized aorta, a VL 4 is more appropriate for patients with larger aortic roots. Figure A9-2B shows the Voda catheter reaching across to the opposite aortic wall. Both a Q4 and AL 0.75 might cannulate the LM but would likely be too short to buttress against the opposite aortic wall. An HS guide is rarely used for left coronary interventions but is useful for some RCA and saphenous vein graft (SVG) interventions.

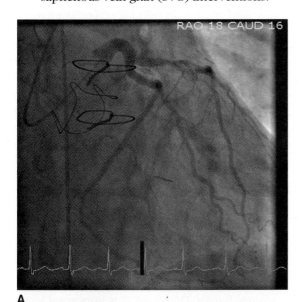

A

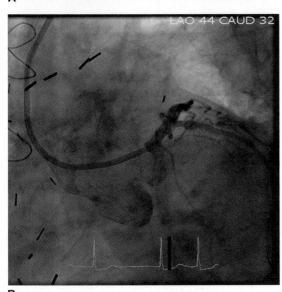

B

Figure A9-2

9.3 **Answer B.** Frequently a JR 4 catheter can be used to cannulate many vein grafts including those to the left or right coronary system. However, vein grafts to the RCA may have an inferiorly directed origin from the aorta, so the distal curve of the JR 4 may not allow selective cannulation. In this case, a catheter with a downward directed and a longer tip is needed and an MP 1 catheter is usually ideal (Fig. A9-3). In this example, it was placed at the ostium, which was adequate for diagnostic angiograms. With rotation, the tip can often be engaged deeper in the graft for more support during PCI. The NTR and IMA have tips of inadequate length and shape to reach the ostium. In a normal aorta, the HS and AL 1 generally have the tip pointed in a cephalad direction and that would not be ideal for this graft origin (Berg R, Lim M. Diagnostic angiographic catheters: coronary and vascular. In: Mukherjee D, Bates ER, Roffi M, Moliterno DJ, eds. *Cardiac catheterization, coronary and peripheral angiography, and interventional procedures.* London: Informa Healthcare, 2009; Baim DS. Coronary angiography. In: Baim DS, ed. *Grossman's cardiac catheterization, angiography, and intervention,* 7th ed. Philadelphia, PA: Lippincott Williams & Wilkins, 2006:191–196.)

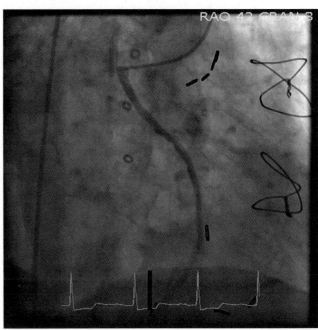

Figure A9-3

9.4 **Answer A.** Radial interventions are commonly performed in Europe and gradually gaining popularity in the US market. With more experience, operators have gradually approached increasingly complex interventions with good success rates, thus immediate conversion to a femoral approach is rarely required. Nonetheless, adequate guide catheter support is required and a 6-F JL 4 is unlikely to provide the necessary support in this case. Radial arteries are smaller than femoral arteries and rarely allow 8-F sheaths without increasing local complication rate (dissection, ischemia, thrombosis, or even vessel rupture). While deep seating the guide catheter can enhance support, it is utilized less frequently now and associated with an increased risk of vessel complication. A "guide within a guide," or telescoping technique, will greatly increase the support that a 6-F guide provides. Currently, this can be achieved using the GuideLiner system (Vascular Solutions, Minneapolis, MN), or the Proxis device (St. Jude Medical, St. Paul, MN, off-label use). With either system, the additional support catheter goes inside of the guide catheter and can be placed within the proximal or even midvessel (Fig. A9-4, notice the GuideLiner placed into the proximal LCX). This not only enhances the performance of the parent guide catheter but also allows enhanced delivery of devices through the proximal and midvessel with less resistance (Mamas MA, Fath-Ordoubadi F, Fraser DG. Distal stent delivery with Guideliner catheter: first in man experience. *Catheter Cardiovasc Interv* 2010;76:102–111. Brilakis ES, Banerjee S. Novel uses of the Proxis embolic protection catheter. *Catheter Cardiovasc Interv* 2009;74:438–445.)

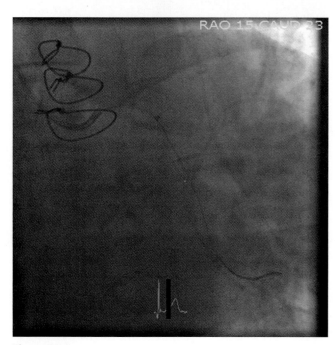

Figure A9-4

9.5 **Answer E.** Larger lumen catheters require larger introducer sheaths and thus have an increased potential for complications at the puncture site as well as the origin of the target vessel. Larger lumen catheters require a larger volume of contrast to fill the catheter and are associated with higher contrast loads. Care should be taken to limit contrast loads in patients with underlying renal dysfunction when larger diameter catheters are needed. Larger lumen catheters, especially 8 F, have been associated with more trauma to the aorta and the potential for producing atherosclerotic debris. This is especially true for certain shapes of catheters including the JL, VL, and multipurpose (Grossman PM, Gurm HS, McNamara R, et al. Percutaneous coronary intervention complications and guide catheter size: bigger is not better. *JACC Cardiovasc Interv* 2009;2:636–644. Eggebrecht H, Oldenburg O, Dirsch O, et al. Potential embolization by atherosclerotic debris dislodged from aortic wall during cardiac catheterization: histologic and clinical findings in 7,621 patients. *Catheter Cardiovasc Interv* 2000;49:389–394. Keeley EC, Grines CL. Scraping of aortic debris by coronary guiding catheters: a prospective evaluation of 1,000 cases. *J Am Coll Cardiol* 1998;32:1861–1865.)

9.6 **Answer D.** Figure Q9-6 shows an anomalous circumflex arising from a separate ostium near the origin of the RCA. An anomalous circumflex is one of the most common coronary anomalies encountered among patients referred for angiography (prevalence 0.18% to 0.67%) and the anomalous vessel may be affected by atherosclerosis. Therefore, it is important to understand guide catheter options that can be used to cannulate this anomalous artery. The anomalous LCX can arise from a separate ostium near the ostium of the RCA, an ostium shared with the RCA, or from the proximal RCA. Its course is posterior to the aorta toward the posterior AV groove. A multipurpose curve or JR catheter often will engage the ostium of the anomalous circumflex although backup support may not be ideal. An Amplatz right (1 or 2 curve) or HS curve is a reasonable option. Although designed for LCX interventions in an anatomically normal LCX, a VL 4 is unlikely to engage this artery adequately. Figure A9-6 shows this artery after successful stent placement through an MP 1 guide catheter (West NE, McKenna CJ, Ormerod MA, et al. Percutaneous coronary intervention with stent deployment in anomalously-arising left circumflex coronary arteries. *Catheter Cardiovasc Interv* 2006;68:882–890.)

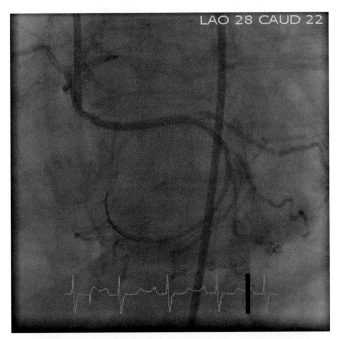

Figure A9-6

There is some variation in the internal diameters from various manufacturers so it is appropriate to anticipate the burr sizes you will need and make certain you are using a guide catheter of sufficient size. Although it is recommended that the I.D. of the guide catheter be 0.004 in. larger than the burr size, practical experience has shown 0.002 in. to be acceptable, although it will be more difficult to advance the burr through the guide catheter.

9.8 **Answer D.** The diagnostic angiogram shows an inferiorly directed origin of the RCA. Of the provided guide catheter choices, the IM, AL 1, and ART 1 are best suited for an RCA with a horizontal or superiorly directed origin. While the JR 4 would likely fit, the need for enhanced backup support in treating the occlusion should be anticipated and would not be provided by a JR catheter. The best selection would be the AR 1, which should fit coaxially and provide adequate support (Fig. A9-8A,B). Other options would include an HS or MP 1 catheters.

9.7 **Answer B.** An essential component in planning a rotational atherectomy case is knowledge of the maximum burr size, which can be used in the chosen guide catheter. Table A9.7 is from the manufacturer and recommends a minimum guide size of 0.004 in. larger than the burr.

Table A9-7. Guide Catheter Selection and Sizing

Burr (mm)	Burr Diameter (in.)	Minimum Manufacturer Recommended Guide Catheter Internal Diameter (in.)	Commonly Used Guide Catheter Sizes
1.25	0.049	0.053	≥5 F
1.50	0.059	0.063	≥6 F
1.75	0.069	0.073	≥6 F
2.00	0.079	0.083	≥7 F
2.15	0.085	0.089	≥8 F
2.25	0.089	0.093	≥8 F
2.38	0.094	0.098	Rarely used
2.50	0.098	0.102	Rarely used

(Adapted from http://www.bostonscientific.com/templatedata/imports/collateral/Coronary/rota_checklist_01_us.pdf, accessed: 1/28/11.)

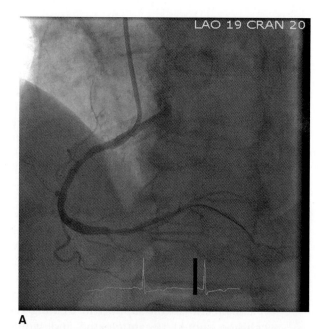

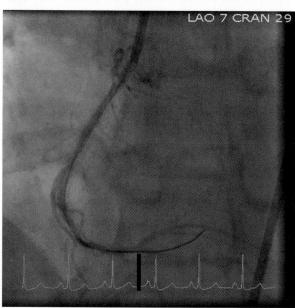

Figure A9-8

9.9 **Answer D.** When choosing Judkins catheters for a right radial approach, traditional teaching is that the Judkins left catheters should be downsized by 0.5 cm (e.g., JL 3.5 in place of the usual JL 4), while the Judkins right should be upsized (JR 4.5 or JR 5 in place of the usual JR 4). Therefore a JR 3.5 is not likely to be a good choice and successful in this case. Alternatively, dedicated radial catheters have been developed, which may allow cannulation of both the left and the right corona ry with the same catheter, such as the Jacky, Kimny, or Barbeau catheters

(Figure A9-9A,B), showing cannulation of the left and RCA with the same Jacky catheter (Terumo Medical Somerset, NJ) (Baim DS, Simon DI. Percutaneous approach, including trans-septal and apical puncture. In: Baim, DS, eds. *Grossman's cardiac catheterization, angiography, and intervention*, 7th ed. Philadelphia, PA: Lippincott Williams & Wilkins, 2006:97–100. Shibata Y, Doi O, Goto T, et al. New guiding catheter for transrad PTCA. *Cathet Cardiovasc Diagn* 1998;43:344–351.)

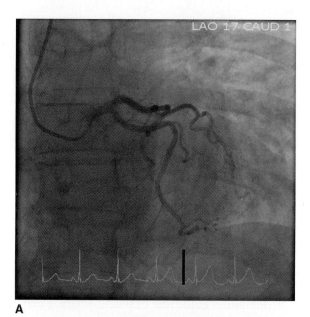

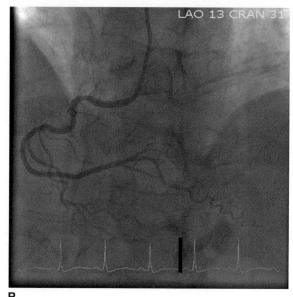

Figure A9-9

9.10 **Answer A.** With the increasing popularity of radial artery interventions, operators have adapted ways to complete many types of complex interventions via 6-F guide catheters. Frequently, radial arteries cannot safely accommodate sheaths larger than 6 F. To complete this procedure with a 6-F guide catheter, monorail or "rapid exchange" equipment would be required. Two monorail balloons or stents systems can simultaneously pass through current generation 6-F guides. In addition to bifurcation stenting, other complex interventions can be performed through 6-F systems (rotational atherectomy up to a 1.75-mm burr, Angiojet with an XMI catheter, manual thrombectomy catheters, etc.). However, opacification of the target vessel may be suboptimal when larger devices are used through a 6-F system.

9.11 **Answer C.** While minimizing vessel trauma is always important, the need for adequate visualization and support may require more aggressive guide catheter size and shape. The slight increased risk of vessel trauma or ischemia should be discussed with the patient before the procedure and, in this case, the unique risk associated with traversing septal collaterals. A larger French size guide catheter and catheters that gain support by bracing themselves against other parts of the aorta are usually necessary. If the distal vessel is best seen with contralateral injections, then dual guide systems can be valuable for proper opacification, which, in turn, can increase the odds of success. Dual-site injections are now common during complex CTO PCI (Thompson CA, Jayne JE, Robb JF, et al. Retrograde techniques and the impact of operator volume on percutaneous intervention for coronary chronic total occlusions: an early U.S. experience. *J Am Coll Cardiol Interv* 2009;2:834–842. Moses JW, Weisz G. Contemporary principles of coronary chronic total occlusion recanalization. *Catheter Cardiovasc Interv* 2010;75(suppl 1):S21–S27.)

9.12 **Answer D.** When treating a stenosis that is very distal in the coronary artery or when it is necessary to approach the stenosis through a bypass conduit, a common technical limitation is the shaft length of the balloon or stent catheter (typically 135 cm). If a 90-cm guide is used, 10 additional centimeters of working length is preserved and may allow successful completion of the procedure. Alternatively, some balloons and stents may be obtained on longer shafts (e.g., 143 to 150 cm). Although not the only route to success, a left radial approach has gained popularity and could be utilized but there would still be the need for a shorter guide catheter.

9.13 **Answer B.** When the tip of a Judkins catheter lies just inferior to the LM ostium, one must recognize that the curve size of the Judkins catheter is too large. This is commonly encountered in patients who are of short stature (regardless of weight). Sometimes gentle rotation of the catheter will allow engagement of the LM especially if the LM ostium is slightly out of the normal plane. A JL 5, AL 2, and Voda 4 are "longer" than the JL 4 and thus are not expected to fit. An MP 1 catheter might work, but the easiest thing to try first is another attempt to engage the LM with the patient taking a deep breath. As the diaphragm moves downward, the heart and aorta also move and the ostium of the LM is "pulled" downward. If the tip of the JL catheter is slightly below the LM, this simple maneuver often allows engagement of the LM.

9.14 **Answer A.** Saphenous vein bypasses to the left coronary (LAD or LCX) most frequently arise from the left anterior surface of the aorta superior to the native vessels. The JR 4 and LCB catheters will often provide adequate backup support when treating left-sided vein graft lesions. An HS and left Amplatz left catheters can be expected to provide additional support and backup compared with the JR 4 and LCB catheters. The NTR catheter (Williams catheter) was designed for the RCA and generally would be directed to the opposite wall of the aorta. Figures A9-14A,B are from a different patient and show a typical superiorly directed origin of a saphenous vein Y-graft anastomosed to branches of the left coronary artery (Berg R, Lim M. Diagnostic angiographic catheters: coronary and vascular. In: Mukherjee D, Bates ER, Roffi M, Moliterno DJ, eds. *Cardiovascular catheterization and intervention*, New York: Informa, 2010:196–198.)

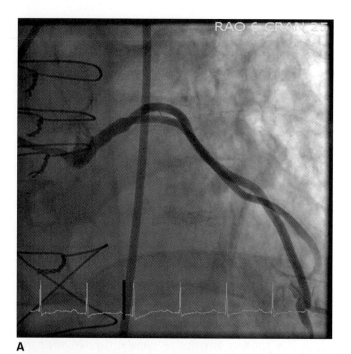

A

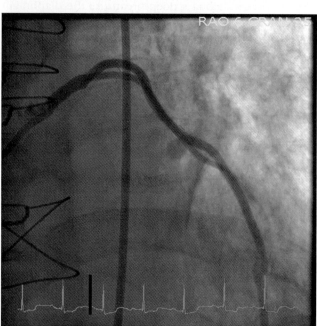

B

Figure A9-14

9.15 **Answer C.** You should recognize this as a type III aortic arch. In this type of arch configuration, a simple (or so-called passive) curve catheter such as J R4, IM, or vertebral catheter will not reach into the ostium of the innominate to allow wire access. An "intermediate" catheter such as a JB 1 is popular for type I and type II arches but is unlikely to allow access to the innominate artery of a type III arch. The best choice would be a Simmons catheter, which comes in various

tip lengths (Simmons 1, Simmons 2, etc.). Such a "reverse angle" (or so-called active) catheter requires re-formation and then manipulation in the aorta to engage the innominate artery. Originally, re-formation was accomplished by placing the catheter tip in the left subclavian artery and then prolapsing the catheter forward to re-create the shape. Subsequently alternate techniques were developed including clockwise rotation in the arch, advancement to the sinus of Valsalva and counterclockwise rotation, or reforming the tip by deflecting the J wire off of the aortic valve and then tracking the catheter over this wire to the proximal ascending aorta (Berg R, Lim M. Diagnostic angiographic catheters: coronary and vascular. In: Mukherjee D, Bates ER, Roffi M, Moliterno DJ, eds. *Cardiovascular catheterization and intervention*, New York: Informa, 2010:202–204. Simmons CR, Taso EC, Thompson JR. Angiographic approach to the difficult aortic arch: a new technique for transfemoral cerebral angiography in the aged. *Am J Roentgenol Radium Ther Nucl Med* 1973;119:605–612. Smith DC, Simmons CR. The quick aortic turn: a rapid method for reformation of the Simmons sidewinder catheter. *Radiology* 1985;155:247–248.)

9.16 **Answer D.** When performing rotational atherectomy, the operator must be aware of certain equipment requirements. The guide catheter must be large enough (French size) to accommodate the needed atherectomy burr. To help facilitate washout of the debris created by the burr, it is important that good flow is maintained down the vessel, so many routinely use a guiding catheter with side holes. Coaxial positioning at the ostium is always important but especially for easy advancement of the burr, and the guide catheter tip should be stiff enough to remain engaged in the ostium throughout the procedure. However, with rotational atherectomy, deep seating is not necessary or particularly desirable. The operator should slowly advance the burr allowing it to engage and debulk the stenosis rather than force the burr into the stenosis using a great amount of forward pressure. Although deep seating of the guide catheter is not necessary for rotational atherectomy, it still may be necessary for subsequent stent placement.

9.17 **Answer D.** When attempting to reach very distal locations, as described in this question, failure to use a shortened guide catheter may result in

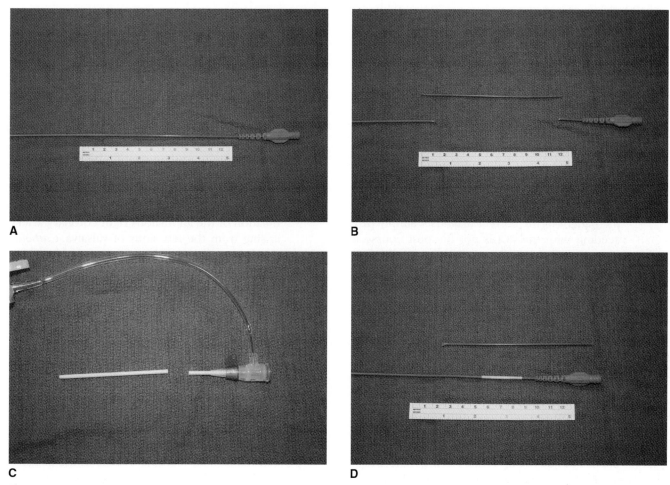

A

B

C

D

Figure A9-17

an inability of standard balloons or stents (typically 135 cm shafts) to reach the target lesion. Shorter guide catheters (90 cm) are available in many of the standard sizes and shapes and are always best to use. However if a shorter guide is unavailable, or a length <90 cm is required, it may be necessary to create one by shortening a 100-cm catheter. This can be done by removing the desired excess length (typically 10 to 20 cm) toward the back end of the catheter. It is best to remove and patch the guide catheter in a location that will not enter the body in the event the catheter disarticulates. The most common method excises the desired length approximately 5 cm from the hub (Fig. A9-17A,B). A piece of sheath 1 F size smaller is used to reconnect the guide (Fig. A9-17C,D). Alternatively, the terminal 10 to 15 cm of the catheter including the hub can be removed and attached to a sheath 1 F smaller using the diaphragm that

is part of the sheath (Thompson CA, Jayne JE, Robb JF, et al. Retrograde techniques and the impact of operator volume on percutaneous intervention for coronary chronic total occlusions: An early U.S. experience. *J Am Coll Cardiol Interv* 2009;2:834–842. Stratienko AA, Ginsberg R, Schatz RA, et al. Technique of shortening angioplasty guide catheter length when therapeutic catheter fails to reach target stenosis. *Cathet Cardiovasc Diagn* 1993;30:331–333. Wu EB, Chan WW, Yu CM. Retrograde chronic total occlusion intervention: Tips and tricks. *Catheter Cardiovasc Interv* 2008;72:806–814.)

9.18 **Answer C.** When angiography is performed with a 4- or 5-F diagnostic catheter, it is possible for important LM disease to be missed. Left main disease may be suspected when a larger French size guide catheter is placed and pressure dampening or "ventricularization" occurs (See

Figure A9-23A for an example of ventricularization). While this can occur in the absence of obstructive disease, such as when the catheter is not coaxial, or when the LM has an angulated takeoff, this should be investigated to assure the patient does not have significant LM disease. IVUS is an excellent way to understand the mechanism of pressure dampening. If significant obstructive disease is identified, the treatment plan for the patient may need to be modified. Changing to a side-hole guide catheter or to a smaller guide system may minimize the ischemia experienced by the patient but could deprive the patient of the correct diagnosis. Simply proceeding with the PCI is not the best course if there is uncertainty about important LM disease (Baim DS. Coronary angiography. In: Baim DS, ed. *Grossman's cardiac catheterization, angiography, and intervention*, 7th ed. Philadelphia: Lippincott Williams & Wilkins, 2006:190–191.)

9.19   **Answer D.** Saphenous vein grafts to the RCA usually have an inferiorly directed origin and arise from the anterior wall of the aorta. The MPA, Judkins right, and RCB catheters have a less acute curve just before the catheter tip and usually allow satisfactory graft cannulation. Occasionally an Amplatz catheter with the proper curve size and the tip rotated to the right side of the aorta will cannulate the graft. The LCB has a more acute angle and usually does not seat coaxially with the right-sided vein graft origin. (Safian RD, Freed MS. Coronary intervention: preparation, equipment and technique. In: Safian RD, Freed MS, eds. *The manual of interventional cardiology*, 3rd ed. Royal Oak, MI: Physicians' Press, 2001:14–17.)

9.20   **Answer D.** The Amplatz catheter shape, the XB family of curves (Cordis), EBU family of curves (Medtronic), or Voda curves (Boston Scientific) should all provide substantial backup for delivery of stents and/or larger devices such as an Angiojet. The JL 4 shape provides modest backup and frequently operators rely on catheter manipulation or support wires to complete even straightforward interventions when a left Judkins guide is used.

9.21   **Answer A.** The anomalous right originating above the usual location and between the left and the right cusps is often very challenging to cannulate. Standard left catheters (JL 3.5, JL 4, JL 5, AL 1, and AL 2) can sometimes be utilized. Both a Voda curve and Q-curve catheters can also be used successfully to cannulate such an anomalous RCA and can provide reasonable backup support. However, Judkins right catheters are least likely to work in this situation. It is important to understand the route of the anomalous RCA as some variants course directly between the aorta and the pulmonary artery and have been associated with sudden cardiac death. While its course may be determined with some certainty in the catheterization laboratory, CT or MR angiography is very helpful in determining the course of an anomalous artery (Qayyum U, Leya F, Steen L, et al. New catheter design for cannulation of the anomalous right coronary artery arising from the left sinus of valsalva. *Catheter Cardiovasc Interv* 2003;60:382–388.)

9.22   **Answer D.** In the presence of a tortuous iliac artery, diagnostic or guide catheters can become kinked when attempting to rotate them into the RCA ostium. This is recognized by dampening or even complete loss of the pressure waveform. If this occurs, the operator should rotate the catheter in the opposite direction (usually counterclockwise) in an attempt to "unkink" the catheter. Once kinking of the catheter has occurred, it is best to remove this catheter often using a stiff wire. Kinking of a catheter can occur with tortuous vessels in the absence of obstructive disease. A possible solution is to place a stiff 0.035-in. wire (Amplatz, SupraCor, or other) through the diagnostic catheter into the aorta and then change the short sheath for a long (45 cm) sheath. This will straighten the iliac vessel and "absorb" the contact of the iliac vessels allowing better movement of the guide catheter. Obviously, if the operator has experience in radial artery catheterization, this route could be chosen.

9.23   **Answer D.** The waveform recorded from the guide catheter should be monitored frequently by the physician as well as the cardiovascular technician monitoring the patient. Particular attention is necessary (a) when first seating the guide catheter, (b) before each injection, and (c) when passing interventional equipment in or out of the guide catheter—all maneuvers that could change the guide position. In this case, the pressure waveform displays a significant loss of systolic pressure, although it does not have the typical shape of "ventricularization" (Fig. A9-23A). While this could represent pressure dampening from placing the catheter in a very small or disease artery, in this case, the pressure did not improve after assuring the catheter was free within the aorta, and it did not correlate with noninvasive pressures. Therefore, this is most likely due to obstruction within the fluid filled pressure line such as can occur when thrombus or air becomes entrapped. An injection should not occur until the catheter is thoroughly aspirated and then flushed, with care taken not to allow air back into the system (see Figure A9-23B for restoration of a normal wave form and pressure after aspirating and flushing the pressure line). A kinked guide catheter will typically have a very low pressure reading with a very narrow "pulse pressure." Deep intubation and an unappreciated ostial stenosis are associated with systolic dampening or "ventricularization," although these possibilities should be considered in all such cases (Baim DS. Coronary Angiography. In: Baim DS, ed. *Grossman's cardiac catheterization, angiography, and intervention*, 7th Ed. Philadelphia: Lippincott Williams & Wilkins, 2006:190–191).

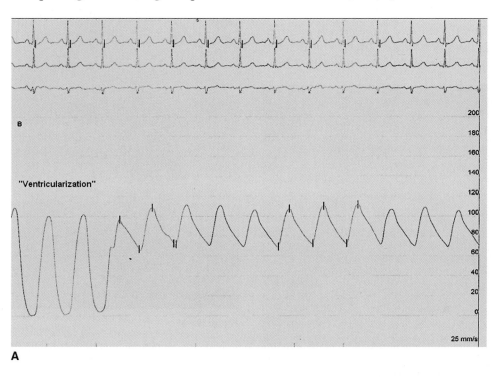

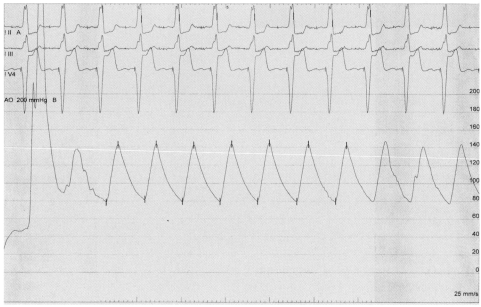

Figure A9-23

9.24 **Answer A.** For enhanced support with a left-sided saphenous vein graft, an Amplatz left guide (AL 1, AL 1.5, or AL 2 depending on the size of the aorta) should allow for adequate support (Fig. A9-24). Alternatively, an LCB or HS catheter may provide additional support. A Judkins right catheter and internal mammary catheter, while having the correct tip shape, are not long enough to rest against the contralateral aortic wall and seat securely in the ostium. The Judkins left catheters are not suitable for SVG cannulation. (Baim DS. Coronary Angiography. In: Baim DS, ed. *Grossman's cardiac catheterization, angiography, and intervention*, 7th ed. Philadelphia: Lippincott Williams & Wilkins, 2006:191–196).

9.25 **Answer C.** An RCA with an upward takeoff can frequently present difficulties in device passage around the proximal bends; thus, optimal coaxial alignment and backup support are desirable. Of the catheters listed, the AL 1 is the best choice (Fig. A9-25). The AR 1 and HS are best suited for a horizontal or downward takeoff. The JR 4 and NTR may seat coaxially but would not provide very much support.

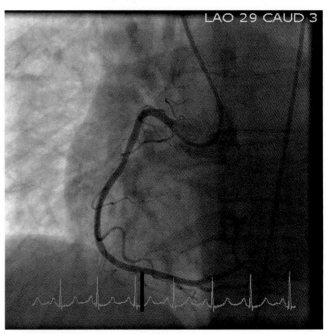

Figure A9-25

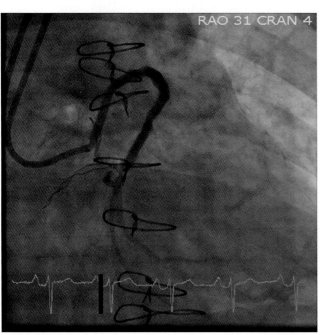

Figure A9-24

10 Intravascular Contrast Agents

Michael C. Reed and Brahmajee K. Nallamothu

QUESTIONS

10.1 A 68-year-old man with a history of four-vessel coronary artery bypass surgery to the right posterior descending artery, the obtuse marginal branch of the left circumflex artery, the left anterior descending artery, and the diagonal branch of the left anterior descending artery presents with progressive stable angina and inferior ischemia on stress testing. His diagnostic angiogram and cardiac rhythm is shown in Figure Q10-1. What is the best next step?

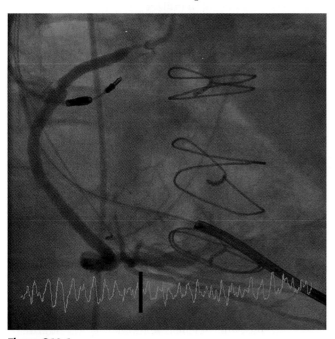

Figure Q10-1

(A) Switch to iso-osmolar contrast in order to minimize contrast cardiotoxicity
(B) Disengage the diagnostic catheter and instruct patient to cough
(C) Switch to power injection in order to optimize bypass graft visualization
(D) Insert a transvenous pacemaker

10.2 A 75-year-old woman with lifestyle-limiting angina, diabetes mellitus, and chronic renal insufficiency with a serum creatinine of 2.3 mg/dL is scheduled for elective cardiac catheterization with possible percutaneous coronary intervention. Which is a preferred contrast agent in this setting?

(A) Ioxaglate (Hexabrix)
(B) Iodixanol (Visipaque)
(C) Diatrizoate (Hypaque, Renografin, Angiovist)
(D) Carbon dioxide

10.3 A 74-year-old man presents with a non–ST-elevation myocardial infarction (non-STEMI). Surface echocardiogram shows an ejection fraction of 25%. His first coronary injection is shown (Fig. Q10-3). What strategy will likely reduce the risk of contrast-related cardiotoxicity in this patient?

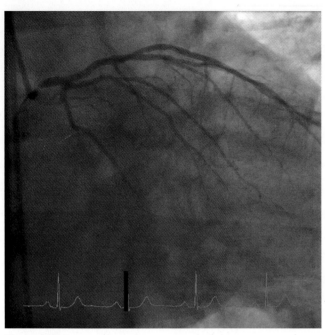

Figure Q10-3

(A) Use of high-osmolar contrast
(B) Limiting the number of injections and volume of contrast per injection
(C) Coronary injection during pressure wave ventricularization
(D) *N*-acetylcysteine

10.4 A 42-year-old woman with stable angina, anterior ischemia on dobutamine stress echocardiogram, asthma, and anaphylaxis to penicillin and peanuts expresses concern about her risk of a contrast reaction during diagnostic cardiac catheterization. Which of the following is the most accurate statement?

(A) Patients with anaphylaxis to penicillin should receive prophylaxis prior to diagnostic cardiac catheterization
(B) Use of biplane coronary angiography and forgoing left ventriculography will minimize her chance of having a hypersensitivity reaction to contrast
(C) Preprocedure skin testing is proven to be beneficial in predicting the occurrence of a hypersensitivity reaction
(D) Bradycardia and nausea are common reactions to contrast and do not typically indicate a hypersensitivity reaction

10.5 A 47-year-old man with diabetes and chronic kidney disease with a baseline serum creatinine of 2.7 mg/dL and a non-STEMI is referred for coronary angiography. Which of the following should the patient receive prior to the procedure?

(A) Fenoldopam
(B) Mannitol
(C) Normal saline
(D) Renal-dose dopamine

10.6 Typical doses of contrast agents for left ventriculography and thoracic aortography during routine cineangiography include:

(A) 30 to 40 mL injected at a rate of 10 mL/s and 80 to 100 mL injected at a rate of 40 mL/s, respectively
(B) 30 to 40 mL injected at a rate of 10 mL/s and 40 to 60 mL injected at a rate of 20 mL/s, respectively
(C) 20 to 30 mL injected at a rate of 5 mL/s and 20 to 40 mL injected at a rate of 20 mL/s, respectively
(D) 60 to 80 mL injected at a rate of 20 mL/s and 40 to 60 mL injected at a rate of 20 mL/s, respectively

10.7 A 52-year-old man with a history of hypertension, diabetes, and unstable angina develops pruritus, urticaria, wheezing, heart rate of 95 bpm, and hypotension with a systolic blood pressure of 70 mm Hg despite a 500-mL IV bolus of normal saline after his first injection of contrast for diagnostic cardiac catheterization. What is the best next step?

(A) Hydrocortisone 200 mg IV
(B) Diphenhydramine 50 mg IV
(C) 0.01 mg of 1:10,000 epinephrine IV
(D) Albuterol nebulizer

10.8 A 49-year-old man with exertional dyspnea, mitral valve prolapse with a flail leaflet, and severe mitral regurgitation confirmed by transesophageal echocardiography is referred for preoperative coronary angiography. Coronary angiogram through the femoral artery is normal. He then develops pruritus, urticaria, and respiratory distress with wheezing, angioedema, and severe stridor. Blood pressure is 120/70 mm Hg and heart rate is 115 bpm. His oxygen saturation is 95% on 3-L nasal cannula. What is the best next step?

(A) Albuterol nebulizer
(B) Intraaortic balloon pump and furosemide IV
(C) Continuous positive airway pressure
(D) Prepare for emergent endotracheal intubation

10.9 A 75-year-old man with an abdominal aortic aneurism and chronic kidney disease with a baseline serum creatinine of 2.3 mg/dL is referred for cardiac catheterization in the setting of unstable angina. Coronary angiography through the femoral artery reveals an 80% focal mid right coronary artery stenosis, which is treated with implantation of a 3.0- × 18-mm everolimus drug-eluting stent. The day following the procedure, his urine output is only 30 mL over 12 hours, and his serum creatinine has increased to 3.0 mg/dL. Which of the following best differentiates contrast-induced nephropathy from atheroembolic renal failure?

(A) Absence of cutaneous findings like livedo reticularis
(B) Absence of hypereosinophilia or hypereosinophiluria
(C) Recovery of serum creatinine within 2 weeks
(D) Presence of a normal urinalysis

10.10 A 49-year-old woman with diabetes and chronic kidney disease with a baseline creatinine of 2.2 mg/dL, stable angina, and inferolateral ischemia on myocardial perfusion is referred for coronary angiography. Which of the following strategies is *least* likely to reduce her risk of contrast-induced nephropathy?

(A) Biplane angiography
(B) Oral *N*-acetylcysteine following the procedure
(C) Preprocedure and postprocedure hydration with intravenous normal saline
(D) Staging percutaneous coronary intervention for at least 72 hours after diagnostic coronary angiography

10.11 When compared to high-osmolar contrast agents, which of the following statements regarding low-osmolar contrast agents is the most CORRECT?

(A) Low-osmolar agents increase the risk of thrombotic complications
(B) Low-osmolar agents reduce the risk of bradyarrhythmias
(C) Low-osmolar agents increase the risk of postprocedure renal failure
(D) Low-osmolar agents increase the risk of anaphylactoid reactions

10.12 A 57-year-old man with diabetes and chronic kidney disease with a baseline creatinine of 1.8 mg/dL undergoes coronary angiography and complex multivessel percutaneous coronary intervention. Two days following the procedure, his serum creatinine has increased to 2.6 mg/dL despite adequate volume repletion. Which of the following is a typical clinical feature of contrast-induced nephropathy?

(A) Serum creatinine usually peaks within 12 to 24 hours
(B) Recovery of serum creatinine within 2 weeks
(C) Transient need for renal replacement therapy with hemodialysis

(D) Fractional excretion of sodium reliably distinguishes contrast-induced nephropathy from prerenal azotemia.

10.13 What is the incidence of life-threatening reactions to contrast agents?

(A) 1:100
(B) 1:1,000
(C) 1:100,000
(D) 1:1,000,000

10.14 Which of the following patients has the highest risk of developing contrast-induced nephropathy following cardiac catheterization and/or percutaneous coronary intervention?

(A) A 72-year-old woman with diabetes mellitus and a serum creatinine of 2.0 mg/dL who presents with STEMI and hypotension
(B) A 48-year-old man without diabetes mellitus and a serum creatinine of 2.6 mg/dL undergoing elective percutaneous coronary intervention
(C) An 80-year-old man with diabetes mellitus and a serum creatinine of 1.0 mg/dL who is also taking metformin
(D) A 45-year-old woman with a history of a solitary kidney and a serum creatinine of 0.9 mg/dL who is undergoing a right- and left-heart catheterization for a suspected atrial septal defect

10.15 A 53-year-old woman with a 50-pack-year smoking history and lifestyle-limiting claudication is referred for peripheral angiography and possible intervention. Her baseline creatinine is 2.0 mg/dL. Which of the following techniques may increase her risk of contrast-induced nephropathy?

(A) Use of interactive mode in runoff studies of the lower extremities with a single bolus injection
(B) Use of nontraditional agents like gadolinium or carbon dioxide
(C) Use of trace subtract fluoroscopy (i.e., road mapping)
(D) Use of a furosemide drip to maintain steady urine output during the procedure

10.16 For which of the following scenarios should a patient receive corticosteroids prior to coronary angiography with low-osmolar contrast?

(A) 43-year-old man with a shellfish allergy
(B) 41-year-old woman with rheumatoid arthritis and a topical iodine allergy
(C) 64-year-old man with diabetes and a serum creatinine of 2.7 mg/dL
(D) 78-year-old woman with hives and wheezing after high-osmolar contrast 15 years ago

10.17 Which is correct regarding the mechanism of action of an anaphylactoid reaction to contrast media?

(A) It is due to immunoglobulin E (IgE)-mediated degranulation of mast cells

(B) It is due to chemokine release from memory T cells, which causes degranulation of mast cells

(C) It involves iodine binding of vitronectin receptors and basophil degranulation

(D) It involves degranulation of basophils and tissue mast cells by direct complement activation

10.18 Which is correct regarding the contrast agent, iodixanol (Visipaque)?

(A) It has consistently been shown to be superior to the low-osmolar, nonionic contrast agent, iopamidol (Isovue), in reducing the incidence of contrast-induced nephropathy

(B) It may cause less discomfort than ionic contrast agents in patients undergoing peripheral angiography

(C) It is a low-osmolar, nonionic contrast agent

(D) It is associated with a higher risk of catheter thrombosis compared to high-osmolar contrast agents

10.19 All of the following are clear indications for using low-osmolar contrast agents for coronary angiography, EXCEPT:

(A) Severe coronary artery disease (e.g., left main disease)

(B) Severe emphysema

(C) Severe aortic stenosis

(D) Moderate-to-severe left ventricular dysfunction

10.20 Side effects of high-osmolar contrast agents, such as a transient decrease in systolic blood pressure, flushing, bradycardia, and nausea, are thought to be mediated by what properties?

(A) Hypertonicity

(B) Sodium concentration

(C) Iodine-mediated vasodilatation

(D) Low viscosity

10.21 In which of the following scenarios should you consider switching from low-osmolar to iso-osmolar contrast medium?

(A) To minimize cardiotoxicity in a patient with severe left ventricular dysfunction

(B) To minimize the risk of an anaphylactoid reaction in a patient with multiple drug allergies

(C) To minimize patient discomfort associated with a peripheral angiogram

(D) To optimize visualization of the coronary arteries in a morbidly obese patient

10.22 The mechanism of contrast-induced nephropathy is thought to be related to which of the following?

(A) Inhibition of preglomerular prostaglandin synthesis

(B) Deposition of T lymphocytes and monocytes in the renal interstitium

(C) Direct cellular toxicity and hypoxia due to renal vasoconstriction and hyperviscosity

(D) Immunoglobulin deposition and complement activation within renal glomeruli

10.23 A 58-year-old man with poorly controlled hypertension presents with acute onset of severe "tearing" chest pain that radiates to his mid back. Electrocardiogram shows sinus tachycardia, left ventricular hypertrophy, and no evidence of myocardial ischemia or injury. Serum creatinine is 3.9. Which test would you order next to establish a diagnosis?

(A) CT aortogram with IV contrast

(B) Transesophageal echocardiogram

(C) MRI of the aorta with and without gadolinium

(D) Coronary angiography

10.24 A 48-year-old man with polycystic kidney disease and a baseline serum creatinine of 3.3 presents to the emergency department with chest discomfort and dyspnea. Dobutamine stress echocardiogram reveals inferior, inferoseptal, and inferolateral ischemia. Coronary angiography reveals one-vessel disease with an ostial 80% stenosis in a dominant right coronary artery with TIMI-3 flow. Which of the following strategies will most likely reduce the risk of contrast-induced nephropathy in this patient?

(A) Prophylactic hemodialysis immediately after the procedure

(B) Use of a guide catheter with side holes

(C) Staging the intervention for 72 hours later

(D) Biplane ventriculography

10.25 A 63-year-old woman suffered bronchospasm during diagnostic coronary angiography with a high-osmolar contrast agent 2 years ago. She presents for repeat coronary angiography secondary to angina and a positive stress test. What is the likelihood of another reaction when exposed to a nonionic low-osmolar contrast agent?

(A) <1%

(B) <10%

(C) <25%

(D) <50%

ANSWERS AND EXPLANATIONS

10.1 **Answer B.** This patient has a severe ostial stenosis of the vein graft to the right posterior descending artery and ventricular fibrillation with contrast injection. The best initial steps are to stop the injection, disengage the catheter, and instruct the patient to cough (if he is still conscious) to clear contrast from the myocardium. The other options do not immediately address the arrhythmia.

10.2 **Answer B.** High-osmolar agents (diatrizoate) cause more contrast-induced nephropathy than low-osmolar or iso-osmolar agents (*Radiology* 1993;188:171–178) and are less commonly used in current practice. The nonionic iso-osmolar iodixanol is one of the preferred agents in this setting. It has been proven to be less nephrotoxic than the ionic low-osmolar ioxaglate, but data in comparison to other ionic low-osmolar agents are less clear (*J Am Coll Cardiol* 2006;48:924–930). There is no role for carbon dioxide above the diaphragm given the risk of cerebral embolization.

10.3 **Answer B.** This patient has critical ostial left main coronary artery disease and is at high risk for cardiotoxicity (myocardial ischemia or arrhythmia) with repeated or large-volume injections. High-osmolar contrast is more cardiotoxic than low- or iso-osmolar contrast. Coronary injection during pressure wave ventricularization may increase the risk of arrhythmia or coronary dissection. *N*-acetylcysteine has no role in minimizing cardiotoxicity.

10.4 **Answer D.** Bradycardia and nausea likely reflect a vagal reaction to contrast. Although patients with multiple drug allergies may be at increased risk of a contrast reaction, pretreating patients with a penicillin allergy is not indicated. Fatal anaphylactoid reactions to contrast have been reported with <4 mL of contrast, so the volume of contrast used may not impact the risk of a hypersensitivity response. Preprocedure skin testing may not identify people at risk for a contrast reaction (*Am J Roentgenol* 2008;190:666–670).

10.5 **Answer C.** Normal saline is the only agent listed that has been definitively established to reduce contrast-induced nephropathy. Fenoldopam dopamine, and mannitol have shown inconsistency in reducing nephrotoxicity.

10.6 **Answer B.** Adequate visualization of the left ventricle and thoracic aorta requires rapid delivery of large amounts of contrast agents through power injectors. Typical rates for these procedures are listed in (B), but these may be modified on the basis of the heart size or cardiac output, the catheter being used (e.g., lower flow rates with end-hole catheters), or the use of digital subtraction imaging in the case of aortic imaging (*Grossman's cardiac catheterization, angiography, and intervention* 2006:225–227, 263).

10.7 **Answer C.** This patient is having a severe anaphylactoid reaction to contrast and should receive IV epinephrine immediately. Corticosteroids are reasonable to help prevent a delayed hypersensitivity reaction but take hours to work. Diphenhydramine and albuterol may also be given, but these are a lower priority than systemic epinephrine.

10.8 **Answer D.** This patient's stridor and angioedema in the setting of a hypersensitivity reaction indicates severe laryngeal edema and impending airway collapse. Delay in endotracheal intubation could result in complete airway collapse and need for emergent cricothyroidotomy. The other options will not treat laryngeal edema.

10.9 **Answer C.** Although cutaneous findings and peripheral eosinophilia or eosinophiluria should raise suspicions for atheroembolic renal failure, they are not consistently present. Skin findings occur in 50% of patients, and peripheral eosinophilia is transient and may be difficult to document. The most consistent clinical finding that favors contrast-associated nephropathy is recovery within 2 weeks. A continuously increasing serum creatinine 3 to 8 weeks following the procedure raises suspicions of atheroembolic renal failure. Active sediment may be present in the urine of patients with either disease (*Medicine Baltimore* 1995;74:350–358).

10.10 **Answer B.** Oral *N*-acetylcysteine has been shown to be beneficial in some small studies if begun 1 day before the injection of intravascular contrast (*Lancet* 2003;362:598–603), but in a more recent large comprehensive randomized trial, the benefit of this medication has not been shown (Acetylcysteine for Contrast-Induced Nephropathy Trial (ACT), American Heart Association (AHA) 2010 Scientific Sessions). Prehydration with normal saline is universally accepted prophylaxis against contrast-induced nephropathy. Minimization of contrast volume with the use of staged interventions and biplane angiography is another effective strategy.

10.11 **Answer B.** Low-osmolar nonionic contrast agents are better tolerated by patients and produce fewer episodes of bradycardia, transient hypotension, renal dysfunction, and both mild and serious anaphylactoid reactions. There are no clear differences in the incidence of thrombotic complications between these agents (*Grossman's cardiac catheterization, angiography, and intervention* 2006:31–33).

10.12 **Answer B.** Creatinine typically peaks at 48 to 72 hours and renal function typically recovers within 2 weeks. Patients require hemodialysis <0.1% of the time (*Kidney Int* 2006;70:1811–1817). The fractional excretion of sodium may be low or high, depending on the degree of prerenal hypoperfusion vs. actual tubular injury, and is not a reliable way to distinguish contrast-induced nephropathy from prerenal azotemia.

10.13 **Answer C.** Fatal reactions to contrast agents are rare and are most often quoted as being between 1:75,000 and 1:170,000 procedures (*Radiology* 1990;175:621–628).

10.14 **Answer A.** Risk factors for contrast-associated nephropathy include preexisting chronic renal insufficiency, diabetes mellitus, advanced age, hemodynamic instability, intraaortic balloon pump placement, congestive heart failure, anemia, volume depletion, and the volume of contrast used. The 72-year-old woman has several of these risk factors (*J Am Coll Cardiol* 2004;44:1393–1399). In addition, it is likely that a serum creatinine of 2.0 mg/dL represents a more substantial decline in glomerular filtration rate in an elderly woman than a higher serum creatinine in a younger (and presumably larger) man. Metformin does not increase the risk of contrast-related nephropathy, but its continued use in that setting is contraindicated due to the risk of metabolic acidosis from impaired renal clearance.

10.15 **Answer D.** Use of furosemide will reduce preload (thus having the opposite effect of normal saline) and consequently may increase risk of contrast nephropathy. All of the other above techniques take advantage of the relatively static nature of many peripheral vascular structures. In road mapping and digital subtraction angiography (DSA), this static nature allows for the generation of baseline images in which radiopaque structures (i.e., bone) are subtracted out. It also permits the interactive mode and limits the need for sequential static imaging of the lower extremity runoff. Finally, this static nature permits the use of nontraditional agents, but vascular imaging may be suboptimal (*Manual of peripheral vascular intervention* 2005:36–38, 44–45).

10.16 **Answer D.** Although the risk of a repeat reaction with low-osmolar contrast is lower, any patient with a prior hypersensitivity reaction to contrast should receive a "prep" that includes corticosteroids. It has been proposed that shellfish allergy confers a higher risk of contrast allergy because shellfish contain iodine. However, the allergen in shellfish is the protein, tropomyosin, not iodine. While atopic individuals are more likely to suffer multiple unrelated allergies, shellfish allergy is not a causative risk factor for contrast allergy. Topical iodine hypersensitivity does not increase the risk of an anaphylactoid reaction to contrast media. Diabetes and renal dysfunction do not increase the risk of a contrast hypersensitivity reaction.

10.17 **Answer D.** Contrast media can cause direct complement activation with the degranulation of basophils and mast cells. This is considered an "anaphylactoid" reaction (*Ann Pharmacother* 1994;28:236–241).

10.18 **Answer B.** Iodixanol is an iso-osmolar, nonionic agent. It causes less discomfort during peripheral angiography than ionic higher osmolar agents. The largest randomized controlled trial comparing iodixanol to iopamidol found no difference in the incidence of contrast-induced nephropathy (*Circulation* 2007;115:3189–3196). There is no increase in catheter thrombosis when compared to high-osmolar agents (*Circulation* 2000;101:131–136).

10.19 **Answer B.** Severe emphysema is not an indication for low-osmolar contrast agents. All other conditions listed in the preceding text make patients more susceptible to the hemodynamic effects associated with high-osmolar contrast agents.

10.20 **Answer A.** The physiologic and adverse effects of high-osmolar contrast agents are largely a result of the hypertonicity and calcium chelating properties of these compounds (*Grossman's cardiac catheterization, angiography, and intervention* 2006:31–33).

10.21 **Answer C.** Of the choices listed, the most clearly established reason to use iso-osmolar contrast media instead of low-osmolar contrast is to minimize discomfort during a peripheral procedure. Iso-osmolar contrast may actually result in *less* optimal visualization than low-osmolar contrast, particularly in a morbidly obese person.

10.22 **Answer C.** Renal hypoperfusion due to renal vasoconstriction and hyperviscosity in the small renal arterials as well as direct renal toxicity are proposed mechanisms of contrast-induced nephropathy. The other choices describe the mechanism of renal injury due to nonsteroidal anti-inflammatory drugs (A), interstitial nephritis (B), and glomerulonephritis (D).

10.23 **Answer B.** The history is consistent with an acute aortic dissection. Transesophageal echocardiography will establish the diagnosis without risk of contrast-induced nephropathy or gadolinium-induced nephrogenic systemic fibrosis.

10.24 **Answer C.** Staging the intervention will allow time for contrast from the diagnostic procedure to clear from this patient's system. Many laboratories enable reference images from diagnostic angiograms to be used at a later date for a staged intervention. Prophylactic hemodialysis following the procedure does not appear to diminish the risk of nephrotoxicity (*Am J Kidney Dis* 2006;48:361–371). Although there is some evidence that continuous venovenous hemofiltration initiated 4 to 8 hours before angiography and continued for 18 to 24 hours after angiography improves outcomes compared to normal saline alone in patients with advanced renal failure, this strategy remains controversial (*N Engl J Med* 2003;349:1333–1340). The use of a guide catheter with side holes may minimize pressure dampening during a percutaneous coronary intervention to an ostial stenosis, but typically results in *more* contrast use because a significant amount of contrast is injected into the aorta. While biplane coronary angiography will reduce procedural contrast volume, ventriculography (whether in biplane or monoplane) will markedly increase procedural contrast volume.

10.25 **Answer A.** Even without pretreatment using steroids and histamine blockers, the incidence of severe cross-reactions between ionic and nonionic contrast agents is extremely low (*J Am Coll Cardiol* 1993;21:269–273).

11 Elective Coronary Intervention

Sunil V. Rao

QUESTIONS

CASE No. 1 (FOR QUESTIONS 11.1 THROUGH 11.11):
A 66-year-old man with progressive exertional angina is transferred to your institution for cardiac catheterization. His past medical history includes an MI with subsequent catheterization and three-vessel coronary artery bypass grafting (CABG) 9 years ago. He is currently taking aspirin and clopidogrel, losartan and diltiazem for hypertension, and simvastatin for hyperlipidemia. He admits to occasionally missing doses of his medications, and he continues to smoke cigarettes. He has normal left ventricular (LV) systolic function by a recent echocardiogram, and his creatinine is chronically elevated in the range of 1.7 to 2.2 mg/dL. Although he gives no history of neurologic problems, a recent carotid Doppler study demonstrated bilateral high-grade internal carotid stenoses (80% to 99%). A recent sestamibi was interpreted as "multiple reversible defects over anterior and lateral walls suggestive of multivessel coronary artery disease (CAD)." He experienced one episode of angina at rest on the day prior to transfer and activated EMS, who took him to his local hospital that does not have catheterization facilities. His chest pain resolved with intravenous nitroglycerin, and he was ruled out for acute MI with serial cardiac markers.

Diagnostic angiography was performed with a total of 80 mL of x-ray contrast after vigorous prehydration with normal saline and bicarbonate. The following findings were obtained:

- Left internal mammary artery (LIMA) to left anterior descending (LAD) was widely patent with good anastomosis and good flow; there was approximately 70% eccentric stenosis of the native LAD shortly after insertion of the LIMA (Fig. Q11-1A)

- Saphenous vein graft (SVG) to the posterior descending was patent with a good distal anastomosis and good flow; the native vessel was <2.0 mm with additional discrete high-grade stenosis downstream from graft insertion (Fig. Q11-1B)

- SVG to obtuse marginal (OM) was shaggy and irregular with angiographic suggestion of thrombus; there were high-grade lesions both in the body of the SVG and at the distal anastomosis; the native vessel was also small caliber (Fig. Q11-1C)

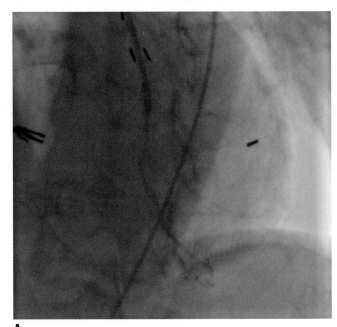

A
Figure Q11-1A

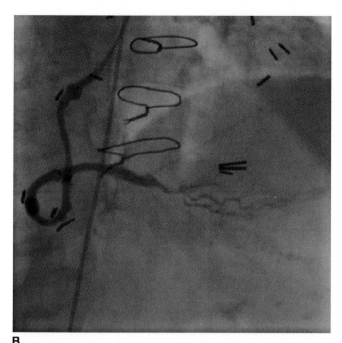

B

Figure Q11-1B

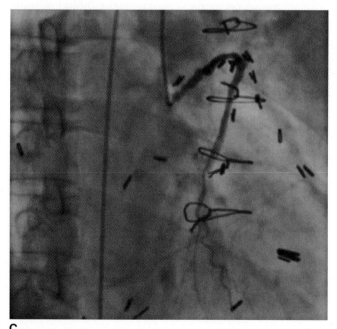

C

Figure Q11-1C

11.1 What clinical and anatomic features weigh against a reoperation (repeat CABG) in this patient?

(A) Patent internal mammary graft to the LAD artery

(B) Three patent grafts

(C) Bilateral severe carotid vascular disease

(D) Chronic renal insufficiency

(E) Risk of second CABG is approximately 3× higher than first CABG

(F) All of the above

11.2 What clinical and anatomic features weigh against PCI for this patient?

(A) Noncompliance causes concern for the use of dual antiplatelet therapy if the patient were to receive DES

(B) Noncompliance with statins and antihypertensive agents increases likelihood of adverse outcomes after PCI

(C) Chronic renal insufficiency increases risk of bleeding and restenosis

(D) Multivessel disease increases likely dye load and attendant contrast-associated nephropathy

(E) SVG disease is associated with decreased likelihood of procedural success and increased likelihood of distal embolization with attendant morbidity and/or mortality

(F) All of the above

11.3 How soon is the creatinine likely to peak from the development of contrast-associated nephropathy?

(A) 1 day

(B) 2 days

(C) 3 days

(D) 5 days

(E) 1 week

11.4 Risk factors for contrast-associated nephropathy after PCI include all of the following, EXCEPT:

(A) Total dye dose from procedure

(B) Multiple dye procedures within 1 week

(C) Diabetes

(D) Elevated creatinine before catheterization

(E) Number of coronary arteries with >70% stenosis

11.5 Which of the following are established means (supported by Class IIa or higher recommendation in published guidelines) of reducing the likelihood of contrast-associated nephropathy?

(A) Hydration with normal saline

(B) Use of iso-osmolar contrast agents

(C) Fenoldopam

(D) *N*-acetyl cysteine

(E) Dopamine infusion in "renal perfusion" dose (<5 $\mu g/kg/min$)

(F) A and B

(G) A and D

11.6 With regard to PCI of the native LAD lesion in this patient, which of the following concepts is usually CORRECT?

(A) PCI through the native LAD (were it possible) would be less likely to injure the internal mammary artery

(B) PCI of the distal LIMA-LAD anastomosis is one of the few anatomic settings where stents have not been shown to reduce restenosis

(C) Straightening of the LIMA with a PCI wire can produce pseudolesions

(D) With a regular-length LIMA guide and a long internal mammary vessel, it is possible to "run out of catheter length" when trying to treat native LAD lesions

(E) All are correct

11.7 With regard to PCI of the SVG-OM artery in this patient, which of the following concepts is CORRECT?

(A) The use of glycoprotein IIb/IIIa inhibitors (GPI) has not been shown to reduce the incidence of major adverse cardiac events after PCI of an SVG

(B) RCT data do not support the use of "distal protection" in old (>3 years) SVG lesions when technically feasible

(C) The use of rotational atherectomy for treating SVG lesions is associated with a reduction in major adverse cardiac events over the use of stents

(D) Thrombectomy devices have been shown to be superior to balloon angioplasty in SVG lesions

(E) Stents have been shown to be superior to balloon angioplasty in SVG lesions

(F) A and E

(G) A, B, and E

11.8 With regard to PCI of the SVG-PDA in this patient, which of the following is likely to be CORRECT?

(A) The posterior descending artery (PDA) is too small for even the smallest BMS

(B) This is not likely the source of anterior or lateral ischemia

(C) There is no "landing zone" for distal protection

(D) All are correct

11.9 What is the most evidence-based approach for this patient?

(A) Smoking cessation clinic

(B) Repeat CABG

(C) PCI of the SVG-PDA and SVG-OM with distal protection to address the anterior ischemia

(D) Optimize doses of β-blocker, ACE-I, and statins, and follow clinically for anginal symptoms

(E) A and D

11.10 If the patient is adherent to your recommendations for maximal medical therapy and lifestyle modifications, the following is/are considered an appropriate indication/indications for PCI:

(A) Class II angina with low-risk findings on noninvasive testing including normal LV function

(B) Class III angina with low-risk findings on noninvasive testing including normal LV function

(C) Class II angina with intermediate-risk findings on noninvasive testing

(D) B and C

11.11 The following findings in a patient with Class II angina on medical management should prompt PCI according to the ACC/AHA/SCAI update to the PCI Guideline:

(A) Only a small area of viable myocardium at risk

(B) No objective evidence of ischemia

(C) Lesions that have a low likelihood of successful dilatation

(D) Mild symptoms that are unlikely to be related to myocardial ischemia

(E) Factors associated with increased morbidity or mortality

(F) Left main disease and eligibility for CABG

(G) Insignificant disease (<50% stenosis)

(H) None of the above

CASE No. 2 (FOR QUESTIONS 11.12 THROUGH 11.17): A 58-year-old man is referred for catheterization and likely revascularization. Three years ago, you performed right coronary artery stenting to treat an acute inferior/STEMI in this patient and he has subsequently done well on a medical regimen that included aspirin, metoprolol, and simvastatin; he does not smoke. After 3 days of severe chest pain, he reported to his local hospital and was found to have anterior ST-segment elevation and positive troponins. Because >24 hours had passed from onset of symptoms, he was given heparin, intravenous nitroglycerin, and eptifibatide, and because of continued pain, he was transferred emergently. He is now pain free >4 days out; he is hemodynamically stable (normal sinus rhythm in the low 70s with blood pressure of 120/78 and respiratory rate of 18 and unlabored with 98% arterial saturation on 2 L, and has clear lung fields without jugular venous distension).

On angiography, you demonstrate that his dominant right coronary artery is free of significant (>50%) narrowing with a widely patent bare-metal stent. The left main is smooth and not narrowed, but the proximal LAD has approximately 80% stenosis; a significant diagonal branch follows the stenosis (Fig. Q11-12). There is a large, tortuous ramus intermedius branch with a diminutive circumflex artery.

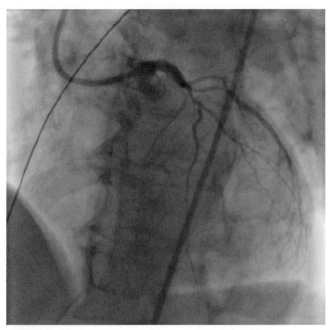

Figure Q11-12

11.12 This patient presented as an STEMI who did not receive reperfusion (because of presentation >24 hours after pain onset). Which of the following are ACC/AHA/SCAI Class I indications for PCI of post-STEMI patients who did not receive thrombolytics?

(A) Recurrent MI
(B) Spontaneous or provocable myocardial ischemia
(C) Cardiogenic shock or hemodynamic instability
(D) All of the above

11.13 The criteria for considering a patient's symptoms as "medically refractory" include continued symptoms and ischemia despite which of the following?

(A) Aspirin, unless contraindicated
(B) Clopidogrel, unless contraindicated
(C) β-Blocker in all post-MI patients and patients with congestive heart failure, unless contraindicated, and to blood pressure and heart rate targets
(D) ACE-I in all patients with LV dysfunction, unless contraindicated, and to blood pressure targets
(E) Statins, unless contraindicated
(F) All of the above

11.14 The lesion involves the proximal LAD. In a patient receiving maximal medical therapy with Class II angina and 1-vessel CAD involving the proximal LAD who has low-risk findings on noninvasive testing, is it appropriate, inappropriate, or uncertain to pursue revascularization?

(A) Appropriate
(B) Inappropriate
(C) Uncertain

11.15 The use of a drug-eluting stent to treat the LAD lesion is a Class I recommendation in which of the following situations?

(A) Known nonadherence with medical therapy
(B) Planned hip replacement surgery in 12 months
(C) A patient with type 2 insulin-requiring diabetes mellitus, adherent to medications, and low risk for bleeding
(D) All of the above

11.16 The patient undergoes coronary stenting with a drug-eluting stent. Which of the following are considered the criteria for angiographic and procedural success?

(A) Angiographic success: <50% residual stenosis, TIMI 2 flow; procedural success: no major complications, asymptomatic elevation of CKMB > 2 times upper limit of normal
(B) Angiographic success: <20% residual stenosis, TIMI 3 flow; procedural success: no major complications, postprocedure chest pain with elevation of CKMB > 5 times upper limit of normal
(C) Angiographic success: <20% residual stenosis, TIMI 2 flow; procedural success: no major complications, no further chest pain, no elevation of CKMB
(D) Angiographic success: <20% residual stenosis, TIMI 3 flow; procedural success: no major complications, no further chest pain, no elevation of CKMB

11.17 Which of the following features of the LAD lesion would make it a high-risk lesion (i.e., ACC/AHA Type C)?

(A) Fibrotic plaque by IVUS imaging with virtual histology

(B) Inability to protect a major side branch

(C) Fractional Flow Reserve (FFR) value of 0.60

(D) 60 degrees angulation from the left main into the LAD

CASE No. 3 (FOR QUESTIONS 11.18 THROUGH 11.23): An 84-year-old male is referred to you for angiography. He has a history of severe peripheral arterial disease with a known infrarenal abdominal aortic aneurysm and complete occlusions of both iliac arteries. In addition, he has a history of diabetes mellitus, hypertension, and oxygen-requiring chronic obstructive pulmonary disease with an FEV1 < 1 L. He is not very active but walks up and down his street, which is approximately the distance of 1 city block. Over the past 3 months, he has noticed exertional chest tightness that has increased in frequency and intensity. A dobutamine MUGA demonstrated a significant decrease in his LV function with stress. You perform angiography via the right radial artery approach that demonstrates a nondominant right coronary artery, a focal 90% stenosis of the distal left main, with nonsignificant disease in the LAD and left circumflex artery (Fig. Q11-18).

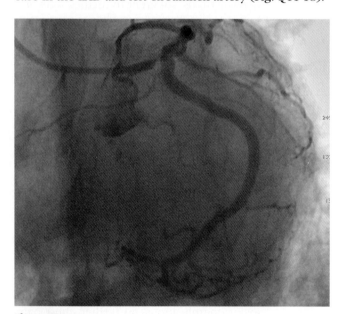

Figure Q11-18

11.18 Under which of the following scenarios is revascularization appropriate in the presence of left main stenosis?

(A) No symptoms

(B) CCS Class I or II angina, low-risk findings on noninvasive imaging

(C) CCS Class III angina

(D) CCS Class III angina, high-risk findings on noninvasive imaging

(E) All of the above

11.19 In the SYNTAX trial, which strategy (CABG or PCI) was associated with a significantly lower rate of major adverse cardiac events (death, MI, stroke, or repeat revascularization) at 12 months for all patients with left main stenosis?

(A) CABG

(B) PCI

(C) PCI was associated with a higher rate of repeat revascularization but a lower rate of stroke, resulting in no significant difference between the two strategies

(D) Hybrid revascularization with a LIMA to the LAD and DES for left circumflex and right coronary artery lesions

11.20 In the SYNTAX trial, PCI was associated with a numerically lower rate of major adverse cardiac events in which subset of patients with left main stenosis?

(A) Isolated left main stenosis, low SYNTAX score

(B) Left main stenosis and significant disease in the LAD, left circumflex, and right coronary arteries

(C) Left main stenosis and high SYNTAX score

(D) High SYNTAX score with aortic stenosis

(E) All of the above

11.21 The ACC/AHA/SCAI 2009 Focused update to the PCI guidelines gives which recommendation to PCI for left main stenosis?

(A) Class I based on randomized clinical trial data that PCI is superior to CABG in patients with left main stenosis

(B) Class IIa based on randomized clinical trial data that PCI is significantly superior to CABG in certain patients with left main stenosis

(C) Class III based on randomized clinical trial data that PCI significantly increases mortality in patients with left main stenosis

(D) Class IIb based on subgroup analyses from the SYNTAX trial showing some trends favoring PCI in patients with left main stenosis and limited CAD

11.22 Which angiographic view is most likely to help assess the left main, LAD, and circumflex anatomic relationships?

(A) LAO caudal

(B) Left lateral

(C) LAO cranial

(D) 60 degrees LAO

(E) All of the above

11.23 You decide to proceed with PCI of this patient's left main stenosis based on the fact that his chronic lung disease makes him a poor surgical candidate. The procedure is successful both angiographically and clinically. At what point should you schedule the patient for repeat angiography?

(A) 2 to 6 months regardless of the patient's symptoms

(B) Routine repeat angiography is no longer recommended by the guidelines

(C) Every 6 months

(D) Annually

(E) As often as his insurance will allow

CASE No. 4 (FOR QUESTIONS 11.24 THROUGH 11.27): A 54-year-old man presents to your catheterization laboratory for diagnostic angiography to evaluate progressive exertional chest pain. He has a history of type 2 diabetes mellitus, hypertension, peripheral arterial disease, and CAD. He underwent CABG 7 years ago with a LIMA to LAD, and SVGs to the left PDA, the Ramus, the third OM artery, and the second Diagonal artery. Three years after his CABG, he developed recurrent angina and underwent angiography that demonstrated a patent LIMA, but complete occlusion of all of his vein grafts. He underwent PCI with bare-metal stents to the proximal, mid, and distal left circumflex artery. He did well without recurrent symptoms until three weeks prior to presentation when he developed exertional angina. He progressed to the point where he was seen by his primary care physician who referred him to you. Based on his prior history of CABG and PCI, you decide to proceed with diagnostic angiography. This reveals a left dominant system, patent LIMA, occluded vein grafts, an occluded mid LAD, a diffuse 50% in-stent restenosis of the proximal left circumflex, and a 90% in-stent restenosis of the mid left circumflex (Fig. Q11-24).

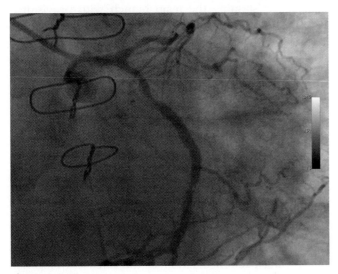

Figure Q11-24

11.24 What would be the BEST approach to revascularizing this patient?

(A) Repeat CABG

(B) PCI of the chronically occluded LAD

(C) PCI of the mid left circumflex artery with FFR assessment of the 50% proximal left circumflex lesion

(D) B and C

11.25 In the FAME trial of FFR-guided PCI vs. conventional angiography-guided PCI, the rate of 12-month death, nonfatal MI, or repeat revascularization showed which pattern between the two arms?

(A) Higher rate of the composite end point among patients assigned to FFR-guided PCI

(B) Significantly lower in the FFR-guided PCI arm

(C) No difference between two arms

(D) Nonsignificantly higher death rate but lower rate of repeat revascularization in the FFR-guided PCI arm resulting in an overall slightly higher event rate in the FFR-guided PCI arm.

11.26 In which of the following instances can PCI of the proximal left circumflex artery stenosis be safely deferred?

(A) Coronary flow reserve (CFR) = 3.0

(B) Relative CRF (rCFR) = 1.9

(C) FFR = 0.86

(D) All of the above

(E) Just stent it in case it might cause problems later

11.27 If the patient has a history of prior MI in the area supplied by the left circumflex, which of the following findings are indications for PCI?

(A) CFR = 3.0, rCFR = 2.0, FFR = 0.86

(B) CFR = 1.5, rCFR = 0.6, FFR = 0.82

(C) CFR = 2.5, rCFR = 0.7, FFR = 0.91

(D) CFR = 2.3, rCFR = 2.0, FFR = 0.70

CASE No. 5 (FOR QUESTIONS 11.28 THROUGH 11.32): A 77-year-old female is scheduled for elective coronary angiography for invasive risk stratification after a non–ST-segment elevation myocardial infarction. She presented yesterday with chest pain at rest. On initial exam, she had a body mass index of 34 (body weight of 90 kg), and her oxygen saturation was 98% on room air. Her vital signs showed a heart rate of 90 beats/min in a regular rhythm, a blood pressure of 180/90 mm Hg, and a respiratory rate of 18 breaths/min. Her initial ECG demonstrated 1 mm of downsloping ST-segment depression in leads I and II and aVF, and her bedside qualitative troponin value was elevated. Her initial laboratory values showed a hemoglobin value of 10 g/dL, creatinine of 1.8 mg/dL, platelet count of 430,000, creatine kinase-MB of 36 ng/mL (upper limit of normal 9 ng/mL), and a troponin I of 4.0 ng/mL (upper limit of normal 0.10 ng/mL). Her medical history is significant for hypertension, hyperlipidemia, ongoing cigarette smoking, and chronic kidney disease with a baseline creatinine of 1.7 to 2.0 mg/dL. Her current medications include aspirin 81 mg daily, furosemide 40 mg daily, simvastatin 40 mg daily, and a multivitamin. She is adherent with her medical regimen. A chest-wall echocardiogram reveals an ejection fraction of 50% with anterior wall hypokinesis.

11.28 What clinical features of the case should prompt consideration of invasive risk stratification?

(A) Low TIMI risk score
(B) Hypertension on admission
(C) Anemia, which could be the cause of her MI
(D) Elevated cardiac markers
(E) None of the above

11.29 The patient is treated initially with two sublingual nitroglycerin tablets, which relieve her chest pain, unfractionated heparin, and 300 mg of clopidogrel orally. What clinical features of this patient are associated with high bleeding risk?

(A) Age
(B) Female sex
(C) Renal insufficiency
(D) Body weight
(E) All of the above
(F) A, B, and C

11.30 You decide to proceed with cardiac catheterization using a 6-French system. This reveals nonsignificant disease in the right coronary artery and the left circumflex artery. The LAD has a complex 70% to 80% lesion that extends from the proximal to the mid segment, across a large second diagonal, which also has a 90% lesion in its ostium (Fig. Q11-30). Based on the available evidence, what is the best treatment for this patient?

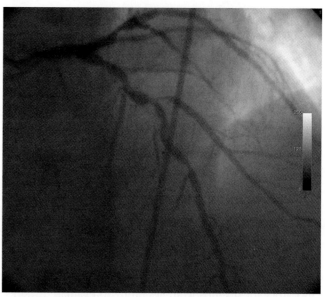

Figure Q11-30

(A) Control of risk factors
(B) Maximal medical therapy, secondary prevention, and revascularization of the LAD system
(C) Smoking cessation, antianginal therapy
(D) FFR of the second diagonal branch

11.31 If you decide to proceed with PCI of the LAD system, what does the totality of the clinical evidence suggest about bifurcation stenting?

(A) The best approach for true bifurcation disease is culotte stenting with drug-eluting stents
(B) Using a drug-eluting stent in the main branch and a bare-metal stent in the side branch is associated with reduced mortality compared with CABG
(C) Most of the evidence supports a strategy of stenting the main branch with provisional stenting of the side branch for dissections, reduced TIMI flow, or symptoms
(D) Simultaneous kissing stents with drug-eluting stents has been proven to be superior to CABG with respect to long-term death, MI, or repeat revascularization

11.32 You decide to proceed with PCI of the LAD-diagonal bifurcation and place a 28-mm drug-eluting stent followed by an 18-mm drug-eluting stent in the LAD. After deployment of the LAD stent, flow in the second diagonal is reduced to TIMI 2, and the patient begins to complain of chest pain. You quickly place a 0.014″ angioplasty wire into the diagonal branch and proceed with kissing balloon inflation of the LAD and diagonal, which reestablishes TIMI 3 flow in the diagonal.

You notice that there is a visible dissection in the proximal portion of the diagonal with contrast staining. You then place a 15-mm drug-eluting stent in the diagonal using a "T" stent technique. After placement of the diagonal stent, the dissection is no longer visible and the result is excellent angiographically. You decide to stop the procedure and remove the guidewires and take your final pictures. Which of the following features of this case are independently associated with increased risk of drug-eluting stent thrombosis?

(A) Radial approach
(B) Bifurcation stenting
(C) Renal failure
(D) Stent length
(E) Age > 70 years
(F) B, C, and D

11.33 Which of the following strategies can be used to facilitate stent delivery through tortuous or calcified coronary arteries?

(A) Upsizing the guide catheter size
(B) Using a stiffer guidewire
(C) Aggressive guide manipulation ("throating the guide")
(D) Using a buddy wire
(E) Using a buddy balloon
(F) All of the above

11.34 The radial approach to PCI has been generally associated with which of the following compared with the femoral approach?

(A) Less bleeding and vascular complications, lower costs, higher radiation exposure, and higher crossover to a different vascular access
(B) No difference in bleeding or vascular complications, lower costs, higher radiation exposure, and higher crossover to a different vascular access
(C) Less bleeding and vascular complications, higher costs, no difference in radiation exposure, and higher crossover to a different vascular access
(D) Higher bleeding and vascular complications, lower costs, higher radiation exposure, and lower crossover to a different vascular access

11.35 Revascularization of chronic total occlusions is considered appropriate under which of the following conditions?

(A) Class II angina, chronic total occlusion of one major epicardial coronary artery without other coronary stenoses, low-risk findings on noninvasive imaging, not receiving maximal medical therapy
(B) Class II angina, chronic total occlusion of one major epicardial coronary artery without other coronary stenoses, low-risk findings on noninvasive imaging, receiving maximal medical therapy
(C) Class III angina, chronic total occlusion of one major epicardial coronary artery without other coronary stenoses, intermediate-risk findings on noninvasive imaging, not receiving maximal medical therapy
(D) Class III Angina, chronic total occlusion of one major epicardial coronary artery without other coronary stenoses, intermediate-risk findings on noninvasive imaging, receiving maximal medical therapy

11.1 **Answer F.** Both a patent LIMA and three patent grafts (to each major vascular territory: anterior, lateral, and inferior) reduce the potential benefit of a reoperation. The CABG Guideline lists the effect of reoperation in terms of operative mortality as threefold. Renal disease and cerebrovascular disease are risk factors for CABG mortality, and cerebrovascular disease is an additional risk for cerebral morbidity with CABG (*Ann Thorac Surg* 1994;57:27–32; *J Am Coll Cardiol* 1996;28:1478–1487; *N Engl J Med* 1996;335:1857–1863).

11.2 **Answer F.** A number of trials, notably intercoronary stenting and antithrombotic results and stent antithrombotic regimen study, demonstrated the superiority of dual antiplatelet therapy over aspirin alone or Coumadin as adjuncts to stenting. Failure to continue taking antiplatelet therapy is potentially a greater problem with DES, which inhibits endothelialization. In addition to the wealth of data showing hard end point clinical benefits in patients with CAD with lipid-lowering and hypertension control, specific evaluation of post-PCI patients, as in the LIPS trial of statins, demonstrates the importance of ongoing medical management. Chronic renal insufficiency is a PCI risk factor for multiple reasons, including both increased bleeding diathesis and increased restenosis. SVG intervention is associated with increased risk of distal embolization, which is part of the rationale for "distal protection," and not necessarily ameliorated by GPI (PCI Guideline Table 10 and Section 3.5.6) (*Circulation* 2001;103:1967–1971; *N Engl J Med* 1998;339:1665–1671; *Am J Med* 2000;108:127–135; *J Am Coll Cardiol* 2004;44:1393–1399; *J Am Coll Cardiol* 2005;45:947–953; *N Engl J Med* 1996;334:1084–1089; *Circulation* 2003;108:548–553).

11.3 **Answer D.** Contrast-associated nephropathy manifest as elevation in the serum creatinine is most likely to appear 5 days after contrast administration (*J Am Coll Cardiol* 2002;39:1113–1119; *Circulation* 2002;105:2259–2264; *Ann Intern Med* 1986;104:501–504).

11.4 **Answer E.** The risk for contrast-associated nephropathy is dependent on the timing and volume of contrast administered and preexisting kidney disease or diabetes. Coronary artery disease burden is not a predictor of contrast_associated nephropathy (*N Engl J Med* 2003;348:491–499; *Lancet* 2003;362:598–603; *J Am Coll Cardiol* 2004;44:1763–1771; *N Engl J Med* 1989;320:143–149; *N Engl J Med* 1994;331:1416–1420; *Ann Intern Med* 1986;104:501–504).

11.5 **Answer F.** Both hydration with normal saline and the use of iso-osmolar contrast agents or low osmolar contrast agents are recommended by the ACC guidelines and SCAI (*J Am Coll Cardiol* 2008;51:172–209; *Catheter Cardiovasc Interven* 2007;69:135–140). Clinical trials of *N*-acetylcysteine have come to conflicting conclusions, and the European guidelines give its use a Class IIb recommendation. Neither fenoldopam nor "renal-dose" dopamine have been found to be beneficial.

11.6 **Answer E.** All of choices are potential issues when performing the PCI of the LAD in the patient with a pre-existing LIMA graft (*J Am Coll Cardiol* 2000;35:944–948).

11.7 **Answer F.** A meta-analysis of randomized trials of GPI in the setting of PCI found no advantage to the addition of GPI to unfractionated heparin (*Circulation* 2002;105:1285–1290; *Circulation* 2002;106:3063–3067; *Circulation* 2003;108:548–553). In addition, a post-hoc analysis from the REPLACE-2 trial showed that bivalirudin is just as efficacious as the combination of heparin and GPI at reducing the composite end point of death, MI, or target vessel revascularization, with a significant reduction in bleeding complications (*Catheter Cardiovasc Interv* 2006;68:352–356). The use of rotational atherectomy or thrombectomy is not recommended for SVG PCI, while the use of distal protection devices when technically feasible has been proven to be associated with significant reductions in MACE.

11.8 **Answer D.** The PDA is <2.25 mm in diameter and the smallest diameter DES available commercially is 2.25 mm. Because the PDA supplies the inferior wall, the presence of stenoses in it would not explain the stress test findings. There is no significant lesion in the vein graft to the PDA; therefore distal protection is not necessary (*Am J Med* 2000;108:176–177).

11.9 **Answer E.** There are no RCT data to support survival benefit or MI reduction from either repeat CABG or PCI in a patient who has already had one or more CABG. PCI of both the SVGs to the circumflex and right coronary artery territories are unlikely to relieve the ischemia documented in the anterior distribution; accordingly, any PCI strategy should likely include the LAD artery stenosis. There are survival benefit data from RCTs of statins, beta-blockers, ACE-I, and smoking cessation (*Lancet* 2002;360:7–22; *N Engl J Med* 1998;339:1349–1357).

11.10 **Answer D.** The appropriate use guidelines for revascularization (*J Am Coll Cardiol* 2009; 53:530–553) underscore the importance of assessing symptoms, maximizing medical therapy, and findings on noninvasive testing in making decisions about revascularization. It is uncertain whether patients with prior CABG, Class II angina, and low-risk findings on noninvasive testing should undergo revascularization.

11.11 **Answer H.** None of these should prompt PCI according to the Guidelines, section 5.1 on patients with asymptomatic ischemia or CCS Class I or II angina.

11.12 **Answer D.** All are indications for PCI in a patient with STEMI who did not receive lytic theraphy.

11.13 **Answer F.** "Medically refractory" symptoms imply the use of maximal medical theraphy, which includes antiplatelet therapies and secondary prevention measures such as beta-blocker, ACE-inhibitors, and statins (*BMJ* 1994;308:81–106; *Circulation* 1998;97:946–952; *Circulation* 1998;97:2202–2212; *Prog Cardiovasc Dis* 1985;27:335–371; *JAMA* 1988;260:2259–2263).

11.14 **Answer A.** See Appropriate Use Guidelines for Coronary Revascularization (*J Am Coll Cardiol* 2009;53:530–553).

11.15 **Answer C.** The ACC/AHA/SCAI guidelines for PCI 2007 Focused update give a Class I recommendation to the use of drug-eluting stents for patients in whom clinical trials indicate a favorable risk/benefit profile. Diabetes mellitus is a major risk factor for in-stent restenosis

and repeat revascularization. Clinical trials have demonstrated a significant advantage of DES over BMS in diabetic patients. Because the use of DES necessitates long-term antiplatelet therapy, patients who are at risk for premature cessation of dual antiplatelet therapy because of nonadherence, invasive procedures that require discontinuation of antiplatelet therapy, or both should not receive DES (*J Am Coll Cardiol* 2008;51:172–209; *JAMA* 2005;293:2126–2130).

11.16 **Answer D.** In the era of coronary stenting, angiographic success is defined as residual stenosis <20% with TIMI 3 flow. The criterion of <50% residual stenosis applies when balloon angioplasty is the primary treatment. Procedural success refers to complications of the procedure. While the clinical impact of post-PCI CKMB elevation is a topic of some debate, elevations 5 times the upper limit of normal are considered to be directly related to the PCI procedure even in the absence of Q waves (*JACC* 2006;47:e1–e21).

11.17 **Answer B.** The following are criteria for a Type C lesion: length >2 cm, excessive tortuosity of the proximal segment, extremely angulated segments (>90 degrees), total occlusions >3 months old and/or bridging collaterals, inability to protect major side branches, and degenerated vein grafts with friable lesions. Remember that these criteria are associated with technical failure and not necessarily acute complications.

11.18 **Answer E.** According to the published Appropriateness Criteria for Revascularization (*J Am Coll Cardiol* 2009;53:530–553), the presence of left main stenosis should prompt consideration of revascularization regardless of symptoms. Importantly, this does not mean PCI; instead, it means either CABG or PCI depending on other issues such as patient comorbidities, anatomical features, etc.

11.19 **Answer C.** The SYNTAX trial randomized 1,800 patients with 3-vessel or left main CAD to either CABG or PCI (*NEJM* 2009;360961–360972). The primary end point was 12-month all-cause death, MI, stroke, or repeat revascularization. PCI failed to meet the noninferiority criteria in comparison with CABG. PCI was associated with a significant reduction in stroke but an increase in repeat revascularization. In the left main subset, a similar pattern was seen resulting in no significant difference between the two strategies. This finding should be interpreted with caution given that it is a subgroup analysis. Hybrid revascularization was not addressed in the SYNTAX trial.

11.20 **Answer A.** Further analyses from the SYNTAX trial showed that among patients with left main stenosis and lower CAD burden as assessed by the SYNTAX score, major adverse cardiac events trended lower with PCI compared with CABG (isolated left main disease: 8.5% CABG vs. 7.1% PCI; left main plus 1-vessel CAD: 13.2% CABG vs. 7.5% PCI) (*NEJM* 2009;360961–360972).

11.21 **Answer D.** Based on the trends seen in the subgroup analyses of the SYNTAX trial, the 2009 Focused Update to the PCI guidelines have upgraded the recommendation for left main PCI in certain patients from Class III to Class IIb (*J Am Coll Cardiol* 2009;54:2205–2241).

11.22 **Answer A.** Of the choices provided, the LAO caudal view provides the best separation of the LAD and left circumflex arteries.

11.23 **Answer B.** Routine angiography is no longer recommended after left main PCI based on the inability of angiography to predict acute, sudden stent thrombosis and the risks associated with repeat angiography in a patient who has undergone placement of a left main stent (*J Am Coll Cardiol* 2009;54:2205–2241).

11.24 **Answer C.** The 2009 Focused Update to the PCI guidelines give a Class IIa (level of evidence A) to use intracoronary physiological measurements (i.e., fractional flow reserve or FFR) as an alternative to noninvasive functional testing to guide PCI. In this patient, the proximal left circumflex artery stenosis is of intermediate severity (defined in the guidelines as 30% to 70%) and should be evaluated further with FFR. This can be done either before stenting of the 90% distal lesion with a "pullback" technique or after stenting of the distal lesion. Repeat CABG is not indicated in this patient with a patent LIMA. Recanalizing the chronically occluded LAD is also not indicated because the LIMA is patent.

11.25 **Answer B.** The FAME trial randomized 1,005 patients with multivessel CAD to PCI guided by conventional angiographic assessment or PCI guided by FFR (*NEJM* 2009;360:213–224). Patients assigned to the angiography-guided PCI had all lesions stented, while patients assigned to the FFR-guided PCI strategy had only those lesions with an FFR value ≤ 0.80 stented. The FFR-guided strategy was associated with a significantly lower rate of death, nonfatal MI, or repeat revascularization at 12 months (13.2% vs. 18.3%, *p* = 0.02).

11.26 **Answer D.** CFR is measured distal to a lesion and is the ratio of the flow distal to a lesion before and after vasodilation ($Q_{dil}/Q_{initial}$). The rCFR compares the CFR in a normal vessel to one that has the lesion of interest. Values below 2.0 for the CFR and below 0.8 for the rCFR indicate a hemodynamically significant lesion. As mentioned above, an FFR value ≤ 0.80 indicates a hemodynamically significant lesion.

11.27 **Answer D.** The key to this question is the history of prior MI in the territory supplied by the artery in question. Only the FFR is reliable in the presence of a prior MI; therefore, the FFR value of 0.70 indicates a hemodynamically significant lesion regardless of the CFR and rCFR values.

11.28 **Answer D.** This patient has a TIMI risk score of 5, giving her a 26% incidence of death, MI, or urgent revascularization within 14 days. This indicates a high-risk situation and the presence of elevated cardiac markers should prompt invasive risk stratification.

11.29 **Answer F.** Several analyses have examined risk factors for bleeding complications in patients with acute coronary syndrome undergoing PCI. These have demonstrated that age, female sex, and renal insufficiency are major risk factors for hemorrhagic complications. Low body weight is also a risk, but the patient described in the case is overweight. (*EHJ* 2007;28:1193–1204; *J Am Coll Cardiol* 2010;55:2556–2566).

11.30 **Answer B.** Revascularization of the presumed culprit artery is indicated in high-risk patients with acute coronary syndrome. This patient has a high TIMI risk score, and the results of her chest wall echo correlate with significant stenosis on the coronary angiogram. Choices A and C are not the best answer because they do not include revascularization. FFR is indicated for lesions of intermediate severity (30% to 70%).

11.31 **Answer C.** Most of the retrospective studies and prospective randomized trials support a strategy of provisional stenting of side branches for true bifurcation lesions (*J Am Coll Cardiol* 2000;35:929–936; *J Am Coll Cardiol* 2005;46:1446–1455).

11.32 **Answer F.** A prospective cohort study of 2,229 patients who underwent drug-eluting stenting demonstrated that independent predictors of cumulative stent thrombosis include premature cessation of antiplatelet therapy, renal failure, bifurcation stenting, diabetes, and LV dysfunction. Age was a univariate predictor, but was not independently associated with stent thrombosis after multivariable adjustment.

11.33 **Answer F.** All are techniques that can facilitate stent delivery through tortuous or calcified coronary arteries.

11.34 **Answer A.** The transradial approach has been compared with the brachial and femoral approaches as well as with femoral approach with vascular closure device. A meta-analysis of these trials demonstrated that the radial approach is associated with a near-70% reduction in bleeding or vascular complications but higher crossover to the femoral approach (*AHJ* 2009;157:132–140). Other trials have shown that the radial approach is associated with significantly lower costs but higher radiation exposure (*Am J Med* 1998;104:343–348; *Ann Intern Med* 1998;128:194–203; *J Card Surg* 1996;11: 128–133; discussion 134–135). Most recently, the RIVAL trial showed lower vascular complications with radial access. Major bleeding rates were similar using the CURRENT trial definitions (*Lancet* 2011;377:1409–1420).

11.35 **Answer D.** The Appropriateness Criteria for Revascularization take into account symptoms, findings on noninvasive testing, and the use of medical therapy. For patients with chronic total occlusion of one major epicardial artery, revascularization is considered appropriate for patients with intermediate-risk findings on noninvasive testing and Class III or IV angina despite maximal medical therapy. Revascularization is also considered appropriate for patients with high-risk findings on noninvasive testing and Class III or IV angina even if they are not receiving maximal medical therapy. Revascularization is considered inappropriate for choice A and is uncertain for choices B and C.

12

Percutaneous Coronary Intervention for Acute Coronary Syndromes

José G. Díez

12.1 A 70-year-old man presents to the emergency room (ER) with complaints of new onset waxing and waning chest pain over the past 4 hours. His initial electrocardiogram ECG is shown in Figure Q12-1. In deciding whether to initiate treatment with a glycoprotein (GP) IIb/IIIa receptor antagonist (and if so, which agent to use), all of the following should influence your decision, EXCEPT:

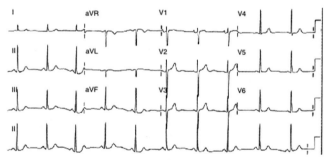

Figure Q12-1

(A) Plans for a conservative or invasive management approach and the timing of any potential invasive approach
(B) Whether the patient has already received 600 mg of clopidogrel from the ER physician
(C) In the setting of a percutaneous coronary intervention (PCI), clinical trials have not found an incremental benefit in decreasing peri-PCI thrombotic events
(D) Troponin status

12.2 For a patient presenting to the catheterization laboratory in the setting of a recent acute coronary syndrome (ACS), which of the following is FALSE regarding the use of aspirin therapy?

(A) To minimize the risk of gastric bleeding, an enteric-coated aspirin should be used long-term
(B) Chewing 160 to 325 mg leads to complete antiplatelet effects within 15 to 20 minutes
(C) In placebo-controlled trials in coronary syndrome and PCI, aspirin decreases death and myocardial infarction (MI) rates by approximately 50%
(D) Patients who have aspirin allergy or intolerance should receive clopidogrel

12.3 An 87-year-old woman is transferred to your facility for catheterization and possible PCI after presenting with chest pain with ST-segment depressions and an elevated troponin level. Her creatinine level is 1.9 mg/dL and she weighs 58 kg. The patient is started on aspirin, 600-mg clopidogrel, enoxaparin, and eptifibatide. All of the following are independently associated with an increased risk of major bleeding, EXCEPT:

(A) Renal dysfunction
(B) Female gender
(C) Previous coronary artery bypass graft (CABG)
(D) Advanced age

12.4 Which of the following is TRUE regarding the use of clopidogrel in a patient presenting with ACS?

(A) A loading dose of at least 300 mg should be used

(B) Clinical outcomes in patients treated with clopidogrel are significantly worse in the setting of concomitant atorvastatin

(C) Doubling the loading dose and maintenance dose of clopidogrel has been shown to be more effective than standard therapy in high-risk patients

(D) A loading dose of clopidogrel is efficacious regardless of the time of dosing as long as it is before the PCI

12.5 A 51-year-old man was admitted the previous day with a troponin-positive non–ST-segment elevation ACS and was started on enoxaparin 1 mg/kg subcutaneously. The patient is now in the catheterization laboratory preparing for coronary angiography and possible intervention. He has received two doses of enoxaparin. His last subcutaneous dose of enoxaparin was documented to have been given 5 hours earlier. Optimizing antithrombotic therapy in the setting of a possible PCI for this patient would require:

(A) No additional anticoagulant is necessary

(B) 50 to 70 U/kg of unfractionated heparin (UFH) titrated to an ACT of >200 if a GP IIb/IIIa inhibitor is being used and to an ACT of 300 if no GP IIb/IIIa inhibitor is planned

(C) Additional intravenous enoxaparin of 0.3 mg/kg

(D) Further use of additional anticoagulant based on whether a GP IIb/IIIa inhibitor is to be used

12.6 A 56-year-old diabetic woman is transferred directly to your catheterization laboratory in the setting of an anterior ST-segment elevation myocardial infarction (STEMI) treated with fibrinolytic therapy at an outside hospital. She has also been treated with aspirin, UFH, and 600-mg clopidogrel. Her ST segments have normalized, and she is pain free and hemodynamically stable. By the time you arrive, the coronary angiography has already been completed by your partner and demonstrates the following: severe stenosis in the LAD but with TIMI 3 flow and severe 90% RCA lesion.

The optimal treatment approach to this patient would be:

(A) PCI with stenting of the left anterior descending (LAD) only

(B) PCI with stenting of the LAD and likely clinically significant right coronary artery (RCA) lesions

(C) Cardiothoracic surgery consults for urgent CABG surgery in this diabetic patient with multivessel disease

(D) Medical stabilization with plans to risk stratify before discharge

12.7 A 48-year-old man presents to your emergency department with substernal chest pain of 8 hours duration. Despite increasing chest pain, the patient worked all day trying to ignore his discomfort. However, the pain increased while he was driving home, and he drove himself to the hospital. Initial ECG demonstrates normal sinus rhythm with 1.5 mm inferolateral ST-segment depression. The patient is administered sublingual nitroglycerin, a single dose of intravenous morphine and metoprolol, and oxygen by nasal cannula. His pain slowly resolves. Initial cardiac enzymes are negative. Follow-up ECG shows resolution of the prior ST-segment depression. What is the best way to proceed with this patient at this point?

(A) Observe the patient in your chest pain unit, give the patient a proton pump inhibitor, and have the patient follow up with his primary care provider as long as you rule out MI and the patient has no further chest pain

(B) Admit the patient to telemetry for medical treatment only, proceeding only to angiography if his chest pain recurs or enzymes become positive

(C) Admit the patient with plans to proceed to angiography only if he has a high-risk noninvasive evaluation

(D) Plan on proceeding to cardiac catheterization regardless of recurrence of chest pain, cardiac enzymes, or ECG changes

12.8 You are called to evaluate a 68-year-old man who presents with 2 hours of crushing substernal chest pain. Initial ECG shows 4-mm anterior ST-segment elevations consistent with acute anterior STEMI. Within 45 minutes of presentation, coronary angiography reveals a totally occluded mid LAD with a long segment of apparent thrombus after the first septal perforator. The patient is hemodynamically stable. Because of the large thrombus burden, you consider whether thrombectomy may be beneficial in this patient. The patient's initial angiogram is shown in the Figure Q12-8. Which of the following is TRUE regarding thrombectomy in this setting?

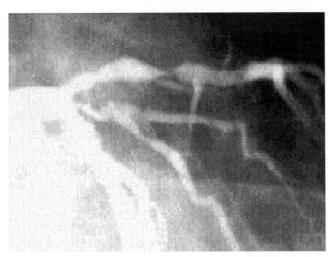

Figure Q12-8

(A) Thrombectomy in the setting of a short ischemic time and large thrombus burden in STEMI has not been shown to improve the postprocedural TIMI flow rates, TIMI blush grade, or ST resolution

(B) Overall major adverse cardiac events (MACE) rates are lower in the patients undergoing thrombectomy before definitive therapy in patients with inferior STEMI only

(C) Mortality might be expected to be decreased in patients undergoing aspiration thrombectomy before definitive therapy in STEMI patients with short ischemic time and large thrombus burden

(D) Thrombectomy in this setting only reduces the future incidence of target lesion revascularization

12.9 A 52-year-old man presents with a 2-week history of increasing exertional chest pain. His past medical history is significant for a 35-year history of ongoing tobacco use, hypertension, and "diet-controlled" diabetes mellitus. He undergoes coronary angiography followed by stenting of a circumflex stenosis. His postintervention course is unremarkable, and he is deemed ready for discharge 36 hours after his presentation. Secondary prevention goals for this patient include all of the following, EXCEPT:

(A) Start drug therapy if blood pressure (BP) is >130/80 mm Hg

(B) Start β-blocker therapy if there are no specific contraindications before discharge

(C) Fasting lipid profiles should be delayed for >48 hours after a patient presents with an ACS

(D) Calculate body mass index (BMI), and encourage diet and exercise to achieve a BMI < 30 kg/m^2

12.10 A 68-year-old woman is sent to you for evaluation of chest pain. She is generally healthy, and has no history of hypertension, hyperlipidemia, or diabetes. She is a lifelong nonsmoker. She reports that over the last several months she has experienced chest pressure associated with exposure to cold, emotional stress, or briskly walking up inclines or stairs. She has undergone stress echocardiography, showing no discrete areas of stress-induced wall motion abnormalities after walking 8 minutes on Bruce protocol, with mild global hypokinesis of the LV at rest. She is very concerned about her chest pain and wishes to have definitive coronary angiography performed. Catheterization reveals near-normal coronary arteries angiographically, except for a discrete focal 50% stenosis in a posterolateral ventricular branch of a dominant RCA. What is the most appropriate course of action for this patient?

(A) Given the patient's concern, proceed with PCI to the focal lesion with a goal of improving her 5-year event-free survival from adverse cardiac events

(B) Proceed with PCI of the lesion with a goal of alleviating the patient's symptoms

(C) Do not proceed with PCI; rather repeat stress testing with nuclear scintigraphy for evaluation with a different modality

(D) Stop the diagnostic case with a goal of aggressive medical therapy as part of a comprehensive risk reduction strategy

12.11 A patient returns to your clinic for follow-up after you performed a PCI for single-vessel CAD in the setting of an NSTEMI. He has done very well, and has had no evidence of recurrent angina or CHF. He is known to have normal left ventricular systolic function following the intervention. He asks about the benefit of future stress testing and wonders if he should periodically have such a noninvasive evaluation performed. What should you tell him?

(A) Stress ECG is a simple and sensitive way to predict and identify the presence of restenosis following PCI

(B) All patients with documented CAD who undergo PCI should have yearly stress testing performed to evaluate functional capacity and to look for objective evidence of ischemia

(C) Stress testing in asymptomatic patients is indicated only for patients with high-risk features when trying to find objective evidence of ischemia

(D) Only the presence of recurrent symptoms justifies periodic stress testing in patients who have undergone PCI

12.12 A 72-year-old woman with known CAD presents to your office for routine follow-up. She underwent stenting for a focal RCA stenosis 5 months ago. Her BP is 145/85 and her pulse is 70 beats/min. She is a known type II diabetic patient with a history of mild renal insufficiency. Today, she complains of increasing frequency and severity of exertional substernal chest pain, CCS Class II. Your preliminary diagnosis is UA perhaps related to in-stent restenosis of her previous stent. An early invasive strategy is a Class I indication in UA/NSTEMI patients who present with certain high-risk features. Which of the following characteristics places this patient in the high-risk group, thereby justifying the early invasive strategy?

(A) Age > 70 years
(B) History of diabetes
(C) BP > 140/80
(D) Presence of renal insufficiency
(E) Recent PCI within the prior 6 months

12.13 One of your long-term patients returns to see you in the clinic 1 month before his scheduled appointment because of chest pain at rest and occasionally with exertion. He is known to have CAD and has had multiple PCIs in the past. In addition, he has been well controlled medically from the standpoint of secondary prevention. His last catheterization was 1 year ago, demonstrating mild in-stent restenosis in a drug-eluting stent (DES) in a large diagonal branch. In your office, his BP is 145/95 and pulse is 88. You advise repeat catheterization because of his history and the severity of his symptoms. Angiography reveals 40% to 50% in-stent restenosis of the diagonal stent; otherwise, no hemodynamically significant disease is noted. A fractional flow reserve (FFR) performed across the lesion is 0.82. What is the most appropriate way to proceed with this patient?

(A) End the procedure and proceed with medical management to ensure the best possible control of risk factors, which may predispose the patient to ischemic chest pain
(B) End the procedure with plans for noninvasive nuclear stress testing in search of objective evidence of ischemia, which you suspect
(C) Given the severity of the patient's symptoms that you feel are highly suggestive of ischemia and without any other coronary culprit, proceed with PCI of the diagonal lesion
(D) Intravascular ultrasound (IVUS) the suspected lesion as you strongly suspect that the lesion is responsible for the patient's chest pain

12.14 You intend to perform an intervention on a complex left circumflex lesion in a 60-year-old man who presented 18 hours ago with a classic history of recent onset angina. His three sets of cardiac enzymes have been abnormal, but he has not had recurrence of chest pain or dynamic ECG changes. You plan to use a GP IIb/IIIa inhibitor for the case. Which of the following agents have been shown to be efficacious in reducing ischemic complications in patients with ACS?

(A) Tirofiban
(B) Abciximab
(C) Eptifibatide
(D) All of the above

12.15 A 59-year-old male bus driver is brought to the ER after developing progressive chest pressure, dyspnea, and diaphoresis. The patient was operating his usual bus route through downtown during the morning rush hour. Symptoms initially developed at 4:30 in the morning, when the patient had to clean the frost covering the windshield. They were initially intermittent but worsened during the next couple of hours. His past medical history is significant for obesity, elevated glucose, and serum lipids being treated with diet, hypertension, and cigarette smoking. On arrival, his physical exam was remarkable for a BP of 156/95 mm Hg, heart rate 102 bpm, and augmented S2 cardiac sound. The electrocardiogram showed sinus tachycardia, voltage criteria for left ventricular hypertrophy, and ST-segment depression in leads V4 to V6. Troponin levels were elevated three times the upper reference value. The variables and risk factors that most likely precipitated the ACS include:

(A) The exposure to cold weather
(B) Hypertension, hyperglycemia, hyperlipidemia, and smoking
(C) The stress generated by driving and exposure to smog
(D) All of the above

12.16 During the night shift, a 69-year-old woman was admitted due to new-onset, intermittent angina. Her past medical history and cardiovascular risk factor profile were significant for hyperlipidemia and hypertension. She had been treated with low-dose aspirin, simvastatin 40 mg daily, and lisinopril 10 mg daily. Since admission to the Emergency Department, she had remained asymptomatic and hemodynamically stable. The physical exam and vital signs were found to be within normal limits. An electrocardiogram showed ST-segment depression in the inferior leads and laboratory tests revealed elevated cardiac enzymes and hemoglobin 14 g/dL; creatinine clearance was calculated as 49.95 mL/min.

The patient was admitted to the coronary care unit. Her admission orders included metoprolol tartrate 25 mg every 6 hours, clopidogrel 600-mg loading dose followed by 75 mg daily, and continuation of statin and ACE inhibitor, and of enoxaparin 1 mg/kg subcutaneous twice a day, which was initiated in the Emergency Department. The last dose of enoxaparin was given at 5:00 AM, with the patient having received a total of 2 doses.

Given a working diagnosis of ACS (non-ST elevation) and following an early invasive pathway, the patient was taken within 48 hours from admission to the cardiac catheterization laboratory for angiography. Access was obtained in the right femoral artery using modified Seldinger technique. A 5-F system was used for the diagnostic angiography. An atherosclerotic, 80% lesion was identified in the mid segment of the right coronary artery. As over 4 hours had elapsed from the last dose of enoxaparin, UFH was given intravenously at 60 U/kg. An ACT of 297 seconds was obtained. PCI was performed, predilating the lesion with a compliant 2.5 × 12 mm balloon and following with DES 2.75 × 16 mm. An excellent angiographic result was obtained.

Fourteen hours after the PCI the patient developed hematemesis, hemoglobin decreased to 9.4 g/dL, heart rate increased to 89 bpm, but BP remained stable without orthostatism. The most likely factor precipitating the bleeding event was:

(A) The administration of enoxaparin
(B) The administration of UFH
(C) The administration of clopidogrel without previous knowledge of the coronary anatomy
(D) The failure to initiate a proton pump inhibitor like lansoprazole to a patient receiving clopidogrel

12.17 A diagnosis of ACS was performed in a very active, 70-year-old woman who still manages her own restaurant. Her cardiovascular risk profile is significant for hypertension well controlled on amlodipine 5 mg daily, and hyperlipidemia on atorvastatin 20 mg daily. During the last 14 months, she has required intermittent antibiotic treatment for recurrent episodes of urinary tract infection. Initial evaluation had revealed a residual

urinary volume of 147 mL, mild prolapsed bladder, and urethral strictures. She was admitted 2 days ago with severe urinary tract infection and temperature of 39°C. Her BP was 137/85 mm Hg, heart rate 100 bpm. Her weight was 52 kg. Laboratory data showed a creatinine 1.5 mg/dL, WBC 12,700, and hemoglobin 12 g/dL. She developed intermittent chest pressure during her first night in the hospital. There were no ST-segment changes on the electrocardiogram. Troponins were followed and found to be abnormal. Following an early invasive pathway, the patient is planned to undergo angiographic evaluation.

In the event a PCI is needed and if the bleeding risk of anticoagulation is to be minimized, which would be the most appropriate antithrombin agent to be used?

(A) UFH at 60 U/kg without concomitant GP IIb/IIIa inhibitor
(B) UFH at 50 U/kg with concomitant GP IIb/IIIa inhibitor but maintaining ACT < 200 seconds
(C) Enoxaparin given intravenously and as a single bolus of 0.75 mg/kg
(D) None of the above

12.18 You are discussing with your colleague which would be the fastest acting thienopyridine to be used in the case of a 52-year-old man, diabetic, admitted with NSTEMI. After evaluating the diagnostic angiogram, a PCI in the mid segment of a dominant right coronary artery was planned. Prasugrel was chosen in combination with aspirin.

Which of the following is the primary reason that prasugrel has a greater and more rapid inhibition of platelet aggregation than does clopidogrel?

(A) Does not need cytochrome P450 for biotransformation to the active metabolite
(B) Has greater affinity for the platelet $P2Y_{12}$ receptor
(C) Is converted to the active metabolite more rapidly
(D) Works primarily through the platelet $P2Y_1$ rather than the $P2Y_{12}$ receptor

12.19 During the evening shift, a 67-year-old man presented to the ER with a 2-day history of recurrent chest discomfort. His symptoms initiated after helping his neighbor clean the yard. The chest discomfort was described as pressure-like, lasted between 2 and 5 minutes, and was relieved by rest. The evening of admission, the pressure presented at rest and was associated with dyspnea.

His past medical history and risk factor profile were significant for hypertension and hyperlipidemia.

On arrival the physical exam was only significant for an augmented second aortic sound. The electrocardiogram showed a normal sinus rhythm and nonspecific repolarization changes. The cardiac enzymes were elevated, and the patient was admitted with a diagnosis of NSTEMI to the coronary care unit. Appropriate antiplatelet and antithrombin therapies were initiated, in addition to continuing metoprolol, lisinopril, and atorvastatin. A 2D echocardiogram performed while in the emergency department documented inferolateral hypokinesis, EF 45% to 49%, and mild mitral regurgitation (MR).

The following morning a coronary angiogram was performed documenting an 80% stenosis in the mid segment of long ramus branch perfusing most of the lateral wall as the other obtuse marginal branches were small and diffusely diseased. There were no obstructive lesions in the other main epicardial vessels. It was decided to perform PCI with angioplasty and stent.

A DES that interferes with the polymerization of tubulin and microtubule disassembly was chosen. Which stent was used?

(A) Everolimus
(B) Paclitaxel
(C) Sirolimus
(D) Zotarolimus

12.20 During a diagnostic coronary angiogram, the patient complained of severe discomfort at the access site. The procedure was performed for evaluation of NSTEMI in a 64-year-old woman with BMI 32, creatinine clearance 32 mL, and baseline anemia. The angiogram in Figure Q12-20 was obtained. The most appropriate access site management, in order to prevent this angiographic finding would have been:

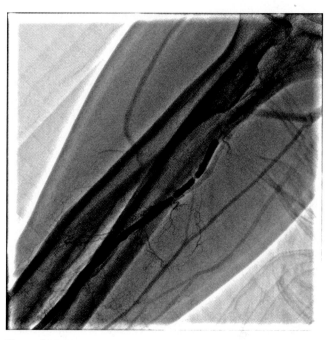

Figure Q12-20

(A) Previous evaluation with ankle-brachial index (ABI) for severe peripheral arterial disease and consideration for limb surgical revascularization
(B) Previous evaluation with ABI for severe peripheral arterial disease and consideration for limb percutaneous revascularization
(C) The use of a long, coating-free sheath for arterial access
(D) The use of preventive measures for access management

12.21 The angiographic sequence in Figure Q12-21 describes the percutaneous revascularization of a 67-year-old man with previous surgical revascularization and known ischemic cardiomyopathy with EF 25% to 29%. He presented with an ACS and hemodynamic instability. The culprit vessel was found to be a complete occlusion of the circumflex artery. The left internal mammary artery to LAD artery was patent. So was the vein graft to posterior descending artery. A DES was used in order to provide the best long-term outcome.

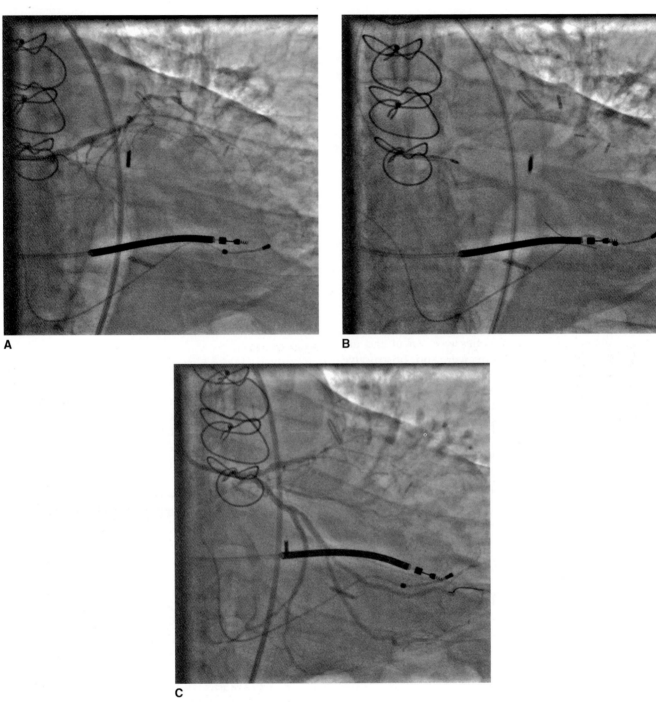

Figure Q12-21

The most likely sequence of events during the procedure and lesion characteristics include:

(A) IVUS, followed by intraaortic balloon pump (IABP), and then stenting in a long thrombotic lesion

(B) IABP, followed by IVUS, and then stenting in a nondilatable lesion

(C) IABP, followed by rotational atherectomy, and then stenting in a nondilatable lesion

(D) Acute hemodynamic decompensation after DES thrombosis requiring IABP and then rotational atherectomy in a long thrombotic lesion

12.22 A DES (paclitaxel) was deployed for a severe and long stenosis identified to be the culprit lesion in an NSTEMI. In reference to Figure Q12-22, the finding depicted has been associated with:

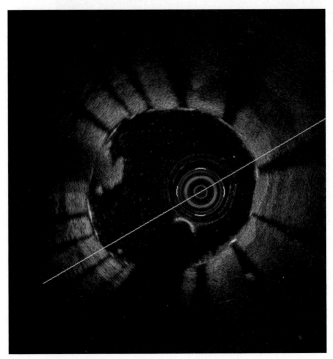

Figure Q12-22 (see color insert)

(A) Lower incidence of restenosis

(B) Higher incidence of restenosis

(C) Lower incidence of late acquired stent malapposition

(D) Higher incidence of late acquired stent malapposition

QUESTIONS 23 THROUGH 28. The following are intravascular images (Fig. Q12-23 through Q12-28). Match the image with the most appropriate answer:

12.23

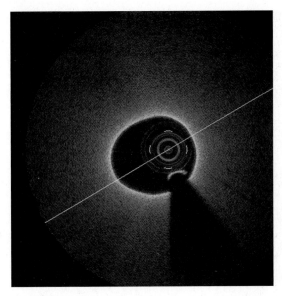

Figure Q12-23

(A) Normal vessel anatomy

(B) Unstable angina

(C) Guiding catheter

(D) Stable angina

(E) Side branch

(F) ACS if rupture occurs

12.24

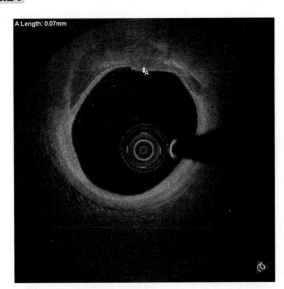

Figure Q12-24 (see color insert)

(A) Normal vessel anatomy

(B) Unstable angina

(C) Guiding catheter

(D) Stable angina

(E) Side branch

(F) ACS if rupture occurs

12.25

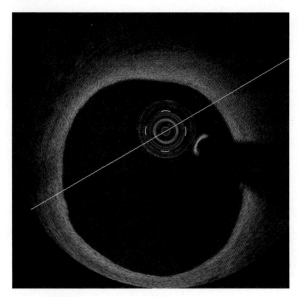

Figure Q12-25 (see color insert)
- (A) Normal vessel anatomy
- (B) Unstable angina
- (C) Guiding catheter
- (D) Stable angina
- (E) Side branch
- (F) ACS if rupture occurs

12.26

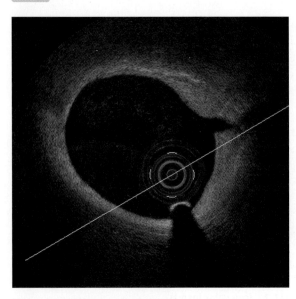

Figure Q12-26 (see color insert)
- (A) Normal vessel anatomy
- (B) Unstable angina
- (C) Guiding catheter
- (D) Stable angina
- (E) Side branch
- (F) ACS if rupture occurs

12.27

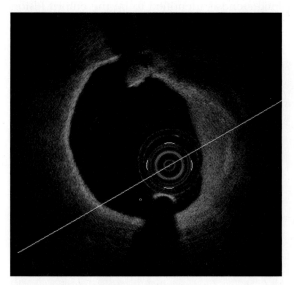

Figure Q12-27
- (A) Normal vessel anatomy
- (B) Unstable angina
- (C) Guiding catheter
- (D) Stable angina
- (E) Side branch
- (F) ACS if rupture occurs

12.28

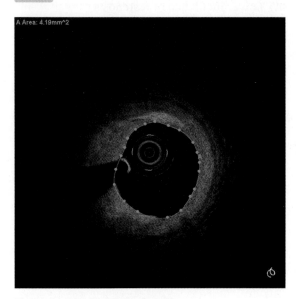

Figure Q12-28 (see color insert)
- (A) Normal vessel anatomy
- (B) Unstable angina
- (C) Guiding catheter
- (D) Stable angina
- (E) Side branch
- (F) ACS if rupture occurs

12.1 **Answer C.** In the setting of PCI, clinical trials have shown benefit of the three available GP IIb/IIIa inhibitors in decreasing periprocedural ischemic events. The timing for PCI is important. Abciximab is not recommended for use in a noninvasive approach or when a delayed (>24 hours) invasive approach is planned based on the GUSTO IV result that found no benefit of abciximab vs. placebo in this population (*Lancet* 2001;357:1915–1924). The addition of a GP IIb/IIIa antagonist to a 600-mg loading dose of clopidogrel was found to significantly reduce peri-PCI events compared with 600-mg loading dose of clopidogrel alone in the ISAR-REACT 2 trial, with the difference confined to troponin-positive patients (*JAMA* 2006;295:1531–1538). Finally, post hoc analysis (Fig. A12-1) of placebo-controlled trials of GP IIb/IIIa antagonists in ACS patients (CAPTURE, PRISM, and PARAGON-B) have consistently found a marked benefit for these agents in troponin-positive patients, and no difference in outcomes compared with placebo in troponin-negative patients (*N Engl J Med* 1999;340:1623–1629; *Lancet* 1999;354:1757–1762; *Circulation* 2001;103:2891–2896).

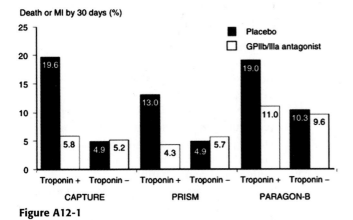

Death or MI by 30 days (%)

Figure A12-1

12.2 **Answer A.** Enteric-coating or buffered aspirin preparations do not appear to influence the risk of a major upper gastrointestinal bleeding (*Lancet* 1996;348:1413–1416). A wide range of aspirin doses, preparations, and methods of ingestion have been evaluated to determine the best way to achieve maximal antiplatelet activity in an acute setting. Chewing an aspirin or drinking solubilized aspirin (e.g., Alka-Seltzer)

significantly shortens aspirin absorption and the onset of antiplatelet activity. A study of 12 volunteers compared 325 mg of buffered aspirin, either chewed or swallowed, with Alka-Seltzer. Chewing the pill or drinking the solution resulted in maximal inhibition of serum TXB2 production within 20 to 30 minutes of ingestion, whereas just swallowing the pill required approximately 60 minutes (*Am J Cardiol* 1999;84:404–409). In another study of 18 volunteers, chewing an 81-, 162-, or 324-mg aspirin pill led to equivalent reduction in TXB2 production, but maximal inhibition within 15 minutes of ingestion was achieved only after the 162- and 324-mg doses (*Am J Cardiol* 1994;74:720–723). The results of these and other studies suggest that to achieve the maximal effects of aspirin rapidly (within approximately 15 minutes), at least 162 mg should be chewed and swallowed.

Four placebo-controlled trials found a consistent 50% or greater risk reduction in the combined end point of death or MI through the early initiation of aspirin therapy in patients with an NSTEMI ACS (*N Eng J Med* 1983;309:396–403).

12.3 **Answer C.** The best data evaluating the risk of in-hospital bleeding in an ACS population come from an analysis of over 24,000 patients in the Global Registry of Acute Coronary Events (*Eur Heart J* 2003;24:1815–1823). The analysis showed an incidence of major bleeding in 4.7% of the NSTEMI population and identified four independent predictors of an increased risk of major bleeding: advanced age, female gender, a history of bleeding, and renal insufficiency. As has been found in the subsequent studies, major bleeding was associated with a significant increase in mortality.

12.4 **Answer A.** The ACC/AHA/ACS and PCI guidelines both recommend a 300-mg loading dose of clopidogrel, although the PCI guidelines suggest a 600-mg loading dose (*Circulation* 2006;113:e166–e286). Although some *ex vivo* studies have found that concomitant atorvastatin therapy influences the level of platelet function achieved with clopidogrel (some findings showed decreased platelet inhibition, others showed increased platelet inhibition), the bulk of the clinical data have found no clinically important interaction (*Circulation* 2003;108:921–924). In the most recent PCI guidelines, a recommendation is made to consider doubling the maintenance dose of clopidogrel in high-risk patents if their measured inhibition of platelet aggregation is >50% (*Circulation* 2006;113:e166–e286). The new 2011 ACC/AHA guideline takes into account data from OASIS 7 and gives broad range for loading. Plavix loading of 300 or 600 mg is recommended (2011 ACCF/AHA Focused Update of the Guidelines for the Management of Patients With Unstable Angina/Non–ST-Elevation Myocardial Infarction [Updating the 2007 Guideline], *J Am Coll Cardiol* 2011;57:1920–1959).

12.5   Answer A. The pharmacokinetics of enoxaparin allow for what is generally considered to be therapeutic levels of anti-Xa activity within 30 to 60 minutes of a subcutaneous dose that is maintained for 8 hours (*Catheter Cardiovasc Interv* 2003;60:185–193).

Therefore, it is recommended that no additional anticoagulant be given unless it has been 8 hours or more since their last dose, and in that case a booster dose of 0.3 mg/kg IV should be given. This was the peri-PCI treatment regimen utilized in the SYNERGY trial that involved over 10,000 high-risk ACS patients randomized to either enoxaparin or UFH (*JAMA* 2004;292:45–54). Overall, the trial found no difference in efficacy between enoxaparin and UFH. One important outcome of SYNERGY was the knowledge that combined anticoagulant therapies (e.g., giving UFH to an enoxaparin-treated patient) was associated with a substantial increase in bleeding complications and no improvement in efficacy.

12.6   Answer D. The patient has multivessel disease with an angiographically severe LAD stenosis, but successful reperfusion following lytic therapy in the setting of an acute anterior STEMI. Emergent PCI is not indicated following thrombolysis and successful reperfusion as indicated in this patient by resolution of ST-segment elevation and restoration of normal flow in the LAD by angiography despite the presence of an angiographically severe lesion. The potential harm of routine PCI following thrombolytic therapy was confirmed recently in the ASSENT-4 study in which patients with STEMI randomized to lytics followed by PCI

had significantly higher mortality than patients randomized to primary PCI alone (*Lancet* 2006;367:569–578). Similarly, there is no clear indication for percutaneous treatment of this patient's RCA lesions at this time. In fact, the ACC/AHA guidelines make this a Class III recommendation even in the setting of a primary PCI, stating that a PCI should not be performed in a noninfarct artery at the time of primary PCI in patients without hemodynamic compromise (*J Am Coll Cardiol* 2004;44:671). Urgent CABG is also contraindicated in patients with successful epicardial reperfusion and no mechanical complications.

12.7   Answer D. This situation must be tempered by the nuances of the patient presentation, and many would argue that the decision regarding when to proceed to catheterization varies from patient to patient. However, this patient presents with clear high-risk features, particularly dynamic ECG changes in the setting of anginal chest pain. As it is clear that an unstable coronary process must be evaluated, the essential part in decision making in this patient is determining whether one should pursue an "early invasive" or "early conservative" strategy. The early conservative strategy reserves coronary angiography for UA/NSTEMI patients who have evidence of recurrent ischemia or high-risk stress testing despite optimal and aggressive medical therapy. High-risk features that support an "early invasive" strategy include:

- Recurrent angina/ischemia at rest or with low-level activities despite intensive anti-ischemic therapy
- Elevated TnT or TnI
- New or presumably new ST-segment depression
- Recurrent angina/ischemia with congestive heart failure symptoms, an S_3 gallop, pulmonary edema, worsening rales, or new or worsening mitral regurgitation
- High-risk findings on noninvasive stress testing
- Depressed systolic function (e.g., ejection function < 0.40 on noninvasive study)
- Hemodynamic instability
- Sustained ventricular tachycardia
- PCI within 6 months
- Prior CABG

In the absence of these high-risk features in the setting of UA/NSTEMI, either the early invasive or conservative strategy is acceptable in hospitalized patients. Although the trial designs differed, the two most recent clinical trials comparing early invasive vs. early conservative strategies in UA/NSTEMI patients were TACTICS-TIMI 18 and FRISC II. In TACTICS-TIMI 18, 2,200 patients with UA/NSTEMI were treated with aspirin, heparin, and an "upstream" GP IIb/IIIa inhibitor (tirofiban) (*N Engl J Med* 2001;344:1879–1887). They were then randomized to an early invasive strategy including routine angiography within 48 hours, or a more conservative symptom-driven approach. In the latter, catheterization was performed only if the patient had recurrent ischemia or a positive stress test. Death, MI, or rehospitalization for ACS at 6 months occurred in 15.9% of the patients assigned to the invasive strategy vs. 19.4% assigned to the more conservative strategy ($p = 0.025$). Death or MI was also reduced at 6 months (7.3% vs. 9.5%, $p < 0.05$). Interestingly, if the patient did not have high-risk features, the outcomes between the two groups were similar. In FRISC II, more than 3,000 patients were randomized in a 2 × 2 fashion with one arm being an early invasive vs. early conservative approach (*Lancet* 1999;354:708–715). At 6 months, death or MI occurred in 9.4% of the patients assigned to the invasive strategy and in 12.1% of those assigned to the noninvasive strategy ($p < 0.031$). During the first year, the mortality rate in the invasive strategy group was 2.2% compared with 3.9% in the noninvasive strategy group ($p = 0.016$) (*Lancet* 2000;356:9–16).

12.8 **Answer C.** Expeditious restoration of coronary blood flow is the primary goal of all revascularization strategies, and time-to-reperfusion is the best correlate with most outcome measures in patients presenting with acute STEMI. Rheolytic thrombectomy was developed out of concern for protection of distal vessels and microvasculature when patients present with apparent large thrombus burden. In the VEGAS-1 and 2 trials, efficacy of thrombectomy in patients with STEMI and large thrombus burdens in vein grafts was established. (*Am J Cardiol* 2002;89:326–330). However, thrombectomy was compared with intracoronary infusion of urokinase, and the rates of adjunctive therapy such as GP IIb/IIIa inhibitor were low. In 2004, the AiMI trial sought to determine whether thrombectomy plus "definitive therapy" was superior to "definitive therapy" alone in patients presenting with anterior STEMI or large inferior STEMI (*Eur Heart J* 2006;27:1139–1145). This trial was a multicenter, prospective, randomized, and controlled trial that included 480 such patients presenting within 12 hours of symptom onset. Interestingly, the primary end point of final infarct size as measured by SPECT imaging at 14 to 28 days was significantly larger in the subset of patients receiving thrombectomy. In addition to infarct size, mortality was also shown to be significantly higher in the thrombectomy arm (4.6% vs. 0.8%; $p < 0.02$). Secondary end points including postprocedural TIMI flow and MACE (death, new Q wave MI, stroke, target lesion revascularization) showed no difference between the two treatment arms. Unlike VEGAS, patients with vein grafts were excluded in the AiMI trial, and the rate of GP IIb/IIIa use was much higher in AiMI (eptifibatide use > 90%). The AiMI trialists concluded that their data do not support routine use of rheolytic thrombectomy in STEMI. However, more recent trials exploring the use of thrombectomy are available. The new 2011 guideline takes into account new data from TAPAS and EXPIRA trial as well as a meta-analysis study and states that it is "reasonable to assume" that thrombectomy is useful in STEMI patients with short ischemic time and large thrombus burden (*J Am Coll Cardiol* 2011;57:1920–1959). The Thrombus Aspiration During Percutaneous Coronary Intervention in Acute Myocardial Infarction Study (TAPAS) randomized 1,071 STEMI patients to aspiration thrombectomy followed by stenting vs. stenting alone. Aspiration was successfully performed in 90% of patients, thrombus or atheroma was retrieved in 72% of patients, and direct stenting (without predilatation) was performed in 59% of patients. The frequency of myocardial blush grade 3 (the primary end point) and complete STR—the secondary end point—was significantly higher with aspiration thrombectomy. These improved results in myocardial reperfusion were associated with clinical benefit at 1 year, with a lower incidence of cardiac death (3.6% vs. 6.7%, $p = 0.02$) and cardiac death or MI (5.6% vs. 9.9%, $p = 0.008$) (*N Engl J Med* 2008;358:557–567; *Lancet* 2008;371:1915–1920).

Bavry and Bhatt evaluated 13 randomized trials with manual thrombectomy and found that thrombectomy improved myocardial perfusion, measured both by MBG and STR, and was associated with lower mortality (*Eur Heart J* 2008;29:2989–3001). A separate meta-analysis evaluated 9 randomized trials comparing PCI with aspiration thrombectomy vs. PCI alone and found that patients treated with thrombectomy had less distal emboli, a higher frequency of TIMI 3 flow and MBG 3 post-PCI, and lower 30-day mortality (*Eur Heart J* 2008;29:3002–3010).

12.9   **Answer C.** As part of a comprehensive risk reduction strategy after PCI, the guidelines from the ACC/AHA/SCAI state that all post-MI and acute patients be started on β-blocker therapy before discharge if there are no specific contraindications (*Circulation* 2006;113:e166–e286). In regard to drug therapy for hypertension for secondary prevention of events, it is recommended that therapy be initiated for individuals with BP > 140/90 mm Hg. However, if patients have chronic kidney disease or diabetes, drug therapy should be started if BP is > 130/80 mm Hg (*Circulation* 2006;113:2363–2372). Although there has been historical controversy over when to obtain lipid profiles in patients presenting with ACSs, the published guidelines state that lipid profiles should be obtained in all patients, preferably within 24 hours of an acute event. With mounting evidence suggesting that lower low-density lipoprotein cholesterol (LDL-C) portends better outcomes, statins are still preferred in post-PCI patients even with LDL-C < 100 mg/dL at baseline. Regular exercise should be encouraged, with a minimum of 30 to 60 minutes at least five times weekly. BMI should be calculated and documented, with the desirable approximate range of 18.5 to 24.9 kg/m². The table summarizes the ACC/AHA recommendations regarding appropriate secondary prevention in these patients.

Table A12-9.   Intervention Recommendations with Class of Recommendation and Level of Evidence

Smoking Goal: Complete cessation; no exposure to environmental tobacco smoke	• Ask about tobacco use status at every visit. I (B) • Advise every tobacco user to quit. I (B) • Assess the tobacco user's willingness to quit. I (B) • Assist by counseling and developing a plan for quitting. I (B) • Arrange follow-up, referral to special programs, or pharmacotherapy (including nicotine replacement and bupropion). I (B) • Urge avoidance of exposure to environmental tobacco smoke at work and home. I (B)
BP control Goal: <140/90 mm Hg or <130/80 mm Hg if patient has diabetes or chronic kidney disease	For all patients: • Initiate or maintain lifestyle modification—weight control; increased physical activity; alcohol moderation; sodium reduction; and emphasis on increased consumption of fresh fruits, vegetables, and low-fat dairy products. I (B) For patients with BP ≥ 140/90 mm Hg (or ≥ 130/80 mm Hg for individuals with chronic kidney disease or diabetes): • As tolerated, add BP medication, treating initially with β-blockers and/or ACE inhibitors, with addition of other drugs such as thiazides as needed to achieve goal BP. I (A) (For compelling indications for individual drug classes in specific vascular diseases, see Seventh Report of the Joint National Committee on Prevention, Detection, Evaluation, and Treatment of High BP [JNC 7].)[a]
Lipid management Goal: LDL-C < 100 mg/dL If triglycerides are ≥200 mg/dL, non-HDL-C should be <130 mg/dL[b]	For all patients: • Start dietary therapy. Reduce intake of saturated fats (to <7% of total calories), *trans*-fatty acids, and cholesterol (to <200 mg/d). I (B) • Adding plant stanol/sterols (2 g/d) and viscous fiber (>10 g/d) will further lower LDL-C. • Promote daily physical activity and weight management. I (B) • Encourage increased consumption of omega-3 fatty acids in the form of fish[c] or in capsule form (1 g/d) for risk reduction. For treatment of elevated triglycerides, higher doses are usually necessary for risk reduction. IIb (B) For lipid management: Assess fasting lipid profile in all patients, and within 24 h of hospitalization for those with an acute cardiovascular or coronary event. For hospitalized patients, initiate lipid-lowering medication as recommended below before discharge according to the following schedule: • LDL-C should be <100 mg/dL I (A), and • Further reduction of LDL-C to <70 mg/dL is reasonable. IIa (A) • If baseline LDL-C is ≥ 100 mg/dL, initiate LDL-lowering drug therapy.[d] I (A) • If on-treatment LDL-C is ≥ 100 mg/dL, intensify LDL-lowering drug therapy (may require LDL-lowering drug combination[e]). I (A)

Table A12-9. Intervention Recommendations with Class of Recommendation and Level of Evidence *(Continued)*

	• If baseline LDL-C is 70 to 100 mg/dL, it is reasonable to treat to LDL-C <70 mg/dL. IIa (B) • If triglycerides are 200 to 499 mg/dL, non-HDL-C should be <130 mg/dL. I (B), and • Further reduction of non-HDL-C to <100 mg/dL is reasonable. IIa (B) • Therapeutic options to reduce non-HDL-C are • More intense LDL-C-lowering therapy I (B), or • Niacin*f* (after LDL-C-lowering therapy) IIa (B), or • Fibrate therapy*g* (after LDL-C-lowering therapy) IIa (B) • If triglycerides are ≥ 500 mg/dL,*g* therapeutic options to prevent pancreatitis are fibrate*f* or niacin*f* before LDL-lowering therapy; and treat LDL-C to goal after triglyceride-lowering therapy. Achieve non-HDL-C <130 mg/dL if possible. I (C)
Physical activity Goal: 30 min, 7 d/wk (minimum 5 d/wk)	• For all patients, assess risk with a physical activity history and/or an exercise test, to guide prescription. I (B) • For all patients, encourage 30 to 60 minutes of moderate-intensity aerobic activity, such as brisk walking, on most, preferably all, days of the week, supplemented by an increase in daily lifestyle activities (e.g., walking breaks at work, gardening, household work). I (B) • Encourage resistance training 2 d/wk. IIb (C) • Advise medically supervised programs for high-risk patients (e.g., recent acute coronary syndrome or revascularization, heart failure [HF]). I (B)
Weight management Goal: BMI: 18.5 to 24.9 kg/m² Waist circumference: men <40 in, women <35 in.	• Assess BMI and/or waist circumference on each visit and consistently encourage weight maintenance/reduction through an appropriate balance of physical activity, caloric intake, and formal behavioral programs when indicated to maintain/achieve a BMI between 18.5 and 24.9 kg/m². I (B) • If waist circumference (measured horizontally at the iliac crest) is ≥ 35 in. in women and ≥ 40 in. in men, initiate lifestyle changes and consider treatment strategies for metabolic syndrome as indicated. I (B) • The initial goal of weight loss therapy should be to reduce body weight by ~10% from baseline. With success, further weight loss can be attempted if indicated through further assessment. I (B)
Diabetes management Goal: HbA$_{1c}$ < 7%	• Initiate lifestyle and pharmacotherapy to achieve near-normal HbA$_{1c}$. I (B) • Begin vigorous modification of other risk factors (e.g., physical activity, weight management, BP control, and cholesterol management as recommended above). I (B) • Coordinate diabetic care with patient's primary care physician or endocrinologist. I (C)
Antiplatelet agents/anticoagulants	• Start aspirin 75 to 162 mg/d, and continue indefinitely in all patients unless contraindicated. I (A) • For patients undergoing coronary artery bypass grafting, aspirin should be started within 48 hours of surgery to reduce saphenous vein graft closure. Dosing regimens ranging from 100 to 325 mg/d appear to be efficacious. Doses higher than 162 mg/d can be continued for up to 1 y. I (B) • Start and continue clopidogrel 75 mg/d in combination with aspirin for up to 12 mo in patients after ACS or PCI with stent placement (≥ 1 mo for bare-metal stent (BMS), ≥ 3 mo for sirolimus-eluting stent, and ≥ 6 mo for paclitaxel-eluting stent [PES]). I (B) • Patients who have undergone PCI with stent placement should initially receive higher dose aspirin at 325 mg/d for 1 mo for BMS, 3 mo for sirolimus-eluting stent, and 6 mo for PES. I (B) • Manage warfarin to international normalized ratio = 2.0 to 3.0 for paroxysmal or chronic atrial fibrillation or flutter, and in post-MI patients when clinically indicated (e.g., atrial fibrillation, left ventricular thrombus). I (A) • Use of warfarin in conjunction with aspirin and/or clopidogrel is associated with increased risk of bleeding and should be monitored closely. I (B)

(Continued)

Table A12-9. Intervention Recommendations with Class of Recommendation and Level of Evidence *(Continued)*

Renin-angiotensin-aldosterone system blockers	ACE inhibitors: • Consider for all other patients. I (B) • Among lower-risk patients with normal left ventricular EF in whom cardiovascular risk factors are well controlled and revascularization has been performed, use of ACE inhibitors may be considered optional. IIa (B) Angiotensin receptor blockers: • Start and continue indefinitely in all patients with left ventricular ejection fraction (EF) ≤40% and in those with hypertension, diabetes, or chronic kidney disease, unless contraindicated. I (A) • Use in patients who are intolerant of ACE inhibitors and have HF or have had an MI with left ventricular EF ≤40%. I (A) • Consider in other patients who are ACE inhibitor intolerant. I (B) • Consider use in combination with ACE inhibitors in systolic-dysfunction HF. IIb (B) • Aldosterone blockade: • Use in post-MI patients, without significant renal dysfunction[h] or hyperkalemia,[i] who are already receiving therapeutic doses of an ACE inhibitor and β-blocker, have a left ventricular EF ≤40%, and have either diabetes or HF. I (A)
β-blockers	• Start and continue indefinitely in all patients who have had MI, ACS, or left ventricular dysfunction with or without HF symptoms, unless contraindicated. I (A) Consider chronic therapy for all other patients with coronary or other vascular disease or diabetes unless contraindicated. IIa (C)
Influenza vaccination	Patients with cardiovascular disease should have an influenza vaccination. I (B)

[a]Patients covered by these guidelines include those with established coronary and other atherosclerotic vascular disease, including peripheral arterial disease, atherosclerotic aortic disease, and carotid artery disease. Treatment of patients whose only manifestation of cardiovascular risk is diabetes will be the topic of a separate American Health Association scientific statement. ACE, angiotensin-converting enzyme; HDL, high-density lipoprotein.
[b]Non-HDL-C, total cholesterol minus HDL-C.
[c]Pregnant and lactating women should limit their intake of fish to minimize exposure to methylmercury.
[d]When LDL-lowering medications are used, obtain at least a 30% to 40% reduction in LDL-C levels. If LDL-C <70 mg/dL is the chosen target, consider drug titration to achieve this level to minimize side effects and cost. When LDL-C <70 mg/dL is not achievable because of high baseline LDL-C levels, it generally is possible to achieve reductions of >50% in LDL-C levels by either statins or LDL-C–lowering drug combinations.
[e]Standard dose of statin with ezetimibe, bile acid sequestrant, or niacin.
[f]The combination of high-dose statin + fibrate can increase risk for severe myopathy. Statin doses should be kept relatively low with this combination. Dietary supplement niacin must not be used as a substitute for prescription niacin.
[g]Patients with very high triglycerides should not consume alcohol. The use of bile acid sequestrant is relatively contraindicated when triglycerides are >200 mg/dL.
[h]Creatinine should be <2.5 mg/dL in men and <2.0 mg/dL in women.
[i]Potassium should be <5.0 mEq/L.
(Adapted from AHA/ACC Guidelines for Secondary Prevention for Patients With Coronary and Other Atherosclerotic Vascular Disease: 2006 Update. *Circulation*. 2006;113:2363–2372.)

12.10 **Answer D.** This patient probably should not have undergone coronary angiography in the first place, given her presentation, paucity of risk factors for CAD, and her otherwise low-risk stress test. Once the diagnostic images have been obtained, however, the interventionalist is faced with a dilemma—whether to proceed with an intervention or to choose the primary medical management approach. Many factors are involved in this decision, but ultimately it is the interventionalist's job to integrate the entirety of the patient's presentation and make informed, conscientious decisions in the patient's best interest. PCI in this case may be a Class III recommendation according to the 2005 ACC/AHA/SCAI guidelines regarding PCI if the lesion is not hemodynamically significant (*Circulation* 2006;113:2363-2372). A Class III recommendation implies that based on the best available evidence, the intervention would extend more risk than benefit to the patient, and therefore should not be performed. This patient has Canadian Cardiovascular Society (CCS) Class II angina on presentation, and there is no objective evidence of ischemia based on available information. Furthermore, the particular location of this lesion would place only a small area of myocardium at risk. Should the operator demonstrate a focal lesion in this patient that is well suited for PCI and that places a moderate or large-sized area of myocardium at risk, then proceeding with PCI would become a Class I recommendation. It is left to the discretion of the interventionalist to make these decisions with competence on behalf of each individual patient. One option would be doing FFR of the 50% stenosis to ascertain hemodynamic significance.

12.11 **Answer C.** Routine periodic stress testing of patients who have undergone PCI with no high-risk features and who are asymptomatic received a Class III recommendation from the ACC/AHA in 2002 (*J Am Coll Cardiol* 2002;40:1531–1540). High-risk patients generally include those with decreased left ventricular function, multivessel CAD, proximal LAD disease, previous sudden death, diabetes mellitus, hazardous occupations, and suboptimal percutaneous transluminal coronary angioplasty PCI results. In the presence of such high-risk features, exercise testing within 12 months of PCI to detect restenosis is a Class IIb recommendation, indicating additional studies are needed to confirm efficacy and safety of this approach. The only Class I recommendation for stress testing after revascularization is for recurrent symptoms that suggest ischemia. Another potential use for postrevascularization stress testing is to assist with activity counseling and to guide exercise training as part of a comprehensive cardiac rehabilitation program.

12.12 **Answer E.** Because this patient has undergone PCI within the last 6 months, she should be considered in the high-risk group, thereby making an early invasive strategy a Class I indication in managing her disease (*Available at:* http://www.acc.org/clinical/guidelines/unstable/unstable.pdf 2002). The ACC/AHA/SCAI 2005 Guideline Update for PCI identifies nine such features that help identify patients as high risk and therefore more likely to benefit from an early invasive strategy when presenting with UA/NSTEMI (*Circulation* 2006;113:e166–e286) and include:

- Recurrent ischemia despite intensive anti-ischemic therapy
- Elevated troponin level
- New ST-segment depression
- HF symptoms or new or worsening MR
- Depressed LV systolic function
- Hemodynamic instability
- Sustained ventricular tachycardia
- PCI within 6 months
- Prior CABG

Many clinical trials (e.g., TIMI-IIIB, VANQWISH, and FRISC II) have evaluated different strategies for managing patients presenting with UA or NSTEMI, including both invasive and medical strategies to compare outcomes. More recent trials, such as RITA III, ISAR-COOL, and TACTICS-TIMI 18, suggest that patients who are treated with an early invasive strategy have reduced incidence of recurrent angina, and a combined end point of death and MI. On the basis of data compiled from these various trials, the most recent guidelines suggest that an early invasive approach is the preferred strategy in patients presenting with UA/NSTEMI with high-risk features.

12.13 **Answer A.** In this scenario, you are faced with a patient with known CAD and a chest pain syndrome consistent with escalating angina. Diagnostic coronary angiography reveals a moderate lesion in the large diagonal branch and no other potential "culprit" lesions. Appropriately, FFR is done to assess the hemodynamic significance of the lesion but fails to demonstrate it. Using the technique of determining FFR to establish the hemodynamic significance of intermediate coronary lesions (30% to 70%) has been proved to be beneficial in many circumstances (*Circulation* 2006;113:e166–e286). At this point, careful consideration must be given to the entirety of the patient's condition, and not just the angiographic appearance of the suspected culprit lesion. Most would agree that IVUS has no added benefit to the initial FFR determination in this situation. Although, depending on the interventionalist's interpretation of the significance of the angiographic appearance of the lesion, IVUS of the potential culprit lesion could be a Class IIa, IIb, or even Class III indication (if the angiographic appearance of the lesion is clear and no intervention is planned). It has been shown that deferring PCI for intermediate coronary lesions with normal physiology (i.e., normal FFR determination) produces similar results to intervening on such lesions with respect to event-free survival and freedom from anginal symptoms (*J Am Coll Cardiol* 1998;31:841–847; *Circulation* 2001;103:2928–2934; *J Am Coll Cardiol* 1995;25:178–187). Proceeding with nuclear imaging once the FFR determination has been done is also unappealing, primarily because of the wealth of evidence, which correlates abnormal FFR determination with nuclear stress testing. In fact, an FFR of <0.75 has been consistently shown to identify physiologically significant stenosis associated with inducible myocardial ischemia with high sensitivity (88%), specificity (100%), positive predicted value (100%), and overall accuracy (93%). One must be impressed that the patient presented with poorly controlled BP and elevated resting pulse rate from the available information and physiologic data would be the more beneficial target for the physician to focus.

12.14   **Answer D.** In the EPIC trial with abciximab, high-risk patients (including severe UA patients) had 35% lower incidence of ischemic complications (death, MI, revascularization) at 30 days compared with placebo (12.8% vs. 8.3%, $p = 0.0008$) (*N Engl J Med* 1994;330:956-961). A 13% benefit was seen at 3 years, mainly attributable to decreased need for bypass surgery or repeat PCI in the group treated with abciximab (*JAMA* 1997;278:479-484). Showing even greater benefit, patients with UA in the EPILOG trial demonstrated a 64% reduction (10.1% to 3.6%, $p = 0.001$) in the composite occurrence of death, MI, or urgent revascularization to 30 days with abciximab therapy compared with placebo (standard-dose weight-adjusted heparin) (*N Engl J Med* 1997;336:1689-1696). Tirofiban was evaluated in the PRISM-PLUS trial, which included patients with UA and NSTEMI presenting within 12 hours of symptom onset (*N Engl J Med* 1998;338:1488-1497). Here, the 30-day incidence of death, MI, refractory ischemia, or rehospitalization for UA was 15.3% in the group that received heparin alone compared with 8.8% in the tirofiban/heparin group. After PCI, death or nonfatal MI occurred in 10.2% of those receiving heparin vs. 5.9% in those treated with tirofiban. Eptifibatide has been evaluated in two randomized clinical trials and has also demonstrated efficacy in reducing ischemic complications in patients with UA. In the PURSUIT trial, such patients were randomized to receive placebo or eptifibatide in addition to standard therapy of aspirin with or without UFH. (*N Engl J Med* 1998;339:436-443). In patients undergoing PCI within 72 hours of randomization, eptifibatide administration resulted in a 31% reduction in the combined end point of nonfatal MI or death at 30 days (17.7% vs. 11.6%, $p = 0.01$). Other GP IIb/IIIa trials are summarized in Figure A12-14.

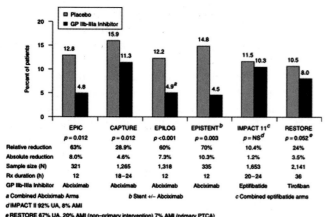

Figure A12-14

12.15   **Answer D.** Both an abrupt decline in air temperature and poor air quality (increased exposures to carbon monoxide as is typically generated by traffic, fine particulate matter, and cigarette smoke) have been reported to trigger ACS. Diet-related issues that increase cardiovascular risk include high dietary salt intake, lack of moderate alcohol consumption, and development of the metabolic syndrome.

12.16   **Answer B.** In the STACKENOX (STACK-on to ENOXaparin) trial (*Am Heart J* 2009;158:177-184), the addition of 70 U/kg of UFH 4 to 10 hours after the last dose of enoxaparin 1 mg/kg resulted in supratherapeutic anti-Xa and anti-IIa levels and complete inhibition of thrombin generation for 2 hours, despite an activated clotting time that was <270 seconds. This addition increased the risk of periprocedural and postprocedural bleeding. Therefore, to avoid excess bleeding, UFH should not be administered routinely in the catheterization laboratory <10 hours after administration of 1 mg/kg enoxaparin, unless factor Xa activity levels are low.

12.17   **Answer D.** None of the above. Bivalirudin would be the most appropriate anticoagulant agent, given the patient's renal insufficiency. The calculated creatinine level is 28.65 mL/min.

Further analyses of the ACUITY (Acute Catheterization and Urgent Intervention Triage strategY) trial compared various antithrombotic strategies in patients with NSTE-ACS in two important subgroups of patients, namely those managed without revascularization (*Circulation* 2010;121:853-862) and patients with chronic kidney disease (*J Am Coll Cardiol Intv* 2009;2:748-757). Large and consistent reductions in bleeding complications with bivalirudin monotherapy compared with heparin with a GPI, without loss of ischemic protection through 1 year, were reported. In the ISAR-REACT (Intracoronary Stenting and Antithrombotic Regimen: Rapid Early Action for Coronary Treatment) 3 trial (*Eur Heart J* 2010;31:582-587), bivalirudin was compared with UFH (140 U/kg, a dose in excess of current guideline recommendations and that used in the ACUITY trial) in 4,570 patients with stable or UA and normal levels of troponin T and creatine kinase myocardial band who underwent PCI. Patients randomized to bivalirudin experienced less bleeding and had similar rates of ischemic complications through 1 year compared with those who received UFH. Of note, in this trial all patients were pretreated with clopidogrel 600 mg more than 2 hours before PCI, and no GPI was used.

12.18 **Answer C.** Prasugrel is a prodrug that is metabolized to one active metabolite (R-138727) and numerous inactive metabolites. Absorption is complete and rapid, with mean time to peak plasma concentration of approximately 30 minutes for R-138727. The pharmacokinetics of prasugrel metabolites were linear and dose proportional in healthy volunteers. Median plasma half-life of the active metabolite is approximately 4 hours, and excretion is mainly urinary. Plasma clearance data suggest that prasugrel metabolism does not vary significantly among individuals. Pharmacodynamic studies have shown potent and selective P2Y$_{12}$ blockade and dose-dependent inhibition of platelet aggregation with prasugrel (or R-138727). Onset of antiplatelet action is within 30 minutes, and steady state is reached in 3 days. Inhibition of platelet aggregation by prasugrel has been shown to be more rapid, more potent (on a mg/body-weight basis), and more consistent than that with clopidogrel (*Pharmacotherapy* 2009 Sep;29(9):1089–1110).

12.19 **Answer B.** Paclitaxel is a microtubule-stabilizing agent with potent antiproliferative and antimigratory activity for multiple cell types, including fibroblasts, epithelial cells, and tumor cells (*Nature* 1979;277:665–667). The drug does not inhibit polymerization of tubulin into microtubules, but enhances microtubule assembly into stable polymerized structures. This decreases the concentration of tubulin required for new microtubule formation (*Int J Cancer* 1995;63:688–693). Microtubules are components of the cytoskeleton and mitotic spindle, being required for both cell division and motility. The activation of MAP-kinase signaling by growth factors associates with microtubule depolymerization and is inhibited by paclitaxel (*Int J Cancer* 1995;63:688–693). By stabilizing cytoplasmic microtubules and blocking microtubule disassembly, paclitaxel prevents DNA synthesis initiated by growth factors (*Exp Cell Res* 1984;155:1–8).

12.20 **Answer D.** Radial artery spasm (RAS) is frequently associated with transradial coronary access. Incidence varies around 10% and is caused by many factors. Spasm rarely leads to serious complications such as eversion atherectomy. It is commonly associated with procedural failure and patient discomfort. With "RAS" one usually means the considerable amount of friction—along with the associated patient discomfort—encountered when manipulating the arterial sheath or guide catheter in a radial artery. This friction is caused by mismatch between the outer diameter of the sheath or guide and the inner diameter of the radial artery. Several preventive measures have been described and reviewed (*J Invasive Cardiol* 2006 Apr;18:159–160). These include the use of an intra-arterial cocktail (5 mg of verapamil plus 200-g nitroglycerin in 10 mL of normal saline) described to decrease spasm when compared to placebo. A hydrophilic-coated sheath may additionally reduce the force required to remove a radial sheath. In a study comparing coating-free vs. hydrophilic coated sheaths, the latter reduced the required force and discomfort associated with removal of a radial sheath following transradial coronary intervention. A combination of an intra-arterial cocktail described above with a short (10 to 15 cm) hydrophilic sheath, reduced the clinical incidence of spasm to 5% (including patients with small arteries). Others propose the simple intra-arterial administration of nitroglycerin 100 µg together with heparin.

12.21 **Answer C.** A nondilatable lesion was identified. The patient was initially stabilized with IABP and vasopressor support. Heavy coronary calcification may not yield to balloon angioplasty and may limit stent expansion. Modifying the calcified plaque by rotational atherectomy followed by drug-eluting stenting may provide the best long-term outcome. In an observational study, at a mean follow-up period of 15 months (range 1 to 54), the total cardiac death rate was 4.9%, target lesion revascularization was 8.8%, and the incidence of MI was 3.9%. The combined end point occurred in 12.7% of cases.

DES following rotational atherectomy for heavily calcified coronary lesions is a safe and effective procedure that provides good long-term clinical outcomes (*J Invasive Cardiol* 2011 Jan;23:28–32). The combination of rotablation and DES implantation (Rota-DES) has a favorable effect on clinical and angiographic outcomes at 9 months when treating heavily calcified lesions compared to rotablation followed by BMS implantation. (*J Interven Cardiol* 2007 Apr;20:100–106).

12.22 **Answer D.** The OCT image shows plaque/thrombus protrusion through a recently implanted DES. The Harmonizing Outcomes with Revascularization and Stents in Acute Myocardial Infarction (HORIZONS-AMI) trial was a dual-arm, factorial, randomized trial comparing PES and otherwise equivalent BMS in STEMI patients. The intravascular ultrasound substudy enrolled 241 patients with 263 native coronary lesions (201 PES, 62 BMS) with baseline and 13-month follow-up imaging. At follow-up, a higher frequency of late stent malapposition was detected in PES-treated lesions (46.8%) mainly because of more late acquired stent malapposition (30.8%) compared with BMS-treated lesions. Independent predictors of late acquired stent malapposition were plaque/thrombus protrusion (OR, 5.60; 95% confidence interval [CI], 2.32 to 13.54) and PES use (OR, 6.32; 95% CI, 2.15 to 18.62).

The incidence of acute stent malapposition was similar in PES- and BMS-treated lesions, but late acquired stent malapposition was more common in PES-treated lesions. Late acquired stent malapposition was due mainly to positive remodeling and plaque/thrombus resolution. (Guo, N et al., Incidence, mechanisms, predictors, and clinical impact of acute and late stent malapposition after primary intervention in patients with acute myocardial infarction: an intravascular ultrasound substudy of the Harmonizing Outcomes with Revascularization and Stents in Acute Myocardial Infarction (HORIZONS-AMI) trial, *Circulation* 2010 Sep 14;122:1077–1084).

12.23 **Answer C.** Guiding catheter. There are no vessel wall structures seen.

12.24 **Answer F.** Evidence of thin fibrotic cap, large atheromatous burden. Most likely would provoke an acute coronary syndrome in the event of rupture.

12.25 **Answer A.** Normal anatomy with very mild atherosclerotic changes.

12.26 **Answer E.** Side branch.

12.27 **Answer B.** Unstable angina. Shows plaque rupture/dissection.

12.28 **Answer D.** Significant atheromatous burden with a decrease in mean lumen area. Most likely would be associated with stable angina.

QUESTIONS

13.1 The currently accepted maximum medical contact-to-balloon or door-to-balloon time for patients with ST-segment elevation myocardial infarction (STEMI) is:

(A) 30 minutes
(B) 60 minutes
(C) 90 minutes
(D) 120 minutes
(E) 360 minutes

13.2 A 76-year-old man presents with an acute anterior wall myocardial infarction (MI). Emergency coronary angiography reveals a completely occluded left anterior descending (LAD) artery with thrombolysis in myocardial infarction (TIMI) 0 flow (Fig. Q13-2A) and a 70% to 80% stenosis of the right coronary artery (RCA) with TIMI 3 flow (Fig. Q13-2B). Left ventriculogram shows anterolateral hypokinesis. His heart rate is 88 and blood pressure (BP) is 127/78 with an oxygen saturation of 98% on room air. Optimal management of this patient will include:

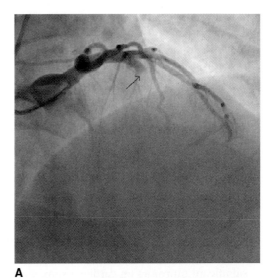

A

B

Figure Q13-2

(A) Bypass surgery because he has two-vessel disease involving the LAD artery

(B) Percutaneous coronary intervention (PCI) of the LAD artery only and consideration of PCI of the RCA at a later date (staged PCI) or non-invasive evaluation to assess RCA territory ischemia postdischarge, and PCI if indicated

(C) PCI of the LAD and the RCA

(D) PCI of the LAD and measurement of fractional flow reserve of the RCA to assess hemodymanic significance followed by PCI if indicated

13.3 A 69-year-old man presents to the emergency room of a community hospital without a PCI facility with an acute ST-segment elevation anterior wall MI. He is tachycardic and tachypneic with a heart rate of 112 and BP of 76/43 and has rales in both lung fields. Optimal management of this patient includes:

(A) Immediate administration of full-dose fibrinolysis

(B) Immediate administration of half-dose fibrinolysis with full-dose abciximab

(C) Immediate administration of half-dose abciximab with full-dose fibrinolysis

(D) Arrangement for transfer to the nearest hospital with PCI facility that is 70 minutes away

13.4 A 68-year-old woman presents to your office for evaluation of chest discomfort she had the previous evening. The discomfort lasted for approximately 30 to 40 minutes and subsequently resolved. Currently, she is pain free with a heart rate of 74 and a BP of 118/71. Her lungs are clear to auscultation and you do not hear any significant murmurs on cardiac exam. Electrocardiogram (ECG) reveals an evolving STEMI. On further questioning, she states discomfort started at approximately 7:00 PM last evening and lasted till 7:45 PM or so. It is now 10:00 AM the next morning. Appropriate management would include:

(A) Admission to the hospital and treatment with aspirin, heparin, clopidogrel, statins, and β-blockers

(B) Admission to the cardiac catheterization laboratory for emergency angiography with a goal of primary PCI

(C) Administration of full-dose fibrinolysis, admission to hospital, and treatment with aspirin, heparin, clopidogrel, statins, and β-blockers

(D) Administration of full-dose fibrinolytics and then admission to the catheterization laboratory for emergency angiography

13.5 Transfer of patients with STEMI to a PCI-capable center rather than immediate fibrinolysis should be considered in all of the following situations, EXCEPT:

(A) When fibrinolytic therapy is contraindicated or unsuccessful

(B) When cardiogenic shock ensues

(C) When the anticipated delay to PCI is 90 to 120 minutes

(D) When symptoms have been present for > 2 to 3 hours

13.6 In patients with STEMI, compared with fibrinolysis, primary PCI lowers the (relative) odds of death at 1 year by:

(A) 5%

(B) 10%

(C) 15%

(D) 20%

(E) 25%

13.7 The role of embolic protection devices in primary PCI is BEST characterized as being:

(A) Strongly recommended for all patients undergoing primary PCI (Class I recommendation)

(B) Strongly recommended for primary PCI only in patients with large thrombus burden (Class I recommendation)

(C) Currently not recommended for primary PCI

(D) Recommended for patients with no reflow after PCI

13.8 A 67-year-old man undergoes bypass surgery for severe three-vessel coronary artery disease. Approximately 12 hours after the surgery he becomes short of breath and has 3-mm ST elevation in the inferolateral leads. The BEST management strategy at this time is:

(A) Conservative management without coronary angiography

(B) Coronary angiography, intending to manage the patient with a catheter-based treatment strategy (i.e., immediate PCI)

(C) Coronary angiography, intending to manage the patient with a surgical-based treatment strategy (i.e., emergency redo coronary artery bypass graft surgery)

(D) Coronary angiography followed by conservative treatment

13.9 Predictors of 1-year mortality among 30-day survivors after primary PCI include all, EXCEPT:

(A) Age > 70 years

(B) Any tachyarrhythmia during index hospital-ization (defined as ventricular or supraven-tricular tachycardia that required treatment)

(C) Weight < 80 kg

(D) Number of diseased coronary arteries

(E) Left ventricular ejection fraction (LVEF)

(F) Female gender

13.10 Among patients undergoing primary PCI, out-comes are BEST in those who are:

(A) Underweight or thin (body mass index [BMI] < 18 kg/m²)

(B) Normal weight (BMI < 25 kg/m²)

(C) Overweight (≥25 to <30 kg/m²)

(D) Obese (≥30 kg/m²)

13.11 A 44-year-old man presents with chest heaviness and 0.5-mm ST-segment elevation in ECG leads I and aVL. Coronary angiogram is performed (Fig. Q13-11). The most likely etiology of his chest pain is:

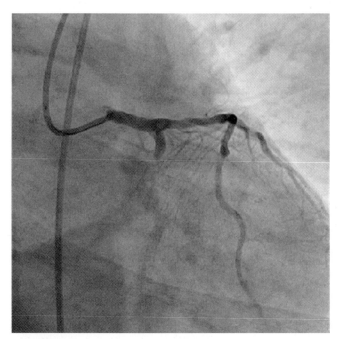

Figure Q13-11

(A) Pericarditis

(B) Occluded coronary artery

(C) Anomalous coronary artery

(D) Kawasaki's disease

(E) Congenital coronary artery fistula

13.12 A 63-year-old woman presents with an acute STEMI. Emergency coronary angiography reveals a completely occluded RCA with large thrombus burden (Fig. Q13-12). Optimal management of this lesion includes:

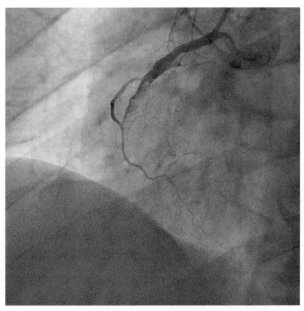

Figure Q13-12

(A) Rheolytic thrombectomy

(B) Emboli protection device

(C) Balloon angioplasty followed by stenting

(D) Medical therapy

13.13 A 57-year-old man presents with an acute ante-rior wall MI. The patient is administered aspirin, clopidogrel, and abciximab and undergoes emer-gency coronary angiography (Fig. Q13-13). The BEST management strategy in this individual is:

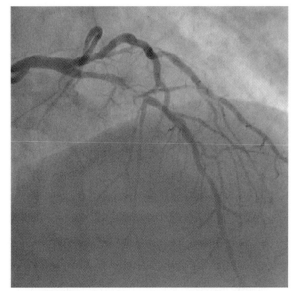

Figure Q13-13

(A) Balloon angioplasty

(B) Fibrinolytic therapy followed by PCI in 3 to 4 days

(C) Bare-metal stent (BMS) implantation

(D) Drug-eluting stent (DES) implantation

13.14 A 34-year-old woman lawyer presents with chest discomfort after a particularly challenging tennis match. ECG reveals a 1-mm ST-segment elevation in leads II, III, and aVF. An emergency coronary angiogram is performed (Fig. Q13-14). The most likely etiology of her chest pain is:

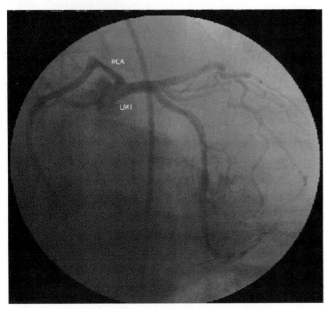

Figure Q13-14

(A) Anomalous coronary artery

(B) Musculoskeletal chest pain

(C) Coronary artery dissection

(D) Coronary embolus

13.15 You are asked to consult on an 83-year-old woman for possible PCI. Eight days ago, she was admitted to the hospital with chest pain and ST elevation in leads V2 to V4. She was diagnosed with an acute anterior MI. However, she was not given thrombolytic therapy because of her history of stroke 4 months before admission and she refused cardiac catheterization. She was treated with aspirin, heparin, clopidogrel, simvastatin, metoprolol, and lisinopril. She responded well to the treatment, and her chest pain eventually resolved. Her ECG now has Q waves in the anterior leads. She has been free of chest pain since hospital day 1 and hemodynamically stable without any arrhythmias. Her echocardiogram on hospital day 4 was unremarkable except for anterior wall hypokinesis and LVEF of 35%. Her physician son has come in from out of town

and wants her to undergo cardiac catheterization and possible PCI. What will be the effect of delayed PCI of a persistently occluded IRA in this setting?

(A) Delayed PCI will result in long-term improvement in the LVEF, greater freedom from adverse in-hospital clinical events, and a reduced incidence of long-term MI and death from CAD

(B) Delayed PCI will result in long-term improvement in the LVEF and greater freedom from adverse in-hospital clinical events but will not decrease the incidence of subsequent MI or death from CAD

(C) There are no convincing data to support the routine use of late PCI days after MI in patients who did not receive reperfusion therapy

(D) There are no convincing data to support the routine use of late PCI days after MI in patients who did not receive reperfusion therapy, but it does reduce recurrent angina

13.16 A 61-year-old woman is brought to the emergency room by paramedics with chest pain for 2 hours. She is found to have ST elevation anteriorly. Her initial BP is 95/60 with a heart rate of 100. The closest hospital with an interventional catheterization laboratory is 2 hours away. Which of the following options is the most appropriate initial strategy?

(A) Reteplase plus abciximab and transfer for PCI only if ongoing chest pain

(B) Abciximab alone with subsequent transfer for PCI

(C) Reteplase with transfer for PCI as soon as possible

(D) Half-dose reteplase plus abciximab and transfer for PCI

13.17 Each community should develop a STEMI system of care that follows standards at least as stringent as those developed for the AHA's national initiative (Mission: Lifeline) to include which of the following?

(A) Multidisciplinary team meetings

(B) A process for prehospital identification and activation

(C) Destination protocols for STEMI receiving centers

(D) Transfer protocols for patients arriving at STEMI referral centers

(E) All of the above

13.18 A 52-year-old woman with cardiac risk factors including diabetes, hypertension, and tobacco use presents with an acute inferior MI. She is hemodynamically stable. Emergency cardiac catheterization reveals diffuse (but non–flow restricting) disease in the left coronary distribution. A right coronary guide is advanced, and the first image of the RCA documents a 3.5-mm vessel with a proximal occlusion just past the first bend in the RCA. You request a coronary guidewire and what additional interventional device?

(A) 3.0-mm balloon
(B) 3.5-mm balloon
(C) 3.5-mm stent
(D) Aspiration catheter
(E) End-hole infusion catheter

13.19 A 71-year-old man is admitted to the hospital after promptly receiving a fibrinolytic agent, heparin, aspirin, and clopidogrel for an inferior wall MI. Primary angioplasty was not performed because the catheterization laboratory was not readily available at 2:00 AM when he presented. The patient's chest pain gradually resolved over several hours, and you see him later that morning when making rounds. He remains free of chest pain though he complains of dyspnea. His BP is 110/68, with a pulse rate of 92 and a respiratory rate of 20. On physical examination, a third heart sound is faintly heard, and crackles are noted over the lower third of the posterior lung fields. Although he is free of chest pain, you decide to urgently send him for coronary angiography. In the catheterization laboratory, the RCA is found to be completely occluded with faint left-to-right collateral. No other severe coronary artery disease is noted, and the LVEF is 40% to 45%. Which of the following would be the appropriate treatment?

(A) The MI is completed, therefore place a Swan-Ganz catheter and return the patient to the intensive care unit for diuretic therapy and initiation of angiotensin-converting enzyme inhibitors
(B) Perform PCI and give an appropriate anticoagulant plus antiplatelet agent
(C) Begin intravenous IIb/IIIa inhibition and have the patient return tomorrow for follow-up angiography and possible PCI
(D) Consult cardiothoracic surgery for consideration of bypass grafting to the RCA

13.20 The Middlesbrough Early Revascularization to Limit INfarction (MERLIN) trial enrolled 307 patients with STEMI and failed thrombolytic therapy. They were randomized to an emergency coronary angiography with or without rescue PCI, or to conservative treatment. Thirty-day all-cause mortality was similar in the rescue and conservative groups. According to the subgroup analysis, which group had the highest rate of 30-day all-cause mortality?

(A) Rescue PCI with resolution of ST elevation
(B) Rescue PCI without resolution of ST elevation
(C) Conservative therapy with resolution of ST elevation
(D) Conservative therapy without resolution of ST elevation

13.21 In the REACT trial, patients presenting with failed pharmacologic reperfusion therapy were randomized to repeat thrombolysis, conservative therapy, or rescue PCI. Which of the following best describes the statistical findings of this study?

(A) Significant reduction in all-cause mortality with rescue PCI compared with repeat thrombolysis
(B) A several fold reduction in recurrent MI with rescue PCI vs. repeat thrombolytic therapy
(C) More cerebrovascular accidents and major bleeding events in the rescue PCI group compared with the other groups
(D) Highest cost associated with PCI

13.22 Nearly 20 years ago, the TIMI 2 investigators randomized patients with STEMI receiving thrombolytic therapy to immediate vs. delayed (18 to 48 hours) angiography and possible angioplasty (TIMI 2A phase, $n = 391$). They observed a similar rate of mortality between the two groups though a higher rate of bleeding among those randomized to early catheterization. Recently, the ASSENT-4 investigators performed a similar study whereby patients unable to promptly (1 to 3 hours) undergo primary PCI were randomized to standard PCI or to PCI preceded by full-dose tenecteplase. With 1,320 patients enrolled, what did the ASSENT-4 investigators observe among patients randomized to the facilitated strategy of routine PCI urgently after thrombolytic therapy?

(A) Similar mortality and similar non-central nervous system (CNS) major bleeding rates
(B) Higher mortality and similar non-CNS major bleeding rates
(C) Similar mortality and higher non-CNS major bleeding rates
(D) Higher mortality and higher non-CNS major bleeding rates

13.23 A 34-year-old woman who had a healthy baby 12 days prior via spontaneous vaginal delivery develops unrelenting substernal chest pain while doing the laundry. She presents to the emergency department 90 minutes later where she is found to be hypotensive with a BP of 82/44 and a pulse of 120. ECG documents 8-mm anterior ST elevation. The STEMI team is activated and she undergoes emergency cardiac catheterization documenting a 100% occlusion of the proximal LAD with TIMI 0 flow. A guidewire easily crosses the occlusion, almost immediately restoring antegrade perfusion. A hazy linear filling defect with residual thrombus is apparent. The reference vessel diameter proximal to the lesion is approximately 3.4 mm, and the coronary vessel both proximal and distal to the filling defect appears clean and free of disease. What is the appropriate next step?

(A) Aspiration thrombectomy, followed by stent implantation

(B) Intracoronary injection of nitroglycerin to improve distal perfusion and more accurately assess the reference vessel diameter

(C) Administration of a β-blocker, aspirin, clopidogrel, and a platelet glycoprotein IIb/IIIa inhibitor, with no intervention planned

(D) Direct stent implantation

13.24 According to the 2009 ACC/AHA guidelines for the management of patients with STEMI, which of the following clinical scenarios is the most appropriate for immediate primary PCI?

(A) A 77-year-old female with 4 hours of chest pain and 2-mm of anterior ST elevation

(B) A 67-year-old man with 8 hours of chest pain and 3-mm of inferior ST elevation

(C) An 80-year-old female with chest pain that started 2 hours ago and a new LBBB

(D) A 76-year-old man with ongoing chest pain for the last 14 hours with 4-mm ST elevation in leads V2 to V6

13.25 You have been recruited by a growing community hospital to assist them in improving their hospital quality standards and to establish a "24/7" primary PCI program. The hospital does not have a cardiothoracic surgeon on staff. Which of the following recommendations is most appropriate?

(A) The hospital's catheterization laboratory must perform at least 150 PCI procedures per year, of which at least 36 are primary PCI for STEMI

(B) The hospital's catheterization laboratory must perform at least 200 PCI procedures per year, of which at least 36 are primary PCI for STEMI, but cardiac surgery backup is not essential

(C) Each interventional cardiologist credentialed to perform primary PCI at the hospital must have an annual volume of ≥75 PCI procedures (ideally with ≥11 primary PCIs for STEMI) and plans for immediate on-site cardiothoracic surgical support should be made

(D) Each interventional cardiologist credentialed to perform primary PCI at the hospital must have an annual volume of ≥75 PCI procedures (ideally with ≥11 primary PCIs for STEMI) and plans for rapid transportation to a regional cardiothoracic surgical facility must be in place should the need arise

13.26 A 65-year-old man presents with 2 hours of crushing substernal chest pressure to the emergency room. ECG reveals complete AV block and ST elevation in leads I, II, III, aVF, aVL, and V5 to V6. On physical examination, he is cool, diaphoretic, and hypotensive with a systolic BP 80 mm Hg. Appropriate pharmacotherapy is administered and you place a transvenous pacemaker and perform emergency coronary angiography. This reveals a RCA that is occluded in its midportion, normal left main and LAD arteries, and an occluded mid circumflex artery. Which of the following is the best therapeutic option?

(A) IABP placement and referral for bypass surgery

(B) Primary PCI of the circumflex artery with staged PCI of the RCA in 30 days

(C) Primary PCI of the RCA, followed by attempted PCI of the LCX artery if chest pain and hemodynamic instability continue after RCA PCI

(D) Primary PCI of the RCA only, with IABP support for continued chest pain and hemodynamic instability after RCA PCI

13.27 A 46-year-old woman with Stage IV pancreatic cancer presents with 10/10 chest pain and 2-mm ST elevation in leads I and aVL to a local community hospital that does not have primary PCI capability. She receives full-dose thrombolytic therapy, and 90 minutes later has 60% resolution of ST segments with (2/10) residual chest pain. The emergency room physician treating the patient consults you for further management. You recommend:

(A) Repeat thrombolysis at half dose

(B) Immediate transfer to the nearest catheter-ization laboratory for coronary angiography and rescue PCI if needed

(C) Heparin bolus followed by infusion and gly-coprotein IIb/IIIa inhibition

(D) Conservative management and usual post-MI care

13.28 A 54-year-old type 1 diabetic (HbA1c 7%) without other known medical problems presents with an acute anterior ST elevation MI. He is a Medicaid-receiving patient. Following emergency coronary angiography and subsequent thrombus aspira-tion of the LAD artery, you are about to select a stent. Assessment of the proximal LAD lesion by quantitative coronary angiography suggests a reference vessel diameter of 2.4 mm and lesion length of at least 15 mm. Which of the following devices is most appropriate?

(A) 2.5- × 15-mm BMS

(B) 2.5- × 18-mm BMS

(C) 2.5- × 18-mm DES

(D) 2.25- × 18-mm DES

13.29 An emergency room physician calls you about a 72-year-old female with diabetes mellitus, hyper-tension, and a history of embolic stroke 2 years ago, who has presented to the emergency room with several hours of crushing substernal chest discomfort. Physical examination reveals a thin woman (weight 58 kg) with ongoing chest pain, tachycardia (rate 110), and BP 100/70 mm Hg. ECG demonstrates ST elevation in the anterior precordial leads. The ER physician has already given aspirin 325 mg, morphine 2 mg IV, and a heparin bolus and has started a nitroglycerin drip. He is now asking for advice on which thi-enopyridine regimen you would like the patient to receive before you perform cardiac catheter-ization. You recommend:

(A) Prasugrel 60-mg loading dose, followed by 10 mg daily

(B) Clopidogrel 75 mg daily

(C) Prasugrel 10 mg daily

(D) Clopidogrel 600-mg loading dose, followed by 75 mg daily

13.30 All of the following are absolute contraindi-cations to thrombolytic therapy for STEMI, EXCEPT:

(A) History of intracranial hemorrhage

(B) Intrascapular pain associated with hypoten-sion and >60 mm Hg BP differential between the left and the right arm

(C) Bronchial carcinoma with intracranial meta-static disease

(D) Traumatic and prolonged cardiopulmonary resuscitation lasting >30 minutes

(E) Significant facial trauma 2 weeks ago

13.31 A 47-year-old male presents with chest pain to his local community ER. A 12-lead ECG shows 4-mm ST elevation in the inferior leads. He is tachycardic and his systolic BP is 90 mm Hg. The nearest PCI facilities are 3 hours away. What is the next most appropriate step in the manage-ment of this patient?

(A) Full-dose thrombolysis followed by transfer to the nearest PCI facility only if ongoing chest pain or <50% resolution of the ST seg-ments at 60 to 90 minutes

(B) Full-dose thrombolysis followed by immedi-ate transfer to the nearest PCI facility

(C) Half-dose thrombolysis plus abciximab fol-lowed by PCI

(D) Full-dose abciximab followed by PCI

13.32 A 47-year-old single male truck driver presents to the emergency room. You initially saw him 2 years ago in clinic, at which time you advised him to return for follow-up after prescribing anti-hypertensive medication and a lipid-lowering agent. His BMI at that time was 42. Your records show that he has missed multiple appointments and has not returned phone calls from your office. In the ER, it becomes evident that he is having an acute inferior wall MI. You take him to the catheterization laboratory, where he has a proximal occlusion of a large, dominant RCA. One pass with an aspiration thrombectomy device is performed restoring TIMI 2 flow and revealing a focal lesion with a large amount of residual thrombus. The distal vessel size is approximately 3.3 mm. What is the most appro-priate next step in this patient's management?

(A) 3.5-mm BMS deployed without predilatation

(B) 3.0-mm DES deployed at high pressure and grown to 3.5 mm

(C) Additional aspiration thrombectomy followed by 3.0-mm BMS

(D) Additional aspiration thrombectomy followed by 3.5-mm DES

(E) Additional aspiration thrombectomy followed by 3.5-mm BMS

13.33 You are asked to see a 68-year-old female who describes an episode of chest pressure, which radiated to her jaw, diaphoresis, and shortness of breath that occurred 29 hours ago at home.

She did not seek medical attention at the time but now presents to the ER at the insistence of her husband. She is currently pain free with an ECG that demonstrates normal sinus rhythm with 2-mm ST elevation in leads II, III, and aVF and pathologic Q waves. Her BP is 110/70 mm Hg and her O_2 saturations are 98% on room air. You recommend diagnostic angiography, which demonstrates a RCA that is occluded in its mid segment with some left to right collaterals. She is also found to have an 80% lesion in her mid LAD. What is the most appropriate next step in the management of this patient?

(A) Aspiration thrombectomy of the RCA followed by PCI
(B) Balloon angioplasty followed by stenting of the LAD
(C) Medical management
(D) Aspiration thrombectomy of the RCA followed by PCI of RCA and LAD

13.34 In the TRANSFER-AMI trial, 1,059 high-risk STEMI patients who presented to a non-PCI hospital and were treated with tenectaplase thrombolysis within 12 hours of chest pain were randomized to either urgent transfer for cardiac catheterization (PCI within 6 hours after fibrinolysis) or to standard care (transfer for rescue and/or urgent PCI or for routine catheterization after 24 hours). Patients were eligible for inclusion in the study either if they had ST-segment elevation of ≥2 mm in two anterior leads or if they had ST-segment elevation of ≥1 mm in two inferior leads and at least one of the predefined high-risk characteristics. High-risk features in this trial included all of the following, EXCEPT:

(A) Systolic BP < 100 mm Hg
(B) Prior CABG
(C) Killip Class 2 or 3
(D) Heart rate > 100 bpm
(E) ≥2-mm anterior ST depression or ≥1-mm ST elevation in V_4R

13.35 In patients with STEMI with known chronic kidney disease (not on hemodialysis) undergoing coronary angiography for primary PCI, which of the following contrast media is recommended?

(A) Ioxaglate
(B) Iohexol
(C) Iodixanol
(D) A nonionic hyperosmolal agent
(E) An ionic hyperosmolal agent

ANSWERS AND EXPLANATIONS

13.1 **Answer C.** The 2005 ACC/AHA guidelines recommend that PCI for acute STEMI should be performed as quickly as possible, with a goal of a medical contact-to-balloon or door-to-balloon time within 90 minutes (*J Am Coll Cardiol* 2006;47:216–235). This recommendation has not been revised in the most recent 2009 Focused Updates of the STEMI/PCI guidelines (*J Am Coll Cardiol* 2009;54:2205–2241). Time from symptom onset to reperfusion remains an important predictor of patient outcome even with PCI.

13.2 **Answer B.** The 2005 ACC/AHA guidelines clearly state that elective PCI should not be performed in a non–infarct-related artery at the time of primary PCI of the infarct-related artery in patients without hemodynamic compromise and is considered a contraindication (*J Am Coll Cardiol* 2006;47:216–235). This recommendation has not been revised in the most recent 2009 Focused Updates of the STEMI/PCI guidelines (*J Am Coll Cardiol* 2009;54:2205–2241). The elective PCI of the noninfarct artery may actually worsen the outcomes in this setting. Although bypass surgery is an alternative in elective patients with severe multivessel disease, particularly diabetes, waiting for bypass is not an option in this patient with an occluded LAD artery and a large amount of myocardium at jeopardy.

13.3 **Answer D.** Primary PCI should be performed for patients younger than 75 years old with ST elevation or presumed new left bundle-branch block (LBBB) who develop shock within 36 hours of MI and are suitable for revascularization that can be performed within 18 hours of shock, unless further support is futile because of the patient's wishes or contraindications/unsuitability for further invasive care (*J Am Coll Cardiol* 2006;47:216–235). PCI appears to have its greatest mortality benefit in high-risk patients. In patients with cardiogenic shock, an absolute 9% reduction in 30-day mortality with mechanical revascularization instead of immediate medical stabilization was reported in the SHOCK trial (*N Engl J Med* 1999;341:625–634). Fibrinolysis is not very effective in patients with cardiogenic shock, and there are no data to support combination therapy in these patients. Consideration

should be given to the placement of an intraaortic balloon pump (IABP) before transfer if feasible.

13.4 **Answer A.** 2005 guidelines state that primary PCI should not be performed in asymptomatic patients who are hemodynamically and electrically stable more than 12 hours after the onset of STEMI (*J Am Coll Cardiol* 2006;47:216–235). This recommendation has not been revised in the most recent 2009 Focused Updates of the STEMI/PCI guidelines (*J Am Coll Cardiol* 2009;54:2205–2241). She should be admitted for management of MI and be referred for semielective cardiac catheterization. However, she does not meet criteria for either emergency cardiac catheterization or fibrinolytic therapy for management of an acute STEMI.

13.5 **Answer C.** The time from symptom onset to reperfusion is an important predictor of patient outcome. After adjustment for baseline characteristics, the time from symptom onset to balloon inflation is significantly correlated with 1-year mortality in patients undergoing primary PCI for STEMI (relative risk of 1.08 for each 30-minute delay from symptom onset to balloon inflation, $p = 0.04$) (*Circulation* 2004;109:1223–1225). Delays in door-to-balloon time vs. door-to-needle time of >60 minutes because of interhospital transfer might actually negate the potential mortality benefit of transfer for primary PCI over immediate intravenous fibrinolysis demonstrated in these trials (*Am J Cardiol* 2003;92:824–826). Transfer of patients to PCI-capable centers should be considered when fibrinolytic therapy is contraindicated or unsuccessful, when cardiogenic shock ensues, when the anticipated delay is <60 minutes, or when the symptoms have been present for >2 to 3 hours.

13.6 **Answer E.** Primary PCI with stenting has been compared with fibrinolytic therapy in 12 randomized clinical trials. These investigations demonstrate that PCI-treated patients experience lower mortality rates (5.9% vs. 7.7%, OR 0.75, 95% CI 0.60 to 0.94, $p = 0.013$), fewer reinfarctions (1.6% vs. 5.1%, OR 0.31, 95% CI 0.21 to 0.44, $p = 0.0001$), and fewer hemorrhagic strokes than those treated by fibrinolysis (Fig. A13-6) (*Lancet*

2003;361:13–20). Compared with percutaneous transluminal coronary angioplasty alone, intracoronary stents achieve a better immediate angiographic result with a larger arterial lumen, less reclosure of the infarct-related artery, and fewer subsequent ischemic events.

with acute perioperative myocardial ischemia because of early graft failure following CABG (*Eur J Cardiothorac Surg* 2006). When technically feasible, percutaneous revascularization of the native coronary vessel affected by the acutely occluded graft vessel should be considered.

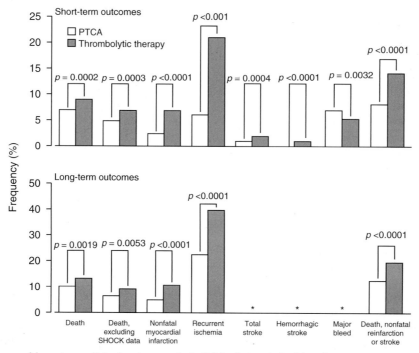

Figure A13-6.   Short-term and long-term clinical outcomes in individuals treated with primary percutaneous coronary interventions vs. fibrinolytic therapy. (Adapted from Keely EC, Boura JA, Grines CL. Primary angioplasty versus intravenous thrombolytic therapy for acute myocardial infarction: a quantitative review of 23 randomised trials. *Lancet* 2003;361:13–20.)

13.7   **Answer C.** Embolic protection devices have not shown benefit in the setting of primary PCI for STEMI, as noted in the Enhanced Myocardial Efficacy and Recovery by Aspiration of Liberated Debris (EMERALD) trial (GuardWire) (*JAMA* 2005;293:1063–1072). The subsequent trials such as the PCI Treatment of Myocardial Infarction for Salvage of Endangered Myocardium (PROMISE) study have also failed to show benefit with these devices (*Circulation* 2005;112:1462–1469). Embolic protection devices are not currently recommended for native-vessel primary PCI.

13.8   **Answer B.** The best approach to managing acute graft failure after CABG has been unclear for some time. However, a 2006 study compared primary PCI, emergency reoperation, and conservative therapy in a cohort of patients who developed an acute MI shortly after bypass surgery. The study reported that re-revascularization with emergency PCI may limit the extent of myocardial cellular damage compared with the surgical-based treatment strategy in patients

13.9   **Answer F.** An analysis from the CADILLAC trial using a multivariate logistic regression model identified age > 70 years (OR, 3.3; 95% CI, 1.9 to 5.7), weight < 80 kg (OR, 1.9; 95% CI, 1.1 to 3.6), any tachyarrhythmia during index hospitalization (defined as ventricular or supraventricular tachycardia that required treatment) (OR, 2.4; 95% CI, 1.2 to 4.8), number of diseased coronary arteries (OR, 1.5; 95% CI, 1.1 to 2.1), and LVEF (each 10% decrease, OR, 1.5; 95% CI, 1.2 to 1.8) as factors independently associated with risk of death at 1 year among 30-day survivors. Female gender was not a multivariate predictor of outcomes (*Am J Cardiol* 2006;97:817–822).

13.10   **Answer C.** A recent study analyzed the impact of BMI on the outcome of patients with AMI. Obese patients compared with normal-weight patients had lower V-hospital mortality (0.9% vs. 2.7%, *p* = 0.03) at 30 days (1.1% vs. 3.8%, *p* = 0.02) and 1 year (1.8% vs. 7.5%, *p* < 0.0001). Obese patients with AMI have an improved prognosis after primary PCI compared with normal-weight patients, a finding most likely related to AMI onset at younger age, with better renal function and less anterior infarction (*Am Heart J* 2006;151:168–175).

13.11 **Answer B.** The coronary angiogram reveals acute occlusion of the left circumflex (LCX) artery consistent with his symptoms and a (relatively) electrocardiographically silent lateral MI. ECG changes are often subtle in patients with LCX artery disease. Although pericarditis should be considered in the differential diagnosis of chest pain in a relatively young individual, the presence of an occluded coronary artery rules out this diagnosis. The angiogram does not reveal any coronary anomalies or arteriovenous fistula. Patients with Kawasaki's disease are younger and typically have coronary artery aneurysms rather than occlusions.

13.12 **Answer C.** There is no consistent evidence that rheolytic (AngioJet) thrombectomy or the emboli protection devices are useful in native coronary arteries with thrombus. A study conducted using AngioJet in acute STEMI failed to demonstrate a reduction in infarct size or other improvement in clinical outcome measures (the AngioJet Rheolytic Thrombectomy in Patients Undergoing Primary Angioplasty for STEMI [AiMI] trial). Regarding embolic protection devices, neither the EMERALD nor PROMISE trials demonstrated a benefit in thrombus-containing native coronary arteries. Of note, several trials of thrombus aspiration have been positive, and this should be strongly considered whenever technically feasible and meta-analysis has supported aspiration thrombectomy (*Eur Heart J* 2008;29;3002–3010). Regardless, an attempt at revascularization is indicated in all patients with STEMI and medical therapy alone would not be appropriate in this situation.

13.13 **Answer D.** Available data suggest that compared with conventional BMS, DES implantations are not associated with increased risk when used for primary PCI in patients with STEMI. Postprocedure vessel patency, biomarker release, and the incidence of short-term adverse events were similar in patients receiving sirolimus-eluting stent (SES) or BMS. Thirty-day event rates of death, reinfarction, or revascularization were 7.5% vs. 10.4%, respectively ($p = 0.4$) (*J Am Coll Cardiol* 2004;43:704–708). Hofma et al. reported the safety and efficacy of currently available DES in patients with acute MI and demonstrated that there were no significant differences in major adverse cardiac outcomes-free survival at 1 year between SES and paclitaxel-eluting stents for the treatment of AMI with very low rates of reintervention for restenosis with both (*Heart* 2005;91:1176–1180). In this patient with a relatively proximal LAD artery stenosis, absent a contraindication, a DES rather than BMS or balloon angioplasty is the best option. There is no reason to administer fibrinolytic therapy after performing coronary angiography in this patient.

13.14 **Answer A.** The angiogram reveals an anomalous RCA. Subsequent CT angiogram revealed a

Table A13-14. Common Coronary Artery Anomalies and their Potential Clinical Manifestations

Coronary Artery Anomaly	Incidence (%)	Potential Clinical Manifestations
Separate origin of the LAD and LCX	0.31	—
Ectopic origin of the LCX from the RCA	0.25	—
Ectopic origin of the LCX from the right sinus	0.13	—
Myocardial bridge	0.11	UA, AMI, MA, SD
Ectopic origin of the LCA from the right sinus	0.098	UA, AMI, MA, SD
Single coronary artery	0.098	SA, UA, SD
Atresic coronary artery	0.039	SI
Dual LAD type IV	0.039	—
Ectopic origin of the RCA from the left sinus	0.039	UA, AMI, MA, SD
Coronary artery fistula	0.039	HF, UA, AMI, SYC
Ectopic origin of the RCA from the PA	0.020	SD
Ectopic origin of the LCA from the PA	0.020	HF, SA, UA
Total	1.21	

LAD, left anterior descending coronary artery; LCX, left circumflex coronary artery; RCA, right coronary artery; UA, unstable angina; AMI, acute myocardial infarction; MA, malignant arrhythmias; SD, sudden death; LCA, left coronary artery; SA, stable angina; SI, silent ischemia; HF, heart failure; SYC, syncope; PA, pulmonary artery.

course between the aorta and pulmonary artery. She developed ST-segment elevation on vigorous exercise with a treadmill. Table A13-14 lists the common congenital coronary anomalies and their clinical manifestations.

13.15 **Answer C.** There are no data to support the routine use of late (days to weeks) PCI days after MI in patients who did not receive reperfusion therapy. This patient had her event 8 days ago and is now stable without recurrent ischemic symptoms, hemodynamic compromise, or arrhythmia. Specifically, the Occluded Artery Trial documented no difference, with a trend toward harm, in stable patients post-STEMI who were randomized to reperfusion of an occluded artery 3 to 30 days following the STEMI. Cardiac catheterization is thus not indicated in this patient (*N Engl J Med* 2006;355:2395–2407).

13.16 **Answer C.** Based on results from the FINESSE trial (*N Engl J Med* 2008;358:2205–2217), the use of a facilitated pharmacologic strategy for reperfusion, with either abciximab alone or abciximab plus reduced-dose reteplase, in anticipation of urgent PCI for patients with STEMI, did not improve clinical outcomes. Primary PCI with abciximab administered in the catheterization laboratory provided a better benefit-to-risk ratio than the two facilitated strategies among patients with STEMI who underwent PCI within 4 hours after the first medical contact.

It is worth noting that the 2007 STEMI Focused Update (*J Am Coll Cardiol* 2008;51:210–247) described several strategies for reperfusion, among them *facilitated* PCI and *rescue* PCI. These terms are no longer used for the recommendations in the most recent guideline update (*J Am Coll Cardiol* 2009;54:2205–2241), so that the contemporary therapeutic choices that lead to reperfusion as part of the treatment of patients presenting with STEMI can be described without these potentially misleading labels.

13.17 **Answer E.** The 2009 STEMI/PCI Guidelines (*J Am Coll Cardiol* 2009;54:2205–2241) underline the importance of regional systems of STEMI care to include encouraging the participation of key stakeholders in collaborative efforts to evaluate care, measuring outcomes and adherence to evidence-based processes (Class I recommendation). The AHA has also promoted its "Mission: Lifeline" initiative, which was developed to encourage closer cooperation and trust among prehospital emergency services and cardiac care professionals.

13.18 **Answer D.** A series of clinical trials have documented that manual intracoronary aspiration thrombectomy with various devices such as the Export and Pronto systems improves myocardial perfusion during primary PCI for acute STEMI. A key trial is the TAPAS trial (*N Engl J Med* 2008;358:557), with a recent meta-analysis documenting an overall survival benefit (*Eur Heart J* 2008;29:2989–3001), resulting in a Class IIa recommendation for the performance of aspiration thrombectomy as the first treatment device in primary PCI.

13.19 **Answer B.** According to the 2009 joint STEMI/PCI Focused Update Recommendations (*J Am Coll Cardiol* 2009;54:2205–2241), it is reasonable for high-risk patients who receive fibrinolytic therapy as primary reperfusion therapy to undergo early PCI with an appropriate antithrombotic regimen. The most recent trials to support this recommendation include the CARESS-in-AMI trial (*Lancet* 2008;371:559–568) and the TRANSFER-AMI trial (*N Engl J Med* 2009;360:2705–2718), both of which defined patients with Killip class II as high risk.

13.20 **Answer B.** As has been reported in previous post hoc analyses of primary angioplasty studies, patients who undergo emergency PCI for AMI and who do not achieve TIMI 3 flow or do not have resolution of their ST-segment elevation have a particularly poor outcome. In the MERLIN trial, patients undergoing rescue PCI who failed to have resolution of their ST-segment elevation had a 30-day all-cause mortality of 20% as compared with 6% for those who were treated conservatively, but who attained resolution of their ST-segment elevation, and compared with 3% for those who had rescue PCI and also attained resolution of their ST-segment elevation. It is not clear which pharmacologic adjuncts may best benefit patients at increased risk for failed reperfusion following rescue angioplasty. Several small trials have shown benefit from intracoronary vasodilators such as nitroprusside, while others have shown improved reperfusion with the use of intravenous GP IIb/IIIa inhibitors. In the MERLIN trial, only 3% of patients undergoing rescue angioplasty received a GP IIb/IIIa inhibitor, and 12% were treated with an IABP.

13.21 **Answer B.** Although the rescue PCI group did have a numerically lower rate of all-cause mortality compared with repeat thrombolysis (6.2% vs.

12.7%),this did not reach statistical significance. On the other hand, there was a significantly lower rate of recurrent MI and a halving of the composite of death, repeat MI, stroke, and severe heart failure (15.3% vs. 31.0%) with PCI vs. repeat thrombolytic therapy. There was no difference in the rate of stroke or major bleeding among the groups. The REACT study did not assess the financial implications of the treatment groups (*N Engl J Med* 2005;353:2758-2768).

13.22 **Answer B.** Early and late follow-up in the TIMI 2 study (*JAMA* 1988;260:2849-2858; *J Am Coll Cardiol* 1993;22:1763-1772) showed similar mortality between the treatment groups randomized to aggressive vs. conservative strategies. The higher bleeding rates, particularly in TIMI 2A portion of the study, resulted from the close time pairing of the thrombolytic therapy and the relatively large arterial access sheaths (≥8 F) used in the TIMI 2 era. More recently, with the use of smaller access sheaths and newer thrombolytic regimens, it was hoped that bleeding and mortality would be improved with a contemporary facilitated PCI approach among patients unable to quickly undergo primary PCI. The ASSENT-4 study (*Lancet* 2006;367:543-546) was discontinued well before the planned enrollment of 4,000 patients because of a higher mortality rate in the group undergoing facilitated PCI (6% vs. 3%). Several other adverse end points (e.g., reinfarctions, stroke, and repeat revascularization) were also higher in the facilitated PCI group though the rate of non-CNS major bleeding was similar in both the groups.

13.23 **Answer C.** This is a classic presentation for spontaneous coronary dissection without significant atherosclerotic coronary disease. Coronary intervention, even if performed by direct stent implantation, can cause propagation of the dissection and is relatively contraindicated. With restoration of flow, even aspiration thrombectomy is not needed. The appropriate course of management is medical therapy, particularly focusing on reducing the workload of the heart and the propensity for rethrombosis. Depending on the recovery of perfusion and the underlying anatomy, some interventionalists proceed with stent placement, though randomized data are not available.

13.24 **Answer B.** The 2005 ACC/AHA practice guidelines for the management of patients with STEMI (*J Am Coll Cardiol* 2006;47:216-235) give a

Class I (level of evidence: B) recommendation for primary PCI in patients with ST elevation within 12 hours of symptom onset in patients <75 years. Primary PCI for STEMI in patients ≥75 years of age is a Class IIa (level of evidence: B) recommendation since there are not as much data supporting benefit in primary PCI in the older age group. These recommendations have not been revised in the most recent 2009 Focused Updates of the STEMI/PCI guidelines (*J Am Coll Cardiol* 2009;54:2205-2241).

13.25 **Answer C.** Ideally, primary PCI for STEMI should be performed by interventionalists who perform ≥75 PCI procedures per year (including ≥11 primary PCIs per year for STEMI), in a catheterization laboratory that performs ≥200 PCI procedures per year, of which at least 36 are primary PCI for STEMI, and have on-site cardiac surgery capability. This is a Class I (level of evidence: B) recommendation (*J Am Coll Cardiol* 2006;47:216-235).

13.26 **Answer C.** In general, PCI should not be performed in a noninfarct artery at the time of primary PCI (Class III, level of evidence: C). However, in patients with more than one potential infarct-related artery and evidence of hemodynamic compromise or cardiogenic shock, multivessel PCI may be considered.

13.27 **Answer D.** Although data from the CARESS-in-AMI (*Lancet* 2008;371:559-568) and TRANSFER-AMI (*N Engl J Med* 2009;360:2705-2718) studies have added further support to the strategy of immediate transfer to a PCI center even before waiting to establish whether reperfusion has occurred, a strategy of coronary angiography with intent to perform PCI (or emergency CABG) is not recommended in patients who have received fibrinolytic therapy if further invasive management is contraindicated (Class III, level of evidence C) (*J Am Coll Cardiol* 2008;51:210-247). In this specific scenario, there is sufficient evidence to suggest reperfusion (>50% ST segment resolution and minimal chest pain), but more importantly, a strategy of coronary angiography and possible revascularization is unlikely to provide significant morbidity or mortality benefit in a patient with end-stage metastatic pancreatic cancer.

13.28 **Answer C.** There does not appear to be a significant difference between BMS and DES in mortality rates of MI or stent thrombosis with DES having the advantage of a reduction in TVR rates as compared to BMS. It is reasonable to use a DES as an alternative to BMS for primary PCI in STEMI (Class IIa, level of evidence B) especially if clinical and anatomic considerations such as small vessel diameter, longer lesion length, or diabetes mellitus are present. The most significant practical challenge is usually trying to determine, in an emergency setting, if the patient is a candidate for dual antiplatelet therapy. If there is evidence of financial limitations, patient noncompliance, increased bleeding risk, and upcoming surgical procedures, DES should be avoided. In this case, however, the patient is insured and, at least by HbA1c, the patient appears to be compliant and without any obvious bleeding concerns. A DES would be preferred given the lesion location and length, vessel diameter, and history of diabetes.

13.29 **Answer D.** A loading dose of thienopyridine is recommended for STEMI patients in whom PCI is planned (Class I, level of evidence C). Clopidogrel at a loading dose of 300 to 600 mg or prasugrel 60 mg should be given as soon as possible before or at the time of primary PCI. However, prasugrel is relatively contraindicated in patients ≥75 years of age and with a body weight <60 kg or those with a history of TIA or stroke. Patients weighing <60 kg have an increased exposure to the active metabolite of prasugrel and an increased risk of bleeding. Data from the TRITON-TIMI 38 trial (*N Engl J Med* 2007;357:2001–2015) that randomized high-risk ACS/STEMI patients to prasugrel 60-mg load, 10-mg maintenance vs. clopidogrel 300-mg load, and 75-mg maintenance dose showed superior efficacy in major predefined subgroups. However, a post hoc analysis suggested that patients with prior CVA/TIA had net harm from prasugrel and patients with a body weight <60 kg and ≥75 years of age had no net benefit from prasugrel.

13.30 **Answer D.** Traumatic or prolonged (>10 minutes) cardiopulmonary resuscitation is a relative contraindication. All other responses are absolute contraindications to thrombolytic therapy.

13.31 **Answer B.** High-risk STEMI patients (≥2 mm of ST-segment elevation in two anterior leads or ST elevation of at least 1 mm in inferior leads with at least one of the following: systolic BP < 100 mm Hg, heart rate ≥ 100 bpm, Killip class II to III, ≥2 mm of ST-segment depression in the anterior leads, or ≥1 mm of ST elevation in right-sided lead V4 indicative of right ventricular involvement) presenting to non–PCI-capable facilities who are not close enough to be transferred for primary PCI within 90 minutes should receive thrombolytic therapy as the primary reperfusion strategy and then be moved immediately to a PCI-capable facility for diagnostic catheterization and consideration of PCI without waiting to determine whether reperfusion has occurred. This strategy is based on evidence from both the CARESS-in-AMI trial (*Lancet* 2008;371:559–568) and the TRANSFER-AMI trial (*N Engl J Med* 2009;360:2705–2718). Data from both trials support early diagnostic angiography and possible revascularization (Class IIa, level of evidence B).

13.32 **Answer E.** Consideration for choosing stents (DES vs. BMS) in STEMI should include the ability of the patient to comply with prolonged dual antiplatelet therapy, the bleeding risk, and the possibility that the patient may need surgery during the ensuing year, which may require cessation of dual antiplatelet therapy. This patient has a history of noncompliance both with follow-up appointments and with medicines suggesting that he may not take a thienopyridine for ≥1 year if directed, making the use of a DES less appealing. In general, studies have found that the rate of death or MI is similar with the use of BMS vs. DES in patients presenting with AMI. The major advantage of a DES is in its ability to decrease restenosis and reduce the risk of repeat TVR. In this case, since the lesion is focal in a large-diameter vessel, the restenosis rate is unlikely to be high, and the advantage of using a DES over a BMS is diminished. Aspiration thrombectomy is reasonable for patients undergoing primary PCI (Class IIa, level of evidence B) and particularly in this case where there is a large thrombus burden.

13.33 **Answer C.** PCI of a totally occluded infarct artery >24 hours after STEMI is not recommended in asymptomatic patients with one- or two-vessel disease if they are hemodynamically and electrically stable and do not have evidence of severe, ongoing ischemia (Class III, level of evidence B). Further, in the absence of hemodynamic compromise or cardiogenic shock, PCI should not be performed in a noninfarct artery in the acute setting (Class III, level of evidence C) (*J Am Coll Cardiol* 2008;51:210–247).

13.34 **Answer B.** Key exclusion criteria for the TRANSFER-AMI trial included cardiogenic shock before randomization, PCI within the previous month, previous coronary artery bypass surgery, and the availability of primary PCI with an anticipated door-to-balloon time of less than 60 minutes. All other options were inclusion criteria for the trial. Among high-risk STEMI patients who were treated with fibrinolysis, transfer for PCI within 6 hours after fibrinolysis was associated with significantly fewer ischemic complications than standard treatment (*N Engl J Med* 2009;360:2705–2718).

13.35 **Answer C.** In patients with chronic kidney disease undergoing angiography who are not undergoing chronic dialysis, either an isosmolar contrast medium, that is, iodixanol, (Class I, level of evidence A) or a low-molecular-weight contrast medium other than ioxaglate or iohexol is indicated (Class I, level of evidence B). This is based on a number of trials including the moderate-sized randomized clinical trial RECOVER (*J Am Coll Cardiol* 2006;48:924–930) that compared the isosmolar agent iodixanol and ioxaglate and favored the former as well as the CARE trial (*Circulation* 2007;115:3189–3196) that compared iodixanol and the low-osmolar agent iopamidol and found no difference. However, several larger randomized trials have been published more recently that reported no difference in contrast-induced nephropathy when iodixanol was compared with various other low-osmolar contrast media other than iohexol (*Am J Roentgenol* 2008;191:151–157; *Am Heart J* 2008;156:776–782; *Invest Radiol* 2008;43:170–1788). A pooled comparison of iodixanol with all nonionic low-osmolar contrast media indicated equivalent safety (*J Am Coll Cardiol Intv* 2009;2:645–654).

QUESTIONS

14.1 Cardiac catheterization performed on a 69-year-old female who presented with unstable angina revealed a long diffuse lesion extending from mid to distal atrioventricular left circumflex coronary artery (Fig. Q14-1A). The first angiogram after balloon angioplasty and stenting is shown (Fig. Q14-1B). Which of the following mechanisms explains the findings seen on this angiogram?

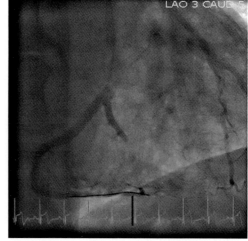

B

Figure Q14-1

(A) Side-branch closure with embolization
(B) Occlusive dissection
(C) Microvascular obstruction due to embolization
(D) Epicardial obstruction due to thrombus formation

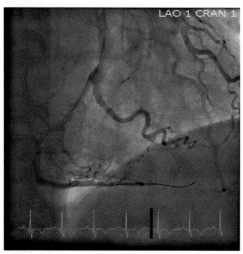

A

14.2 Compared to balloon angioplasty alone, which of the following has the highest risk of embolization following percutaneous coronary intervention (PCI)?

(A) Extraction atherectomy
(B) Rotational atherectomy
(C) Directional coronary atherectomy (DCA)
(D) All of the above

14.3 All of the following are likely to increase the risk of embolization during PCI, EXCEPT:

(A) Large plaque burden
(B) Use of DCA
(C) Calcification requiring rotational atherectomy
(D) Saphenous vein graft (SVG) interventions
(E) Use of glycoprotein IIb/IIIa (G PIIb/IIIa) inhibitors

14.4 The use of distal embolic protection device during PCI of saphenous vein aortocoronary bypass grafts has been shown to reduce which of the following?

(A) Death
(B) MI
(C) Emergency bypass
(D) All of the above
(E) None of the above

14.5 Which of the following treatments has been shown to significantly reduce the risk of periprocedural MI?

(A) Rotational atherectomy if performed for less than 2 minutes
(B) Pretreatment with intragraft verapamil before SVG intervention
(C) Thrombectomy using AngioJet device before stent implantation in SVG intervention
(D) Pretreatment with atorvastatin before elective coronary intervention
(E) Intracoronary urokinase when given 15 minutes before PCI

14.6 Which of the following interventions has been shown to reduce the rate of periprocedural MI associated with percutaneous transluminal angioplasty, elective stenting, and DCA?

(A) Atorvastatin
(B) Clopidogrel
(C) Aspirin
(D) Prasugrel
(E) Abciximab

14.7 All of the following have been shown to reduce distal embolization during percutaneous intervention of SVG, EXCEPT:
(A) Distal filter-based catheter
(B) Angioguard device
(C) DCA
(D) Use of distal balloon occlusion and aspiration system
(E) None of the above

14.8 A 69-year-old male with prior coronary bypass surgery presents with unstable angina. Angiography reveals a relatively normal SVG with severe narrowing at the distal graft 4 mm from the anastomosis of the SVG to posterior descending artery (PDA). Which of the following would be the BEST embolic protection device (EPD) for this patient?

(A) Angioguard
(B) FilterWire
(C) Accunet
(D) SPIDER
(E) Proxis

14.9 Use of an EPD during PCI has a guideline-recommended class I indication for which of the following interventions?

(A) Direct stenting of the left main trunk
(B) PCI of native coronary artery in the setting of ST-segment elevation myocardial infarction (STEMI)
(C) PCI of native coronary artery in the setting of non-STEMI
(D) PCI of native coronary artery in the setting of unstable angina
(E) PCI of SVG to left circumflex artery

14.10 The likelihood of an adverse event occurring at 30 days when using EPD during PCI of SVG is around:

(A) >60%
(B) 46% to 60%
(C) 31% to 45%
(D) 16% to 30%
(E) 0% to 15%

14.11 Which of the following patient characteristics may increase the risk of periprocedural myonecrosis?

(A) Increased arterial inflammation
(B) Aspirin resistance
(C) Clopidogrel resistance
(D) Genetic predisposition
(E) All of the above

14.12 In clinical practice, CK-MB elevations (<5 times the upper normal limits) occur after what percentage of technically successful PCIs?

(A) 0% to 15%
(B) 15% to 30%
(C) 31% to 45%
(D) 46% to 60%
(E) >60%

14.13 There is a dose–response relationship between periprocedural CK elevation and mortality.

(A) True
(B) False

14.14 All of the following outcomes listed below are associated with periprocedural myonecrosis, EXCEPT:

(A) Immediate in-hospital mortality
(B) Short-term (<30 days) mortality
(C) Long-term (>1-year) mortality
(D) Stroke
(E) All of the above

14.15 Which of the following factors is associated with a decreased risk of periprocedural MI?

(A) Statin therapy
(B) Clopidogrel therapy
(C) Aspirin therapy
(D) Prasugrel therapy
(E) All of the above

14.16 You are planning an elective intervention on an 82-year-old male with a 90% mid right heavily calcified mid right coronary artery lesion. In order to assess the likelihood of distal embolization, you perform an intravascular ultrasound (IVUS) assessment. All of the following findings by IVUS have been shown to be associated with higher periprocedural CK elevations, EXCEPT:

(A) Plaque burden
(B) Lesion site calcification
(C) cross-sectional narrowing at the lesion site by IVUS
(D) Lumen dimension at the lesion site
(E) Positive remodeling

14.17 In the setting of STEMI, which of the following approaches has been shown in randomized clinical trials to lower mortality?

(A) Aspiration
(B) Distal filters
(C) Distal balloon occlusion
(D) None of the above
(E) All of the above

14.18 All of the following factors have been shown to be independent predictors of distal embolization during SVG interventions, EXCEPT:

(A) Undersizing of stents
(B) Presence of thrombus
(C) Diffusely diseased vein grafts
(D) Use of DCA
(E) Balloon angioplasty followed by stenting

14.19 A 78-year-old female underwent PCI of a totally occluded right coronary artery (RCA) (Fig. Q14-19A). After percutaneous intervention is performed on the occlusion, the patient is discovered to have another abnormality in the RCA (Fig. Q14-19B). What is the abnormality shown at the arrow in Figure Q14-19B?

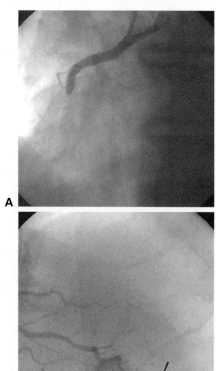

Figure Q14-19

(A) Vasospasm
(B) Dissection
(C) Perforation
(D) Distal embolization and cutoff
(E) Stenosis

14.20 Match the following items listed with the appropriate image in Figure Q14-20A–E.

1. PercuSurge GuardWire device
2. Angioguard device
3. Boston Scientific FilterWire
4. Guidant ACCUNET
5. IntraTherapeutics IntraGuard

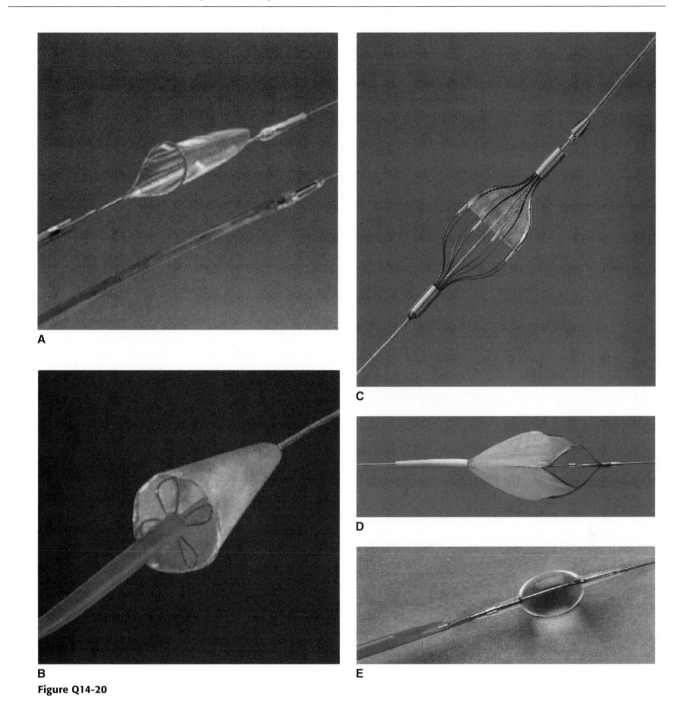

Figure Q14-20

14.21 In randomized clinical trials, mechanical thrombectomy for STEMI has been shown to reduce the risk of which of the following?

(A) Death
(B) Reinfarction
(C) Congestive heart failure
(D) Hospital length of stay
(E) Low myocardial blush score

14.22 All of the following are manual aspiration devices, EXCEPT:

(A) Export
(B) Fetch
(C) Pronto LP
(D) AngioJet
(E) Zeek

14.23 In the TAPAS Trial, atherothrombotic material was retrieved in what percentage of cases?

(A) 10% to 20%
(B) 30% to 40%
(C) 50% to 60%
(D) 60% to 70%
(E) 70% to 80%

14.24 Manual aspiration may result in which of the following?

(A) Increased door-to-balloon (D2B) time
(B) Improved myocardial perfusion
(C) Less flow-limiting dissection
(D) Lower number of stents used
(E) Reduced side-branch occlusion

14.25 All of the following trials evaluated the utility of thrombus aspiration in the setting of primary PCI, EXCEPT:

(A) EMERALD
(B) REMEDIA
(C) AIMI
(D) TAPAS
(E) BOOST

14.1 **Answer A.** This angiogram shows abrupt closure with embolization of the obtuse marginal branch after stenting the AV left circumflex artery. The other answers are known causes of periprocedural myocardial infarction (MI). The major mechanism for periprocedural MI is embolization of microscopic debris with subsequent platelet activation and inflammation leading to impairment in microvascular flow (*Textbook of interventional cardiology* 2003:251–266).

14.2 **Answer D.** The CAVEAT trial (*N Engl J Med* 1993;329:221–227), showed a significant increase in death and MI at 6 months associated with DCA when compared with balloon angioplasty alone. Patients with high-risk lesions in SVG and native coronary arteries who underwent transluminal extraction atherectomy in the New Approaches to Coronary Interventions registry had a high rate of distal embolization at 8.3%. Distal embolization was associated with an in-hospital mortality of 18.5% vs. an in-hospital mortality of 3.0% in patients without distal embolization (*Catheter Cardiovasc Interv* 1999;47:149–154).

14.3 **Answer E.** Antiplatelet agents such as GP IIb/IIIa inhibitors have been shown to decrease the rate of death and MI associated with any percutaneous device (*Am J Cardiol* 2000;85:1060–1064). The exact mechanism is unknown, but it is likely related to GP IIb/IIIa inhibitors ability to preserve microvascular flow by minimizing the response to distal embolization. All other answers have been shown to increase the risk of distal embolization. SVG interventions without EPD are known to be associated with up to 20% risk of distal embolization (*Circulation* 2002;105(11):1285–1290). As noted previously more invasive methods of revascularization, such as DCA or rotational atherectomy, are associated with increased embolization (*Textbook of interventional cardiology* 2003:251–266).

14.4 **Answer B.** The randomized trial of a distal embolic protection device during percutaneous intervention of saphenous vein aortocoronary bypass grafts (*Circulation* 2002;105(11):1285–1290) showed a significant reduction in the composite end point of death, MI, emergency bypass, or target lesion revascularization at 30 days among those who received distal protection (9.6%) compared to the control group (16.5%) (*p* = 0.004). However, this was mainly driven by lower MI and "no-reflow" phenomenon (3% distal embolic protection vs. 9% control, *p* = 0.02).

14.5 **Answer D.** In the Atorvastatin for Reduction of Myocardial Damage During Angioplasty (ARMYDA) trial (*Circulation* 2004;110:674–678), atorvastatin (40 mg/day) administered 7 days before elective coronary intervention had a significant reduction in all markers for myocardial injury, including CK-MB, troponin I, and myoglobin measured at 8 and 24 hours after the procedure when compared with patients who did not receive atorvastatin. Postprocedural MI measured by CK-MB occurred in 5% of patients who received atorvastatin vs. 18% in patients in the placebo group (*p* = 0.025). Intragraft verapamil before PCI in SVG was examined in a small study and verapamil was shown to decrease the rate of "no reflow" and improve flow rate in the vessel; however, there was no difference in postprocedural cardiac enzyme release (*J Invasive Cardiol* 2002;14:303–304). In a study of 797 patients with diseased SVG or thrombus-containing native coronary arteries, routine thrombectomy before stent implantation did not decrease the incidence of periprocedural MI when compared with stent implantation without thrombectomy (*J Am Coll Cardiol* 2003;42:2007–2013). Many studies have shown the increased rates of distal embolization and periprocedural MI with directional and rotational atherectomy.

14.6 **Answer E.** Abciximab, a GP IIb/IIIa inhibitor, has been shown to reduce periprocedural MI and death regardless of the device used (*Am J Cardiol* 2000;85:1060–1064). GP IIb/IIIa inhibitors, through their antiplatelet effect, have been shown to reduce microvascular occlusion and the subsequent left ventricular dysfunction that occurs with distal embolization. While ARMYDA trial (*Circulation* 2004;110:674–678) showed a reduction in MI with PCI, the role of statins in the setting of DCA has not been evaluated. Similarly, in multiple trials clopidogrel has shown to reduce short- and long-term clinical events in those undergoing PCI; however, its role in the setting of DCA is not known.

14.7   Answer C. Distal embolization can occur in up to 20% of percutaneous intervention of SVGs. In the SAFER trial (*Circulation* 2002;105:1285–1290), the use of the PercuSurge GuardWire system (a distal balloon occlusion and aspiration system) was associated with a 42% relative risk reduction in composite end point of death, MI, emergency bypass, or target lesion revascularization at 30 days, which included a significant reduction in MI and "no reflow" phenomenon. In the CAVEAT I trial (*Circulation* 1995;91:1966–1974), DCA of de novo vein graft lesions was associated with increased rates of distal embolization when compared with angioplasty alone. The Symbiot trial (*J Invasive Cardiol* 2005;17:609–612.) failed to show any decrease in the rate of distal embolization with the use of the Symbiot, a PTFE-covered stent as compared with bare-metal stents during PCI of SVGs. Angioguard is a filter-based distal embolic protection device.

14.8   Answer E. The three basic types of EPDs are the distal filter and balloon occlusion devices and proximal occlusion devices. Of the devices shown, Proxis is the only proximal protection device. The balloon occlusion device prevents flow to the distal circulation and traps all embolic debris. The disadvantage of preventing all distal flow is that it prohibits visualization of the vessel beyond the device. However, one potential benefit of preventing distal flow is the prevention of the passage of cytokines and other vasoactive substances.

14.9   Answer E. In the SAFER trial (*Circulation* 2002;105:1285–1290), 801 patients undergoing percutaneous intervention to stenotic SVGs were randomly assigned to stent placement over the shaft of the PercuSurge GuardWire balloon occlusion and aspiration system versus stent placement over a conventional angioplasty guidewire. Use of the distal protection device resulted in a 42% relative risk reduction in the primary end point, which was a composite of death, MI, emergency bypass, or target lesion revascularization by 30 days. Analysis of the individual components of the primary end point revealed a statistically significant reduction in

MI and "no reflow." Therefore, the use of EPD for SVG intervention has a class I indication by the current guidelines. EPD is not indicated for any of the other interventions listed.

14.10   Answer E. The MACE rate with use of the current EPDs (including distal filters, proximal devices, and distal balloon occlusion/aspiration systems) is 7% to 12% depending upon the device. The SAFER trial, which evaluated a distal balloon occlusion and aspiration system (PercuSurge GuardWire), had a 9.6% MACE rate at 30 days. In the FilterWire EX Randomized Evaluation (FIRE) trial (*J Am Coll Cardiol* 2002;40:1882–1888), which assessed the utility of a distal filter device (FilterWire EX), there was a 30-day MACE rate of 11.3%. The Protection Devices in PCI Treatment of Myocardial Infarction for Salvage of Endangered Myocardium (PROMISE) trial (*unpublished, presented at TCT 2005 meeting*), examining the efficacy of a proximal balloon and occlusion system (Proxis), had a 9.2% MACE at 30 days. The Protection During Saphenous Vein Graft Intervention to Prevent Distal Embolization (PRIDE) trial (*J Am Coll Cardiol* 2005;46:1677–1683), which examined the use of a balloon-protection flush and extraction system (TriActiv System), found an 11.2% MACE at 30 days.

14.11   Answer E. Genetic predisposition, aspirin and clopidogrel resistance, and increased arterial inflammation are factors believed to increase the risk of periprocedural myonecrosis (*Circulation* 2005;111:906–912).

14.12   Answer A. In clinical practice, asymptomatic CK-MB elevations (<5 times the upper normal limits) occur after 3% to 11% of technically successful PCIs (*Circulation* 2007;116:2634).

14.13   Answer A. The EPIC trial (*JAMA* 1997;278:479–484) was one of the first trials to demonstrate the association between periprocedural MI and increased mortality in the intermediate period after percutaneous intervention. The study demonstrated a direct relationship between degree of CK elevation postprocedure and 3-year mortality. Patients with CK elevations 10×, 5×, and 3× the normal CK level had an estimated mortality rate at 3 years of 16.5%, 14.8%, and 13.1%, respectively. As compared with those with normal CK levels, patients with CK levels greater than once the upper limit of normal also had an increased mortality rate at 3 years (10.2% vs. 7.3%).

14.14 **Answer D.** The association between periprocedural MI and PCI has been established by numerous studies and meta-analysis (*Circulation* 2005;112:906–915; discussion 923). However, periprocedural MI has not been linked to increased stroke risk.

14.15 **Answer E.** Antiplatelet and antithrombotic therapies including aspirin, clopidogrel, prasugrel, and G PIIb/IIIa inhibitors have been shown to attenuate the impact of embolization during PCI leading to reductions in periprocedural MI. Similarly, as noted previously, statins have also been shown to significantly reduce the risk of periprocedural MI when given before PCI.

14.16 **Answer D.** IVUS assessment of 2,256 patients undergoing PCI of native coronaries identified plaque burden at the lesion, lesion site calcification, positive remodeling, cross-sectional narrowing at the lesion, and reference sites to be associated with periprocedural CK-MB elevations. In the multivariable analysis, age, sex, diabetes mellitus, and lumen dimension at the lesion site before and after intervention were not predictive of CK-MB elevation (*Circulation* 2000;101:604–610).

14.17 **Answer A.** In a meta-analysis of all randomized clinical trials that evaluated EPDs or aspiration catheters, only aspiration showed a significant reduction in mortality (HR: 0.49, 95% CI: 0.29–0.82) (*Circulation* 2008;118:S974).

14.18 **Answer A.** Observational studies and case reports have shown lower distal embolization with less aggressive stent sizing in SVGs. However, the long-term safety and efficacy of this approach are not well established. The CAVEAT-II was a prospective, multicenter trial comparing percutaneous transluminal coronary angioplasty vs. DCA in patients with SVG lesions. The use of DCA and the presence of thrombus in this clinical trial were both independent predictors of distal embolization (*Circulation* 1995;92:734–740). Other angiographic predictors of distal embolization after balloon angioplasty of SVGs included diffusely diseased vein grafts and large plaque volume (*Am J Cardiol* 1993;72:514–517). Graft age is also a predictor of distal embolization.

14.19 **Answer D.** The angiogram shows distal embolization and cutoff in the distal PDA after intervention was performed to the complete occlusion in the midsegment of the RCA.

14.20 **Answers.** A-3, B-5, C-2, D-4, E-1.

14.21 **Answer E.** The TAPAS (Thrombus Aspiration during Primary Percutaneous Coronary Intervention) trial examined the utility of manual aspiration using 6-F Export Aspiration Catheter (Medtronic) (*N Engl J Med* 2008;358:557–567). The primary end point was the postprocedural frequency of a myocardial blush grade of 0 or 1. In this study, Export Aspiration Catheter was shown to be superior to conventional treatment for primary end point. While there was a trend towards lower clinical events with manual aspiration, this did not reach statistical significance.

14.22 **Answer D.** AngioJet, unlike those listed, is a powerful rheolytic thrombectomy system. It was evaluated in the JETSTENT trial (Comparison of AngioJet Rheolytic Thrombectomy Before Direct Infarct Artery Stenting with Direct Stenting Alone in Patients with Acute Myocardial Infarction). The study failed to meet primary end point; however, overall there was a trend towards lower clinical event with AngioJet device.

14.23 **Answer E.** In the TAPAS (Thrombus Aspiration during Primary Percutaneous Coronary Intervention) trial (*N Engl J Med* 2008;358:557–567), 73% of those who underwent manual aspiration had atherothrombotic material extracted.

14.24 **Answer B.** D2B time is typically calculated from arrival to emergency room to "device" activation. Therefore, manual thrombectomy does not prolong D2B time. As noted previously, the TAPAS trial has shown improved myocardial perfusion with manual thrombectomy compared to conventional treatment. Similarly, in the TAPAS trial no significant differences were seen for the rate of side-branch closure, number of stents used, or flow-limiting dissection between the conventional approach and manual aspiration.

14.25 **Answer E.** The EMERALD trial (*JAMA* 2005;293:1063–1072) randomized 501 patients presenting with ST-segment MI to receive PCI with a balloon occlusion and aspiration distal microcirculatory system versus angioplasty without any distal protection. There was no difference among the treatment groups with respect to either of the co-primary end points, which were ST-segment resolution measured 30 minutes after PCI by continuous Holter monitoring and infarct size measured by single photon emission computed tomography imaging between days 5 and 14. There was also no improvement in microvascular flow or success of reperfusion. The Randomized Evaluation of the Effect of Mechanical Reduction of Distal Embolization by Thrombus-Aspiration in Primary and Rescue Angioplasty (REMEDIA) trial was a single-center, prospective, randomized study that was designed to determine the safety and efficacy of the *Diver CE* catheter for thrombus aspiration in ST-segment elevation AMI patients vs. standard PCI. The primary end point was myocardial blush score > 2 and ST-segment resolution > 70%. REMEDIA

showed that thrombus aspiration prior to PCI resulted in an improvement in myocardial blush score and ST resolution compared to PCI alone. The AIMI (AngioJet Rheolytic Thrombectomy In Patients Undergoing Primary Angioplasty for Acute Myocardial Infarction) trial evaluated 480 patients and failed to show a significant difference in ST resolution. Furthermore, those who underwent thrombectomy had a larger infarct size and 1-month MACE rate. The TAPAS trial has been described above. BOOST (Intracoronary autologous bone-marrow cell transfer after MI) randomized controlled clinical trial did not test thrombus aspiration.

15 Chronic Total Occlusions

David E. Kandzari and Dimitri Karmpaliotis

QUESTIONS

15.1 Compared with percutaneous revascularization of nonocclusive coronary lesions, which statement best characterizes outcomes among patients with chronic total occlusions when using bare-metal stents (BMS)?

(A) Chronic total occlusions have higher rates of restenosis and reocclusion

(B) Restenosis is higher with total occlusions, but reocclusion rates are similar

(C) Reocclusion is more frequent among total coronary occlusions, but restenosis rates are similar

(D) Rates of both restenosis and reocclusion are similar

15.2 Which variable best predicts improvement in left ventricular function following successful recanalization of a chronic total occlusion?

(A) History of prior myocardial infarction (MI)

(B) Baseline left ventricular dysfunction

(C) Angiographic presence of collateral flow

(D) Duration of occlusion

15.3 Compared with conventional BMS, treatment with drug-eluting stent (DES) following recanalization of chronic total occlusions is associated with all of the following, EXCEPT:

(A) Reductions in restenosis

(B) Decrease in repeat target lesion revascularization

(C) Improved survival

(D) Decreased rates of reocclusion

15.4 Compared with procedural failure to recanalize chronic total occlusions, successful percutaneous revascularization of chronic total occlusions is associated with all of the following, EXCEPT:

(A) Improved long-term survival

(B) Increased need for repeat revascularization procedures

(C) Reduced angina

(D) Improved left ventricular function

15.5 The most common reason for failure of percutaneous revascularization of chronic total occlusions is:

(A) Guidewire entry into a subintimal dissection plane

(B) Inability to cross the occluded segment

(C) Inability to deliver an angioplasty balloon

(D) Coronary artery perforation

15.6 Which of the following statements regarding coronary perforation in revascularization of total coronary occlusions is TRUE?

(A) In-hospital mortality is similar among patients who do and do not experience cardiac tamponade

(B) Cardiac tamponade often develops hours following the interventional procedure

(C) Guidewire perforation most commonly occurs distal to the occluded segment

(D) Absence of angiographic evidence of contrast extravasation excludes the diagnosis of cardiac tamponade

15.7 A 73-year-old Caucasian male is referred to you for percutaneous coronary intervention (PCI) of a chronically occluded right coronary artery (RCA) (Fig. Q15-7A). The procedure is successful (Fig. Q15-7B), and the interventional cardiology fellow asks you which of the following statements regarding collateral flow in chronic total occlusions is NOT true?

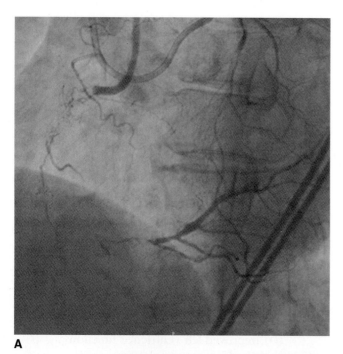

A

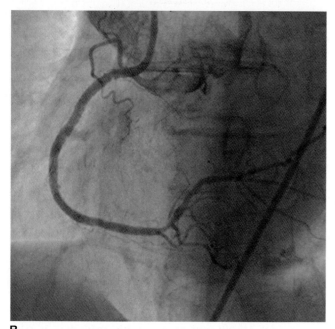

B

Figure Q15-7 A: Chronic total occlusion of the right coronary artery. B: Right coronary artery following PCI.

(A) Collateral function is worse in patients with impaired regional wall motion

(B) The presence and extent of collateral flow predicts improvement in ventricular function following revascularization

(C) Collateral function regresses after recanalization of chronic total occlusions

(D) Growth factor expression is related to collateral function and the duration of occlusion

15.8 Which of the following technologies/strategies has demonstrated significantly higher procedural success over coronary guidewires in a randomized trial?

(A) Excimer laser guidewire

(B) Fibrinolytic infusion

(C) Optical coherence tomography guidewire

(D) None of the above

15.9 Advances in coronary guidewires for chronic total occlusions include all of the following, EXCEPT:

(A) Tapered tip

(B) Hydrophilic coating

(C) Increased tip stiffness

(D) Absence of coiled tip

15.10 Which characteristic is NOT a predictor of procedural failure in chronic total coronary occlusion revascularization?

(A) Presence of side branch at the site of occlusion

(B) Tapered stump of occlusion

(C) Bridging collaterals

(D) Duration of total occlusion

15.11 Compared with the treatment of nonocclusive lesions, percutaneous revascularization of chronic total occlusions is characterized by all of the following procedural characteristics, EXCEPT:

(A) Increased use of iodinated contrast

(B) Increased exposure to ionizing radiation

(C) Increased stent length and number

(D) Increased risk of in-hospital death and MI

15.12 Chronic total occlusions:

(A) Are present in approximately one-half of patients with other severe coronary artery disease

(B) Are identified in approximately one-third of all diagnostic coronary angiograms following abnormal stress testing

(C) Account for approximately 10% of all percutaneous revascularization procedures

(D) All of the above

15.13 Chronic total coronary occlusions are most prevalent in which vessel?

(A) Left anterior descending artery
(B) Left circumflex artery
(C) RCA
(D) Left main artery

15.14 The pathophysiology of chronic total occlusions includes which of the following?

(A) Adventitial neovascularization
(B) Expression of collagen types I and III
(C) Organized thrombus
(D) All of the above

15.15 Angiographic collateral flow is a predictor of:

(A) Improvement in left ventricular function
(B) Restenosis
(C) Reocclusion
(D) None of the above

15.16 Before crossing a total coronary occlusion with a guidewire, appropriate adjunctive pharmacology includes treatment with which agent?

(A) Bivalirudin
(B) Unfractionated heparin
(C) Glycoprotein IIb/IIIa inhibitor
(D) Low-molecular-weight heparin

15.17 Which statement best characterizes the histology of chronic total coronary occlusions?

(A) Approximately one-half of chronic total occlusions are <99% stenotic despite their angiographic appearance
(B) The severity of lumen stenosis is related to lesion age
(C) Collagen-rich fibrous tissue is most dense in the mid segment of the total occlusion
(D) Inflammation is most prevalent in the adventitia

15.18 In patients with ST-segment elevation MI who do not receive reperfusion therapy, a total occlusion is identified in approximately what percent of patients at 1 month?

(A) 10%
(B) 25%
(C) 50%
(D) 75%

15.19 In patients with chronic total occlusions who undergo attempted revascularization, which factor is most predictive of increased long-term mortality risk?

(A) Chronic kidney disease
(B) Diabetes mellitus
(C) Multivessel coronary disease
(D) Procedural failure

15.20 Technical maneuvers to confirm guidewire placement in the distal true lumen may include all of the following, EXCEPT:

(A) Use of contralateral angiography
(B) Ability to deliver angioplasty balloon
(C) Use of intravascular ultrasound
(D) Contrast injection through end-hole catheter

15.21 Among patients presenting with acute ST-elevation MI, the presence of a CTO in a non–infarct-related artery (non-IRA) is:

(A) A stronger predictor of 5-year mortality than the presence of multivessel disease (MVD)
(B) Less predictive of 5-year mortality after ST-elevation MI than the presence of MVD and diabetes mellitus
(C) Not independently associated with increased 5-year mortality after adjustment for other angiographic and clinical variables
(D) A predictor of late-term (>1 year) mortality, but not at earlier time points

15.22 Among patients with MVD and a CTO, successful CTO PCI ("complete" revascularization) compared to no CTO revascularization is associated with:

(A) Neutral effect on long-term survival but lower incidence of MI at 2 years
(B) Improved 2-year survival in patients with MVD
(C) Worse 2-year survival in patients with MVD
(D) Improved 2-year survival only in patients with CTO involvement of the RCA

15.23 Grade III coronary perforation is:

(A) Most commonly caused by a guidewire
(B) Associated with a high rate of in-hospital adverse cardiovascular events, but not late-term events following hospital discharge
(C) Associated with high in-hospital and late-term adverse cardiovascular events
(D) Most commonly treated with emergency coronary bypass surgery

ANSWERS AND EXPLANATIONS

15.1 Answer A. Chronic total occlusion revascularization with BMS is associated with considerably higher rates of restenosis and reocclusion compared with stenting of nonocclusive lesions. In the Total Occlusion Study of Canada (TOSCA)-1 (*Circulation* 1999;100:236–242), the rates of restenosis and reocclusion at 6-month angiographic follow-up were 55% and 11%, respectively, among patients assigned to treatment with BMS. In the Stenting in Chronic Coronary Occlusion trial (*J Am Coll Cardiol* 1996;28:1444–14451), the reocclusion rate was 16% in the stent cohort.

15.2 Answer B. Compared with patients with normal or regional impairment of left ventricular function and chronic total occlusions, patients with global left ventricular dysfunction derive the greatest relative improvement in the percent ejection fraction (EF) and decrease in wall motion severity index following successful revascularization. In a recent study of patients with angiographic follow-up, baseline left ventricular dysfunction was an independent predictor of improvement in left ventricular function (*Am Heart J* 2005;149:129–137). Variables including angiographic collateral flow, duration of occlusion, or history of MI were not predictive of improvement. Recent studies with cardiac magnetic resonance angiography have also identified dysfunctional but viable myocardium as the most significant predictor of improvement in the left ventricular EF and wall motion severity index (*Am Heart J* 2005;96:165H; *J Am Coll Cordiol* 2006;47:721–725). Finally, TOSCA examined the influence of successful revascularization on left ventricular EF and regional wall motion (*Am Heart J* 2001;142:301–308). Although an occlusion duration ≤6 weeks was independently predictive of a significant increase in the percent EF, the greatest improvement was among patients with baseline EF < 60%.

15.3 Answer C. Several recent studies have examined the safety and efficacy of DES in chronic total occlusion revascularization. In most instances, nonrandomized observational studies have compared angiographic and clinical outcomes with historical controls of patients with total coronary occlusions treated with BMS. A consistent finding among these trials is a significant reduction in angiographic binary restenosis, reocclusion, and the need for repeat target vessel revascularization. In the only randomized trial to date comparing sirolimus-eluting stents and BMS, treatment with sirolimus-eluting stents was associated with an 81% relative reduction in in-stent restenosis at 6-month angiographic follow-up (36% vs. 7%, $p < 0.0001$) *Circulation* 2006;114:921–928. There were no differences in survival between patients treated with BMS or DES.

15.4 Answer B. Several observational studies examining the influence of attempted percutaneous revascularization of chronic total occlusions have demonstrated that compared with failed attempts, successful revascularization is associated with improved long-term survival, reduced angina, and improvements in left ventricular EF and regional wall motion (*J Am Coll Cardiol* 2003;41:1672–1678; *Circulation* 2001;104:2–415; *J Am Coll Cardiol* 2001;38:409–414). Successful total occlusion revascularization is not associated with an increased need for repeat revascularization but instead with a significant improvement in event-free survival from bypass surgery (*Circulation* 2001;104:2–415).

15.5 Answer B. The most common mode of failure is inability to successfully pass a guidewire across the occluded segment into the distal true lumen of the vessel. Among 397 patients undergoing attempted total occlusion revascularization (*J Am Coll Cardiol* 1995;26:409–415), the most common reasons for procedural failure were inability to cross the lesion with a guidewire (63% of cases), long intimal dissection with creation of a false lumen (24%), dye extravasation (11%), failure to cross with a balloon or dilate (2%), and thrombus formation (1.2%).

15.6 Answer B. In a series of patients who developed cardiac tamponade from complications related to PCI, cardiac tamponade was diagnosed on an average of 4.4 hours following completion of the procedure (*Am J Cardiol* 2002;90:1183–1186). The occurrence of cardiac tamponade is associated with a high likelihood of in-hospital death and MI. Guidewire perforation typically occurs at the site of the occluded segment; however, perforation may occur in the distal segment of the vessel, underscoring the need to exchange stiff, tapered, or hydrophilic guidewires for soft, less traumatic guidewires after successful crossing. Absence of contrast extravasation does not exclude the possibility of cardiac tamponade. Therefore, if perforation is suspected although not angiographically evident, important measures include serial echocardiography and hemodynamic monitoring.

15.7 **Answer B.** Recovery of impaired left ventricular function after revascularization of a chronic total occlusion is not directly related to the extent of collateral function (*Am Heart J* 2005;149:129–137). Growth factor expression, in particular, fibroblast growth factor, has been related to both the duration of occlusion and collateral function (*Circulation* 2004;110:1940–1945). Collateral function is better in patients with a total coronary occlusion and normal regional wall motion than in patients with impaired regional function (*Circulation* 2001;104:2784–2790). Collateral function also regresses during long-term follow-up after successful recanalization and may not be readily recruitable in the event of acute occlusion (*Circulation* 2003;108:2877–2882).

15.8 **Answer D.** Of the techniques listed, only the laser wire has been compared with conventional coronary guidewires in a randomized trial. In the Total Occlusion Trial with Angioplasty by using a Laser Wire trial (*Eur Heart J* 2000;21:1797–1805), 303 patients with chronic total occlusions were randomized to treatment with either the laser wire or conventional wire technique. Successful lesion crossing was achieved in 53% of the laser wire cohort versus 47% in the conventional wire group ($p = 0.33$).

15.9 **Answer D.** Guidewires with a tapering tip diameter of 0.009 to 0.011 in. may facilitate wire engagement in microchannels of chronic total occlusions. Similarly, guidewires with incremental tip stiffness may penetrate the occluded segment more easily and provide greater shape retention. Hydrophilic wires typically advance with minimal resistance and are easily maneuverable in tortuous vessels, and are therefore used by some operators in chronic total occlusions. However, hydrophilic wires must also be used with caution because they are more likely to penetrate beneath the plaque and cause dissection and more frequently select small vessel

branches, increasing the likelihood of perforation (*Catheter Cardiovasc Interv* 2005;66:217–236).

15.10 **Answer B.** Compared with a blunted appearance of the occlusion or side branch presence at the site of occlusion, angiographic appearance of a tapered occlusion has been associated with an increased likelihood of procedural success (*Catheter Cardiovasc Interv* 2000;49:258–264; *J Am Coll Cardiol* 2003;41:1672–1678; *Catheter Cardiovasc Interv* 2005;66:217–236; *Br Heart J* 1993;70:126–131). Increasing duration of the occlusion and the presence of bridging collaterals are also associated with increased procedural failure (*Catheter Cardiovasc Interv* 2000;49:258–264; *J Am Coll Cardiol* 2003;41:1672–1678; *Catheter Cardiovasc Interv* 2005;66:217–236; *Br Heart J* 1993;70:126–131).

15.11 **Answer D.** Attempted total occlusion revascularization is associated with increased use of iodinated contrast and exposure to ionizing radiation. Because significant disease distal to the occluded segment may not be readily visible on the initial angiogram, successful recanalization is often associated with considerably greater stent length and number compared with the treatment of nonocclusive disease.

Among 2,007 procedures for chronic total occlusion revascularization over a 20-year period, the annualized in-hospital major adverse event rate was 3.8%, which did not statistically differ from the major complication rate from a matched cohort of 2,007 patients undergoing treatment during the same period for nonoccluded vessels (*J Am Coll Cardiol* 2001;38:409–414). However, compared with those patients in whom the procedure was successful, the in-hospital occurrence of major adverse cardiac events was significantly higher among patients with procedural failure (3.2% vs. 5.4%, $p = 0.02$).

15.12 **Answer D.** Overall, a chronic total occlusion is identified in approximately one-third of all diagnostic coronary angiograms, yet attempted percutaneous revascularization of a total occlusion accounts for <10% of all PCIs (*Am Heart J* 1993;126:561–564; *Circulation* 2002;106:1627–1633). However, in a summary of 8,004 patients presenting for diagnostic cardiac catheterization over a 10-year period, a chronic total occlusion was identified in 52% of patients with significant disease (≥70% stenosis) in another major epicardial vessel (*Am J Cardiol* 2005;95:1088–1091).

15.13 **Answer C.** According to the National Heart, Lung and Blood Dynamic Registry (*Circulation* 2002;106:1627–1633), chronic total occlusions are most prevalent in the RCA and least common in the left circumflex artery. The frequency of total occlusions also increases with advancing age. Total occlusion of the RCA was identified in 18.2%, 21.3%, and 22.8% of patients <65 years, 65 to 79 years, and ≥80 years of age, respectively (*Am Heart J* 2003;146:513–519).

15.14 **Answer D.** Chronic total occlusions most commonly develop from thrombotic occlusion followed by thrombus organization and collagen deposition (in particular, types I and III) (*J Am Coll Cardiol* 1993;21:604–611). Neovascularization is also prominent and begins within the adventitia. As total occlusions age, angiogenesis becomes more extensive, and the number and size of capillaries in t he intima and adventitia become similar.

15.15 **Answer D.** The presence and extent of angiographic collateral flow has been associated with the presence of viable and functional myocardium, but it does not predict the improvement in regional wall motion or occurrence of restenosis or reocclusion following successful revascularization (*Am Heart J* 2005;149:129–137).

15.16 **Answer B.** Attempted revascularization of chronic total occlusions is best performed using unfractionated heparin to achieve an activated clotting time of at least 250 seconds for antegrade procedures and at least 300 seconds for retrograde procedures. (*Catheter Cardiovasc Interv* 2005;66:217–236). If the lesion is successfully crossed, additional heparin and/or a glycoprotein IIb/IIIa antagonist may be administered.

However, if a complication (e.g., coronary perforation) occurs, unfractionated heparin may be readily reversed with intravenous protamine sulfate. In contrast, antithrombin agents such as direct thrombin inhibitors (e.g., bivalirudin) and glycoprotein IIb/IIIa inhibitors are not readily reversible and, therefore, present increased risk of bleeding complications if coronary perforation occurs.

15.17 **Answer A.** By histology, approximately one-half of chronic total occlusions are <99% stenotic despite the angiographic appearance of thrombolysis in myocardial infarction-0 flow. Inflammation is most prevalent in the intima of chronic total occlusions, regardless of the lesion age (*J Am Coll Cardiol* 1993;21:604–611). No relationship exists between the severity of stenosis and either plaque composition or lesion age. The concentration of collagen-rich fibrous tissue is particularly dense at the proximal and distal ends of the lesion with a mid segment characterized by soft lipid core and organized thrombus.

15.18 **Answer C.** In patients with ST-segment elevation MI not treated with reperfusion therapy, an occluded infarct-related artery has been identified in 87% of patients within 4 hours, 65% within 12 to 24 hours, 53% at 15 days, and 45% at 1 month (*Am Heart J* 1979;97:61–69; *Circulation* 1982;65:1099–1105; *N Engl J Med* 1980;303:897–902).

15.19 **Answer D.** Several observational studies have demonstrated increased long-term mortality among patients with failed attempts at total occlusion revascularization compared with successful revascularization (*Eur Heart J* 2005;26:2630–2636; *J Am Coll Cardiol* 2003;41:1672–1678;

Table A15-19.

Trial	Success (N)	Failure (N)	Follow-up Duration (years)	Mortality (%) Success	Failure	*p* Value
British Columbia Cardiac Registry[a]	1,118	340	6	10.0	19.0	<0.001
Suero et al.[b]	1,491	514	10	26.0	35.0	0.001
TOAST-GISE[c]	286	83	1	1.1	3.6	0.13
Aziz et al.[d]	377	166	2.4	2.5	7.3	0.049
Hoye et al.[e]	568	306	5	6.5	12.0	0.02

[a]*Am Heart J* 1979;97:61–69.
[b]*Circulation* 1982;65:1099–1105.
[c]*Circulation* 1999;100:236–242.
[d]*Am J Cardiol* 2005;95:1088–1091.
[e]*Am Heart J* 2003;146:513–519.

Circulation 2001;104:2–415; *J Am Coll Cardiol* 2001;38:409–414). In a multivariable model in 1,118 patients with chronic total occlusions in the British Columbia Cardiac Registry (*Circulation* 2001;104:2–415), only the factors of end-stage renal disease and left ventricular dysfunction were more predictive of late mortality than procedural failure. Table A15-19 shows consistently higher mortality among patients undergoing failed versus successful percutaneous revascularization of chronic total occlusions.

15.20 **Answer B.** Use of contralateral angiography is essential to identify the distal true lumen through collateral vessels (Figure 15-7A). Intravascular ultrasound may help distinguish a false passage into a subintimal dissection from the true lumen. Removal of the guidewire from an end-hole catheter placed distal to the occluded segment and contrast injection may help confirm placement into the true lumen if flow is observed without adventitial staining with contrast. Ability to deliver an angioplasty balloon past the occluded segment should not be interpreted as passage into the distal true lumen because the catheter may be easily advanced into a false lumen.

15.21 **Answer A.** The presence of a CTO in a non-IRA is a strong and independent predictor of 5-year mortality. Particularly in the high-risk subgroup of STEMI patients with DM, MVD has prognostic significance only if a concomitant CTO is present (*Heart* 2010;96:1968–1972). During the first 30 days following ST-elevation myocardial infarction (STEMI), the presence of a CTO (hazard ratio [HR] 3.6, 95% confidence interval [CI] 2.6–4.7) was the strongest predictor of mortality only after the presence of cardiogenic shock (HR 7.4, 95% CI 5.8–9.6) (*J Am Coll Cardiol Cardiovasc Interv* 2009;2:1128–1134).

15.22 **Answer B.** In a retrospective analysis of 486 patients with MVD, Valenti et al. (*Eur Heart J* 2008;29:1336–1342) reported a survival advantage for patients undergoing "complete" revascularization that involved successful treatment of the CTO. In an analysis of 2,608 patients undergoing attempted CTO revascularization, Safley and colleagues reported that successful CTO recanalization of the left anterior descending artery—but not the left circumflex or RCA—was associated with improved survival (*J Am Coll Cardiol Interv* 2008;1.295–1.302).

15.23 **Answer C.** Among 24,465 patients undergoing PCI, Carlino et al. described outcomes among 56 patients who had grade III coronary perforation (*J Am Coll Cardiol Interv* 2011;4:87–95). The device causing perforation was intracoronary balloon in 50%, intracoronary guidewire in 17.9%, rotablation in 3.6%, and directional atherectomy in 3.6%. Following perforation, immediate treatment and success rates, respectively, were prolonged balloon inflation 58.9%, 54.5%; covered stent implantation 46.4%, 84.6%; coronary artery bypass graft surgery and surgical repair 16.0%, 44.4%; and coil embolization 1.8%, 100%. In-hospital mortality was 14.8%. The combined procedural and in-hospital MI rate was 42.9%, and major adverse cardiac event rate was 55.4%. At late-term clinical follow-up (median: 38.1 months), 4.3% of patients experienced MI, 4.3% required coronary bypass surgery, and 15.2% died. The target lesion revascularization rate was 13%, with target vessel revascularization in 19.6%, and major adverse cardiac events in 41.3%.

16 Ostial and Bifurcation Lesions

Antonio Colombo and Azeem Latib

QUESTIONS

16.1 The operator performing percutaneous coronary intervention (PCI) on this right coronary artery (Fig. Q16-1) utilized a 6-F Judkins right guiding catheter with side holes. Which of the following would be very suggestive of an aorto-ostial lesion?

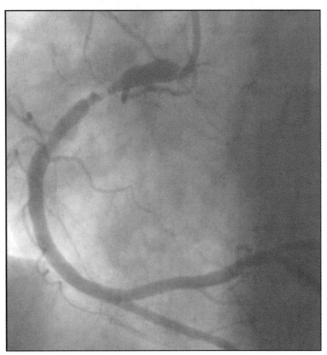

Figure Q16-1

(A) Pressure damping
(B) Absence of backflush of dye into the aorta
(C) Fractional flow reserve (FFR) measurement after intracoronary adenosine
(D) Angiographically visible stenosis

16.2 Directional coronary atherectomy remains an important technique to be used for ostial lesions located in the left anterior descending (LAD) artery (Fig. Q16-2):

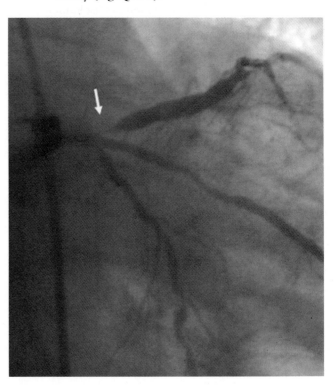

Figure Q16-2

(A) Only registries and single-center experiences support this statement

(B) A study evaluating the outcome of directional atherectomy vs. drug-eluting stent (DES) confirmed the superiority of the second approach

(C) The combination of directional atherectomy and drug-eluting stenting is the most effective one

(D) None of the above

16.3 Among the devices listed, which one has been proposed as the most suitable device to treat calcified non-aorto-ostial lesions?

(A) Cutting balloon

(B) Excimer laser

(C) Rotational atherectomy

(D) Compliant balloon

16.4 A 57-year-old man presenting with chest pain, an elevated troponin, and inferior T-wave inversion on ECG underwent coronary angiography. The left coronary artery was without significant stenosis, and the right coronary artery is shown in Figure Q16-4. The main difference between stent treatment of this aorto-ostial lesion and a non–aorto-ostial stenosis is:

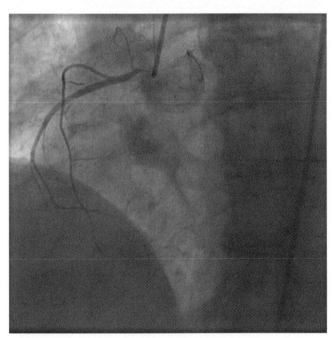

Figure Q16-4. (Courtesy of Dr. Andrew MacIsaac)

(A) There is no specific difference

(B) When treating a lesion located at the aorto-ostial location, the stent should protrude a few millimeters into the aorta

(C) The need to have the stent protrude proximally a few millimeters applies also for non–aorto-ostial lesions

(D) Non–aorto-ostial lesions should be treated routinely with a cutting balloon

16.5 The lesion in the above question was treated with implantation of 3.0/12 mm DES inflated to 14 atmospheres, utilizing an Amplatz left 1 guide catheter. Which of the following is the best description for the angiographic and intravascular ultrasound (IVUS) result at the ostium shown in Figure Q16-5?

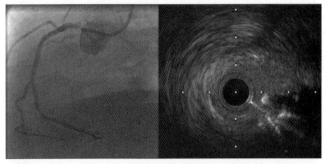

Figure Q16-5. (Courtesy of Dr. Andrew MacIsaac)

(A) The stent is underexpanded at the ostium

(B) Satisfactory stent deployment

(C) Stent strut malapposition

(D) Another stent is required

16.6 The _____ classification of bifurcation lesions is shown in Figure Q16-6:

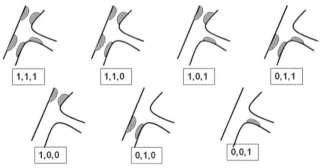

Figure Q16-6 (see color insert)

(A) Lefevre

(B) Medina

(C) Duke

(D) Sanborn

16.7 A 68-year-old patient with new onset chest pain during moderate effort undergoes stress echocardiography that demonstrates inducible ischemia of the anterior wall. Coronary angiography demonstrates the following bifurcation lesion (Fig. Q16-7). Based on the Nordic Bifurcation Study, which of the following would be true about the interventional strategy in this patient?

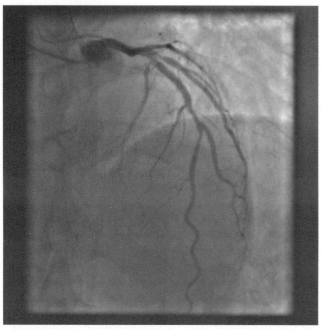

Figure Q16-7

(A) Stenting both branches of the bifurcation is associated with reduced target lesion revascularization rates during follow-up

(B) A provisional side-branch stenting approach is associated with lower side-branch restenosis at angiographic follow-up

(C) Elective stenting of both branches of the bifurcation is associated with higher rates of stent thrombosis

(D) A provisional side-branch approach is associated with lower contrast volumes and fluoroscopy time but similar event rates at follow-up, as compared to an elective two-stent approach

16.8 The bifurcation in the previous question was treated with a provisional approach and the main branch was stented with a 3.0/24 mm zotarolimus-eluting stent. Coronary angiography

reveals a residual stenosis at the side-branch ostium (Fig. Q16-8). The operator decided to perform FFR to evaluate this stenosis. Which of the following statements is true about the measurement of FFR on side branches with >50% angiographic residual narrowing after stent implantation on the main branch?

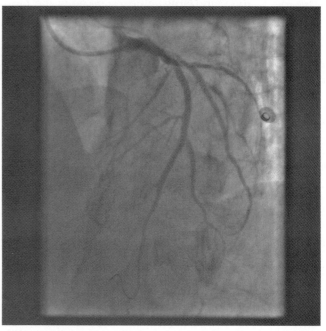

Figure Q16-8

(A) All the lesions have a reduced value of FFR (<0.75), indicating the functional significance of the narrowing in all cases

(B) Angiographic evaluation is sufficient and the residual stenosis in the side branch should be treated further

(C) Most lesions have normal values of FFR (>0.75), indicating the absence of functional significance of the narrowing in the majority of cases

(D) The measurement of FFR in this setting should be avoided due to the high rate of complications when recrossing through stent struts with the pressure guidewire

16.9 FFR evaluation of the jailed side branch in the previous question after adenosine-induced maximal hyperemia is shown (Fig. Q16-9). Based on this finding, what would be the most appropriate strategy for the side branch?

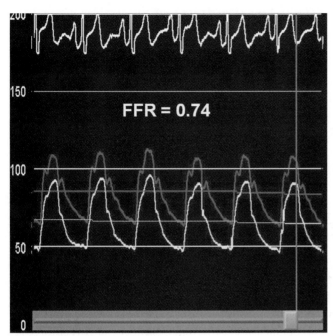

Figure Q16-9

(A) Stent implantation
(B) Kissing balloon inflation
(C) Medical therapy
(D) None of the above

16.10 A 60-year-old man with hypertension and dyslipidemia undergoes coronary angiography for effort-induced angina and a positive exercise stress test. On angiography, the right coronary artery shows no significant stenosis, and the left coronary artery is shown (Fig. Q16-10). Based on the findings of the CACTUS study, which of the following is correct about the percutaneous strategy in this patient?

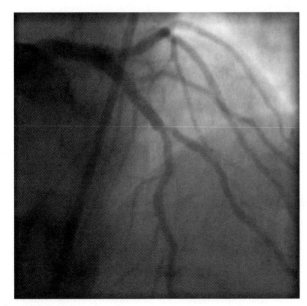

Figure Q16-10

(A) Provisional side-branch stenting is associated with a lower rate of myocardial infarction (MI) and death during follow-up
(B) Additional stenting on the side branch in the provisional group occurred in 50% of lesions
(C) Final kissing inflation was performed in less than half of bifurcations treated in this study
(D) Implantation of two stents in this bifurcation is not associated with a higher incidence of adverse events at 6 months

16.11 When performing the crush technique with sirolimus-eluting stents, which of these is important?

(A) Always deploy the stents using an 8-F guiding catheter
(B) Perform two-step final kissing-balloon inflation
(C) Restenosis and thrombosis rates are influenced by the performance of final kissing balloon inflation
(D) The most frequent site for restenosis is the body of the side branch

16.12 A 55-year-old man with a long-standing smoking history presenting with angina at rest but normal troponin undergoes coronary angiography. For the lesion shown (Fig. Q16-12), which is the best treatment strategy?

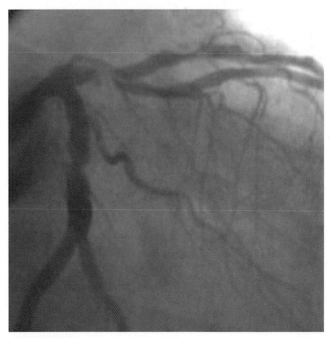

Figure Q16-12

(A) Culotte stenting
(B) Crush stenting
(C) Provisional side-branch stenting
(D) Any of the above

16.13 Which of the following is true about Culotte stenting?

(A) It does not provide complete coverage of the carina and side-branch ostium

(B) In the Nordic Stent Technique Study, Culotte stenting was associated with lower in-stent restenosis rates as compared to crush stenting

(C) Culotte stenting is associated with lower major adverse cardiac event rates as compared to crush stenting

(D) It can be performed in all types of bifurcation anatomy

16.14 A 55-year-old man undergoes coronary angiography and PCI via the right radial artery using a 6-F guiding catheter that demonstrates the following Medina 1,1,1 bifurcation lesion with marked angulation of the side branch (Fig. Q16-14). A floppy workhorse guidewire is placed in the main branch, and after great difficulty, the side branch was eventually wired. What would your bifurcation strategy be to this lesion?

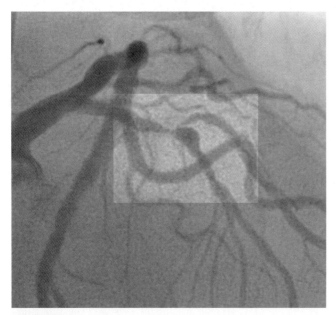

Figure Q16-14

(A) Provisional stenting

(B) V-stenting

(C) Culotte stenting

(D) Classical crush stenting

16.15 The angiographic images show a preintervention and postintervention images of a Medina 1,1,0 bifurcation treated with DES implantation on the main branch (Fig. Q16-15). What would your approach be toward the side branch?

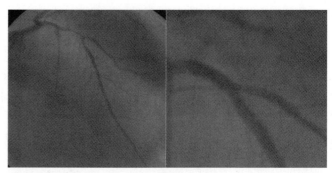

Figure Q16-15

(A) No further treatment of the side branch

(B) Routine final kissing inflation

(C) Side-branch–only dilatation

(D) Elective double stent implantation

16.16 A 65-year-old man presents with exertional angina and anteroapical ischemia on stress echocardiography. Coronary angiography demonstrates a critical stenosis of the mid LAD involving the bifurcation with a large second diagonal (Fig. Q16-16). What would your interventional approach be to this lesion?

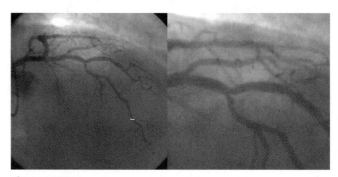

Figure Q16-16

(A) Elective double stenting of the LAD-diagonal bifurcation

(B) Placing a guidewire only in the LAD, followed by stenting across the ostium of the diagonal

(C) Wire both branches, followed by stenting of the LAD across the bifurcation

(D) Placing a guidewire only in the LAD, followed by stenting of the LAD distal to the ostium of the diagonal

16.17 Figure Q16-17 (*Circ Cardiovasc Interv* 2010;3:113–119) demonstrates the angiogram (left), cross-sectional IVUS image at the level of the carina (middle), and longitudinal IVUS image (right) before (upper panels) and after (lower panels) main-branch stent implantation. What is the explanation for the angiographic and IVUS findings of aggravation of the side-branch ostial stenosis after main-branch stent implantation?

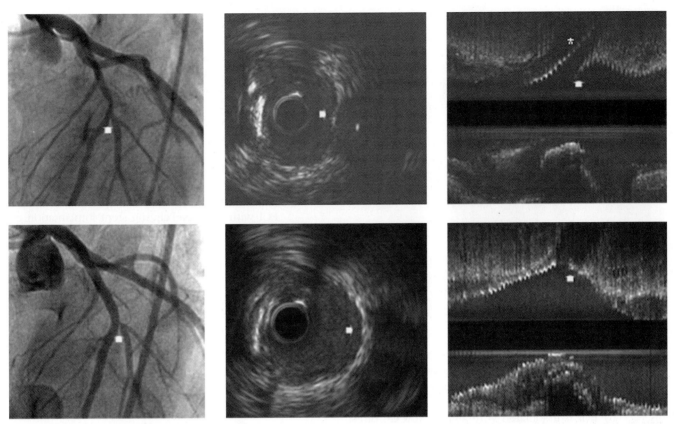

Figure Q16-17. (Courtesy of Dr. Bon-Kwon Koo)

(A) Plaque shift
(B) Thrombus
(C) Dissection
(D) Carina shift

16.18 If stent implantation is considered a clinically appropriate procedure in a patient with the lesion involving an unprotected left main coronary artery shown (Fig. Q16-18), the best approach is:

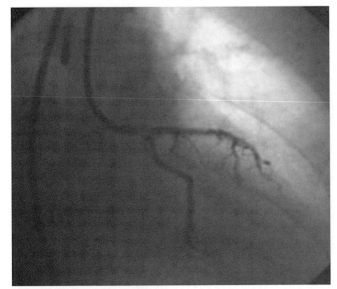

Figure Q16-18

(A) Perform directional atherectomy and then implant two bare-metal stents (BMS)
(B) Implant a DES toward the LAD artery leaving the implantation of a second stent toward the circumflex a possible option
(C) Proceed with implantation of two BMS, one in the LAD artery and the other in the circumflex
(D) Perform balloon angioplasty only in this lesion given its unique complexity

16.19 A 65-year-old male with dyslipidemia, hypertension, and effort angina (CCS 2) with a positive stress test underwent coronary angiography (Fig. Q16-19) that showed critical ostial stenosis of the left main and a focal stenosis of the midobtuse marginal (Syntax score 13). Based on the results of the SYNTAX Trial, which of the following would be true about the expected 12-month event rates in this patient?

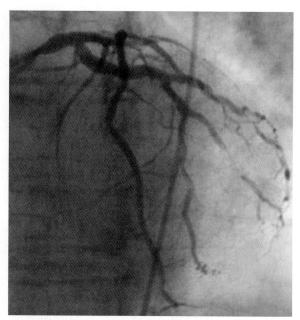

Figure Q16-19

(A) PCI is associated with higher major adverse cardiac and cerebrovascular event (MACCE) rates as compared to coronary artery bypass grafting (CABG)

(B) PCI is associated with similar MACCE rates as CABG

(C) PCI is associated with better outcomes compared to surgery

(D) PCI is associated with lower repeat revascularization rates

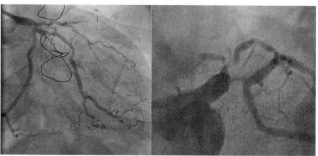

A
Figure Q16-20

16.20 A 72-year-old man with a history of previous coronary artery bypass graft (CABG) and occluded bypass grafts (2 vein grafts and left internal mammary artery) presented with an acute coronary syndrome. Baseline coronary angiography (Fig. Q16-20A) demonstrated a severe stenosis of the distal left main coronary artery (LMCA) bifurcation involving both the LAD and the left circumflex (LCX), a subtotally occluded and diffusely diseased LAD, and severe stenosis of the first diagonal branch (D1). An intra-aortic balloon pump (IABP) was electively inserted and the patient underwent PCI with paclitaxel-eluting stent implantation on the mid-LAD, first diagonal, and crush stenting of the LMCA bifurcation with two 3.5/32 mm stents. Two-step kissing inflation was performed with two 3.5/15 mm noncompliant balloons. The angiographic and IVUS images (Fig. Q16-20B) taken after final kissing inflation demonstrate:

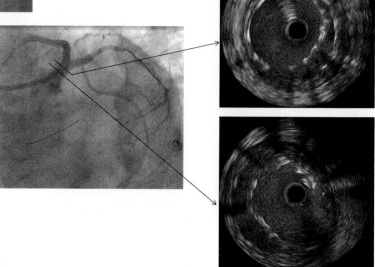

B

(A) Dissection
(B) Thrombus
(C) Stent underexpansion
(D) Stent malapposition
(E) Good final result

16.21 In an important report by Al Suwaidi and colleagues from the Mayo Clinic (*J Am Coll Cardiol* 2000;35:929–936) considering the outcomes following bifurcational bare-metal stenting, the authors conclude:

(A) Acute procedural success was higher in the group treated with two stents
(B) There was a lower incidence of in-hospital major adverse cardiovascular event (MACE) (0% vs. 13%, $p < 0.05$) in patients treated with only one stent
(C) There was a significantly lower restenosis rate when only one stent was implanted in the main branch
(D) The authors conclude that selective implantation of two stents may be advantageous

16.22 Among the most likely causes of restenosis at the ostium of the side branch when two DES are implanted on a bifurcation, the most likely explanation is:

(A) Flow dynamics involving the bifurcation with low shear stress in some sections
(B) The operator left a gap between the main-branch and the side-branch stent
(C) The stent on the side branch has been underdilated
(D) All the above are true

16.23 In a bench model evaluating flow dynamics in bifurcations, which of the following findings is TRUE?

(A) Platelet activation but not leukocyte recruitment was directly influenced by changes in flow pattern
(B) Optimal side-branch lumen will eliminate flow disturbances in the main branch
(C) The pattern of flow in the main branch was directly affected by alterations in the side branch alone
(D) All the above are true

16.24 The concept of "stent deformation" in the context of bifurcation stenting has been put forward to:

(A) Explain the coverage of the ostium of the side branch and the importance of kissing balloon inflation
(B) Explain some insufficient results obtained with culottes stenting
(C) Explain some cases of stent recoil in bifurcation located in tortuous segments
(D) Support the need for final kissing inflation when performing crush stenting

16.25 What is the role of IVUS-guided DES implantation in coronary bifurcation lesion treatment?

(A) IVUS-guided PCI has no role in bifurcation PCI
(B) IVUS-guided PCI is associated with higher periprocedural complication rates
(C) IVUS-guided PCI has been shown to reduce revascularization rates and restenosis after DES in randomized trials
(D) IVUS-guided PCI may improve long-term outcomes in coronary bifurcations, especially if involving the LMCA

16.1 **Answer B.** On the baseline image, there is clearly a proximal lesion, but the ostial lesion is not clearly evident. However, the absence of a good backflush into the aorta during contrast injection is suggestive of an ostial lesion. Pressure damping is also valuable but may be misleading when utilizing a guiding catheter with side holes. The presence of a pressure gradient after adenosine may be useful but is difficult to interpret in the presence of the proximal lesion and when utilizing a guiding catheter with side holes. Figure A16-1 shows the final angiogram after implantation of a 4-× 24-mm drug-eluting stent (DES) to treat the ostial and proximal lesion. The presence of backflow at the final angiogram is an important sign supporting a good final result and satisfactory treatment of the aorto-ostial lesion.

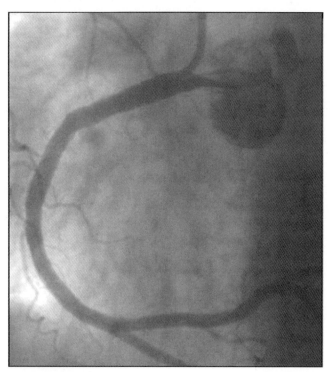

Figure A16-1

16.2 **Answer A.** Directional atherectomy can be used to treat ostial LAD lesions, and some centers still apply this technique with or without subsequent stenting (*Heart* 2003;89:1050–1054; *Am J Cardiol* 2002;90:1074–1078). Despite favorable results, there are no strong data to support a specific advantage of atherectomy compared with stenting with a DES, an approach with favorable registry results (*J Am Coll Cardiol* 2005;46:787–792).

16.3 **Answer C.** The cutting balloon as a stand-alone device is very unlikely to cross the lesion. A number of single-center studies (*J Invasive Cardiol* 1999;11:231–232; *Heart* 1997;77:350–352; *J Invasive Cardiol* 1999;11:201–206) have reported the feasible combination of stenting when preceded by cutting balloon dilatation. In bifurcation lesions, in which there is a large fibrotic plaque at the ostium of the side branch, use of the cutting balloon as a predilatation strategy before stenting does seem reasonable. The Restenosis reduction by Cutting balloon Evaluation (REDUCE) III trial evaluated the role of cutting balloon predilatation before stenting vs. standard balloon predilatation in a variety of lesions. This trial reported a lower restenosis rate when lesions were predilated with the cutting balloon. The Excimer laser is not effective in severely calcified lesions. Even if more specifically applied for calcific lesions, rotational atherectomy (rotablator) is the most appropriate answer (*Textbook of interventional cardiology.* 1999:345–366).

16.4 **Answer B.** Aorto-ostial lesions are more frequently difficult to dilate and are more prone to recoil than non–aorto-ostial lesions. This is due to more fibrous and elastic tissue in the aortic wall than within the coronary arteries. High-speed rotational atherectomy and cutting balloon have been advocated for difficult-to-dilate ostial lesions, especially when they are calcified. Precise stent placement is critical to ensure a satisfactory procedural outcomes. Determining the exact location of the vessel ostium can prove difficult especially after predilatation of the lesion. Appropriate guide catheter positioning is critical. Deep engagement of the vessel ostium may lead to distal stent deployment, that is, geographical miss. Alternatively, disengaging the guide catheter from the vessel ostium can result in poor vessel opacification, poor guide catheter support, and geographic miss. The most appropriate way to treat lesions located at the aorto-ostial location is to place a stent, which will slightly protrude into the aorta. This approach will guarantee adequate coverage of the ostium. Protrusion of more than a few millimeters increases the risk of stent embolization as well difficulty in re-engaging the vessel ostium for future angiography. Geographic miss of the ostium may predispose to stent recoil and restenosis.

16.5 **Answer D.** The angiogram demonstrates a hazy appearance of the right coronary ostium post-stent deployment. The IVUS demonstrates that there are no stent struts at the vessel ostium that has significant concentric plaque, thus confirming geographic miss of the ostial lesion. Another stent is required to cover the aorto-ostial lesion and protrude a few mm into the aorta. In this case, the position of the ostium was clarified by the IVUS ensuring that the second stent was accurately positioned. Figure A16-5 demonstrates the final angiographic result and the IVUS confirming that stent struts are protruding into the aorta.

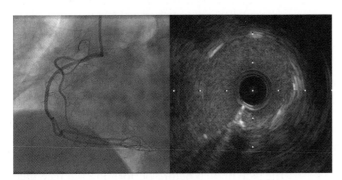

Figure A16-5

16.6 **Answer B.** The classification shown is the Medina classification (*Rev Esp Cardiol* 2006;59:183). Currently, there are at least seven classifications that have been proposed for bifurcation lesions (*J Am Coll Cardiol Interv* 2008;1:218–226). The Medina is the only classification that indicates the position of lesions and does not require memorization. It is comprised of three numbers separated by two commas. The first number represents the proximal main branch, the second number is for the distal main branch, and the third number is for the side branch. The number may either be "1" or "0" indicating the presence or absence of a >50% lesion.

16.7 **Answer D.** The Nordic Bifurcation Study randomized 413 patients to DES implantation in both branches (*n* = 206) with crush, culotte,

Y, or other techniques vs. provisional stenting (*n* = 207). At 8-month angiographic follow-up, there was no significant difference in restenosis of the bifurcation (22.5% vs. 16%, *p* = 0.15) or side branch (19.2% vs. 11.5%, *p* = 0.062) in the 1 vs. 2 stent group, respectively. At 6 months, the rates of major adverse cardiac events (3.4% vs. 2.9%) and stent thrombosis (0% vs. 0.5%) were similar between the double stenting and provisional groups, respectively. A two-stent strategy was associated with higher contrast usage (283 mL of contrast vs. 233 mL with one stent, *p* < 0.0001) and longer fluoroscopy times (21 minutes vs. 15 minutes with one stent, *p* < 0.0001).

16.8 **Answer C.** Angiographic evaluation overestimates the severity of jailed side branches during the provisional strategy, and thus FFR evaluation is recommended in important side branches with significant residual stenosis. Indeed, many lesions at the ostium of a side branch do not demonstrate signs of ischemia. Among 97 bifurcation lesions evaluated with FFR on both branches, none of the 21 lesions with <75% stenosis had FFR < 0.75, and among the 73 lesions with >75% stenosis, only 20 were functionally significant (*J Am Coll Cardiol* 2005;46:633–637). The unreliability of angiography in estimating the severity of side-branch stenosis was highlighted by the same group in a recent study in which FFR assessment of the side branch after intervention revealed that a hemodynamically significant side-branch stenosis was present only in 54.5% of lesions classified as severe by angiography and that 29.4% of angiographically nonsignificant side-branch lesions were associated with an abnormal FFR. Furthermore, in both of these studies, FFR measurement in jailed side-branch lesions was shown to be safe and feasible.

16.9 **Answer B.** In a study by Koo et al. (*Eur Heart J* 2008;29:726–732), kissing balloon angioplasty performed in 26 of 28 side-branch lesions with an FFR < 0.75 was successful in improving FFR to ≥0.75, even though the final mean residual stenosis was 69 ± 10%. During follow-up, there were no changes in side-branch FFR, and the rate of functional restenosis (FFR < 0.75) at 6-month follow-up was only 8%. In this patient, kissing balloon angioplasty was performed and resulted in an excellent angiographic and hemodynamic result (Fig. A16-9).

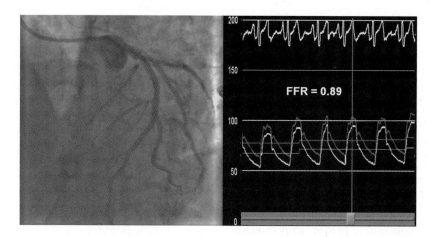

Figure A16-9

16.10 **Answer D.** The CACTUS (Coronary bifurcations: Application of the Crushing Technique Using Sirolimus-eluting stents) trial randomized 350 patients with true bifurcation lesions to either elective crush stenting or provisional side-branch stenting. The rates of angiographic restenosis at 6 months was similar between the crush (4.6% and 13.2% in the main branch and side branch, respectively) and the provisional stenting groups (6.7% and 14.7% in the main branch and side branch, respectively; P = NS). Furthermore, the rates of major adverse cardiac events (15.8% vs. 15%, P = NS), MI (10.7% vs. 8.6%, P = NS), death (0% vs. 0.5%), and TLR (7.3% vs. 6.3%, P = NS) were similar between the crush and the provisional groups. This study, in conjunction with other randomized trials, confirmed that provisional side-branch stenting is effective in most true non replace/with-left main bifurcations. The need to implant a second stent on the side branch occurred in 31% of cases, and we believe that in a real world setting, additional side-branch stenting is required in 20% to 30% of cases. Final kissing inflation was mandatory in CACTUS and successfully performed in over 90% of cases in both groups. A subanalysis suggested that kissing inflation was associated with a lower incidence of angiographic restenosis at the main and side branch of the bifurcation.

16.11 **Answer B.** The classical crush technique in which stents are positioned on the side branch and main branch, simultaneously, requires at least a 7-F guiding catheter, although we prefer using an 8-F guiding catheter. However, when there is the need to perform the minicrush technique and a 6-F guiding catheter is the only available approach (e.g., radial approach), the "step crush" or "the modified balloon crush" techniques can be used. The final result is basically similar to that obtained with the standard crush technique, with the only difference that each stent is advanced and deployed separately, with the side-branch stent crushed by a balloon placed on the main branch prior to side-branch stent deployment. When performing the crush technique, it is important to perform final kissing inflation following recrossing into the side branch. This maneuver lowers the risk of restenosis at the ostium of the side branch but does not seem to affect the risk of thrombosis (*J Am Coll Cardiol* 2005;46:613–620). When performing the crush technique, it is very important to perform the so called two-step kissing inflation that consists of high-pressure balloon inflation in the side branch before performing the true final kissing inflation at medium pressures. Ormiston et al. (*J Am Coll Cardiol Interv* 2008;1:351–357) have recently demonstrated through imaging of bench deployments that (1) recrossing the crushed stent for kissing postdilation, the most difficult part of the procedure, is technically easier with minicrush than with classical crush; (2) traditional one-step kissing postdilation leaves considerable residual metallic stenosis that may not be visible on angiography and may predispose to thrombosis because of eddy currents, stasis, altered shear stress, and foreign body presence; (3) side-branch ostial coverage and residual stenosis by metal struts is significantly reduced by two-step kissing inflation (Fig. A16-11). Finally, irrespective of the bifurcation technique utilized, the most frequent site of bifurcation restenosis remains the ostium of the side branch.

2-Step Kiss

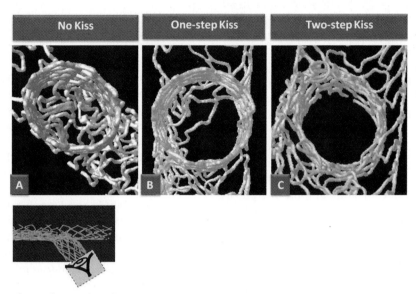

Figure A16-11. (Courtesy of Dr. John Ormiston)

16.12 **Answer D.** There is no recognized standard approach in the treatment of bifurcation lesions except for the preference of provisional side-branch stenting with final kissing balloon when possible (*J Am Coll Cardiol Interv* 2008;1:218–226). In this specific example, there is significant stenosis involving both branches with a reasonable reference vessel diameter (3.0 mm or more). In such a lesion, the usage of two DES as intention to treat appears a reasonable approach.

16.13 **Answer B.** The culotte technique provides near-perfect coverage of the carina and side-branch ostium at the expense of an excess of metal covering the proximal end. It will give the best immediate angiographic result, and theoretically, it may guarantee a more homogeneous distribution of struts and drug at the site of the bifurcation. The only anatomic limitation to the culotte technique is when there is a large mismatch between the proximal main-branch and the side-branch diameters due to the risk of incomplete side-branch stent apposition to the proximal main-branch. The Nordic Stent Technique Study is the only randomized trial comparing two different double stent techniques that result in complete coverage of the side-branch ostium (*Circ Cardiovasc Interv* 2009;2:27–34). In this study, 424 patients were randomized to either crush or culotte stenting utilizing sirolimus-eluting stents (77% of which were true bifurcation lesions). At 6-month clinical follow-up, there were no significant differences between the two groups in terms of death, MI, or revascularization (crush 4.3% vs. culotte 3.7%, $p = 0.87$). Procedure and fluoroscopy times and contrast volumes were also similar in the 2 groups. Angiographically, there was a trend toward less in-segment restenosis (6.6% vs. 12.1%; $p = 0.10$) and significantly reduced in-stent restenosis following culotte stenting (4.5% vs. 10.5%; $p = 0.046$).

16.14 **Answer C.** There are no certain data supporting a specific technique over another in this type of bifurcation. The unfavorable takeoff angle of the side branch may impede recrossing into the side branch with a wire, balloon, or stent after main-branch stenting, and thus the majority of operators would favor a two-stent approach with stenting of the side branch first, rather than a provisional stenting. As this procedure is being performed via the radial artery with a 6-F guiding catheter, two-stent techniques such as V-stenting and classical crush stenting that require the placement of a stent in the side and main branch simultaneously are not possible. The culotte stenting technique can be performed via a 6-F guiding catheter and would be the preferable approach. However, if the operator wants to perform one of the other bifurcation techniques described above, the guiding catheter could be upsized to 7 F, which would allow implantation of the newer second generation DES.

16.15 **Answer A.** In this nontrue bifurcation (i.e., no disease in the side branch), the result in the side branch after main branch is good without any evidence of side-branch compromise. The decision to perform no further treatment on the side branch is supported by the Nordic-Baltic Bifurcation Study III (*Circulation* 2011;123:79–86), which randomized 477 patients with bifurcation lesions undergoing main vessel stenting to final kissing inflation (*n* = 238) or no final kissing inflation (*n* = 239). The 6-month major adverse cardiac event rates were 2.1% and 2.5% (*p* = 1.0) in the final kissing and no final kissing groups, respectively. At 8 months, the rate of angiographic restenosis in the entire bifurcation lesion was 11.0% vs. 17.3% (*p* = 0.11), 3.1% vs. 2.5% in the main vessel (*p* = 0.68), and 7.9% vs. 15.4% in the side branch (*p* = 0.039), in the final kissing vs. no final kissing groups, respectively. The lower restenosis rate in the side branch was due to the efficacy of final kissing inflation in reducing angiographic restenosis in true bifurcation lesions, where the side-branch restenosis rate was 7.6% vs. 20.0% (*p* = 0.024) in the final kissing and no final kissing groups, respectively. This study supports the simple approach of only main vessel stenting without routine final kissing inflation in nontrue bifurcation lesions. However, in true bifurcation lesions that are treated with the provisional approach, routine final kissing inflation should be performed as it is associated with improved angiographic outcomes in the side branch.

16.16 **Answer C.** The most appropriate strategy in this patient would be to place a guidewire in both branches of the bifurcation and stent across the ostium of the diagonal. Stenting distal to the ostium would risk a suboptimal result in the LAD as well as in the diagonal branch. In this particular case, the operator only placed a guidewire in the main branch and not the side branch. Figure A16-16 shows the result after main vessel stenting with occlusion of the side branch (arrow). This case highlights the importance of protecting side branches with guidewires to prevent their closure as it has been shown that side-branch compromise is not inconsequential. Occlusion of side branches >1 mm can be associated with 14% incidence of MI (*Cathet Cardiovasc Diagn* 1989;18:210–212) and compromise of large side branches (≥2 mm) during a provisional approach can be associated with a large periprocedural MI (*J Thromb Thrombolysis* 2007;24:7–13). This approach of wiring both branches during bifurcation stenting is important in protecting the side branch from closure due to plaque shift, carina shift, and/or stent struts during main vessel stenting. The jailed side-branch wire also facilitates rewiring of the side branch (if side branch postdilatation/stenting or final kissing inflation is needed, or if the side branch occludes) by widening the angle between the main branch and the side branch, by acting as a marker for the side-branch ostium, and by changing the angle of side-branch takeoff. Finally, in the case of side-branch occlusion, the side-branch wire can be used to reopen the side branch by pushing a small balloon between the stent and the wall of the vessel. Interestingly, in the French multicenter TULIPE study, the absence of this jailed wire was associated with a higher rate of reinterventions during follow-up (*Catheter Cardiovasc Interv* 2006;68:67–73). There is no need to remove the jailed wire during high-pressure stent dilatation in the main vessel. It is preferable to avoid jailing hydrophilic guidewires as there is a risk of removing the polymer coating. Accurate handling of the guiding catheter to prevent migration into the ostium of the coronary vessel will allow removal of the jailed wire.

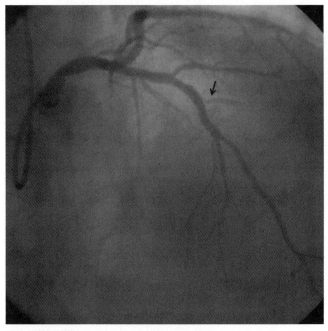

Figure A16-16

16.17 **Answer D.** The images demonstrate there is an alteration in the location and geometry of the carina. The carina is shifted to the side-branch side, and this shift results in an eccentric luminal narrowing of the side-branch ostium. There has been considerable debate as to whether the appearance of a new stenosis or aggravation of an existing stenosis at the side-branch ostium after main-branch stenting is due to plaque shift or carina shift. A recent study by Koo et al. (*Circ Cardiovasc Interv* 2010;3:113–119) of IVUS evaluation after main-branch stent implantation showed (1) a significant increase in the vessel and lumen volume index in both the proximal and the distal segments of the main branch, (2) a significant decrease in the plaque volume index in the proximal segment of the main branch, and (3) no change in the plaque volume index in the distal segment of the main branch after stenting. These results suggest that the lumen increase in the distal main branch is primarily due to enlargement of the vessel and not plaque shift, supporting the concept that part of the luminal narrowing of a side branch after stenting the main branch (MB) is explained by carina shift. However, in the proximal main branch, plaque area changed significantly after stent implantation, particularly in the region closest to the ostium of the side branch. Although, plaque shift to the side-branch ostium was not observed directly, these data provide indirect evidence of plaque shift from the proximal segment of the main branch into the side-branch ostium after main vessel stent implantation. Thus both plaque shift from the main branch and carina shift contribute to the creation/aggravation of a side-branch ostial lesion after main vessel stent implantation. Carina shift resulting in side-branch occlusion may be prevented by selecting the main-branch stent diameter according to the distal main-branch diameter.

16.18 **Answer B.** The lesion presented is a complex stenosis involving a left main coronary artery. Presently these lesions can be treated with stenting only in selected conditions such as the presence of a contraindication to the standard approach for left main stenosis, which is coronary artery bypass grafting (CABG). If the patient needs to be treated with a percutaneous technique, the most favored approach is for a DES (*Circulation* 2005;111:791–795; *J Am Coll Cardiol* 2005;45:351–356). While some operators may perform directional atherectomy, this approach is not considered standard in most coronary lesions; in addition, the stenosis presented here is likely to be calcific, a feature that makes directional atherectomy likely to fail.

16.19 **Answer B.** Current guidelines recommend CABG as the most appropriate strategy of treatment for patients with unprotected left main coronary artery (ULMCA) disease. However, since the introduction of DESs, the use of PCI has steadily expanded into more complex patient and lesion subsets, including patients with left main disease. The Synergy Between Percutaneous Coronary Intervention With TAXUS and Cardiac Surgery (SYNTAX) trial (*N Engl J Med* 2009;360:961–972) was the first large trial (1,800 patients) to randomize the revascularization strategy in patients with ULMCA and/or multivessel disease by either CABG or PCI with DES implantation. Althrough only hypothesis generating, the analysis of the ULMCA subgroup of patients ($n = 705$) enrolled in SYNTAX (*Circulation* 2010;121:2645–2653) showed comparable overall 12-month rates of MACCE with PCI vs. CABG (16% vs. 14%, $p = 0.44$). The rates of MI (4.3% vs. 4.1%; $p = 0.97$) and death (4.2% vs. 4.4.%; $p = 0.88$) were similar for PCI and CABG, while the rate of CVA was lower with PCI (0.3% vs. 2.7%; $p = 0.009$). However, PCI was associated with higher repeat revascularization rates (12% vs. 6.7%; $p = 0.02$). Subgroup analyses by left main in the presence or absence of multivessel disease suggest that the outcomes of PCI compared to CABG are good in patients with isolated left main or left main plus one-vessel disease. In contrast, outcomes in patients with ULMCA plus two- or three-vessel disease demonstrated equivalent safety but higher rates of repeat revascularization in the PCI group. The variability within these subgroup analyses suggested that lesion complexity has a great effect on outcomes in these patients. In this regard, the SYNTAX score may help to stratify the patients according to risk. Indeed analyses of SYNTAX score by baseline tercile demonstrated the concordance between clinical outcomes and baseline score (≤22: 13% CABG vs. 7.7% PCI, $p = 0.19$; 23–32: 15.5% CABG vs. 12.6% PCI, $p = 0.54$; ≥32: 12.9% CABG 25.3% PCI, $p = 0.008$). The available evidence was substantial enough to recently advance guidelines recommendations for ULMCA revascularization with PCI. In Europe, the recommendation for PCI in ULMCA disease was changed to Class IIa B in ostial/shaft lesions that are isolated or associated with single-vessel disease, whereas the indication for more complex ULMCA lesions (bifurcation lesions or ostial/shaft lesions plus two- or three-vessel disease) remained as Class IIb B. In the United States, the guidelines have also been recently modified with the class of recommendation for PCI to ULMCA changing from Class III to Class IIb B.

16.20 **Answer D.** Although the angiographic result appeared good, the IVUS images demonstrated marked malapposition of the stent in the distal LMCA. We thus performed further postdilatation with noncompliant balloons: 4.0 × 15 mm at 18 atm toward LAD, 3.5 × 12 mm at 18 atm toward LCX, and 4.5 × 20 mm at 18 atm on the LMCA. Repeat angiography and IVUS confirmed good stent apposition (Fig. A16-20). This case highlights the value of IVUS in complex lesions such as bifurcations, in particular the LMCA bifurcation.

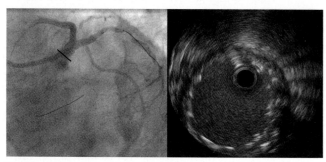

Figure A16-20

16.21 **Answer C.** This study, while nonrandomized, has received a lot of citations in the literature dealing with stenting bifurcational lesions; therefore, the reader needs to be familiar with this paper. In this report, the technique of implanting two stents was associated with more in-hospital MACE compared with the one-stent approach. All other comparisons favored the one-stent approach without reaching statistical significance. The difference in the acute MACE is most probably related to old stent delivery systems and it is unlikely to hold true with current stents, including DES.

16.22 **Answer D.** We do not know why, despite usage of DES, we still see side-branch restenosis in approximately 15% of the cases when two stents are implanted on a bifurcation. This finding is an improvement compared with results obtained following implantation of BMS where the restenosis on the side branch was two times higher or more. All hypotheses presented as answers to the question are potentially correct. A recent study evaluating the results of implantation of two DES (sirolimus) in bifurcational lesions proposed that the underexpansion or underdilatation of the side-branch stent is the main reason for a higher incidence of restenosis at this site (*J Am Coll Cardiol* 2005;46:599–605). Low shear stress and oscillatory shear stress are frequently present in bifurcation lesions and are known to promote intimal hyperplasia.

16.23 **Answer C.** Richter and others conducted a study with an in-vitro model and in an animal model of coronary bifurcations to evaluate the dynamics flow alterations and leukocyte adhesion as triggers for intimal hyperplasia. The main results of this study show that the flow dynamics in the side branch are a major determinant of the flow and patency of the main branch. The study evaluated leukocyte adhesion and not platelet activation. Contrary to the main findings of this study, an optimal side-branch lumen may disturb the flow pattern in the main branch (*J Clin Invest* 2004;113:1607–1614).

16.24 **Answer A.** The concept of stent deformation and side-branch coverage is important when performing provisional side-branch stenting. Some struts of the stent positioned in the main branch will slightly prolapse to partially stent the ostium of the side with balloon dilatation through the struts toward the side branch. If no final kissing balloon inflation is performed, the stent will be unfavorably deformed in the main branch (*Catheter Cardiovasc Interv* 2000;49:274–283; *Heart* 2004;90:713–722).

16.25 **Answer D.** Although the repeat revascularization rates at coronary bifurcations have significantly decreased after the introduction of DES, there still remain many challenges in optimizing outcomes in this complex lesion subset, which may be related to factors such as the variability in bifurcation anatomy and large number of possible anatomical permutations, the dynamic changes in anatomy during treatment, and the flow dynamics and shear stresses related to a bifurcation.

Although majority of IVUS studies have been underpowered or otherwise limited by selection bias or suboptimal technique, the collective results from numerous randomized and registry BMS studies (with rare exception) have demonstrated that IVUS guidance compared with angiographic guidance alone likely results in improved freedom from target vessel revascularization and MACE. Indeed, IVUS-guided PCI may be more beneficial if limited to complex lesions. Park SJ et al. (*Circ Cardiovasc Interv* 2009;2:167–177) have reported the findings from a post hoc analysis from the MAIN-COMPARE (revascularization for unprotected left MAIN coronary artery stenosis: COMparison of Percutaneous coronary Angioplasty vs. surgical REvascularization) multicenter registry in which the nonrandomized outcomes of IVUS guidance and angiography guidance for LMCA stenting were evaluated in 975 patients. Among 145 propensity-matched pairs of patients receiving DES, the 3-year incidence of mortality was 61% lower with IVUS guidance as compared with angiographic guidance. After multivariable adjustment this difference just missed statistical significance ($p = 0.055$). However, the risk of MI and target lesion revascularization was not lowered by the use of IVUS guidance. Furthermore Kim SJ et al. (*Am Heart J* 2011;161:180–187) showed that in patients treated with DES for bifurcation lesions, IVUS-guided PCI was associated with a lower incidence of death and MI at 3-year follow-up compared to angiography guided PCI. Although the exact mechanisms of eventual clinical benefits using IVUS at bifurcation lesions is not clearly explained, this imaging modality may help to better define bifurcation morphology, geometry, and plaque distribution for selecting an optimal stenting strategy. Furthermore IVUS may help to obtain an optimal final result after stent implantation by ensuring optimal stent expansion, adequate lesion coverage, and full stent apposition. The meticulous approach to these procedural aspects may help to reduce future adverse clinical events (i.e., stent thrombosis, MI, and death). Although these data are promising, they have been derived exclusively from retrospective observational studies and no amount of statistical adjustment can correct for major imbalances in unmeasured confounders. Only one randomized trial has been performed in the DES era in complex lesions (AVIO: Angiographic vs. IVUS optimization) and that was underpowered to show reductions in clinical outcome.

17

Long Lesions and Diffuse Disease

Joel A. Garcia and Ivan P. Casserly

QUESTIONS

17.1 What is the American College of Cardiology (ACC)/American Heart Association (AHA) criteria for the definition of a "long" lesion in the coronary circulation?

(A) <5 mm of length
(B) >5 mm of length
(C) >20 mm of length
(D) >10 mm of length

17.2 Which of the following statements is TRUE regarding the influence of lesion length on the AHA/ACC classification of lesion type?

(A) A lesion >2 cm in length represents an AHA/ACC Type B1 lesion
(B) A lesion <10 mm in length represents an AHA/ACC Type A lesion
(C) A lesion >2 cm in length represents an AHA/ACC Type B2 lesion
(D) A lesion 10 to 20 mm in length represents an AHA/ACC Type C lesion

17.3 The relationship between flow across a lesion and lesion length is governed by Poiseuille's law. Which of the following statements describes the relationship between these two variables?

(A) Flow is inversely related to lesion length
(B) Flow is directly related to lesion length
(C) Flow is directly related to the square of lesion length
(D) Flow is inversely related to the square of lesion length

17.4 The interventional treatment of long lesions may be impacted by significant vessel tapering along the length of the vessel. Which of the following statements regarding coronary vessel tapering is FALSE?

(A) Coronary artery lumen tapering is equal in the three major coronary arteries (left anterior descending [LAD], left circumflex [LCX], and right coronary artery [RCA])
(B) Coronary artery lumen tapering is dependent on anatomic vessel tapering (i.e., tapering in the external elastic media [EEM] between the proximal and distal vessels)
(C) In patients with documented coronary artery disease, coronary artery lumen tapering may be dependent on differential plaque accumulation (i.e., greater accumulation of plaque in distal compared with proximal segments)
(D) In patients with coronary artery disease, reverse coronary artery lumen tapering may occur in approximately 10% of coronary arteries
(E) Average coronary artery lumen tapering is 0.22 mm/10 mm of arterial length

17.5 A 58-year-old male who underwent heart transplantation 5 years ago due to an ischemic cardiomyopathy has a recent coronary angiogram characterized by diffuse and severe concentric narrowing of the coronary arteries. Regarding the diagnosis, prognostic significance, and treatment of this condition, all of the following statements are true, EXCEPT:

(A) Intravascular ultrasound (IVUS) offers earlier detection and better characterization when compared with routine angiography

(B) The presence of angiographic coronary disease posttransplantation is highly predictive of subsequent coronary disease–related events

(C) Flow-limiting lesions requiring intervention generally occur >5 years posttransplantation

(D) Primary procedural success for the interventional treatment of transplant vasculopathy lesions is less than for the treatment of native atherosclerosis

(E) Transplant vasculopathy is the second leading cause of death in cardiac transplant patients beyond 1 year from the time of transplantation

17.6 A 50-year-old female with a history of heart transplantation presents with evidence of heart failure and chest pain. The coronary angiogram (Fig. Q17-6) is consistent with which of the following diagnoses?

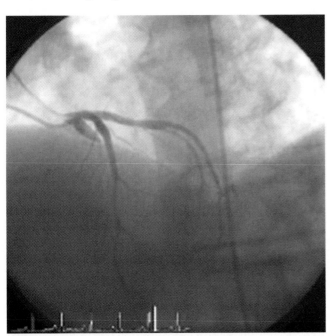

Figure Q17-6

(A) Normal vessel tapering
(B) Allograft vasculopathy in the LCX
(C) Diffuse coronary atherosclerosis
(D) Allograft vasculopathy in the LAD
(E) None of the above

17.7 A 57-year-old woman presented with 2 hours of substernal chest pain, anterior ST elevation, and elevated cardiac biomarkers. On engagement of the left coronary artery (LCA), the following angiographic image (Fig. Q17-7) was obtained. The angiographic appearance is most consistent with which of the following diagnoses?

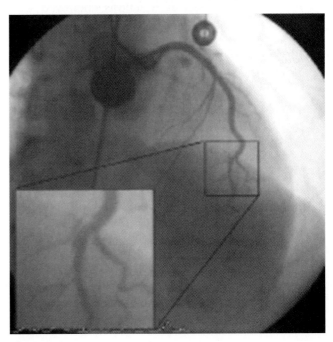

Figure Q17-7

(A) LAD dissection
(B) Unstable plaque in mid-LAD
(C) Diffuse LAD atherosclerosis
(D) Nonocclusive thrombus in the LAD
(E) None of the above

17.8 Regarding the impact of lesion length on clinical outcomes with the use of balloon angioplasty, which of the following statements is TRUE?

(A) Lesion length is a predictor of acute procedural success
(B) Lesion length is a predictor of acute procedural complications
(C) Lesion length is a strong predictor of late lumen loss and restenosis
(D) All of the above

17.9 Comparing stand-alone angioplasty, rotational atherectomy, and excimer laser angioplasty for the treatment of long coronary lesions, which of the following statements is FALSE?

(A) Rotational atherectomy is associated with a higher rate of initial procedural success
(B) Rotational atherectomy is associated with lower rates of restenosis compared with stand-alone angioplasty

(C) The incidence of periprocedural ischemic complications is equivalent for all treatment modalities

(D) Excimer laser angioplasty is associated with higher rates of restenosis compared with stand-alone angioplasty

17.10 Which of the following statements regarding the use of bare-metal stents (BMS) for the treatment of long coronary lesions is FALSE?

(A) The incidence of delivery failure is related to increased stent length

(B) Compared with stenting for treatment of focal lesions, stenting of long lesions is associated with significantly increased rates of lesion restenosis

(C) Compared with stenting for treatment of focal lesions, stenting of long lesions is associated with significantly increased rates of target lesion revascularization (TLR)

(D) Restenosis following stenting of long coronary lesions has been correlated with both lesion length and total stent length

(E) Treatment of long lesions with a single long stent has been proven superior to treatment with multiple overlapping stents

17.11 Regarding the strategy of angioplasty with provisional spot stenting (SS) for the treatment of long lesions, which one of the following statements is TRUE?

(A) The rate of major procedural complications with SS is higher when compared with traditional stenting (TS) of long lesions

(B) The composite incidence of death, myocardial infarction (MI), or target lesion revascularization (TLR) at 6 months is lower with SS compared with TS

(C) The rates of angiographic restenosis are less favorable with SS when compared with TS

(D) IVUS-guided SS has been proved to improve clinical outcomes over non–IVUS-guided SS in randomized studies

17.12 Comparing a strategy of angioplasty alone vs. angioplasty and bare-metal stenting for the treatment of long coronary lesions, which of the following statements is FALSE?

(A) Bailout stenting is required in up to one-third of patients treated with angioplasty alone

(B) Both strategies may have a similar acute angiographic result

(C) Angiographic restenosis is lower with stents

(D) Bailout stenting led to a threefold increase in periprocedural infarction

(E) Major adverse cardiovascular event (MACE) at 9 months favors the stented group

17.13 The Taxus V trial randomized patients with complex coronary lesions to treatment with a paclitaxel-eluting stent vs. a bare-metal stent (BMS). A subset of patients in this trial ($n = 379$) with a mean lesion length of approximately 25 mm required placement of multiple stents. Which of the following statements regarding clinical outcomes in this important subset is FALSE?

(A) In-stent restenosis rates were significantly reduced with the paclitaxel-eluting stent

(B) The use of multiple stents was associated with a significantly increased risk of periprocedural MI

(C) The use of multiple stents was associated with a significantly increased risk of significant side-branch stenosis

(D) The incidence of stent thrombosis was significantly increased in patients receiving multiple stents

17.14 Match the following angiograms (Fig. Q17-14A–D) with the most likely clinical diagnosis.

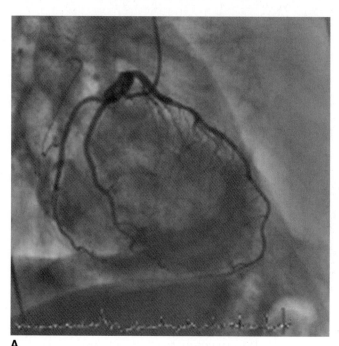

A
Figure Q17-14A

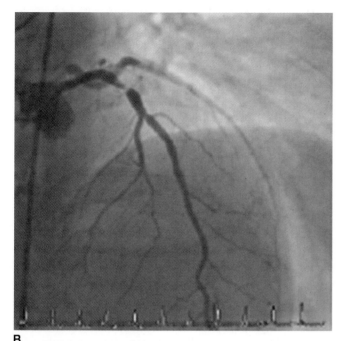

B
Figure Q17-14B

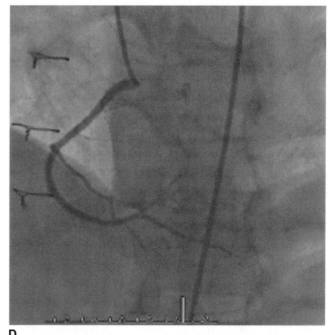

D
Figure Q17-14D

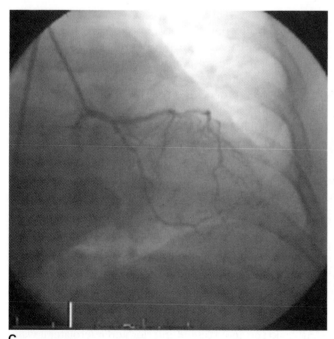

C
Figure Q17-14C

(A) Normal coronary lumen tapering
(B) Diabetic atherosclerosis
(C) Transplant vasculopathy
(D) Nondiabetic atherosclerosis

17.15 Regarding the relationships between the incidence of stent thrombosis and both stent length and lesion length, which of the following statements is TRUE?

(A) With the use of BMS, increased stent length is not predictive of an increased risk of stent thrombosis
(B) With the use of BMS, increased lesion length is predictive of an increased risk of stent thrombosis
(C) With the use of drug-eluting stents (DES), increased lesion length is predictive of an increased risk of stent thrombosis
(D) With the use of DES, increased stent length is predictive of an increased risk of stent thrombosis

17.16 Which of the following statements regarding the randomized efficacy of adjunctive pharmacologic therapies during PCI for the treatment of long lesions is TRUE?

(A) Preloading with a 300-mg dose of clopidogrel load is associated with a decreased rate of periprocedural MI

(B) Preloading with a 600-mg dose of clopidogrel load is associated with a decreased rate of periprocedural MI

(C) Bivalirudin is superior to unfractionated heparin in this cohort

(D) Adjunctive glycoprotein IIb/IIIa inhibition with abciximab decreases the risk of acute procedural complications in this cohort

(E) None of the above

17.17 A 65-year-old male with unstable angina is found to have a 23-mm-long lesion with an associated 90% stenosis in the mid RCA. You tell the patient that the length of the lesion favors the use of a DES as opposed to a BMS due to the risk of restenosis. The patient has concerns about the stent choice and asks for more information regarding current recommendations of BMS and DES. Based on the most recent American College of Cardiology (ACC), American Heart Association (AHA)/Society of Coronary Angiography and Interventions (SCAI), which of the following statements is TRUE?

(A) A DES should be considered as an alternative to a BMS in those patients for whom clinical trials indicate a favorable effectiveness/safety profile

(B) Before implanting a DES, the interventional cardiologist should discuss with the patient the need for and duration of dual antiplatelet therapy (DAT) and confirm the patient's ability to comply with the recommended therapy for DES

(C) In patients who are undergoing preparation for PCI and are likely to require invasive or surgical procedures for which DAT must be interrupted during the next 12 months, consideration should be given to implantation of a BMS or performance of balloon angioplasty with a provisional stent implantation instead of the routine use of a DES

(D) None of the above

(E) All of the above

17.18 A 36-year-old female of childbearing age presents with substernal chest pressure, electrocardiographic evidence of anterior injury, and elevated cardiac biomarkers. She has no significant risk factors. There is angiographic evidence of an LAD artery dissection (>30 mm) extending from the mid to distal preapical segment. There is TIMI I flow in the mid to distal vessel. PTCA was performed resulting in no flow, worsening chest

pressure, and hemodynamic instability. The operator rapidly places a long stent but no-reflow persists. Which of the following statements is TRUE?

(A) Propagation of intramural hematoma may have compromised the distal vessel resulting in a worsening lesion distal to the stent

(B) The operator should question the position of the wire in the true lumen vs. the false lumen

(C) There may be severe spasm at the distal edge of the stent, and coronary vasodilators may help

(D) Ineffective anticoagulation may have resulted in thrombosis

(E) All of the above

17.19 A 61-year-old diabetic male presents with stable angina refractory to standard medical therapy. Myocardial perfusion imaging shows a large defect in the anterior wall of moderate severity. Angiography reveals a long LAD lesion with diffuse disease. Prior to stenting, your interventional colleague prompts you to use IVUS. Which of these arguments is CORRECT?

(A) IVUS evaluation is a very useful tool for selecting the most appropriate sized stent

(B) IVUS allows the operator to discern negative vessel remodeling from plaque burden in diffuse disease

(C) IVUS decreases the risk of undersizing a stent

(D) IVUS decreases the risk of oversizing a stent and thus reduces the risk of vessel rupture

(E) In the context of diffuse disease, it is common to see segments with negative and positive remodeling

(F) All of the above

17.20 A very compliant 59-year-old diabetic presents with worsening angina despite aggressive medical therapy prompting further evaluation. An exercise perfusion imaging test showed an electrocardiographically and clinically positive result at 5 minutes. The imaging portion of the test showed transient ischemic dilatation and areas of ischemia in the anterolateral, inferior, and inferolateral walls. There was movement during the test, increasing the chances of artifact. The angiographic evaluation shows a 20% left main lesion, 22-mm-long 60% lesion in the mid LAD, a 50% 12-mm-long first diagonal lesion, a 12-mm-long 70% circumflex lesion, and a 25-mm-long 70% to 80% RCA lesion. While your colleague calculates the SYNTAX score, you think of the potential lesion evaluation techniques, revascularization strategies, and medical therapy. Which of the following statements is CORRECT?

(A) In the SYNTAX study, the adverse event rates at 3 years were not significantly different for patients with a low (0 to 22) baseline score; for patients with intermediate (23 to 32) or high SYNTAX scores (33) for patients treated with CABG, but adverse events increased with higher scores in patients treated with PCI

(B) Among the SYNTAX randomized patients, 3-year adverse events remained significantly higher for PCI than CABG, mainly driven by higher repeat revascularization in the PCI arm

(C) The 3-year SYNTAX results suggest that CABG remains the standard of care for patients with complex disease (intermediate or high scores); however, PCI may be an acceptable alternative revascularization method to CABG in patients with lower SYNTAX scores

(D) Routine measurement of FFR in the FAME study in patients with multivessel disease who are undergoing PCI with DESs significantly reduces the rate of the composite end point of death, nonfatal MI, and repeat revascularization at 1 year

(E) All of the above

(F) None of the above

17.21 A 47-year-old Caucasian male presents with unstable angina. He has a strong family history for atherosclerosis. His electrocardiogram shows 1 mm of ST-segment depression in V2 to V6. After initial management, his symptoms improve and the electrocardiographic changes improve. Hours after the discontinuation of nitroglycerin due to a headache, his symptoms come back as well as the electrocardiographic changes. A coronary angiogram is completed, and the following image is obtained (Fig. Q17-21). The RCA is normal. Which of the following statements is the most CORRECT?

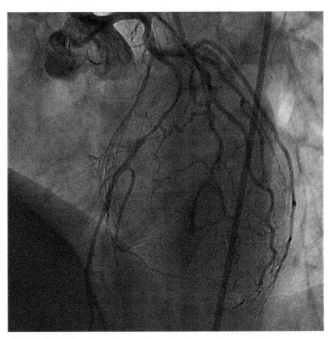

Figure Q17-21

(A) This is an obvious atherosclerotic lesion requiring percutaneous coronary intervention given the unstable angina presentation

(B) Medical management is recommended as the lesion does not appear severe

(C) Administration of an intra-arterial vasodilator is recommended to rule out vasospasm

(D) A fractional flow reserve evaluation should be completed with subsequent intervention if the value is <0.75

17.22 A 73-year-old male with angina pectoris presents to your office with a diagnostic angiogram showing a 31-mm-long diffuse lesion in the mid LAD. He asks you about relative efficacy of currently available DES for this lesion. Based on a subgroup analysis of the ZEST 2-year follow-up you tell him:

(A) Zotarolimus (ZES) results in similar rates of MACE compared with sirolimus (SES)

(B) ZES results in similar rates of MACE compared with paclitaxel (PES)

(C) SES results in similar rates of MACE compared with PES

17.23 The Long DES–II trial had suggested that:

(A) For patients with long native coronary artery disease, SES implantation was associated with a reduced incidence of angiographic restenosis and a reduced need for target lesion revascularization compared with PES implantation

(B) For patients with long native coronary artery disease, SES implantation was associated with a higher incidence of angiographic restenosis and a reduced need for target lesion revascularization compared with PES implantation

(C) For patients with long native coronary artery disease, SES implantation was associated with a similar incidence of angiographic restenosis and a reduced need for target lesion revascularization compared with PES implantation

17.1 **Answer C.** According to the ACC/AHA and the Society for Coronary Angiography and Interventions lesion classifications system, lesions <10 mm in length are discrete, lesions of 10 to 20 mm in length are referred to as tubular, and lesions >20 mm in length are considered long (*Am J Cardiol* 2003;92:389–394).

17.2 **Answer B.** Type A lesions are considered discrete and are <10 mm in length. In terms of lesion length, both Type B1 and B2 lesions are 10 to 20 mm in length. Type B2 lesions have two or more Type B characteristics (e.g., eccentricity, moderate tortuosity, moderate angulation, moderate to heavy calcification, ostial location, bifurcation lesions, presence of thrombus, total occlusion <3 months old). Finally, Type C lesions are considered diffuse and have a length of ≥2 cm (*Am J Cardiol* 2003;92:389–394).

17.3 **Answer A.** According to Poiseuille law, flow = π $(\Delta P)(r^4)/8(\eta)(l)$ where
P = the pressure difference across the lesion
r = minimal lumen radius of the stenotic segment
η = blood viscosity
l = lesion length

The lesion length is inversely related to translesional flow. Therefore, for short, discrete lesions, length exerts relatively little impact on translesional flow, but for longer lesions (>20 mm), length can make a significant impact on translesional flow (*Topol Textbook of Interventional Cardiology* 2003;367–379).

17.4 **Answer A.** In two separate series (*Am J Cardiol* 1992;69:188–193; *Am J Cardiol* 1995;75:177–180) the mean coronary artery lumen tapering was found to be approximately 0.22 mm over a 10-mm length of coronary arterial length. In the series of patients with documented coronary artery disease reported by Javier et al., there was a subset of coronary arteries (11%) that demonstrated reverse coronary artery lumen tapering (i.e., distal lumen CSA greater than proximal lumen CSA). In this same series, coronary artery lumen tapering was significantly greater in the LAD as compared with the LCX and RCA. Using IVUS, Javier examined the mechanism of coronary artery lumen tapering. It appears that in patients with coronary artery disease,

lumen tapering is dependent on both anatomic vessel tapering (i.e., decrease in EEM between proximal and distal segments) and differential plaque accumulation (i.e., greater accumulation of plaque in distal compared with proximal segments). Coronary artery lumen tapering is important in the treatment of long lesions because of the difference in vessel diameter at the proximal and distal margins of the lesion. Balloon and stent sizing to the vessel diameter at the proximal margin of the lesion may increase the risk of dissection at the distal margin of the lesion. In contrast, sizing of balloon and stents to the vessel diameter at the distal margin of the lesion may result in inadequate lumen expansion proximally and a suboptimal result.

17.5 **Answer D.** Traditional noninvasive modalities are insensitive in the detection of transplant vasculopathy. Although conventional coronary angiography is the most commonly employed method for the detection of transplant vasculopathy, it is less sensitive than IVUS, which is the gold standard for the detection of this pathology (*Circulation* 1998;98:2672–2678; *J Am Coll Cardiol* 2005;45:1538–1542; *Circulation* 1999;100:458–460). Significant flow-limiting lesions due to transplant vasculopathy are unusual in the first 5 years posttransplantation but show an exponential rise after this time point. Interventional strategies including angioplasty and stenting have been reported for the treatment of these lesions, with similar primary procedural success compared with the treatment of native coronary atherosclerosis. There is a high rate of repeat procedures in this group, due to a combination of late restenosis at the treatment site and progression of transplant vasculopathy. Beyond 1 year from the time of cardiac transplantation, transplant vasculopathy is the second leading cause of death, with malignancy being the most common cause (*J Heart Lung Transplant* 2005;24:945–955). In patients with end-stage transplant vasculopathy, the only treatment option currently is repeat transplantation.

17.6 **Answer D.** The figure shows a left anterior oblique (LAO) cranial angiogram from the LCA approximately 6 years after cardiac transplantation. It demonstrates a decrease in the lumen caliber of the LAD that is significantly greater than one would expect due to normal vessel tapering. The circumflex is of normal caliber and shows normal vessel tapering. The angiographic findings are most consistent with the diagnosis of significant transplant vasculopathy in the LAD, which was confirmed by IVUS examination.

17.7   Answer A. The angiogram demonstrates a normal-caliber proximal LAD with an abrupt decrease in caliber at the level of the third diagonal branch followed by diffuse narrowing of the distal LAD. Also note the prominent tortuosity of the distal LAD. This angiographic appearance is most consistent with a coronary dissection in the mid-LAD which propagated distally, resulting in diffuse luminal narrowing. The abrupt nature of the luminal diameter change differentiates this pathology from that of diffuse coronary atherosclerosis, and from normal vessel tapering. The presence of an unstable plaque alone would not be expected to be associated with diffuse narrowing distal to the lesion.

17.8   Answer D. In the balloon angioplasty era, acute procedural success with short (<10 mm) lesions was 95%, with tubular lesions (10 to 20 mm) was 85%, and with long lesions (>20 mm) was 74%. Similarly, there was a significant increase in acute procedural complications such as abrupt vessel closure and dissection, and restenosis rates with increasing lesion length. The mechanism of these adverse outcomes with angioplasty alone is likely multifactorial, and is due to an association between increased lesion length and adverse morphologic characteristics (e.g., angulated segments, bifurcation points), and heterogeneity in composition of plaque resulting in uneven distribution of shear stresses during balloon dilatation and predisposition to dissection (*Topol Textbook of Interventional Cardiology* 2003;367–379).

17.9   Answer B. Two randomized studies provide comparative data regarding the treatment of long lesions with angioplasty, rotational atherectomy, and excimer laser. The Excimer laser, Rotational Atherectomy, and Balloon Angioplasty Comparison (ERBAC) trial (*Circulation* 1997;96:91–98) compared all three modalities for treatment of patients with complex lesion morphology (approximately 50% were >10 mm in length). This study showed a higher initial procedural success with rotational atherectomy (89% vs. 80% for angioplasty vs. 77% for Excimer laser). Periprocedural ischemic complications were equivalent for all treatment modalities. Despite

the higher initial procedural success with rotational atherectomy, 6-month restenosis rates were significantly higher in the rotational atherectomy compared with angioplasty (42.4% vs. 31.9%). Similarly, restenosis rates with excimer laser were significantly higher than with angioplasty (46% vs. 31.9%).

The AMRO trial randomized patients with lesions >10 mm in length and stable angina to treatment with excimer laser or angioplasty. The findings mirrored those of the ERBAC trial, with similar initial angiographic success rates and incidence of periprocedural complications for the two treatment modalities, but a higher late lumen loss in the excimer laser–treated patients (*Lancet* 1996;347:79–84).

17.10   Answer E. The use of BMS for the treatment of long lesions is associated with significantly higher rates of restenosis and TLR compared with the treatment of focal disease. In various series, restenosis rates for the treatment of long lesions varies from 20% to 40%, with TLR rates of 15% to 25% (*Circulation* 1997;96:1–472; *J Am Coll Cardiol* 1995;25:156A; *Am Heart J* 2001;141:971–976; *Catheter Cardiovasc Interv* 1999;48:287–293 discussion 294–295; *Circulation* 1996;94:I–685). This compares with a restenosis rate of 11.4% and TLR rate of 8% in the STRESS and BENESTENT trials of stenting of focal lesions (*N Engl J Med* 1994;331:496–501; *N Engl J Med* 1994;331:489–495). A large number of studies have examined the relationship between the rates of restenosis and both lesion length and total stent length. The data are conflicting, but in summary, there is evidence to suggest that both variables impact rates of restenosis. There are no randomized data demonstrating the superiority of a single long BMS vs. multiple overlapping BMS for the treatment of long lesions. In practice, most operators prefer the approach of using a single long stent, since this reduces catheterization time, contrast load, and radiation exposure. However, in some cases, (e.g., because of difficulties with stent delivery, significant mismatch in the diameter between proximal and distal reference segments, lesion length greater than available stent lengths) multiple overlapping stents may be required to treat a long lesion.

17.11   Answer B. Colombo et al. showed that long-term outcomes with IVUS-guided SS (131 lesions in 101 patients), including angiographic restenosis and follow-up MACE, are superior to the outcomes achieved in a matched group of patients treated with TS in an observational study. Although IVUS-guided SS has been associated with good outcomes for the treatment of long lesions, there are no randomized studies to determine the superiority of an IVUS-guided vs. non-IVUS-guided strategy (*J Am Coll Cardiol* 2001;38:1427–1433).

17.12 **Answer E.** Serruys et al. reported a randomized comparison angioplasty with provisional stenting for suboptimal angiographic results vs. angioplasty and elective stenting (using NIR stent) in 437 patients with long lesions (mean length 27 ± 9 mm). The strategy of angioplasty with provisional stenting resulted in bailout stenting in one third of patients (34%), with a threefold increase in periprocedural infarction. Angioplasty followed by elective stenting yielded a lower angiographic restenosis rate, but no reduction in MACE at 9 months (*J Am Coll Cardiol* 2002;39:393–399).

17.13 **Answer D.** Taxus V was a randomized trial of DES vs. BMS for the treatment of complex coronary lesions, including longer lesions (*JAMA* 2005;294:1215–1223). A subset of patients in this trial received multiple stents (either planned for treatment of long lesions or as a bailout for treatment of complications or a suboptimal result). In this subset, although restenosis and TLR rates were significantly reduced in the paclitaxel-eluting stent group, there was an excess of procedure-related MIs in this group (8.3% vs. 3.3%, mainly non–Q wave MIs). The use of multiple stents was also associated with a significant increase in significant side-branch stenosis and occlusion (42.6% vs. 30.6%). The rate of stent thrombosis was not significantly different between the groups (1% in DES group vs. 0.5% in BMS group).

17.14 **Answer 1 = A, 2 = C, 3 = D, 4 = B.** Option A shows an angiographically normal LCA with normal vessel tapering. Option B represents focal nondiabetic atherosclerosis of the proximal LAD. Option C is an example of diabetic atherosclerosis. Note the severe diffuse vessel atherosclerotic narrowing evident in all vessel segments. Option D shows a case of severe transplant vasculopathy in the RCA. Note that there is concentric narrowing of the distal epicardial vessel with prominent involvement of the small side branches, which is the characteristic angiographic appearance of transplant vasculopathy.

17.15 **Answer D.** Increased stent length, both with BMS and DES, predicts an increased risk of stent thrombosis. In an analysis of six BMS trials, Cutlip

et al. demonstrated a 30% increase in the risk of stent thrombosis per 10 mm of BMS (*Circulation* 2001;103:1967–1971). In a large prospective observational series of patients receiving DES, Iakovou et al. demonstrated a similar magnitude of risk of increased stent thrombosis per 10 mm of DES length (*JAMA* 2005;293: 2126–2130). Lesion length does not appear to predict an increased risk of stent thrombosis (*J Am Coll Cardiol* 2005;45:954–959).

17.16 **Answer E.** There are no randomized data regarding the use of antiplatelet or anticoagulant agents in the interventional management of long lesions. Despite the absence of such data, most operators are more aggressive with the use of antiplatelet and anticoagulant agents in the treatment of long lesions.

17.17 **Answer E.** These are all Class I recommendations from the Focused update of the ACC/AHA/SCAI 2005 Guideline Update for Percutaneous Coronary Intervention (*J Am Coll Cardiol* 2008;51:172–209).

17.18 **Answer E.** All are possible explanations as to why stenting resulted in no-reflow in this case. It is not uncommon for propagation of an intramural hematoma to worsen the outflow of the treated segment after stenting. Operators should be very careful in dissected coronary segments not to expand the dissection plane by careful and meticulous evaluation of the wire position (false lumen vs. true lumen). Spasm is not uncommon and, while easily treated (vasodilators), may compromise the outflow of a stented segment. Finally it is very important to consider thrombosis as the possible explanation of reduced flow due to insufficient anticoagulation or antiplatelet therapy.

17.19 **Answer F.** In the context of diffuse disease, IVUS evaluation is a useful tool for selecting an appropriate stent. Visual estimation of a long lesion in diffuse disease does not allow for an accurate evaluation of negative remodeling vs. plaque burden. This visual estimation may result in the undersizing of the stent. Long diffuse disease can have areas of negative and positive remodeling.

17.20 **Answer E.** In the SYNTAX study, the adverse event rates at 3 years were not significantly different for patient with a low (0 to 22) baseline score; for patients with intermediate (23 to 32) or high SYNTAX scores (33) with CABG, but adverse events increased with higher scores in patients treated with PCI. In the SYNTAX randomized patients, 3-year adverse events remained significantly higher for PCI than CABG, mainly driven by higher repeat revascularization in the PCI arm. (The 3-year SYNTAX results suggest that CABG remains the standard of care for patients with complex disease (intermediate or high scores); however, PCI may be an acceptable alternative revascularization method to CABG in patients with lower SYNTAX scores (*N Engl J Med* 2009; 360:961–972). In the FAME study, routine measurement of FFR in patients with multivessel disease who are undergoing PCI with DES significantly reduces the rate of the composite end point of death, nonfatal MI, and repeat revascularization at 1 year (*N Engl J Med* 2009;360:213–224).

17.21 **Answer C.** This is a long LAD artery lesion. Although risk factors are present, it is always a good practice to administer intra-arterial vasodilators to rule out spasm. In this case, the administration of vasodilators resulted in disappearance of the lesion (Fig. A17-21). The use of FFR may have resulted in resolution of the spasm by the administration of adenosine but is clearly more invasive and expensive when compared to the administration of intracoronary nitroglycerin (NTG). FFR should be considered if the lesions does not resolve with NTG.

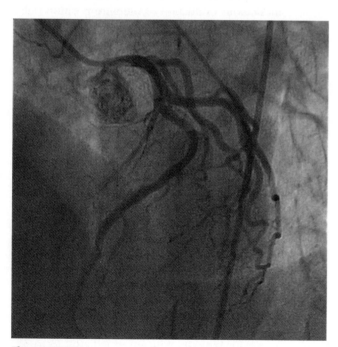

Figure A17-21

17.22 **Answer B.** In the Zotarolimus-Eluting Stent vs. Sirolimus-Eluting Stent and PacliTaxel-Eluting Stent for Coronary Lesions (ZEST) trial, a total of 960 patients with very long coronary lesions were treated with zotarolimus (ZES, 322 patients), sirolimus (SES, 317 patients), or paclitaxel-eluting stents (PES, 321 patients). All patients with very long lesions were available for 2-year clinical follow-up. At 24 months, the ZES group showed similar rates of MACE compared with the PES group (16.1% vs. 17.4, $p = 0.58$), but trend toward higher rates of events compared with the SES group (16.0% vs. 11.0%, $p = 0.059$). These differences were mainly driven by TVR (SES vs. ZES, $p = 0.059$; ZES vs. PES, $p = 0.37$; SES vs. PES, $p = 0.006$). There was no significant difference of death or MI among the groups. Overall, for patients with very long coronary artery disease, PCI with ZES results in similar rates of MACE compared with PES, but trends toward higher rates of MACE compared with SES at 2-year follow-up (*Circulation* 2010;122:A15245).

17.23 **Answer A.** The long DES-II, prospective study compared the use of long (32-mm) SES with PES in 500 patients with long (25-mm) native coronary lesions. The primary end point of the trial was the rate of binary in-segment restenosis according to follow-up angiography at 6 months. The SES and PES groups had similar baseline characteristics. Lesion length was 33.9 ± 11.6 mm in the SES group and 34.5 ± 12.6 mm in the PES group ($p = 0.527$). The in-segment binary restenosis rate was significantly lower in the SES group than in the PES group (3.3% vs. 14.6%; relative risk 0.23; $p < 0.001$). In-stent late loss of lumen diameter was Z 0.09 ± 0.37 mm in the SES group and 0.45 ± 0.55 mm in the PES group ($p < 0.001$). In patients with restenoses, a pattern of focal restenosis was more common in the SES group than in the PES group (100% vs. 53.3%, $p = 0.031$). Consequently, SES patients had a lower rate of target lesion revascularization at 9 months (2.4% vs. 7.2%, $p = 0.012$). The incidence of death (0.8% in SES vs. 0% in PES, $p = 0.499$) or MI (8.8% in SES vs. 10.8% in PES, $p = 0.452$) at 9 months of follow-up was not statistically different between the 2 groups. The trial suggested that for patients with long native coronary artery disease, SES implantation was associated with a reduced incidence of angiographic restenosis and a reduced need for target lesion revascularization compared with PES implantation (*Circulation* 2006;114:2148–2153).

18 Restenosis and Percutaneous Options

Craig R. Narins

QUESTIONS

18.1 A 61-year-old woman with diabetes mellitus and hypertension presented with unstable angina. Coronary angiography demonstrated single-vessel coronary artery disease as displayed in Figure Q18-1. A 2.5/12-mm sirolimus-eluting stent was placed at the ostium of the right coronary artery. Which of the following factors is NOT a predictor of higher restenosis following drug-eluting stent (DES) placement in this patient?

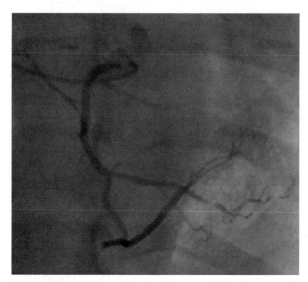

Figure Q18-1

(A) Ostial lesion location
(B) Diabetes mellitus
(C) Smaller reference vessel diameter
(D) Use of a sirolimus-eluting rather than a pacli-taxel-eluting stent
(E) Native vessel rather than vein graft lesion location

18.2 Which of the following statements regarding the pathogenesis of coronary atherosclerosis vs. coronary restenosis is true?

(A) Vessel wall inflammation, which is a major component in the formation of coronary atherosclerosis, plays little role in the development of restenosis
(B) Lipid-rich pools are commonly found in both atherosclerotic and restenotic lesions
(C) Genetic susceptibility plays a role in the occurrence of both atherosclerosis and restenosis
(D) Plaque rupture and acute thrombosis serve as predominant mechanisms for clinical events caused by both atherosclerotic and restenotic lesions

18.3 Which of the following statements is true regarding the use of animal models for the study of restenosis?

(A) Smooth muscle cell proliferation and migration from media to intima is a feature of all animal models of restenosis
(B) Animals subjected to hyperlipidemic diets typically demonstrate histologic features of atherosclerosis identical to those seen in human atherosclerosis including ulceration, intraplaque hemorrhage, and thrombosis
(C) The use of large mammals (particularly canine and porcine models) permits accurate study of complex human phenotypes that predispose to restenosis, such as diabetes
(D) Development of hemodynamically significant lesions following balloon-induced vascular injury is a feature common to all animal models of restenosis

18.4 A 57-year-old man is referred for coronary angiography following a non–ST-elevation MI. The angiogram demonstrates a severe stenosis of the mid-right coronary artery, and a 3.5/18-mm sirolimus-eluting stent is placed. Online quantitative coronary angiography (QCA) performed before and after stenting reveals the measurements listed below (Table Q18-4). Six months later, the patient experienced two episodes of chest discomfort, and an exercise nuclear stress test suggested mild ischemia of the inferior wall. Angiography with QCA demonstrated a patent stent with measurements as described. What is the in-stent late loss in this individual?

Table Q18-4. Quantitative Coronary Angiography (QCA) Post Stenting

	Prestent	Poststent	6-Month Follow-up
Vessel reference diameter (mm)	3.52	—	3.68
Minimum luminal diameter (mm)	1.08	3.40	2.98

(A) 0.32 mm
(B) 1.90 mm
(C) 0.54 mm
(D) 0.16 mm
(E) 0.42 mm

18.5 What is the late loss index for the patient described in Question 18.4 (Table Q18.4)?

(A) 0.18
(B) 3.49
(C) 1.90
(D) 0.66
(E) 0.39

18.6 Compared to balloon angioplasty, bare-metal stent (BMS) implantation is associated with a lower likelihood of restenosis as a result of which one of the following biologic mechanisms?

(A) Reduced degree of neointimal formation
(B) Reduced vascular smooth muscle cell proliferation
(C) Increased collagen deposition
(D) Reduced degree of negative remodeling
(E) All of the above

18.7 A 44-year-old man who underwent orthotopic heart transplantation 6 years ago for treatment of dilated cardiomyopathy presents with increasing dyspnea on exertion and fatigue. He denies chest discomfort, and he has been compliant with his immunosuppressant medications. Coronary angiography demonstrates a severe focal stenosis in the proximal left circumflex artery (Fig. Q18-7) that is treated with stent placement. Which of the following statements regarding restenosis following PCI among patients with transplant arteriopathy is correct?

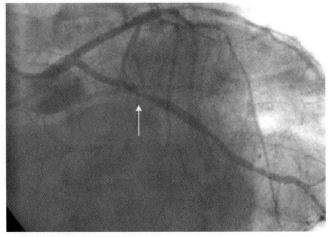

Figure Q18-7

(A) Restenosis rates following balloon angioplasty are equivalent to those following stent placement
(B) Successful PCI is associated with increased longevity of the transplanted heart
(C) The likelihood of restenosis following PCI is reduced with higher doses of antiproliferative immunosuppressant drugs
(D) Restenosis rates following PCI are similar in the setting of transplant arteriopathy and native atherosclerotic disease

18.8 Which one of the following best describes the biologic mechanism of action of paclitaxel for the prevention of restenosis?

(A) Blocks cell cycle progression at the G1 to S phase transition in vascular smooth muscle cells
(B) Stabilizes microtubule assembly
(C) Enhances microtubule breakdown
(D) Functions as a macrolide antibiotic

18.9 A 70-year-old woman underwent sirolimus-eluting stent placement in her right coronary artery 5 months earlier. She returns now with recurrent low-level angina, and coronary angiography demonstrates in-stent restenosis (Fig. 18-9). Which of the following statements regarding the treatment of in-stent restenosis within a DES is true?

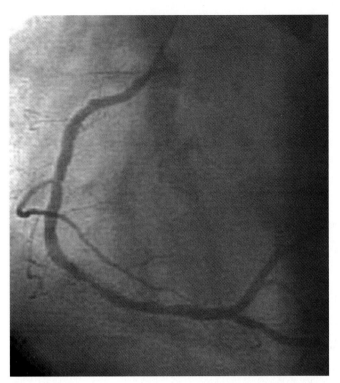

Figure Q18-9

(A) DES placement for treatment of in-stent restenosis is associated with greater long-term patency rates when the originally placed stent was also a drug-eluting rather than a BMS

(B) When in-stent restenosis occurs within a sirolimus-eluting stent, placement of paclitaxel-eluting within the original stent is associated with lower recurrent restenosis rates than placement of another sirolimus-eluting stent

(C) In-stent restenosis following sirolimus-eluting stent placement typically demonstrates a focal rather than a diffuse pattern

(D) In-stent restenosis occurring within a DES is associated with lower long-term clinical event rates (death and MI) than in-stent restenosis involving BMS

18.10 Compared to standard balloon angioplasty for the treatment of in-stent restenosis, which one of the following features is associated with the use of cutting balloon angioplasty?

(A) Increased likelihood of balloon slippage during inflation

(B) Less recoil at the angioplasty site within the first 24 hours

(C) Less late luminal loss

(D) Lower rates of clinical restenosis

18.11 The following figure is a frequency distribution curve from a hypothetical trial comparing two stents, "Stent A" and "Stent B" (Fig. Q18-11). Based on the figure, which one of the following statements is TRUE?

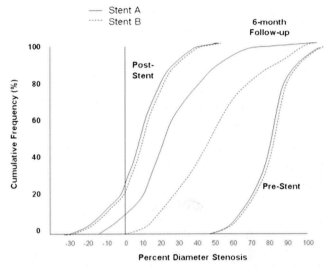

Figure Q18-11

(A) Late loss is greater for stent B than for Stent A

(B) The incidence of angiographic restenosis, defined as a stenosis severity of ≥50% at 6-month follow-up, is approximately 25% for Stent B

(C) The differences in 6-month restenosis rates between the two stents can be attributed to better acute gain with Stent A

(D) The median stent length was greater for patients treated with Stent A than Stent B

18.12 Which of the following statements regarding the time course of restenosis within BMS is TRUE?

(A) The degree of intimal hyperplasia within a stent usually reaches its peak within the first 3 months following stent implantation

(B) Between 6 months and 3 years following stent implantation, there is often lessening in the degree of luminal narrowing within the stent

(C) Early stent recoil is a phenomenon that often contributes to the development of in-stent restenosis

(D) Patients presenting with in-stent restenosis <3 months following initial stent placement have a more favorable response to repeat PCI than patients presenting with restenosis at a later time

18.13 A 66-year-old woman presented with an acute lateral wall STEMI 5 months earlier and underwent bare-metal stenting of the proximal left circumflex with a 3.0/18-mm cobalt–chromium stent. She returns with medically refractory angina and angiography demonstrates severe diffuse in-stent restenosis (Fig. Q18-13). Her left ventricular systolic function is normal, and she has no obstructive coronary disease elsewhere. Which of the following treatment strategies is preferred and why?

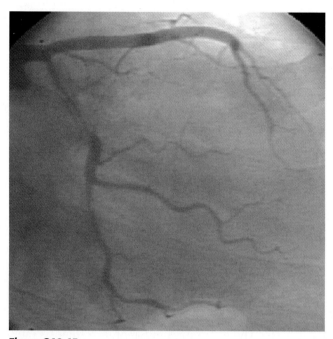

Figure Q18-13

(A) Coronary artery bypass surgery, because the likelihood of recurrent in-stent restenosis with PCI is >50% in this patient regardless of treatment approach

(B) Placement of a BMS, because this approach carries a similar likelihood of recurrent restenosis as DES placement in a vessel of this size, but does not require long-term thienopyridine therapy

(C) Balloon angioplasty followed by intracoronary brachytherapy, because while technically more cumbersome, this approach is associated with lower rates of recurrent restenosis than DES placement

(D) DES placement, because this strategy is associated with the lowest likelihood of recurrent in-stent restenosis

18.14 A 76-year-old man with diabetes mellitus, hypertension, and renal insufficiency (GFR = 46 mL/min) presented with an acute anterior wall STEMI and underwent successful primary PCI with placement of a 3.0/18-mm BMS in his proximal LAD. Angiography at the time of the MI

also demonstrated a 70% proximal stenosis of a large OM-1 branch and proximal occlusion of a dominant right coronary artery, which received brisk collateral flow from the LCX artery. A postdischarge thallium SPECT scan showed mild inferior ischemia, a small anterior fixed perfusion defect, no transient ischemic dilation, and a LVEF = 50%. He was treated medically and completed phase-2 cardiac rehabilitation without angina. Four months following his MI, he experienced two episodes of chest discomfort at rest of similar quality and location as the pain associated with his MI. He was hospitalized and his troponin I level was elevated at 1.1 ng/mL. A coronary angiogram demonstrated diffuse severe in-stent restenosis of the LAD (Fig. Q18-14). There was no change in the severity of the LCX or RCA disease, and the LVEF had decreased to 40% with hypokinesis of the anterolateral and apical segments. Which of the following is the preferred treatment strategy at this time?

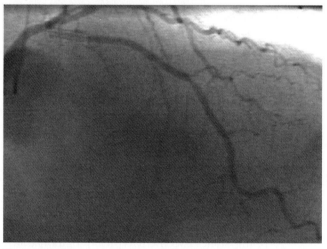

Figure Q18-14

(A) Treatment of the in-stent lesion in the LAD with a DES and continued medical management of the LCX and RCA disease

(B) Treatment of the LAD, LCX, and RCA lesions with DES

(C) Augmented medical therapy, with provisional DES placement in the LAD if his anginal symptoms are refractory to medications

(D) Referral for coronary artery bypass surgery

18.15 Which of the following patterns of bare-metal in-stent restenosis is associated with the highest likelihood of recurrent restenosis following percutaneous intervention? The margins of the stents are indicated by the white lines (Fig. Q18-15).

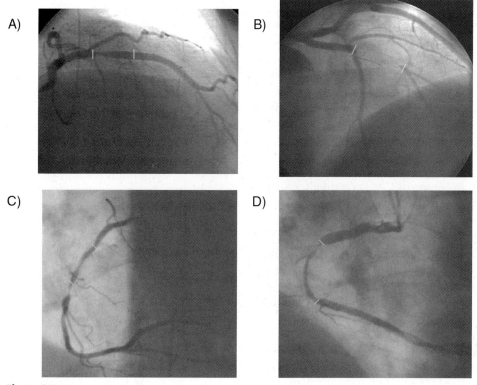

Figure Q18-15

(A) Panel A
(B) Panel B
(C) Panel C
(D) Panel D

18.16 A 54-year-old man underwent placement of a 3.0/23-mm BMS in the mid-RCA. Six months later he presented to the emergency room with chest pain. The ECG showed no interval changes, and his serum troponin I concentration was within normal limits. Coronary angiography demonstrated diffuse restenosis within and proximal to the previously placed stent, and he underwent placement of a 3.0/32-mm paclitaxel-eluting stent. Now, 10 months after the DES was placed, he again presents with angina, and coronary angiography is repeated. Figure Q18-16 is an image of the right coronary artery in the left anterior oblique projection. Which one of the following statements is true regarding the use of DES for the treatment of in-stent restenosis within a BMS?

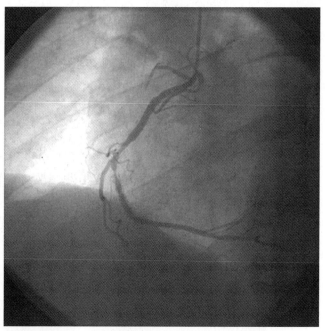

Figure Q18-16

(A) Underexpansion of DES used to treat in-stent restenosis is a common cause of recurrent restenosis
(B) For treatment of BMS restenosis, DES are associated with less late loss but similar clinical event rates compared to balloon angioplasty

(C) DES placement is associated with similar restenosis rates whether used for treatment of in-stent restenosis or for de novo lesions
(D) While DES are associated with lower rates of recurrent restenosis compared to balloon angioplasty at 1-year follow-up, the advantage is no longer present on late follow-up at 4 years

18.17 A 73-year-old woman with hyperlipidemia, ongoing tobacco use, hypertension, and intermittent claudication presents with a 4-week history of left shoulder and upper back discomfort with exertion. An adenosine SPECT study demonstrated normal myocardial perfusion at rest with extensive stress-induced ischemia involving the anterior, apical, lateral, and inferior segments associated with transient ischemic dilation. Coronary angiography is performed and demonstrates severe multivessel disease, as displayed in Figure 18-17). According to current evidence-based standards, which of the following statements is CORRECT regarding therapy for this patient?

(A) The likelihood of repeat revascularization at 1 year is greater with percutaneous revascularization than coronary bypass surgery if BMS are used, but not if paclitaxel-eluting stents are used

(B) The likelihood of repeat revascularization at 1 year is greater with percutaneous revascularization than coronary bypass surgery regardless of whether bare-metal or paclitaxel-eluting stents are used

(C) The likelihood of death and/or MI at 1 year is greater with percutaneous intervention using paclitaxel-eluting stents than with coronary bypass surgery

(D) The likelihood of stroke at 1 year is equivalent regardless of whether percutaneous coronary intervention or coronary bypass surgery is undertaken

18.18 Which of the following statements regarding the biologic characteristics of BMS vs. DES restenosis is TRUE?

(A) On pathologic examination, BMS restenosis is more likely to be associated with organized thrombus and fibrinous material than DES restenosis

(B) Elevated pre-PCI serum inflammatory marker levels such as C-reactive protein are predictive of restenosis following drug-eluting but not BMS placement

(C) Eosinophil infiltrates, indicative of allergic hypersensitivity, are often observed within restenotic tissue surrounding struts of drug-eluting but not BMS

(D) Late development of neointimal hyperplasia ≥1 year following stent placement has been observed in multiple studies of DES placement

18.19 A 57-year-old woman with morbid obesity, hypertension, and a family history of premature coronary artery disease is scheduled to undergo bariatric surgery for weight reduction. During a preoperative evaluation, she described substernal chest pressure with small amounts of activity. On a pharmacologic nuclear stress study, she developed transient ischemic dilatation of her left ventricle and evidence of anterior and inferior ischemia. Coronary angiography demonstrated a focal eccentric 90% proximal LAD stenosis and an 80% concentric mid-RCA stenosis. Both lesions were treated successfully with BMS placement. Following PCI, when is the

Left Coronary System   Left Coronary System   Right Coronary Artery

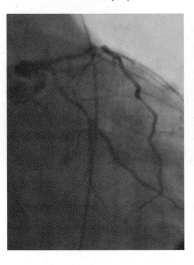 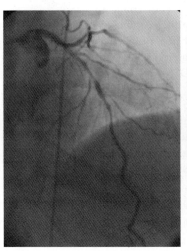 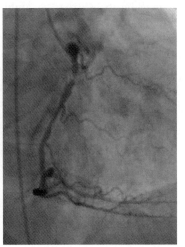

AP Caudal   AP Cranial   Right Anterior Oblique

Figure Q18-17

most appropriate time for performance of her bariatric surgery?

(A) 2–4 weeks
(B) 6–12 weeks
(C) 6 months
(D) ≥12 months

18.20 A 52-year-old man presented with low threshold exertional chest discomfort. During an exercise stress echocardiogram he developed his typical angina during stage 2 of the standard Bruce Protocol associated with 1.5-mm horizontal ST-segment depression in the inferolateral leads and transient hypokinesis of the inferior wall. Subsequent angiography demonstrated a lengthy 90% stenosis of the proximal-to-mid RCA that was treated successfully with slightly overlapping 3.5- × 30-mm and 3.5- × 18-mm zotarolimus-eluting stents. His angina resolved after the intervention, and he returns to your office for follow-up 6 months later. He remains angina free during normal daily activities, and exercises on a treadmill three times a week for 30 minutes without symptoms. Which of the following would constitute the most appropriate means to screen for stent patency at this time?

(A) No testing is indicated
(B) Exercise stress echocardiogram
(C) Exercise treadmill test without adjunctive imaging
(D) Multislice CT angiogram

18.21 Which one of the following modifications to stent design had been associated with increased rates of in-stent restenosis?

(A) Use of a slotted tubular rather than a coil design
(B) Use of a cobalt chromium platform instead of stainless steel
(C) Heparin coating
(D) Gold coating
(E) Thinner stent struts

18.22 Which of the saphenous vein graft lesions depicted below is associated with the lowest likelihood of restenosis following BMS placement (Fig. Q18-22)?

(A) Panel A
(B) Panel B
(C) Panel C
(D) Panel D

A)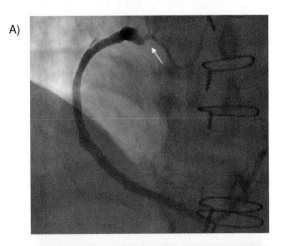

B)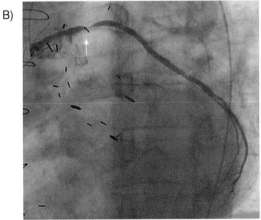

C)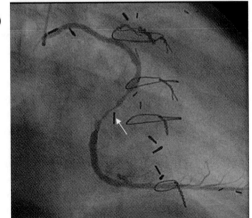

D)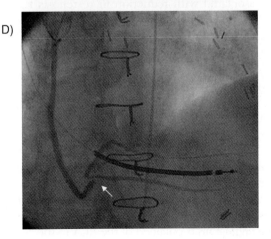

Figure Q18-22

18.23 Which statement is true regarding the use of DES placement vs. vascular brachytherapy for the treatment of restenosis within a BMS?

(A) Unlike DES, intracoronary brachytherapy is ineffective for treatment of diffuse (>30 mm in length) in-stent restenosis

(B) Brachytherapy is associated with similar efficacy as DES placement for the treatment of in-stent restenosis

(C) "Geographic mismatch" is a potential mode of failure for both DES and vascular brachytherapy

(D) There is a 4% to 5% incidence of late aneurysm formation following coronary brachytherapy for in-stent restenosis, which is substantially greater than that observed following drug-eluting stenting

18.24 Which of the following statements is true regarding restenosis following carotid artery stenting?

(A) Significantly, lower rates of repeat target vessel revascularization have been reported among patients treated with carotid stenting compared to carotid endarterectomy in some randomized trials

(B) Among individuals with asymptomatic carotid artery in-stent restenosis of >70% in severity, clinical trials have demonstrated reduced stroke rates with repeat stenting compared to medical therapy

(C) Minimizing residual stenosis during carotid stenting by aggressive postdilation (balloon to artery ratio >1:1) is the preferred approach to reduce the likelihood of subsequent restenosis

(D) Restenosis following carotid bifurcation stenting is more likely when self-expanding stents are used instead of balloon-expandable stents

18.25 Which of the following antiplatelet therapies is associated with reduction in restenosis rates compared to placebo following coronary bare-metal stenting?

(A) Abciximab

(B) Clopidogrel

(C) Cilostazol

(D) Eptifibatide

(E) None of the above

18.26 A 53-year-old woman underwent primary PCI for treatment of an acute inferior MI with placement of a 3.0- × 28-mm BMS in the mid-RCA. She returned 5 months later with low threshold and rest angina despite medical therapy, and the following angiogram is obtained of the RCA in the right

anterior oblique projection (Fig. Q18-26). Because of a history of ulcerative colitis with recurrent gastrointestinal bleeding, long-term thienopyridine therapy is contraindicated. Which of the following therapies is associated with a reduced likelihood of recurrent restenosis compared to stand-alone balloon angioplasty in this patient?

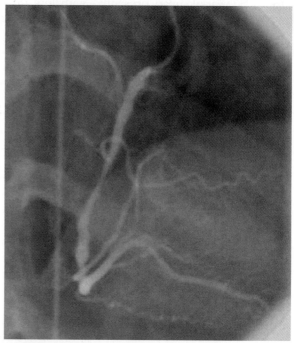

Figure Q18-26

(A) Rotational atherectomy

(B) Directional coronary atherectomy

(C) Excimer laser assisted coronary angioplasty

(D) BMS implantation ("stent within a stent")

(E) None of the above

18.27 Which of the following statements is true regarding the treatment of in-stent restenosis with intracoronary brachytherapy?

(A) The placement of additional stents during the brachytherapy procedure reduces the risk of recurrent restenosis

(B) The presence of thrombus within a restenotic stent is considered a contraindication for the use of brachytherapy

(C) Recurrent angiographic restenosis rates of <10% at 6 to 9 months following brachytherapy have been observed in the majority of randomized clinical trials assessing brachytherapy

(D) Late recurrent restenosis, occurring between 6 months and 5 years following treatment of in-stent restenosis, is uncommon and no more likely to occur following brachytherapy than stand-along balloon angioplasty

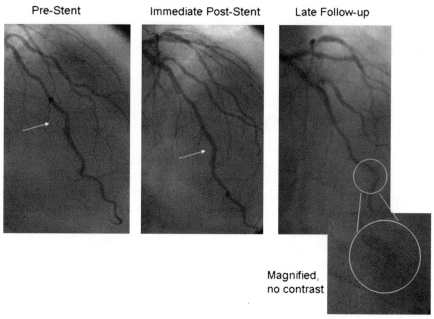

Pre-Stent   Immediate Post-Stent   Late Follow-up

Magnified, no contrast

Figure Q18-29

18.28 Sirolimus, Everolimus, and Zotarolimus, used for the prevention of in-stent restenosis, are associated with which of the following biologic characteristics?

(A) Inhibition of vascular smooth muscle cell migration

(B) Inhibition of vascular smooth muscle cell proliferation

(C) Immunosuppression

(D) Anti-inflammatory

(E) All of the above

18.29 A 71-year-old man underwent implantation of a sirolimus-eluting stent in his mid-to-distal LAD for treatment of unstable angina. He returns 9 months later with a NSTEMI and angiography is performed as demonstrated in Figure 18-29. Which of the following statements regarding late stent fracture following DES implantation is true?

(A) The incidence of late stent fracture is <1%

(B) The probability of stent fracture is significantly greater for stents placed in the left anterior descending artery than for stents placed in the left circumflex or right coronary arteries

(C) The presence of a stent fracture is associated with increased rates of both in-stent restenosis and target lesion revascularization

(D) Shorter stent length is a risk factor for stent fracture

18.30 A 69-year-old woman developed recurrent low threshold angina 5 months following BMS placement in her mid-left anterior descending coronary artery. Coronary angiography demonstrated diffuse in-stent restenosis and IVUS interrogation of the stent was performed. Which of the following statements regarding the IVUS image in Figure Q18-30 is TRUE?

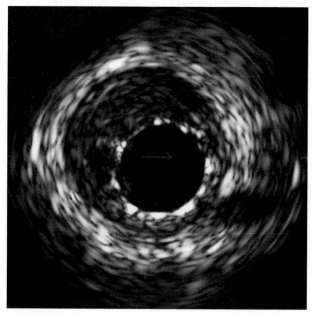

Figure Q18-30

(A) Incomplete apposition of several stent struts is apparent

(B) Heavy vessel wall calcification is present

(C) The stent is well-apposed but under-expanded relative to the size of the vessel

(D) Negative vascular remodeling is the likely cause of restenosis in this patient

18.1 **Answer D.** Most of the clinical and anatomical predictors of restenosis following BMS placement also serve as risk factors for restenosis after DES implantation. Such variables include diabetes mellitus, ostial or saphenous vein graft lesion location, prior restenosis, smaller reference vessel diameter, smaller postintervention minimum luminal diameter, longer lesions, and greater total stent length. (*J Am Coll Cardiol* 2010;56:1897–1907) In addition, several trials have demonstrated higher rates of target lesion revascularization with paclitaxel compared to sirolimus and everolimus-eluting stents. (*N Engl J Med* 2005;353:653–662) Use of sirolimus if anything should lead to lower restenosis compared to paclitaxel-eluting stents.

18.2 **Answer C.** Inflammation plays a key role in the pathogenesis of coronary restenosis. Angioplasty induced injury leads to deendothelialization of the vascular wall leading to localized platelet and fibrin deposition, which in turn promotes leukocyte and monocyte recruitment via expression of multiple surface adhesion molecules and release of chemokines. This inflammatory response promotes proliferation and migration of vascular smooth muscle cells and fibroblasts from the vessel media, leading to the development of the neointimal tissue that, when excessive, is ultimately responsible for restenosis. Unlike atherosclerotic plaque, which typically demonstrates complex features such as lipid pools, necrotic cores, fibrous caps, and often focal calcification, restenotic lesions usually exhibit more homogenous fibrohyperplastic morphology. For this reason, acute plaque rupture with thrombotic vessel occlusion is a much less common presentation with restenosis than atherosclerosis. (*Circulation* 2005;111:2257–2273) Although still poorly understood, genetic susceptibility appears to play a role in the development of restenosis and may ultimately allow for individually targeted antirestenosis therapy. (*Arterioscler Thromb Vasc Biol* 2009;29:1407–1408.)

18.3 **Answer A.** A wide variety of animal models have been created to assess the pathophysiology, prevention, and treatment of restenosis. Animal models have provided valuable insights regarding the potential safety, efficacy, and mechanism of action of perspective antirestenosis therapies; however, these models are also associated with limitations in their ability to replicate human atherosclerosis and restenosis. (*Vet Pathol* 47(1): 58–76.) The histologic appearance and composition of restenotic and atherosclerotic lesions found in humans differs to varying degrees from that found in all animal models. Likewise, myriad metabolic, physiologic, and hemodynamic differences between animals and humans can affect response to therapeutic agents, and numerous examples exist of therapies that have inhibited neointimal hyperplasia in animals, but have failed to demonstrate efficacy in human clinical trials. (*Toxicol Pathol* 2006;34(1):11–8.)

While various animal models have been developed, no single model can replicate all features of human restenosis. For example, even though smooth muscle cell proliferation and migration from media to intima is a prominent feature of all animal models of restenosis, the degree of neointima formation in response to arterial injury varies widely based on species as many animals (including mouse, pig, and dog) rarely form more than a thin layer of hyperplastic tissue. Likewise, no model can replicate the complex phenotypes associated with clinical conditions that predispose to restenosis, such as diabetes or metabolic syndrome.

18.4 **Answer E.** Late loss is the key angiographic parameter used to quantitate the degree of intimal hyperplasia at the site of PCI between the time of the procedure and subsequent angiographic follow-up. Late loss within a stent is defined as the in-stent minimum lumen diameter immediately following stent placement minus the in-stent minimum lumen diameter on late follow-up angiography. In this example, late loss = 3.40 − 2.98 = 0.42 mm.

18.5 **Answer A.** The amount of late loss following angioplasty can depend on the degree of acute gain achieved during the procedure. For example, using a stent that is oversized for a vessel may result in greater acute gain in luminal diameter than a properly sized stent, but may trigger an exaggerated hyperplastic response resulting in excessive late loss. Late loss can be normalized for acute gain by using the late loss index, which is calculated as late loss divided by acute gain. (*Circulation* 2005;111:321–327.) In this example, the late loss index is late loss/acute gain = (3.40 – 2.98)/(3.40 – 1.08) = 0.42/2.32 = 0.18.

18.6 **Answer D.** Compared to stand-alone balloon angioplasty, stent implantation is associated with an exaggerated vascular smooth muscle cell proliferative response, and consequently, an increased degree of neointima formation. (*Curr Opin Lipidol* 1999;10:499–506.) Stent placement, however, essentially eliminates long-term negative remodeling of the vessel wall, which typically more than compensates for the exaggerated proliferative response and results in the reduced frequency of restenosis observed with stenting compared to balloon angioplasty. (*Circulation* 1997;95:363–370.) Restenotic tissue obtained following balloon angioplasty demonstrates fewer smooth muscle cells and greater collagen deposition than tissue recovered from stents that have developed restenosis. (*Eur Heart J* 2000;21:320–324.)

18.7 **Answer C.** Transplant arteriopathy affects about 50% of individuals who undergo orthotopic heart transplantation, and represents a major cause of morbidity and mortality among transplant recipients. While transplant arteriopathy is often diffuse in nature and therefore not amenable to revascularization, PCI is associated with high procedural success rates when used to treat lesions that are more focal in nature. In-stent restenosis, however, occurs with greater frequency following treatment of transplant arteriopathy than following treatment of atherosclerotic disease. As with native vessel coronary disease, balloon angioplasty in the setting of transplant arteriopathy is associated with higher restenosis rates than bare-metal stenting, and DES placement appears to result in lower recurrence rates than BMS placement. Nevertheless, as a result of continued disease progression outside of the treated segment, PCI has not been shown to ultimately increase longevity of transplanted hearts afflicted by coronary arteriopathy. Several medical therapies have been associated with reduced restenosis rates and improved graft survival following PCI for transplant arteriopathy, including higher antiproliferative immunosuppressant dosing, early reduction of steroid dosing, and use of statins.

18.8 **Answer B.** Microtubules are a fundamental component of the mitotic spindle apparatus, and play essential roles in other cellular functions including migration and growth factor signaling. The assembly and disassembly of microtubules within a cell is maintained in a well-regulated equilibrium. Paclitaxel produces its antiproliferative effects by stabilizing microtubules, thus shifting the dynamic balance toward assembly, which consequently interrupts cellular division. The "limus" class of drugs impairs vascular smooth muscle cell division by blocking cell cycle progression at the G1 to S phase transition. (*J Am Coll Cardiol* 2010;56:1–42.)

18.9 **Answer C.** DES have greatly reduced the likelihood of restenosis relative to BMS placement following PCI for de novo disease; however, when in-stent restenosis does occur within DES, it appears to respond less favorably to repeat PCI than restenosis within a BMS. One analysis that examined DES placement for treatment of in-stent restenosis ("stent-in-stent" technique), for example, demonstrated a twofold greater need for repeat revascularization when the initial restenotic lesion was located in a drug-eluting rather than a BMS. (*Am J Cardiol* 2009;103(4):491–495.) Many practitioners initially suspected that when in-stent restenosis occurred within a DES, treatment with a DES of a different drug class would be preferable. The randomized ISAR-DESIRE 2 trial, however, demonstrated no differences in antirestenotic efficacy or clinical outcomes among 450 patients with sirolimus-eluting stent restenosis who were randomized to reintervention with sirolimus vs. paclitaxel-eluting stenting. (*J Am Coll Cardiol* 2010;55:2710–2716.)

Although a variety of angiographic patterns may occur, a focal pattern is typical after DES placement and is often associated with localized stent underexpansion. Paclitaxel-eluting stents represent an exception, as a diffuse pattern of in-stent restenosis is observed in roughly half of the cases. (*J Am Coll Cardiol* 2010;56:1897–1907.) While potentially more difficult to treat, current data suggest that in-stent restenosis occurring within a DES is associated with similar long-term cardiac outcomes as in-stent restenosis involving BMS (*Catheter Cardiovasc Interven* 2010;75:338–342).

18.10 **Answer B.** While cutting balloon angioplasty for in-stent restenosis is associated with less early recoil at the treatment site than conventional angioplasty (*J Interven Cardiol* 2004;17:197–201), the cutting balloon technique does not appear to reduce the likelihood of recurrent restenosis. In the randomized restenosis cutting balloon evaluation trial, 428 patients with in-stent restenosis were randomized to treatment with either conventional or cutting balloon angioplasty. The cutting balloon was associated with less balloon slippage and a lower number of balloons used during the intervention; however, there were no significant differences in angiographic or clinical measures of restenosis between the conventional and cutting balloons at 7-month follow-up. (*J Am Coll Cardiol* 2004;43:943–949.)

18.11 **Answer A.** Frequency distribution curves are used to evaluate the immediate and late angiographic results of competing therapies in clinical trials of restenosis. The median acute luminal gain for each therapy can be determined by measuring the distance between the present and poststent curve for each stent on a horizontal line drawn at the 50% mark on the Y (cumulative frequency) axis. In the example, this distance is similar for Stents A and B. Late lumen loss can be determined by comparing the distance between the poststent and the 6-month follow-up curve for each stent, which in the example is greater for Stent B. The angiographic restenosis rate for each therapy can be determined by drawing a vertical line upward from the 50% diameter stenosis point on the x (percent diameter stenosis) axis. The point on the Y-axis that corresponds to where this vertical line intersects the 6-month follow-up curve for each stent reveals the percentage of individuals who had a ≤50% stenosis at 6-month follow-up. The frequency of angiographic restenosis for that particular stent is determined by subtracting this number from 100. In the example, the frequency of angiographic restenosis is approximately 10% for Stent A and 40% for Stent B. The frequency distribution curve does not contain information regarding stent length.

18.12 **Answer B.** In-stent restenosis occurs following BMS implantation typically occurs within the first 6 months following stent implantation. After 6 months, serial angiographic follow-up studies have demonstrated a gradual spontaneous improvement in the degree of luminal narrowing within the stent (spontaneous regression). (*N Engl J Med* 334:561–566.) Late stent recoil, while occasionally noted on serial IVUS imaging, is an uncommon occurrence. (*J Am Coll Cardiol* 1998;32:584–589.) Patients presenting with restenosis early (within the first 3 months

following stent implantation) have an increased risk of recurrent restenosis following repeat PCI compared to patients who present later. (*Am J Cardiol* 2000;85(12):1427–1431.)

18.13 **Answer D.** Randomized trials comparing sirolimus and paclitaxel-eluting stents to intracoronary brachytherapy for the treatment of BMS restenosis demonstrated significantly lower recurrent restenosis rates following drug-eluting stenting. (Holmes, Teirstein et al., 2006; Stone, Ellis et al., 2006.) Repeat target vessel revascularization rates following DES placement in these trials was <20% at 2- to 3-year follow-up. Because absent or delayed stent endothelialization occurs following both brachytherapy and DES implantation, dual antiplatelet therapy is advised for at least 12 months following both therapies to reduce the likelihood of late stent thrombosis. (Waksman, Ajani et al., 2002.) DES placement and brachytherapy are associated with lower rates of recurrent restenosis than bare-metal stenting; but, DES is superior to brachytherapy and furthermore brachytherapy is no longer available.

18.14 **Answer D.** While repeat PCI remains the most common treatment approach for symptomatic in-stent restenosis, other strategies including medical therapy or coronary artery bypass surgery should also be considered based on patient and lesion specific factors. The patient in this question presented with a non-ST segment elevation MI related to severe in-stent restenosis of the LAD in the setting of multivessel coronary artery disease, diabetes mellitus, and reduced left ventricular systolic function. Because a routine early invasive strategy is associated with a decreased incidence of major adverse cardiac events compared to a conservative approach among patients presenting with acute coronary syndromes, medical management is not the preferred treatment option for this individual. (*N Engl J Med* 2009;360:2165–2175.) For this patient, if repeat PCI with DES placement were undertaken, the ostial location of the in-stent lesion and the acute angle between the LAD and LCX would require that stent extend into the left main (and potentially compromise of the LCX ostium), which would increase procedural risk and complexity. Based on randomized trial data, bypass surgery is associated with a mortality advantage over PCI using BMS among patients with diabetes and multivessel disease. (*J Am Coll Cardiol* 2007;49:1600–1606.) Studies comparing bypass surgery and multivessel DES in diabetes are ongoing.

18.15 **Answer B.** The patterns of in-stent restenosis demonstrated in the figure are (a) focal, (b) total occlusion, (c) diffuse proliferative, in which the restenotic lesion extends beyond the stent margin, and (d) diffuse intra-stent. Mehran et al. devised a classification system for BMS restenosis based on the likelihood of late patency following repeat percutaneous intervention. In their analysis of 288 in-stent lesions treated with PCI, the focal pattern was associated with the lowest need for repeat revascularization (19%), followed by the diffuse intra-stent (35%), diffuse proliferative (50%), and total occlusion (82%) patterns. (*Circulation* 1999;100:1872–1878.) When in-stent restenosis occurs within a DES, the probability of recurrent restenosis following therapy is likewise significantly greater when the initial pattern of in-stent restenosis is diffuse rather than focal. (*J Am Coll Cardiol* 2006;47:2399–2404.)

18.16 **Answer A.** Following DES placement for the treatment of in-stent restenosis, IVUS studies have shown that underexpansion of the DES represents an important cause of late stent failure due to recurrent restenosis. (*Circulation* 2004;109:1085–1088.) While DES represent the preferred therapy for in-stent restenosis, restenosis rates are higher when DES are implanted for treatment of in-stent restenosis compared to when they are used for de novo lesions. In the setting of in-stent restenosis, DES implantation is associated with improved acute luminal gain, less late loss, less negative remodeling, and fewer subsequent clinical events than balloon angioplasty. (*JAMA* 2005;293:165–171.) The results of DES for treatment of in-stent restenosis appear durable, as sirolimus stent placement was associated with significantly reduced MACE rates compared to balloon angioplasty at both 1 and 4-year follow-up in the randomized RIBS-II (Restenosis Intra-stent: Balloon angioplasty vs. elective sirolimus-eluting Stenting) study. (*J Am Coll Cardiol* 2008;52:1621–1627.)

18.17 **Answer B.** The synergy between percutaneous coronary intervention with TAXUS and cardiac surgery (SYNTAX) trial was a randomized-controlled trial of 1,800 patients with left main or three-vessel coronary artery disease who were randomized to undergo coronary artery bypass surgery or paclitaxel-eluting stenting. (*N Engl J Med* 2009;360(10):961–972.) The combined primary outcome measure was the occurrence of all-cause death, stroke, MI, or repeat revascularization at 1 year. The incidence of the combined

primary end point was significantly greater among patients randomized to PCI rather than bypass surgery (17.8 vs. 12.4%, *p* = 0.002). The difference in the primary outcome measure between the two groups was driven by a higher repeat revascularization rate among the PCI group compared to the CABG group (13.5 vs. 5.9%, *p* < 0.001). The rates of death and MI were similar between the groups at 1 year, and bypass surgery was associated with a greater likelihood of stroke than PCI (2.2 vs. 0.6%). A scoring system (the SYNTAX score) was devised to grade the angiographic complexity of coronary disease among patients enrolled in the trial, and the advantage of bypass surgery at 1 year was confined to the patient subgroup with the highest SYNTAX scores. Among patients with low or intermediate SYNTAX scores, combined MACE rates were equivalent between PCI and CABG.

18.18 **Answer D.** Histologically, DES restenosis is more likely to demonstrate evidence of organized thrombus and fibrin deposition within the stent than BMS restenosis, which typically reveals a more homogenous hypercellular neointima. The tendency toward thrombus deposition within DES may reflect the lack of protective neointima that is nearly ubiquitous following BMS placement. While vascular inflammation plays a pivotal role in the pathogenesis of restenosis following both BMS and DES implantation, serum markers of inflammation, most notably CRP, appear predictive of BMS but not DES restenosis. (*J Am Coll Cardiol* 2010;56(22):1783–1793.) It is hypothesized that the high local concentrations of antiproliferative drug associated with DES placement may overcome the enhanced systemic inflammatory state reflected by elevated serum CRP levels that otherwise would predispose to restenosis. A localized allergic-type hypersensitivity reaction to stent materials (metal, polymer), evidenced by the finding of eosinophil infiltrates in restenotic tissue adjacent to stent struts following both bare-metal and drug-eluting stenting, is also thought to play a potential role in the development of in-stent restenosis. Eosinophil infiltrates are not seen after stand-alone balloon angioplasty. Late development of neointimal hyperplasia 2 to 4 years following DES implantation has been observed in several studies employing serial angiography and IVUS. Despite this "catch-up" phenomenon, the degree of late intimal hyperplasia has not been sufficient to adversely affect the advantages of DES over BMS with respect to target lesion revascularization rates. (*J Am Coll Cardiol* 2010;56:1897–1907.)

18.19 Answer B. Following PCI, elective surgery should be delayed for a sufficient interval to minimize the risk of perioperative stent thrombosis, but not for too lengthy a period such that restenosis becomes a potential concern. After BMS placement, noncardiac surgery should be delayed for 6 weeks to allow time for stent endothelialization and completion of a full course of thienopyridine therapy. Surgery performed earlier than 4 to 6 weeks following BMS placement is associated with a two- to five-fold excess of major adverse cardiac events related to stent thrombosis including death and MI. Surgery, however, should not be delayed for > 12 weeks following BMS placement, if possible, since the possibility of in-stent restenosis must be considered after this interval. DES should be avoided during PCI if noncardiac surgery is anticipated within the next 12 months given the necessity of prolonged dual antiplatelet therapy. If balloon angioplasty without stenting is performed, surgery can be performed after a shorter (2-week) delay since perioperative stent thrombosis is not a concern. (*Circulation* 2009;120:e169–e276.)

18.20 Answer A. The performance of routine stress testing or of other coronary imaging modalities to screen for stent patency among asymptomatic individuals has not been shown to improve clinical outcomes. In the absence of clinical symptoms, such testing is typically not indicated for screening purposes following successful PCI. The current ACC Appropriate Use Criteria for Cardiac Radionuclide Imaging, for example, grades imaging for asymptomatic patients within 2 years of PCI as "inappropriate." (*J Am Coll Cardiol* 2009;53:2201–2229.) ACC/AHA guidelines do suggest, however, that screening may be useful in patients considered to be at particularly high risk, for example those with depressed left ventricular function, multivessel coronary disease, proximal LAD disease, multivessel disease, diabetes, hazardous occupations, or suboptimal PCI results. (*Circulation* 2002;106:1883–1892.)

18.21 Answer D. Two randomized studies have demonstrated that the use of stents with thinner struts is associated with a significant reduction of angiographic and clinical restenosis. (*Circulation* 2001;103:2816; *J Am Coll Cardiol* 2003;41(8):1283–1288.) Heparin-coating has not been shown to affect the likelihood of subsequent in-stent restenosis, and likewise there is no evidence to suggest that the use of cobalt chromium stent platforms is related to higher rates of restenosis than stainless steel. (*Am J Cardiol* 2003;92:463–466.) In fact, because the composition of cobalt chromium allows for thinner strut thickness, these stents may be associated with less risk of restenosis. Stents with a coil design, such as the Gianturco–Roubin stent, are associated with restenosis rates that are significantly greater than slotted tubular stents. (*Circulation* 2000;102:1364–1368; *Circulation* 2001;103:2816–2821.) Randomized studies have shown that gold coating is associated with higher rates of restenosis than implantation of identically designed stents that are not gold-coated. (*Circulation* 2000;101:2478–2483; *Am J Cardiol* 2002;89:872–875.)

18.22 Answer D. The likelihood of restenosis is significantly greater when PCI is performed to treat lesions located at the aorto-ostium or within the body of saphenous vein grafts compared to lesions at the distal anastamosis. (*J Am Coll Cardiol* 1989;14:1645–1660.) This difference is likely a result of differences in plaque composition. It is currently uncertain whether DES are superior to BMS for the prevention of restenosis following vein graft PCI, but a recent analysis suggested improved outcomes with DES. (*Am J Cardiol* 2010;106(7):946–951.)

18.23 Answer C. Intracoronary brachytherapy represented the first effective therapy for in-stent restenosis, with documented efficacy for the treatment of both focal and diffuse in-stent restenosis within native vessels and saphenous vein grafts. (*Circulation* 2000;102:r1–r8.) Because of better ease of use and superior outcomes for prevention of recurrent in-stent restenosis, DES placement has now replaced brachytherapy as first-line therapy for treatment of in-stent restenosis within a BMS. (Ellis, O'Shaughnessy et al., 2008; Holmes, Teirstein et al., 2008.) "Geographic mismatch," in which recurrent restenosis following brachytherapy or drug-eluting stenting develops at the edge of the treated segment, can occur when either the brachytherapy catheter or DES fails to completely cover the length of the vessel segment injured by balloon predilation. (*J Am Coll Cardiol* 2001;37:1026–1030.) Late aneurysm formation is a rare (<1% incidence) complication of both DES placement and brachytherapy.

18.24 Answer A. In the SAPPHIRE Trial, 334 patients with severe symptomatic or asymptomatic carotid stenosis who had features that placed them at increased surgical risk were randomized to undergo carotid stenting or endarterectomy. At 1 year, carotid stenting was noninferior to carotid endarterectomy with respect to the composite primary end point of stroke, MI, or death, however, repeat carotid revascularization occurred in fewer patients treated with stenting vs. endarterectomy (0.6 vs. 4.3%; *p* = 0.04). (*N Engl J Med* 2004;351:1493–1501.) No randomized trials have determined the best treatment option for carotid in-stent restenosis, and while repeat angioplasty or stenting is often the preferred treatment option in practice, it remains uncertain if this approach is associated with better (or worse) clinical outcomes than medical therapy. Because restenosis is uncommon following carotid stenting and the use of aggressive postdilation following stent deployment is associated with an increased risk of procedural stroke, practice guidelines advocate avoiding the use of oversized balloons for this purpose. Balloon-expandable stents are not used for carotid bifurcation stenting given the superficial location of the carotid bifurcation with the possibility of the stent kinking or deformation if subjected to external trauma.

18.25 **Answer C.** Cilostazol was associated with a significant reduction in the incidence of angiographic restenosis compared to placebo (22.0 vs. 34.5%, *p* = 0.002) among a cohort of 705 patients who underwent BMS placement in the randomized Cilastozol for Restenosis Trial (CREST). (*Circulation* 2005;112:2826–2832.) In addition to its platelet inhibitory effects, cilostazol also has been shown to inhibit smooth muscle cell growth by inhibiting DNA synthesis in animal studies. While intriguing, the CREST results were overshadowed by the nearly concurrent release of DESs and cilostazol never entered the clinical mainstream for its potential antirestenosis effects. None of the other antiplatelet agents listed have been associated with reductions in neointimal hyperplasia formation or clinical restenosis. In the ERASER study, for example, abciximab therapy at the time of stent implantation was not associated with significant reductions in either IVUS or angiographic measures of restenosis compared to placebo at 6-month follow-up. (*Circulation* 1999;100:799–806.)

18.26 **Answer E.** Prior to the advent of vascular brachytherapy and DES, which both mandate longer-term thienopyridine use following treatment,

no therapy proved effective in reducing the incidence of recurrent in-stent restenosis compared to stand-along balloon angioplasty. (*Eur Heart J* 2003;24:266–273; *J Am Coll Cardiol* 2004;43:936–942.) In the randomized controlled ARTIST study, rotational atherectomy used to treat in-stent restenosis was associated with an increased likelihood of recurrent clinical and angiographic restenosis compared to balloon angioplasty alone. (*Circulation* 2002; 105:583–588.) The RIBS trial, a randomized study of repeat BMS implantation vs. balloon angioplasty for the treatment of in-stent restenosis, demonstrated no significant differences in angiographic or clinical outcomes between the two strategies. (*J Am Coll Cardiol* 2003;42:796–805.) Predominantly, negative results have been reported in case series of directional atherectomy and excimer laser assisted angioplasty for the treatment of in-stent restenosis.

18.27 **Answer B.** Because of superior clinical outcomes and ease-of-use, DES have replaced intracoronary brachytherapy as the first-line treatment for in-stent restenosis. Because brachytherapy remains available as a treatment option for limited patient subsets, such as those with multiple recurrent episodes of in-stent restenosis, it remains important for the interventional cardiologist to understand the principles surrounding its use.

The placement of additional stents during the brachytherapy procedure has been shown to *increase* the likelihood of subsequent recurrent restenosis, and may also increase the risk of stent thrombosis. (*Am Heart J* 2003;146(1):142–145.) The presence of thrombus within a stent is considered to represent an absolute contraindication to brachytherapy. (*Circulation* 2003;107:1744–1749.) While multiple randomized controlled trials of brachytherapy for in-stent restenosis using both beta- and gamma-emitting isotopes have demonstrated significant reductions in recurrent restenosis compared to placebo, the incidence of recurrent angiographic restenosis following brachytherapy has remained >20% in nearly all of these trials. Interestingly, late follow-up reports from both the Washington Radiation for In-Stent Restenosis Trial (WRIST) and GAMMA-1 trials of brachytherapy vs. placebo for treatment of in-stent restenosis demonstrated an excess need for late target vessel revascularization between 6 months and 5 years among patients who received brachytherapy rather than placebo. Most restenosis events in the placebo arms occurred within the first 6 months. While these findings suggest that in some individuals brachytherapy merely delays rather than prevents the development of recurrent in-stent restenosis, at 5 years the cumulative incidence of major adverse cardiac events remained significantly better among patients treated with brachytherapy vs. placebo in both WRIST (46.2 vs. 69.2%, $p = 0.008$) and GAMMA-1 (38.5 vs. 65.5%, $p = 0.02$). (*Circulation* 2002;105:2737–2740; *Circulation* 2004;109:340–344.)

18.28 Answer E. Rapamycin (Sirolimus) is a macrolide antibiotic that produces its cellular effects by blocking cell cycle progression at the G1 to S phase transition in vascular smooth muscle cells, and possesses all of the listed biologic characteristics that likely contribute to its antirestenosis effects. (*J Am Coll Cardiol* 2010;56:1–42)

18.29 Answer C. Late stent fracture is more common than previously recognized and appears to represent an important risk factor for in-stent restenosis. In a recent meta-analysis of eight studies including a total of >5,000 patients who underwent DES placement, the mean incidence of late stent fracture was 4.0%, with a range of 0.8% to 8.4% among the individual studies. (*Am J Cardiol* 2010;106(8):1075–1080.) Compared to intact stents, stent fracture was associated with significantly increased incidences of angiographic in-stent restenosis (38.0 vs. 8.2%, $p < 0.0001$) and target lesion revascularization (17.2 vs. 5.6%, $p < 0.0001$). Stent fracture was significantly more common in the right coronary artery than in the left anterior descending or circumflex arteries, perhaps resulting from a tendency toward greater tortuosity and dynamic torsion in the RCA. Longer stent length, overlapping stents, and stent overexpansion were also identified as risk factors for stent fracture.

18.30 Answer C. The stent is symmetrically deployed and all of the stent struts appear well apposed to the adjacent intima/neointima; however, the stent is underexpanded relative to the size of the vessel. The stent was likely undersized when initially implanted; however, it is also possible that the stent was appropriately sized when it was deployed 5 months earlier, but the vessel underwent positive remodeling in the interim.

QUESTIONS

19.1 Randomized clinical trials of directional atherectomy vs. balloon angioplasty for de novo lesions in native coronary arteries found which of the following comparing atherectomy with angioplasty?
(A) Higher complication rates, higher restenosis
(B) Higher complications rates, lower restenosis
(C) Lower complication rates, lower restenosis
(D) Lower complication rates, higher restenosis

19.2 A 75-year-old female with chronic kidney disease, stage 3, is admitted with progressive angina. Her biomarkers are not elevated, but she had transient ST segment depression in the anterior precordial leads, with return to baseline after initiation of medical therapy. At catheterization she is found to have a 90% stenosis in the mid-LAD coronary artery, but otherwise diffuse moderate nonobstructive disease. The lesion is successfully crossed with a 0.014-in. guidewire and predilation is attempted with a 2.5/15 mm noncompliant balloon. At 15 atm there is a persistent waist in the balloon. Further attempts to "crack the lesion" using higher pressures are not successful (Fig. Q19-2A). An angiogram reveals that the lesion severity and reference segments are relatively unchanged (Fig. Q19-2B). What would be the most optimal next strategy?

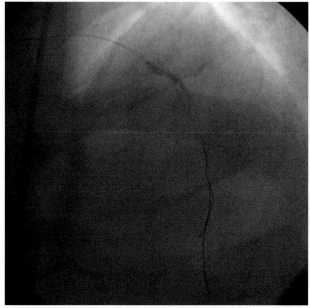

A
Figure Q19-2A

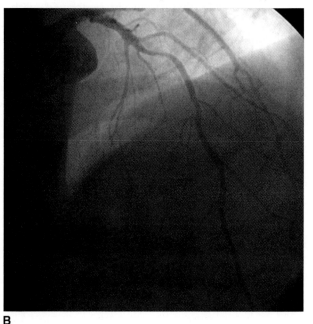

B
Figure Q19-2B

(A) Repeat attempts at predilation with a 3.0/15 mm noncompliant balloon

(B) Exchange the 0.014-in. guidewire for a rotowire, and perform rotational atherectomy with a 1.5-mm burr

(C) Repeat attempts at predilation using a 2.5/10 mm cutting balloon

(D) Stop the procedure and call for a consult for coronary artery bypass graft (CABG)

19.3   Which of the following is TRUE with respect to rotational atherectomy and restenosis?

(A) When compared with balloon angioplasty in randomized clinical trials, restenosis is lower with rotational atherectomy

(B) No randomized clinical trial has shown reduced restenosis rates with rotational atherectomy

(C) Adjunctive use of rotational atherectomy before coronary stenting is associated with lower restenosis rates compared with the use of stenting alone

(D) Restenosis is lower with rotational atherectomy in small vessels compared with balloon angioplasty

19.4   A 72-year-old man develops progressive angina, and undergoes a stress echocardiogram. He develops angina at 4 minutes, and is noted to have inferior and lateral wall hypokinesis on echo. He undergoes elective cardiac catheterization and is found to have diffuse severe coronary calcification, with a significant and lengthy lesion in the midcircumflex coronary artery (Fig. Q19-4A). Rotational atherectomy is performed with a 1.25-mm burr without complications. Rotational atherectomy with a 1.75-mm burr is unsuccessful after multiple attempts, and the angiogram in Figure Q19-4B is obtained. The patient develops chest pain and it is noted that there is ST segment elevation in the inferior leads. What should be the subsequent steps in this case?

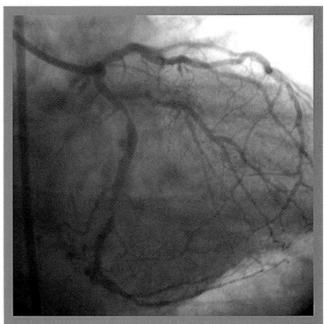

A

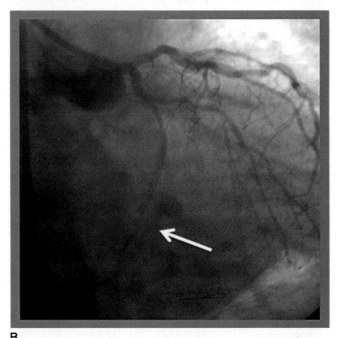

B

Figure Q19-4

(A) Wait a few minutes and then repeat rotational atherectomy

(B) Perform pericardiocentesis

(C) Administer intracoronary vasodilators and maintain adequate blood pressure with pressors as needed

(D) Perform high pressure balloon angioplasty with an oversized balloon at the lesion site

19.5   Which of the following is most likely to lead to potential complications during rotational atherectomy?

(A) Wire bias
(B) Orthogonal displacement of friction
(C) Differential cutting
(D) Microparticulate debris < 12 μm

19.6 Rotational atherectomy of a midcircumflex coronary artery lesion (Fig. Q19-6A) is performed in a stepped fashion with 1.5- and 2.0-mm burrs. The result is shown in Figure Q19-6B. The most likely cause of this result after rotational atherectomy is:

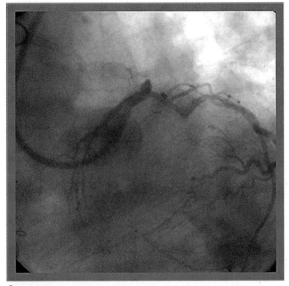

A

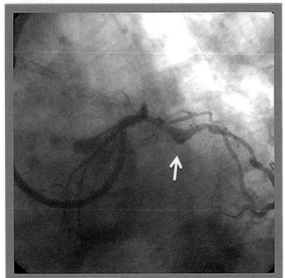

B

Figure Q19-6

(A) Coronary vasospasm
(B) Guide catheter dissection
(C) Centrifugal displacement of friction
(D) Wire bias

19.7 A 52-year-old diabetic man is admitted with recurrent chest pain during hemodialysis. A myocardial infarction is ruled out. A dobutamine echocardiogram reveals inferolateral hypokinesis at peak stress. Cardiac catheterization is advised, and significant stenosis is observed in the proximal portion of a heavily calcified right coronary artery (RCA). Rotational atherectomy of a proximal left circumflex (LCX) lesion was performed using a 1.25-mm burr (Fig. Q19-7A). Some difficulty was encountered in advancing a 1.75-mm burr into the left main coronary artery. During platforming of the burr, the patient complained of chest pain and the angiogram in Figure Q19-7B was obtained. Which of the following is the best option for treatment of this patient at this time?

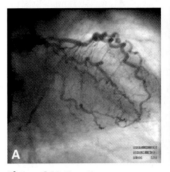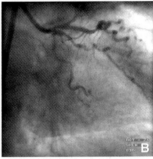

Figure Q19-7

(A) Inject RCA to determine if there is collateral flow to the ramus vessel
(B) Perform immediate pericardiocentesis and prepare the patient for emergency cardiac surgery
(C) Upsize to a 2.25-mm burr and repeat atherectomy
(D) Perform balloon angioplasty and stenting of the proximal ramus

19.8 A 78-year-old man presented with unstable angina. Coronary angiography revealed diffuse, calcific disease of the left anterior descending (LAD) coronary artery as shown in Figure 19-8A. Rotational atherectomy of the LAD coronary artery was performed with a 1.25-mm burr, followed by a 1.75-mm burr. The patient complained of chest pain and the angiogram in Figure 19.8B was obtained. Which of the following is the best treatment for this patient?

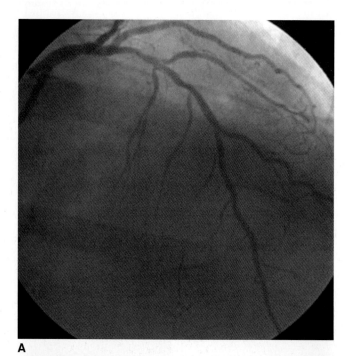

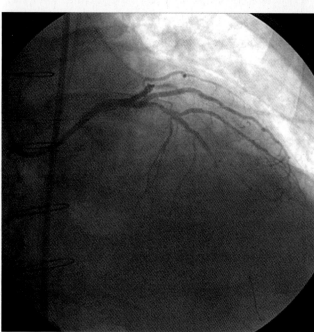

A

B

Figure Q19-8

(A) Intracoronary thrombolytics
(B) Extraction atherectomy
(C) Stenting of the LAD
(D) Low pressure balloon angioplasty with administration of intracoronary vasodilator

19.9 A 69-year-old retired bank president is seen by his primary care provider for progressive angina and dyspnea on exertion. He has had long standing hypertension and poorly controlled diabetes but has been otherwise active. A stress Cardiolyte study reveals a reversible large perfusion defect in the anterior wall. Cardiac catheterization is recommended and a severe, heavily calcified stenosis is found in the proximal LAD coronary artery. Because of the calcification, it is decided to pretreat the lesion with rotational atherectomy. There is a 50% diameter residual stenosis after 1.25- and 1.75-mm burrs. What would be the most optimal next step?

(A) Upsize to a 2.15-mm burr and repeat rotational atherectomy
(B) Perform balloon angioplasty with a 3.0/20 mm noncompliant balloon
(C) Place a 3.0/23 mm cobalt chromium stent
(D) Place a 3.0/23 mm drug-eluting stent

19.10 Compared with balloon angioplasty, with which of the following is laser atheroblation associated?

(A) Decreased complications, decreased restenosis
(B) Increased complications, increased restenosis
(C) Increased complications, decreased restenosis
(D) Decreased complications, increased restenosis

ANSWERS AND EXPLANATIONS

19.1 **Answer B.** The CAVEAT and BOAT trials randomized directional atherectomy vs. balloon angioplasty for de novo lesions in native coronary arteries. (*Circulation* 1998;97:322–331; *N Engl J Med* 1993;329:221–227.) In these trials, directional atherectomy was associated with an increase in creatine phosphokinase (CPK)-MB elevations, which were ≥3 times normal and periprocedural myocardial infarction (MI) compared with balloon angioplasty, and therefore had higher acute complication rates. By contrast, at the time of the angiographic follow-up, there was a statistically lower incidence of restenosis following directional atherectomy compared with balloon angioplasty in the BOAT trial, with a lower rate also observed in the CAVEAT trial ($p < 0.06$). The AMIGO trial was a randomized comparison of "optimal atherectomy" (<20% residual after DCA) followed by bare-metal stenting compared with bare-metal stenting alone. (*Am J Cardiol* 2004;93:953–958.) Despite favorable early reports that debulking and stenting were associated with lower restenosis rates than stenting alone, the randomized trial results indicated equivalent acute gain, similar early complication rates, and no difference in major adverse cardiac events at 8-month follow-up including angiographic restenosis. The benefit of DCA followed by use of drug-eluting stent (DES) has not been evaluated in clinical trials.

19.2 **Answer B.** In the present era rotational atherectomy was used to treat a variety of complex coronary artery lesions including lesions >20 mm in length, calcified lesions, and ostial and bifurcation disease. With the advent of intracoronary stents, in particular DES, use of rotational atherectomy fell dramatically. According to the 2007 update of the ACC/AHA guidelines for coronary interventions, rotational atherectomy is indicated for use in non-dilatable lesions as debulking prior to placement of a stent. In this case, further attempts at predilation would be unhelpful. Cutting balloons have been used with limited success in calcified lesions but are also associated with potential higher rates of dissections, which would preclude use of rotational atherectomy. CABG with a LIMA is an acceptable alternative but would not be preferred by most patients or interventionalists.

19.3 **Answer B.** Although rotational atherectomy has been used extensively in the past to debulk lesions, the STRATAS trial (*Am J Cardiol* 2001;87:699–705) and the DART trial (*Am Heart J* 2003;145:847–854) examined restenosis rates in randomized fashion, comparing rotational atherectomy with balloon angioplasty. Neither study found a lower incidence of restenosis with rotational atherectomy.

19.4 **Answer C.** This patient has developed slow flow vs. no reflow as a result of the high microparticulate burden during multiple burr runs. This leads to microvascular obstruction and ischemia. Prevention of this phenomenon can be achieved by several strategies during rotational atherectomy. Lower burr speeds, short runs <45 to 60 seconds, Rotoglide, aggressive vasodilation with nitroglycerin or nitroprusside, and maintenance of blood pressure with short acting pressors such as neosynephrine have all been used to prevent or minimize slow flow. Continuation of rotational atherectomy without restoring adequate flow would compound the situation. Use of balloon angioplasty may be helpful in this situation to help relieve spasm, but is usually achieved with low pressure inflations.

19.5 **Answer A.** Wire bias refers to the position of the rotational atherectomy wire in an eccentric position within the coronary vessel. In spite of the relatively floppy nature of the rotational atherectomy wire, the physical strength of the wire in an eccentric position leads to atherectomy that follows the position of the wire. If the wire is eccentrically lying against the lesion, this may facilitate the effectiveness of rotational atherectomy. However, if it is against the normal vessel, this may create a track outside of the normal vessel lumen, and may lead to local complications including perforation. Both differential cutting and orthogonal displacement of friction are believed to represent principles that contribute to effective use of rotational atherectomy. The small size of microparticulate debris allows the debris to pass through the distal coronary vasculature and minimizes plugging and vessel obstruction, although inadequate flushing of the vessel during atherectomy may still result in microvascular plugging.

19.6 **Answer D.** In this case, wire bias resulted in rotational atherectomy of the "inner curve" of the bend in the midcircumflex, with a subintimal channel outside of the original coronary lumen. Wire bias represents the phenomenon of eccentric position of a guidewire "cutting the corner" of a tortuous vessel, with subsequent atherectomy within the vessel along this eccentrically positioned guidewire. Although coronary spasm and guide catheters may result in injury to the coronary circulation during rotational atherectomy, they are not likely to have caused this result. Centrifugal displacement of friction is one of the principles that allows movement of the burr over the guidewire with the minimal tolerances between burr lumen and guidewire size.

19.7 **Answer B.** This patient has developed a Type III, free-flowing perforation at the junction of the left main and ramus vessels. This may have occurred as a result of unrecognized wire bias and atherectomy of the carina of the left main and ramus vessels. Additionally, this may have been a result of formation of an unrecognized loop in the guidewire at the tip of the guide catheter during advancement of the burr up the guide catheter. In this situation, platforming of the burr may not have been in a path coaxial with the left main and ramus vessels, resulting in inadvertent atherectomy of the left main. It is unlikely that attempts at balloon tamponade of the perforation would be successful given the location of the perforation. Moreover, prolonged balloon inflation would likely be followed by hemodynamic collapse because of LAD and LCX flow obstruction from the inflated balloon. Reversal of anticoagulation and stopping glycoprotein (GP) IIb/IIIa inhibitors with platelet transfusion would also be reasonable, but are unlikely to adequately treat the perforation without accompanying surgery.

19.8 **Answer D.** This patient has developed either slow flow/no reflow, most likely secondary to excessive microparticulate debris embolization of the distal vasculature, or a dissection.

Intracoronary thrombolytics are unlikely to be of benefit because this complication is not thrombus mediated. Similarly, extraction atherectomy would not be useful, and may also have limited feasibility given the small caliber of the lumen and the presence of diffuse calcific disease. Stenting of the LAD without adequate visualization of the landing zone proximally and distally would be problematic although it may ultimately be an appropriate course of action. Immediate stenting would not address the issue of microvascular plugging. Low pressure balloon angioplasty is a reasonable choice to relieve local spasm or tack up a dissection, and it also provides a means to deliver vasodilators to the distal vascular bed of the LAD. Use of an intraaortic balloon pump to augment coronary perfusion pressures may also be necessary if significant hypotension develops.

19.9 **Answer D.** Most experts agree that the optimal technique of using rotational atherectomy is to perform "facilitated" stenting: lesion preparation with rotational atherectomy aimed at achieving low burr-to-artery ratios, followed by intracoronary artery stenting. In the absence of a contraindication to prolonged use of dual antiplatelet therapy, most experts would recommend use of a DES. However, none of the pivotal randomized clinical trials comparing bare-metal to DES allowed use of atherectomy, thus there are no clinical trials that confirm the effectiveness of this strategy. There are no randomized studies evaluating debulking by rotational atherectomy before use of DES. Therefore, the statement that rotational atherectomy reduces restenosis rates before use of DES is incorrect.

19.10 **Answer B.** In the excimer laser, rotational atherectomy and balloon angioplasty comparison (ERBAC) trial, excimer laser angioplasty was associated with both an increase in coronary complications as well as higher restenosis rate compared with balloon angioplasty. (*Circulation* 1997;96:91–98) In this study, saline flushes were not used and may have been, in part, responsible for this higher rate of local complications.

20

Stents and Stent Thrombosis

Thomas Pilgrim and Stephan Windecker

QUESTIONS

20.1 The first stent implanted in a human coronary artery was implanted in March 1986 by Jacques Puel in Toulouse (France) and was called:

(A) Dotter stent
(B) Wallstent
(C) Palmaz-Schatz stent
(D) Igaki Tamai stent
(E) Cypher stent

20.2 A 78-year-old patient with history of three-vessel coronary artery disease, coronary artery bypass grafting (CABG) 8 years ago, moderately impaired left ventricular ejection fraction, chronic renal failure requiring hemodialysis, chronic obstructive pulmonary disease, and moderate pulmonary hypertension is referred for evaluation of acute chest pain with mild ST-segment depression in leads II, III, aVF, and elevated creatine kinase MB up to four times the upper limit of normal. Coronary angiography 2 years ago had shown a significant stenosis of the distal left main coronary artery, an open LIMA-graft to a proximally occluded LAD, an open saphenous vein graft (SVG) to a large first obtuse marginal branch in the setting of a 90% stenosis of the proximal left circumflex, and an occluded SVG to the distal right coronary artery (RCA) with a 50% calcified lesion of the vertical segment of the native RCA. You decide to repeat coronary angiography. In view of a past medical history notable for a subarachnoid hemorrhage 9 months ago, you decide to use bare-metal stents (BMS). All of the following parameters play an important role in the deliverability, visibility, scaffolding performance, and procedural success of BMS, EXCEPT:

(A) Strut design
(B) Strut thickness
(C) Metal composition
(D) Storing temperature
(E) Delivery system

20.3 A 52-year-old engineer is referred for a staged percutaneous coronary intervention (PCI) of an 80% stenosis of a large first obtuse marginal branch 6 weeks after primary PCI for acute anterior myocardial infarction with thrombotic occlusion of the proximal left anterior descending coronary artery. While providing informed consent for the procedure, the patient is interested in the key prerequisites or attributes for a coronary artery stent. All of the following is correct, EXCEPT:

(A) Tacking of intimal flaps and plaque coverage
(B) Prevention of elastic recoil by scaffolding of the arterial wall
(C) Facilitation of positive arterial remodeling
(D) Ability to fenestrate and access side branches
(E) Favorable deliverability due to a low profile and high flexibility

20.4 The use of covered stents is warranted in which of the following situations depicted in angiograms in Figure Q20-4A–E?

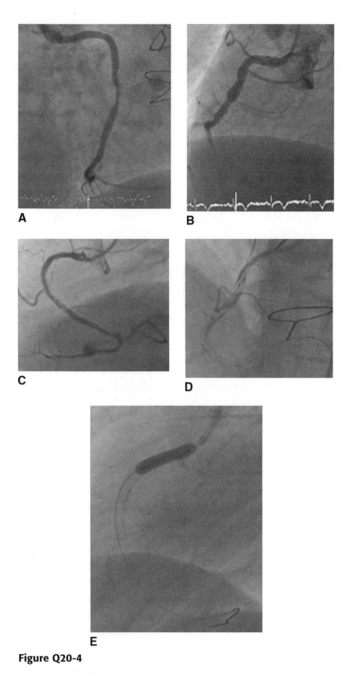

Figure Q20-4

(A) Figure A
(B) Figure B
(C) Figure C
(D) Figure D
(E) Figure E

20.5 A 62-year-old nurse with a past medical history remarkable for PTA and stenting of the left common femoral artery 2 years ago, active tobacco use, and a brother suffering a myocardial infarction at the age of 48 years is referred for coronary angiography due to exertional chest pain and evidence of ischemia during stress echocardiography. Since the peripheral vascular disease had

been treated with a self-expanding (SE) stent, she wishes to know whether you will consider to use a SE stent to treat her coronary artery disease. All statements are correct, EXCEPT:

(A) SE stents are less prone to cause edge dissections
(B) SE stents have been associated with negative recoil due to continued outward radial force after deployment
(C) SE stents have a reduced rate of side branch occlusion and no-reflow
(D) A concern of SE stents is placement accuracy caused by foreshortening on expansion and sudden spring movements
(E) SE stents tend to have a better profile as compared to balloon-expandable (BE) stents

20.6 A 61-year-old female with single-vessel coronary artery disease who suffered a large anterior myocardial infarction as a consequence of very late stent thrombosis 2 years ago is referred for repeat coronary angiography due to a positive stress test. She is interested in the safety and efficacy of novel stent coatings compared with drug-eluting stents (DES). All of the following statements are correct, EXCEPT:

(A) Passive stent coating with titanium-nitride-oxide has been shown to significantly reduce late loss at 6 months as compared to BMS
(B) A titanium-nitride-oxide–coated stent has been shown to reduce cardiac death, myocardial infarction, and stent thrombosis as compared to the TAXUS PES stent
(C) A titanium-nitride-oxide–coated stent has been shown noninferior vis-à-vis a zotarolimus-eluting stent with respect to late lumen loss
(D) Immobilization of antibodies directed against CD34 ligands that allow binding of endothelial progenitor cells may accelerate endothelial coverage of stent struts
(E) Stent coatings using titanium-nitride-oxide, nanothin polyzene-F-polymer, or CD34 antibodies have similar rates of stent thrombosis as DES

20.7 A 57-year-old male with coronary artery disease and multiple PCI of all three coronary vessels is concerned about late consequences of BMS and DES. He inquires about fully bioabsorbable vascular scaffolds. All of the following statements are correct, EXCEPT:

(A) The concept of fully bioabsorbable vascular scaffolds is based on the fact that coronary artery stents do not exert any long-term benefit as acute recoil and neointimal hyperplasia are relatively short-lived phenomena

(B) Early generation DES improve physiologic vasomotion in vessel segments adjacent to the stent

(C) A stent with a biodegradable poly-L-lactide backbone coated with a biodegradable polymer-everolimus mixture is able to normalize vasomotion within the stented segment during long-term follow-up

(D) A stent with a biodegradable poly-L-lactide backbone coated with a biodegradable polymer-everolimus mixture showed promising results with minimal stent recoil and no stent thrombosis in early clinical investigations

(E) A stent with a biodegradable poly-L-lactide backbone coated with a biodegradable polymer-everolimus mixture exerts similar suppression of neointimal hyperplasia as a metallic stent releasing everolimus

20.8 During percutaneous coronary intervention, you implant an adequately sized stent with an implantation pressure of 12 atmospheres. The angiographic results are satisfactory in the absence of edge dissections, and you consider high-pressure postdilatation. Which of the following statements summarizes current evidence most accurately?

(A) Stent underexpansion is associated with restenosis

(B) Stent underexpansion is associated with stent thrombosis

(C) Intramural hematoma and uncovered dissections are associated with abrupt vessel closure

(D) Statements B and C are correct

(E) Statements A, B, and C are correct

20.9 Which statement regarding intravascular ultrasound (IVUS) is CORRECT?

(A) Routine use of IVUS to guide stent implantation has been shown to reduce mortality and the risk of myocardial infarction

(B) IVUS is an adequate tool to assess complete apposition of stent struts to the vessel wall

(C) A minimal stent area of >5 mm^2 is considered satisfactory

(D) Routine use of IVUS reduces the risk of stent thrombosis

(E) IVUS does not allow for tissue characterization

20.10 Which statement is CORRECT regarding the percentages of complications associated with PCI (Fig. Q20-10)?

(A) A denotes in-hospital death, B denotes myocardial infarction, C denotes emergency CABG, and D denotes stroke

(B) A denotes stroke, B denotes myocardial infarction, C denotes emergency CABG, and D denotes in-hospital death

(C) A denotes in-hospital death, B denotes emergency CABG, C denotes myocardial infarction, and D denotes stroke

(D) A denotes myocardial infarction, B denotes severe access site complications, C denotes emergency CABG, and D denotes stroke

(E) A denotes stroke, B denotes emergency CABG, C denotes stroke, and D denotes myocardial infarction

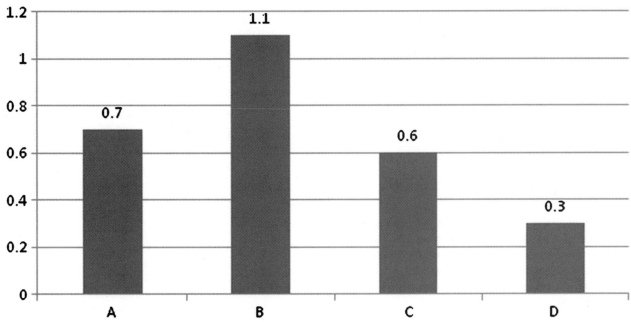

Figure Q20-10

20.11 One of the residents is interested in the risk of PCI periprocedural complications. Which of the following patients has the highest risk of mortality following PCI?

(A) An 82-year-old female with a history of diabetes, a creatinine clearance of 30 mL/min, mild elevation of troponin T, and left ventricular ejection fraction of 40%

(B) An 80-year-old male with a body mass index of 20 kg/m², moderate renal dysfunction, and left ventricular ejection fraction of 35%

(C) A 78-year-old female with a body mass index of 20 kg/m², a creatinine clearance of 60 mL/min, arterial hypertension, and a history of paroxysmal atrial fibrillation

(D) A 62-year-old male with left ventricular ejection fraction of 45% and arterial hypertension who was previously treated with a BMS

(E) A 42-year-old male with a creatinine clearance of 90 mL/min, a body mass index of 39 kg/m², and hypercholesterolemia who is presenting with chest tightness on minimal exertion

20.12 The day after successful percutaneous coronary intervention of a tight stenosis of the mid LAD, a rise in troponin up to two times the upper limit of normal and elevated CK-MB just above the normal range is documented. CK is within normal limits. A 12-lead ECG performed 6 hours after the procedure is without any signs of ischemia. The patient denies having had any episode of chest pain since the procedure. Which of the following statements regarding his subsequent risk of mortality is CORRECT?

(A) Preprocedural troponin elevation is a stronger predictor of short- and long-term mortality than postprocedural troponin elevation

(B) The magnitude of postprocedural biomarker elevation is associated with the likelihood of adverse outcomes in retrospective studies not using high-sensitivity troponin assays

(C) Major lesion-related risk factors for periprocedural myocardial infarction include presence of thrombus, stenosis of SVGs, and type C lesions

(D) Postprocedural elevation of troponin is an independent risk factor for stent thrombosis

(E) Statements A to C are correct

20.13 Repeat coronary angiography 8 months after PCI of the proximal segment of the right coronary artery shows the finding depicted in Figure Q20-13. Which statement is NOT correct regarding the clinical consequences of this finding?

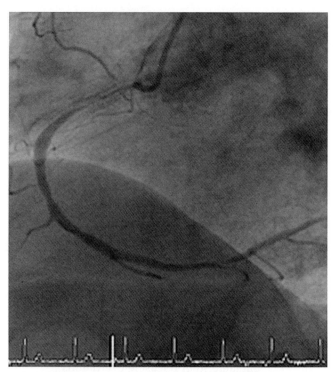

Figure Q20-13

(A) Clinical consequences depend on the following parameters: degree of stenosis, area at risk, recruitable collaterals, and lesion location

(B) This finding is associated with an increased risk of myocardial infarction

(C) Observational studies suggest a negative impact of the finding above on survival

(D) This finding is associated with an increased risk of coronary vasospasm

20.14 A 72-year-old male with three-vessel coronary artery disease s/p CABG 12 years ago presents with typical chest pain and a positive stress test. Coronary angiography shows a patent LIMA-graft to the LAD, a chronic occlusion of the SVG to the circumflex in the setting of a 50% stenosis of the native circumflex, as well as a significant stenosis of the SVG to the chronically occluded right coronary artery. You decide to treat the SVG to the RCA with PCI. Which statement(s) is CORRECT?

(A) PCI of SVGs is associated with an increased risk of periprocedural myocardial infarction

(B) There is no significant difference in the rate of restenosis requiring target lesion revascularization for SVGs and native coronary arteries

(C) Compared with BMS, DES has been associated with adverse clinical outcome in the treatment of SVGs

(D) Embolic protection devices reduce periprocedural myocardial infarctions in PCI for SVGs and their use has a Class IIa recommendation

(E) Statements A and C are correct

20.15 A 75-year-old female with a past medical history remarkable for myocardial infarction of the inferior wall without revascularization complains of angina on moderate exertion and is found to have a left ventricular ejection fraction of 45% on transthoracic echocardiography. She is referred for coronary angiography. Based on the angiogram (Fig. Q20-15), which of the following statements is CORRECT?

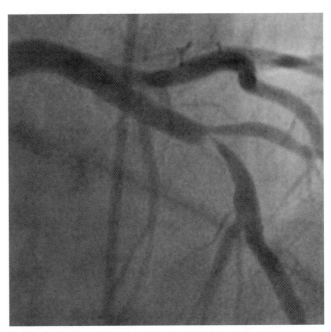

Figure Q20-16

(A) 1,1,1
(B) 0,1,1
(C) 1,0,1
(D) 0,0,1
(E) 1,1,0

20.17 A patient agrees to participate in a randomized stent trial with repeat angiography at 6 to 8 months. How much does repeat angiography impact the rate of target lesion revascularization compared with patients without mandated follow-up angiography?

(A) It is associated with a relative risk increase of TLR of 70%
(B) It does not impact the risk of TLR
(C) It is associated with a relative risk increase of TLR of 35%
(D) It doubles the rate of TLR
(E) It only increases the rate of Non-TLR TVR and Non-TVR

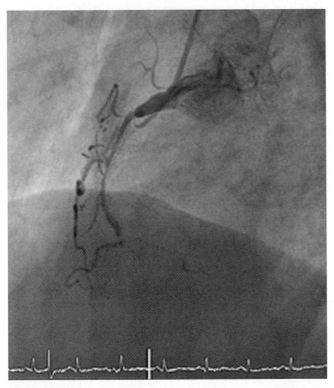

Figure Q20-15

(A) Treatment of the finding shown above may reduce symptoms and improve left ventricular function
(B) Percutaneous coronary intervention in this setting has consistently been demonstrated to improve survival
(C) Percutaneous coronary intervention for lesions as shown above has been shown to reduce the risk of reinfarction and heart failure during 4 years of follow-up as compared to medical treatment
(D) Randomized clinical trials demonstrate a reduction in the rates of death in patients with the finding depicted above treated with SES as compared to BMS
(E) All statements above are correct

20.16 What is the Medina classification of the bifurcation lesion shown in Figure Q20-16?

20.18 An 80-year-old patient with three-vessel coronary artery disease with involvement of the proximal segments of all three coronary arteries asks you whether he should undergo CABG or PCI. He has a history of gastric ulcer with recurrent bleeding and currently has a hemoglobin of 10 g/L. All of the following statements regarding randomized controlled trials comparing PCI with use of BMS vs. coronary artery bypass graft surgery are correct, EXCEPT:

(A) After a mean follow-up of 5 years, no difference in mortality was observed between patients treated with PCI or CABG in a meta-analysis from the ARTS, ERACI II, SOS, and MASSII trials

(B) Randomized trials comparing PCI with BMS vs. CABG demonstrated a roughly four times higher incidence of TLR in disfavor of PCI

(C) The rate of stroke in the ARTS trial was significantly higher for patients treated with CABG

(D) There was no significant difference in the rate of myocardial infarction for PCI and CABG patients in ARTS and ERACI II

(E) A meta-analysis of four randomized trials (ARTS, SoS, ERACI-II, and MASS-II) comparing BMS with CABG showed a similar cumulative incidence of death, MI, and stroke among diabetic patients

20.19 Which of the following mechanisms may lead to the image shown in Figure Q20-19?

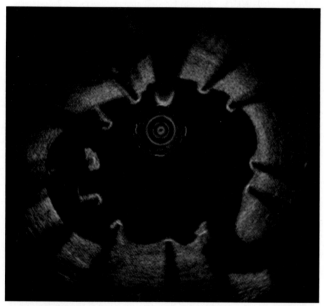

Figure Q20-19

(A) Positive arterial remodeling

(B) A decrease in plaque due to dissolution of jailed material

(C) Stent underexpansion

(D) Statements A, B, and C are correct

(E) None of the statements is correct

20.20 A 57-year-old patient with history of coronary artery disease and PCI of the RCA presents for repeat angiography according to a study protocol. He is asymptomatic and a stress test was inconclusive due to LBBB. Which statement regarding the finding shown in Figure Q20-20A-B is CORRECT?

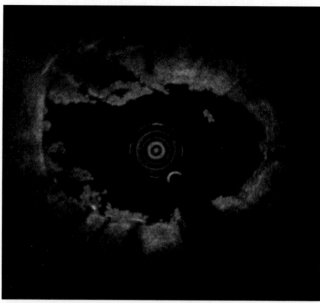

A

B

Figure Q20-20

(A) This finding is most commonly observed with BMS

(B) This angiographic finding is associated with a higher incidence of clinical adverse events

(C) The finding is positively correlated with stent length, stent overlap, and increasing duration after stent implantation

(D) This finding is more commonly observed in the right coronary artery

(E) Statements B, C, and D are correct

20.21 After PCI of a significant stenosis of the mid RCA in a 75-year-old female, you get the following result. Which of the following statements regarding the angiogram shown in Figure Q20-21 is most accurate?

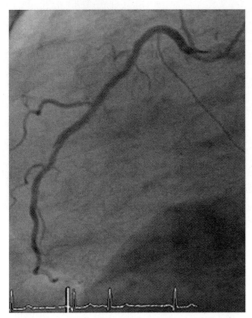

Figure Q20-21

(A) It is safe to leave this finding untreated
(B) It is safe to leave this finding untreated if GpIIb IIIa inhibitors are administered
(C) This finding can adequately be treated with balloon dilatation
(D) This finding is associated with an increased risk of early stent thrombosis
(E) This finding is caused by vasospasm

20.22 Which of the following images obtained with optical coherence tomography (OCT) or angiography after stenting is associated with the greatest risk of early stent thrombosis (Fig. Q20-22A–D)?

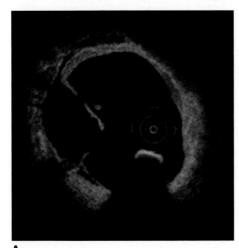

A

Figure Q20-22

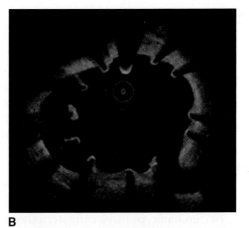

B

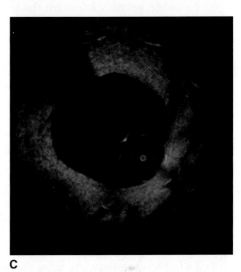

C

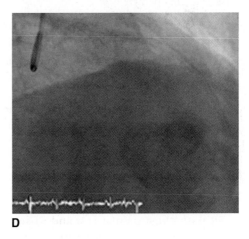

D

QUESTIONS 20.23 THROUGH 20.26. Academic Research Consortium (ARC) definitions of stent thrombosis: Match the following case vignettes with the appropriate term according to the ARC definition of stent thrombosis.

20.23 A 57-year-old male with ST-segment elevation myocardial infarction 35 days after PCI with angiographically proven stent thrombosis:

(A) Definitive, primary, late stent thrombosis
(B) Definitive, primary, early stent thrombosis
(C) Definitive, secondary, late stent thrombosis
(D) Probable, primary, late stent thrombosis
(E) Probable, primary early stent thrombosis

20.24 A 45-year-old male with sudden cardiac arrest 20 days after PCI of a significant ostial LAD lesion:

(A) Definitive, secondary, early stent thrombosis
(B) Probable, primary, early stent thrombosis
(C) Probable, primary, late stent thrombosis
(D) Possible, primary, early stent thrombosis
(E) Possible, secondary, early stent thrombosis

20.25 A 78-year-old female s/p PCI of proximal RCA lesion 2 years ago and PTCA of an in-stent restenosis 1 year ago presenting to a primary care facility in cardiogenic shock with new ST-segment elevations in leads II, III, and aVF who dies before transfer to the catheterization laboratory:

(A) Possible, secondary, very late stent thrombosis
(B) Possible, secondary, late stent thrombosis
(C) Probable, secondary, very late stent thrombosis
(D) Probable, primary, very late stent thrombosis
(E) Definite, secondary, late stent thrombosis

20.26 An 82-year-old female dying in a nursing home 18 months after implantation of a DES:

(A) Possible, primary, late stent thrombosis
(B) Possible, secondary, very late stent thrombosis
(C) Probable, primary, very late stent thrombosis
(D) Possible, primary, very late stent thrombosis
(E) Definite, primary, very late stent thrombosis

20.27 A 59-year-old patient with known coronary artery disease and stent placement to the proximal LAD 9 months ago presents to the ER with chest pain at rest and ST-segment elevations in leads V1-V5. Coronary angiography shows the finding in Figure Q20-27. All of the following are risk factors for the event shown above, EXCEPT:

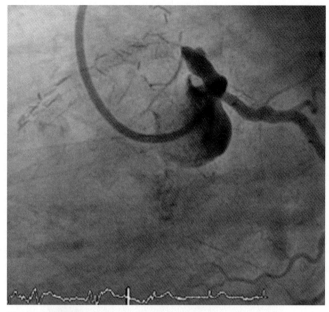

Figure Q20-27

(A) Insulin-dependent diabetes
(B) Impaired left ventricular ejection fraction
(C) Renal failure
(D) Acute coronary syndrome at the time of the index procedure
(E) Male gender

20.28 Which of the following statements regarding the occurrence of stent thrombosis in BMS and DES is most accurate?

(A) Early stent thrombosis occurs more frequently with DES than with BMS
(B) The annual rate of very late stent thrombosis is higher than the rate of early and late stent thrombosis for patients treated with early generation DES and BMS
(C) Secondary stent thrombosis is more common with DES than with BMS
(D) Very late stent thrombosis occurs with similar frequency among patients treated with early generation DES and BMS
(E) The mortality rates for definitive ST range from 9% to 19%

20.29 Which of the following stents has the highest risk for the event occurring 13 months after PCI of the mid LAD depicted in the angiogram in Figure Q20-29?

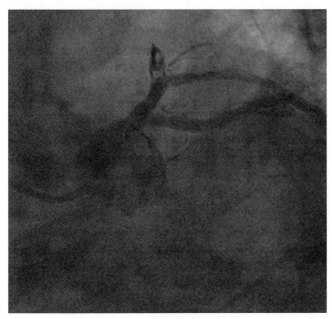

Figure Q20-29

    (A) Early generation DES
    (B) Bare-metal stent
    (C) Stent with passive stent coating
    (D) Newer generation DES
    (E) There are no significant differences in the occurrence of the event depicted above between different stent types

20.30 A 57-year-old diabetic female presents with typical chest pain and a positive stress test. Coronary angiography reveals a bifurcation lesion of the proximal LAD at the take off of the first diagonal branch. The strategy is to perform stenting of the LAD with fenestration of the first diagonal branch. Which of the following statements is CORRECT?

    (A) Final kissing balloon dilatation reduces angiographic side branch stenosis
    (B) Final kissing balloon dilatation is associated with lower risk of death and myocardial infarction at 6 months
    (C) Final kissing balloon dilatation is associated with a longer procedure duration and a greater amount of contrast media use
    (D) Statements A and B are correct
    (E) Statements A and C are correct

20.31 All of the following factors are predictors of early stent thrombosis, EXCEPT:

    (A) Inadequate stent expansion
    (B) Residual dissection
    (C) TIMI 1 flow postprocedure
    (D) Inappropriate inhibition of platelet aggregation
    (E) Body mass index > 30 kg/m^2

20.32 Which of the following statement most accurately summarizes the risk of early stent thrombosis according to clinical presentation?

    (A) The risk of early stent thrombosis is lower with BMS as compared to DES
    (B) Non–ST-elevation myocardial infarction triples the risk of early ST compared to stable angina
    (C) The risk of early stent thrombosis is highest in patients with ST-elevation MI treated with BMS, but not with DES
    (D) The risk of early stent thrombosis in patients with stable angina treated with DES amounts to 0.3% to 0.4%
    (E) Statements B and D are correct

20.33 Which statements regarding applicability of the ARC definition of stent thrombosis is correct?

    (A) Probable and possible stent thrombosis provide a high degree of sensitivity
    (B) The combination of probable and possible stent thrombosis is suitable for the detection of safety signals
    (C) Definite stent thrombosis provides a high specificity but may underestimate the true incidence of stent thrombosis
    (D) The composite of definite and probable stent thrombosis is considered a reasonable balance of specificity and sensitivity
    (E) All of the statements above are correct

20.34 A 52-year-old patient presents with chest pain at rest and inferior ST-segment elevations. Past medical history is significant for PCI of the proximal right coronary artery 14 months ago. Coronary angiography shows a complete occlusion of the RCA; OCT reveals the finding depicted in Figure Q20-34. Which of the following mechanisms may have been associated with the occurrence of the event in question?

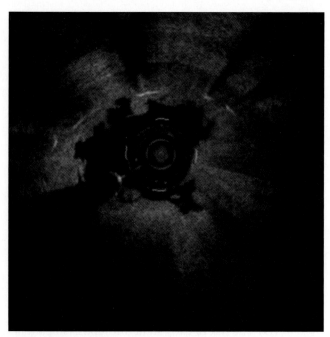

Figure Q20-34

    (A) Delayed healing
    (B) Chronic inflammation
    (C) Hypersensitivity reactions
    (D) Neoatherosclerosis
    (E) All of the above

20.35 Which of the following statements with respect to histologic findings of thrombus aspirates of patients with very late stent thrombosis is CORRECT?

    (A) They may show evidence of severe inflammation with eosinophilic infiltrates
    (B) The eosinophilic infiltrates correlate with the amount of vessel remodeling
    (C) Eosinophilic infiltrates are most commonly found in patients treated with SES
    (D) Both Sirolimus and Paclitaxel have been shown to activate the coagulation cascade
    (E) All of the statements above are correct

20.1 **Answer B.** After Charles Dotter had implanted the first vascular stent in a canine popliteal artery in 1968, the first coronary stent was a self-expanding (SE) stent called *Wallstent* that was implanted for the very first time by Jacques Puel in 1986 in the left anterior descending artery of a 63-year-old patient presenting with restenosis after plain balloon angioplasty. The *Palmaz-Schatz stent* was the first balloon-expandable (BE) (tubular slotted) stent implanted for the first time in December 1987 in Sao Paolo (Brazil). The *Igaki Tamai stent* consisted of poly-l-lactic acid and was the first fully bioabsorbable stent. The Sirolimus-eluting *Cypher stent* was the first DES approved by the FDA in 2002.

20.2 **Answer D.** Strut design (coil, closed-cell slotted tube, open-cell slotted tube, modular), strut thickness, metal composition (stainless steel, cobalt chrome, platinum, nitinol), and delivery system (BE, SE) importantly determine deliverability, visibility, and scaffolding performance. Most stents currently available have a slotted-tube design. Whereas closed cells provide a greater radial strength, open cells allow for greater flexibility. Stents can be stored at room temperature; hence, storing temperature does not determine deliverability, visibility, or radial strength. Conversely, storing temperature plays a role in bioabsorbable vascular scaffolds.

20.3 **Answer C.** Key prerequisites of coronary artery stents are the sealing of coronary artery dissections by tacking of intimal flaps against the arterial wall and the prevention of elastic recoil after balloon angioplasty. Limited deformability is required for bifurcation stenting techniques, and a low profile and high flexibility facilitate stent placement in calcified and tortuous coronary arteries. Positive arterial remodeling is a rare adverse process observed with metallic DES that may lead to late-acquired stent malapposition and may be associated with an increased risk of late stent thrombosis.

20.4 **Answer C.** Image C shows a perforation of a posterior descending coronary artery following plain balloon angioplasty. The use of covered stents is confined to the emergency treatment of coronary perforations or for the exclusion of giant coronary aneurysms (not shown). (*Circ Cardiovasc Interv* 2008;1:85–86). Image A shows a significant stenosis of an SVG. It has been hypothesized that covered stents might decrease distal embolization by entrapping friable degenerated material and reduce neointimal hyperplasia. However, a randomized multicenter trial of 400 patients failed to show any advantage of a polytetrafluoroethylene covered stent compared with a BMS in terms of percent diameter stenosis or major adverse cardiac events at 8 months. (*Catheter Cardiovasc Interv* 2006;68:379–388). Image B shows thrombotic occlusion of a right coronary artery, image D illustrates a periprocedural coronary dissection, and image E demonstrates stent implantation in an ostial lesion.

20.5 **Answer E.** Whereas SE stents and BE stents had been used with similar frequency in the early days of coronary artery stenting, several drawbacks of SE stents, such as less precise placement and negative recoil, have outweighed the potential advantages mentioned in statements B and D. SE stents have been associated with a lower incidence of edge dissections and side branch occlusions (*Catheter Cardiovasc Interv* 2002;56:478–486). However, the mechanism of SE stents is based on the shape memory of nitinol, an alloy of nickel and titanium, which continues to exert an outward radial force after release leading to negative chronic recoil. In contrast to BE stents, deliverability is dictated by the delivery sheath and strut dimensions rather than balloon profile. SE stents are currently being investigated in patients with bifurcation lesions, vulnerable plaques, and small diameter vessels.

20.6 **Answer C.** A titanium-nitride-oxide–coated stent (Titan-2, Hexacath, France) has been shown to be inferior vis-à-vis a zotarolimus-eluting stent in a randomized controlled noninferiority trial (*J Am Coll Cardiol Intv* 2011;4:672–682.). However, passive stent coating with titanium-nitride-oxide has been shown to significantly reduce late loss at 6 months as compared to a BMS (*Circulation* 2005;111:2617–2622) and reduce cardiac death, myocardial infarction, and stent thrombosis as compared to the TAXUS stent (*EuroIntervention* 2010;6:63–68). The Genous Bio-engineered R-Stent (OrbusNeich, Fort Lauderdale, USA) contains antibodies against CD34 ligands on its luminal surface, which may accelerate functional endothelial coverage of stent struts. Limited evidence from clinical trials of novel stents with passive coatings report similar rates of stent thrombosis as observed with DES.

20.7 **Answer B.** Since coronary artery stents do not exert any long-term benefit, both fully biodegradable non–drug-eluting (*Circulation* 2000; 102(4):399–404) and drug-eluting (*Lancet* 2008;371(9616):899–907) scaffolds have been investigated. A stent with a biodegradable poly-L-lactide backbone coated with a biodegradable polymer-everolimus mixture showed promising results with only minimal stent recoil, similar neointimal hyperplasia as a metallic stent releasing everolimus, normalization of coronary vasomotion within the stented segment during long-term follow-up, and absence of stent thrombosis in clinical investigations (*Circulation* 2010;122:2301–2312). DES have been shown to impair but not improve vasomotion in adjacent vessel segments (*J Am Coll Cardiol* 2005;46:231–236).

20.8 **Answer E.** Stent underexpansion has been associated with both restenosis and stent thrombosis after BMS and DES implantation. Residual dissections can lead to abrupt vessel closure (see Answer 20.21 also).

20.9 **Answer B.** Routine intravascular ultrasound-guided percutaneous coronary intervention in the pre–DES era has been shown to improve angiographic minimum lumen diameter and reduce angiographic restenosis and the rate of repeat revascularization in a meta-analysis. However, no effect on death and myocardial infarction was appreciated during a follow-up period of 6 months to 2.5 years (*Am J Cardiol* 2011;107:374–382). A minimal stent area of >5 mm^2 is generally considered satisfactory. Although IVUS can reliably assess stent apposition, no prospective study has proven that routine use of IVUS reduces the incidence of stent thrombosis. IVUS is able to assess tissue characteristics of underlying plaques.

20.10 **Answer A.** An analysis from the ACC/National Cardiovascular Data Registry including 558′273 percutaneous coronary interventions performed between 2001 and 2004 reported an in-hospital mortality of 0.7%, a rate of myocardial infarction of 1.1%, the need of emergency CABG in 0.6%, and stroke ranging from 0.1% to 0.3% during the in-hospital period.

20.11 **Answer A.** Several clinical parameters have been identified to determine the risk of periprocedural mortality including age, female gender, diabetes, renal dysfunction, cardiogenic shock, large area of myocardium at risk, compromised left ventricular ejection fraction, and ST-segment elevation myocardial infarction. The 82-year-old female with a history of diabetes, a creatinine clearance of 30 mL/min, mild elevation of troponin T, and left ventricular ejection fraction of 40% appears to be at the highest aggregate risk.

20.12 **Answer E.** Evidence for the clinical significance of postprocedural elevations of cardiac enzymes is derived from retrospective studies susceptible to potential confounding variables. In a large number of studies, the magnitude of postprocedural biomarker elevation has been associated with an increased likelihood of adverse events. However, most of those studies did either not use high-sensitivity troponin assays or did not apply the currently recommended cutoff value for the upper limit of normal range. Preprocedural elevation in troponin is in general a stronger predictor of short- and long-term mortality than postprocedural troponin elevation. Major lesion-related risk factors for periprocedural myocardial infarction include presence of thrombus, stenosis of SVGs, and type C lesions (*N Engl J Med* 2011;365:453–464). Although postprocedural troponin elevation is associated with an increased risk of adverse events, it has not been shown to be an independent predictor of stent thrombosis.

20.13 **Answer E.** The angiographic image shows a high-grade in-stent restenosis. Clinical consequences depend on the degree of restenosis, the area at risk as determined by lesion location, and the amount of recruitable collaterals. In a retrospective study of 4,503 patients prior to the DES era, restenosis presenting with myocardial infarction was encountered in 2.1% (95% CI, 1.6%–2.6%) of patients; furthermore, restenosis presenting with myocardial infarction was associated with an increased risk of mortality (HR 2.37; *p* < 0.001) (*Circulation* 2007;116:2391–2398). Even though no association of restenosis with survival has been observed in prospective randomized clinical trials, retrospective studies indicate an adverse long-term outcome in patients with restenosis. In a series of 2,272 patients, mortality rate at 4 years amounted to 6.0% in patients with no restenosis as compared to 8.8% in those with restenosis ($p = 0.02$) (*Am Heart J* 2004;147:317–322).

20.14 **Answer A.** PCI for SVGs is associated with suboptimal results due to high rates of periprocedural MI and high rates of restenosis requiring TLR (*N Engl J Med* 1997;337:740–747). Embolic protection devices reduce periprocedural myocardial infarctions in PCI for SVGs and are a Class I recommendation when technically feasible (*J Am Coll Cardiol* 2006;47:e1–e121).In contrast to lesions in native vessels, there is a paucity of data investigating the potential benefits of DES over BMS in SVGs. However, in propensity score matched outcomes in 1,000 patients treated with DES or BMS; DES was associated with a lower rate of MACE (14% vs. 21%, $p = 0.001$), a lower composite of death or MI (8.7% vs. 14%, $p = 0.006$), and a lower rate of TVR (HR:0.36, $p < 0.001$) (*JACC Cardiovasc Interv* 2009;2:1105–1112).

20.15 **Answer A.** The angiographic picture shows a chronic total occlusion (CTO) of the mid to distal right coronary artery. Successful percutaneous recanalization of CTOs is able to reduce symptoms and may improve left ventricular function as compared to a failed attempt in a multicenter prospective observational study (*J Am Coll Cardiol* 2003;41:1672–1678). However, data from the largest randomized controlled trial investigating PCI for persistent occlusion after myocardial infarction showed no reduction in the occurrence of death, reinfarction, or heart failure during 4 years of follow-up as compared with medical treatment (17.2% vs. 15.6%, HR 1.16; 95% CI 0.92–1.45; $p = 0.20$) (*N Engl J Med* 2006;355:2395–2407). Randomized data comparing BMS with SES in the treatment of CTOs demonstrated comparable rates of death (1.3% vs. 2.7%, $p = 0.613$) and myocardial infarction (5.1% vs. 2.7%, $p = 0.682$), whereas the risk of TLR and TVR was significantly reduced in favor of SES (*Eur Heart J* 2010;31(16):2014–2020).

20.16 **Answer B.** The Medina classification of bifurcation lesions indicates the presence or absence of stenosis at the site of bifurcation as 1 or 0 in three segments.The first digit indicates the proximal main vessel, the second digit the distal main vessel, and the third digit the side branch. The stenosis shown in Figure A20-16 involves the distal segment of the main vessel and the side branch (0,1,1).

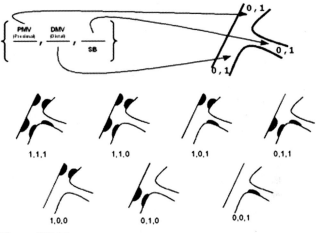

Figure A20-16

20.17 **Answer A.** Serruys et al.(*Lancet* 1998;352:673–681) randomized patients to either clinical and angiographic follow-up or clinical follow-up alone in a stent vs. balloon angioplasty trial. At 6 months, a primary clinical end point had occurred in 12.8% of the stent group and in 19.3% of the angioplasty group ($p = 0.013$). This significant difference in clinical outcome was maintained at 12 months. In the subgroup assigned to angiographic follow-up, restenosis rates occurred in 16% of the stent group and in 31% of the balloon angioplasty group ($p = 0.0008$), with a relative risk increase of TLR of 70% in the angiography group. In the group assigned clinical follow-up alone, event-free survival rate at 12 months was higher in the stent group than in the balloon angioplasty group (0.89 vs. 0.79, $p = 0.004$).

20.18 **Answer C.** Several randomized controlled clinical trials (RCT) have compared PCI in the pre-DES era with CABG. Whereas no significant difference in mortality was observed after 5 years of follow-up in ARTS, ERACI II, and MASS-II, SOS noted a higher rate of death at 6 years of follow-up. However, a meta-analysis of all four RCTs demonstrated no difference in mortality after 5 years between PCI and CABG (8.5% vs.

8.2%, $p = 0.74$). At the same time, repeat revascularization was performed in 25.0% of patients with PCI and in 6.3% of patients undergoing CABG (*Circulation* 2008;118:1146–1154). In the ARTS I trial, no significant difference in the incidence of stroke was seen at 5 years of follow-up between patients treated with PCI or CABG (3.8% vs. 3.5%, $p = 0.76$) (*J Am Coll Cardiol* 2005;46:575–581). Likewise, there was no significant difference in the rate of myocardial infarction for PCI and CABG patients in ARTS I (8.5% vs. 6.4%) and ERACI II (2.8% vs. 6.2%, $p = 0.13$) (*J Am Coll Cardiol* 2005;46:582–588). Randomized controlled trials comparing POBA vs. CABG did not show any difference in mortality between PCI and CABG at 6.5 years in RITA I (7.6% vs. 9.0%), at 8 years in EAST (20.7% vs. 17.3%), at 1 year in CABRI (3.9% vs. 2.7%), at 13 years in GABI (25.0 vs. 21.9%), and at 10 years in BARI (29.0 vs. 26.5%) (*Am J Med* 2009;122:152–161). The cumulative incidence of death, MI, and stroke was similar for diabetic patients undergoing PCI (21.4%) or CABG (20.9%, $p = 0.9$) in a meta-analysis of four trials comparing BMS with CABG (*Circulation* 2008;118:1146–1154).

20.19 Answer D. The cross-sectional OCT image shows incomplete stent apposition at follow-up, which may be the result of positive arterial remodeling, a decrease in plaque due to dissolution of jailed material (i.e., thrombus) at the time of stent implantation, or stent underexpansion (*Circulation* 2007;115:2426–2434).

20.20 Answer E. The image is an example of a stent fracture as late complication of stent implantation with an incidence ranging from 1% to 29% in randomized, observational and autopsy studies (*Catheter Cardiovasc Interv* 2007;69:387–394; *Catheter Cardiovasc Interv* 2007;69:380–386; *Am J Cardiol* 2007;100:627–630; *J Am Coll Cardiol* 2009;54:1924–1931). Stent fractures have predominantly been reported with Cypher stents, whereas stent fractures with TAXUS stents and other stents appear to be less frequent. The risk of stent fracture has been correlated with several mechanical factors and lesions' characteristics such as lesion location in the right coronary artery, severely tortuous vessels, long/overlapping stents, and stent implantation duration (*J Am Coll Cardiol* 2009;54:1924–1931). Approximately three quarters of patients with a stent fracture will present with in-stent restenosis. Some will present with stent thrombosis (*Catheter Cardiovasc Interv* 2007;69:380–386).

20.21 Answer D. The image shows a distal edge dissection. Residual dissections after PCI may cause early stent thrombosis. Whereas it is acceptable to leave mild luminal haziness untreated, intraluminal linear dissection increases the risk of abrupt closure (*Circulation* 2001;103:1967–1971).

Table A20-21. National Heart, Lung and Blood Institute's Classification System of Coronary Dissection

Type	Description	Rate of Acute Closure (%)
A	Mild luminal haziness	0
B	Intraluminal linear dissection	3
C	Extraluminal contrast dye staining or extraluminal cap (with persistence of dye after dye clearance)	10
D	Spiral dissection	30
E	Dissection with filling defects	9
F	Dissection with limited or no flow	69

20.22 Answer A. Images A through C are OCT images. Image A shows a dissection of the intima just distal to the stent edge (no stent struts visible). Image B illustrates strut malapposition between seven and eleven o'clock. Image C shows stent struts covered by neointimal hyperplasia, consistent with in-stent restenosis. In image D from plain fluoroscopy performed without contrast, a long stented segment involving the proximal, mid, and distal segment of the LAD can be appreciated. Both incomplete stent apposition and stent length have been associated with stent thrombosis. An IVUS study showed that incomplete stent apposition was more frequent (77% vs. 12%; $p < 0.001$) and maximal incomplete stent apposition area was larger (8.3 ± 7.5 vs. 4.0 ± 3.8 mm^2; $p = 0.03$) in patients with very late stent thrombosis compared with 144 controls (*Circulation* 2007;115:2426–2434). In a consecutive cohort of 3,145 patients treated with DES, stent lengths ≥ 31.5 mm were associated with higher rates of ST (4.0% vs. 0.7%, $p < 0.001$), death (5.2% vs. 3.0%, $p = 0.005$), and myocardial infarction (2.4% vs. 0.7%, $p = 0.001$) at 3 years, as compared with stent length <31.5 mm (*JACC Cardiovasc Interv* 2010;4:383–389). Nevertheless, intraluminal dissection portends the highest risk for early stent thrombosis.

20.23 Answer A.

20.24 Answer B.

20.25 Answer C.

20.26 Answer D.

The definition of stent thrombosis according to the ARC definition.

Definite stent thrombosis

Either angiographic or postmortem evidence of thrombotic stent occlusion in the presence of symptoms consistent with an acute myocardial infarction

Probable stent thrombosis

Any unexplained death within 30 days of stent implantation, or any myocardial infarction in the territory of the implanted stent irrespective of time

Possible stent thrombosis

Any unexplained death beyond 30 days until the end of follow-up

Early stent thrombosis: ≤1 month

≤1 day: acute stent thrombosis

>1 day: subacute stent thrombosis

Late stent thrombosis: >1 month up to 1 year

Very late stent thrombosis: >1 year

Primary stent thrombosis

Stent thrombosis without intercurrent target lesion revascularization

Secondary stent thrombosis

Stent thrombosis following intercurrent target lesion revascularization

---

20.27 **Answer E.** Several patient- and lesion-related risk factors for stent thrombosis have been identified. Diabetes has been identified as an independent predictor of stent thrombosis in numerous studies. In a registry of more than 15,000 patients treated with SES, DM was associated with a two- to threefold increased risk of ST (OR 2.76, 95% CI 1.71–4.29; $p < 0.0001$) (*Circulation* 2006;113:1434–1441). It also emerged as an independent predictor of early stent thrombosis in a large two-institutional cohort of patients treated with DES (HR: 1.96; 95% CI: 1.18 to 3.28) (*Lancet* 2007;369:667–678). Impaired left ventricular ejection fraction was found to increase the risk of stent thrombosis (HR, 1.09; 95% CI, 1.05–1.36; $p < 0.001$ for each 10% decrease) in a prospective observational cohort study with 2,229 patients undergoing SES or PES implantation. The same study reported an increased risk of stent thrombosis in patients with renal failure (HR, 6.49; 95% CI 2.60–16.15; $p < 0.001$) (*JAMA* 2005;293:2126–2130). Acute coronary syndrome at the time of the index procedure was a predictor for stent thrombosis in the e-Cypher registry (OR 1.75, 95% CI 1.13–2.67; $p < 0.0105$) (*Circulation* 2006;113:1434–1441) and a predictor for early stent thrombosis (HR: 2.21; 95% CI: 1.39 to 3.51) in a two-institutional cohort study by Daemen et al. (*Lancet* 2007;369:667–678). No gender difference in the occurrence of stent thrombosis has been reported.

20.28 **Answer E.** Rates of mortality of stent thrombosis largely depend on the definition of stent thrombosis according to the categories provided by ARC. Definitive stent thrombosis was associated with a 30-day mortality rate of 9% to 19% (*Lancet* 2007;369:667–678; *Circulation* 2006;113:1108–1113). Mortality rates amount to 30% when the definition was extended to cases of probable stent thrombosis (*Lancet* 2007;369:667–678). Current evidence does not indicate a significant difference in the incidence of early ST between patients treated with DES and BMS. Pooled analyses of several trials comparing BMS with SES or BMS with PES reported early ST rates of 0.6% with BMS and 0.5% with SES and PES, respectively (*Am J Cardiol* 2005;95:1469–1472; *J Am Coll Cardiol* 2005;45:941–946). Late stent thrombosis has been reported to occur with a frequency of 0.2–0.3% (*J Am Coll Cardiol* 2005;45:954–959); the risk was increased with PES (HR 2.11, 95% CI 1.19–4.23, $p = 0.017$ vs. BMS; HR 1.85, 95%CI 1.02–3.85, $p = 0.041$ vs. SES) (*Lancet* 2007;370:937–948). Data of early generation DES reported a steady rate of late and very late ST of 0.4% to 0.6% per year between 30 days and 4 years after implantation (*J Am Coll Cardiol* 2008;52:1134–1140). In contrast, the occurrence of stent thrombosis beyond 1 year is exceptionally rare for BMS. Newer generation DES appear to be associated with a lower risk of stent thrombosis than early generation DES. This observation is supported by findings related to surrogate markers of safety such as late-acquired stent malapposition, endothelial function, as well as strut coverage.

20.29 **Answer A.** The image shows a thrombotic occlusion of the stent just distal to the offset of the first diagonal branch. Since the event occurred 13 months after stent implantation, it meets the ARC criteria for very late definite stent thrombosis. A pooled analysis from four double-blind trials comparing sirolimus-eluting stents with BMS and five double-blind trials comparing paclitaxel-eluting stents with BMS showed a significantly higher rate of very late stent thrombosis up to 4 years after implantation for both first-generation DES (SES 0.6% vs. BMS 0%, $p = 0.025$; PES 0.7% vs. BMS 0.2%, $p = 0.028$) (*N Engl J Med* 2007;356:998–1008). Observational data from a large two-center cohort reported an annual occurrence of very late stent thrombosis of 0.4% to 0.6% for first-generation stents (*J Am Coll Cardiol* 2008;52:1134–1140). Somewhat lower numbers (0.3%) have been reported for newer generation DES (*Lancet* 2011;377:1231–1247). There is limited evidence with respect to the occurrence of very late stent thrombosis in stents with passive coating with titanium-nitride-oxide. However, registry data suggest a lower incidence as compared to first-generation DES.

20.30 **Answer E.** In a randomized clinical trial of 477 patients, final kissing balloon dilatation has been shown to reduce angiographic side branch stenosis while being associated with longer procedure times and a greater amount of contrast media use. However, no significant differences in the primary end point of major adverse cardiac events (cardiac death, non–procedure-related index lesion myocardial infarction, target lesion revascularization, or stent thrombosis) were observed at 6 months of follow-up (*Circulation* 2011;123:79–86).

20.31 **Answer E.** Early stent thrombosis is frequently related to procedural factors. The impact of residual dissection on outcome has been illustrated in the Answer 20.21. Stent underexpansion has been identified as an independent predictor of stent thrombosis in an IVUS study of 15 patients with stent thrombosis and 45 controls (*J Am Coll Cardiol* 2005;45(7):995–998). Impaired TIMI flow (<3) has been associated with an increased risk of stent thrombosis in the Dutch stent thrombosis registry, which at the same time correlated with premature discontinuation of clopidogrel within 30 days of the index procedure with an increased risk for stent thrombosis (HR 36.5, 95% CI 8.0–167.8) (*J Am Coll Cardiol* 2009;53:1399–4099). BMI has not been related to early stent thrombosis.

20.32 **Answer E.** Current evidence does not indicate a significant difference in the incidence of early ST between DES and BMS. Pooled analyses of several trials comparing BMS with early generation SES or BMS with early generation PES reported early ST rates of 0.6% with BMS and 0.5% with SES and PES, respectively (*Am J Cardiol* 2005;95:1469–1472; *J Am Coll Cardiol* 2005;45:941–946). Whereas the risk of early stent thrombosis with BMS amounts to 0% to 0.5% for patients undergoing PCI in the setting of stable angina, patients with unstable angina or non–ST-elevation myocardial infarction have a risk of early ST in the range of 1.4% to 1.6%. The risk of early stent thrombosis is highest in patients with ST-elevation myocardial infarction at the time of the index procedure, irrespective of stent type (BMS or DES implantation) (*Circulation* 2009;119:657–659).

20.33 **Answer E.** Whereas definite stent thrombosis may underestimate the true incidence of stent thrombosis, the combination of probable and possible stent thrombosis provides a high sensitivity suitable for the detection of safety signals. The composite of definite and probable stent thrombosis is considered a reasonable balance of specificity and sensitivity and is therefore frequently used as an end point in clinical trials.

20.34 **Answer E.** The OCT image shows stent struts covered by thrombotic debris consistent with the diagnosis of very late stent thrombosis. Several underlying pathophysiologic mechanisms have been suggested and are summarized in statements A through D. In autopsy studies, incomplete reendothelialization and persistent fibrin deposition indicated delayed healing (*J Am Coll Cardiol* 2006;48:193–202). Histologic examination of thrombus aspirates revealed severe inflammation with eosinophilic infiltrates, which correlated with the amount of incomplete stent apposition (*Circulation* 2009;120:391–399). In a registry of 5,783 patients, 17 patients with hypersensitivity symptoms probably or certainly related to DES were found, of which 4 patients had died of coronary stent thrombosis. In histologic examinations, eosinophilic infiltrates and poor intimal healing were demonstrated (*J Am Coll Cardiol* 2006;47:5–81). More recently, Nakazawa and colleagues reported neoatherosclerosis as yet another mechanism of very late stent thrombosis (*J Am Coll Cardiol*, 2011;57:1314–1322)

20.35 **Answer E.** In histologic examination of thrombus aspirates, severe inflammation with eosinophilic infiltrates was demonstrated, which correlated with the extent of incomplete stent apposition. This finding was particularly evident in patients with SES (*Circulation* 2009;120:391–399). Sirolimus and Paclitaxel both activate the coagulation cascade by increasing endothelial tissue factor expression, which is a receptor of factor VII (*Circulation* 2005;112:2002–2011; *Circ Res* 2006;99:149–155).

Drug-eluting Stents and Local Drug Delivery for the Prevention of Restenosis

Peter Wenaweser and Bernhard Meier

QUESTIONS

21.1 Stents eluting drugs of, for example, the limus family reduce the incidence of in-stent restenosis. The main effect of the drugs is on:

(A) Elastic recoil
(B) Arterial remodeling
(C) Smooth muscle cell proliferation/migration
(D) Extracellular matrix production

21.2 Which of the following is true regarding everolimus (Fig. Q21-2)?

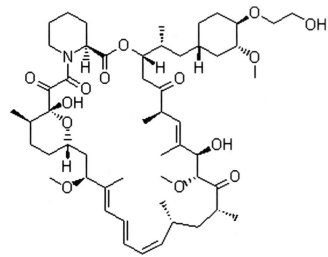

Figure Q21-2. (Atkins MB, Yasothan U, Kirkpatrick P. Everolimus. *Nature Reviews Drug Discovery* **2009; 8: 535-536. Reprinted by permission from Macmillan Publishers Ltd.)**

(A) It is a derivate of sirolimus
(B) It has been tested as immunosuppressive agent reducing the severity of cardiac-allograft vasculopathy

(C) It binds to an intracellular protein, FKBP-12, resulting in an inhibitory complex formation and inhibition of mTOR kinase activity and has been developed for the treatment of advanced renal cell carcinoma
(D) It influences regulator genes that control the cell cycle
(E) A, B, C, and D are correct

21.3 Which of the following statements concerning paclitaxel (Taxol) is INCORRECT?

(A) It is an antimicrotubule drug
(B) It was discovered in a crude extract from the bark of a Pacific yew
(C) It induces disassembly of microtubules
(D) It was first evaluated as an antitumor drug

21.4 Which of the following statements regarding drug-eluting stent (DES) platforms is NOT correct?

(A) The sirolimus-eluting (Cypher) stent is composed of a stainless steel stent, coated with nonerodable polymers
(B) Polymers are long-chain molecules, form a reservoir, and facilitate controlled and prolonged drug delivery
(C) Paclitaxel can only be used in combination with a polymer-based stent platform
(D) Drugs can be released from a stent with and without polymer coating

21.5 Polymeric materials coated on stents:

(A) Allow a controlled and sustained release of agents

(B) Minimize the potential for underdosing or overdosing of drug levels

(C) Serve as drug reservoir

(D) Are potentially toxic and might induce malapposition of a stent

(E) Enhance the radial strength of a stent

(F) A–D are true

(G) A–E are true

21.6 All of the following are true, EXCEPT one. Local drug delivery in humans is successful if:

(A) The appropriate drug is used

(B) The dose needed locally is previously tested in animals

(C) A biocompatible vehicle is able to deliver the drug for the required therapeutic window

(D) The dose applied locally is approximately 5% of the proportion of the systemic drug shown to be effective

21.7 The first randomized comparison of a sirolimus-eluting stent (SES) with a standard bare-metal stent (BMS) reduced the rate of in-stent restenosis after 6 months to:

(A) 20%

(B) 15%

(C) 10%

(D) <5%

21.8 A 49-year-old patient was treated with percutaneous coronary intervention (PCI) and BMS implantation in the setting of an acute coronary syndrome. Seven months later, he complains of recurrent chest pain during minor exertion. The invasive evaluation shows the following (Fig. Q21-8):

For the treatment of this patient with an in-stent restenosis following BMS implantation:

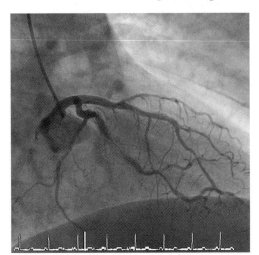

Figure Q21-8

(A) Paclitaxel-eluting stent (PES) implantation appears to be superior to SES implantation

(B) Simple balloon angioplasty is the best option and superior to drug-coated balloon dilatation

(C) A treatment with β-radiation has been shown to be inferior to balloon angioplasty

(D) A treatment with an SES or PES appears to be superior to simple balloon angioplasty

(E) The use of a drug-coated balloon has been shown to be inferior to stent-in-stent implantation

21.9 Experimental models of stent implantation in human coronary arteries show:

(A) That the deployment of sirolimus- or paclitaxel-eluting DES is associated with an increase in neointimal thickness at 28 days in comparison with BMS

(B) Always a greater inflammatory reaction after DES implantation in comparison with BMS within 28 days

(C) A complete healing after BMS implantation within 2 to 4 months

(D) A delayed healing process is also observed with the newer generation DES (e.g., everolimus) in comparison with BMS

21.10 A 45-year-old patient suffers from a stent thrombosis 2.5 years after DES implantation in the left anterior descending (LAD) (Fig. Q21-10). Which of the following statements is wrong?

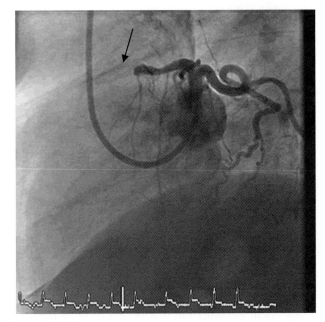

Figure Q21-10

(A) May be associated with chronic inflammation of the arterial wall
(B) May be due to a hypersensitivity reaction to the polymer
(C) Is rare (1% per year)
(D) Can be best avoided by prescribing prolonged dual antiplatelet therapy
(E) Carries a high morbidity and mortality

21.11 Which of the following agents are used or tested on coronary stent platforms?

(A) Everolimus
(B) Biolimus
(C) Zotarolimus
(D) Sirolimus
(E) Paclitaxel
(F) Pimecrolimus
(G) Hirudin
(H) All of the above
(I) All of the above except F and G

21.12 The SIRTAX trial, a randomized, controlled, single-blind study comparing SES with PES in about 1,000 all-comer patients favors a treatment with an SES because of:

(A) A lower incidence of cardiac death
(B) Fewer major adverse cardiac events, primarily by decreasing rates of clinical and angiographic restenosis
(C) A lower incidence of stent thrombosis
(D) Better acute gain and higher success of stent implantation
(E) B and C

21.13 A meta-analysis of randomized trials by Kastrati and coworkers comparing SES with PES in patients with coronary artery disease reported all of the following, EXCEPT:

(A) Target lesion revascularization is less frequently performed in patients treated with an SES
(B) Rate of death is comparable
(C) Rates of myocardial infarction and stent thrombosis are lower in SES-treated patients
(D) Angiographic restenosis is more frequently observed in patients treated with a PES

21.14 A 58-year-old man underwent coronary angiography due to angina pectoris CCS 3. The invasive evaluation showed a subtotal proximal LAD lesion. The result after balloon dilatation and stent implantation is good. Six months later, the patient suffered from acute, ongoing chest pain with anterior ST-segment elevation in the ECG.

The coronary angiography at this point of time is depicted in Figure Q21-14. What is the diagnosis and treatment of choice?

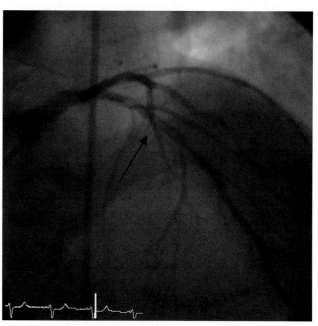

Figure Q21-14

(A) Complete in-stent restenosis with plaque rupture
(B) Late stent thrombosis with a large amount of visible thrombus
(C) Thrombus aspiration/removal, balloon dilatation, and use of abciximab
(D) Balloon angioplasty and additional stent implantation
(E) A and D
(F) B and C

21.15 Evaluation of the cost-effectiveness of DES in an unselected patient population in the year 2003/2004 shows that:

(A) The use of DES in all comers is less cost effective than selective use
(B) A restriction to patients in high-risk groups should be evaluated in further trials
(C) With respect to the current prices of DES, an unrestricted use of these stents is not cost-effective
(D) A–C correct

21.16 Some data suggest that a late loss of more than _____ triggers a target lesion revascularization.

(A) 0.2 to 0.3 mm
(B) 0.5 to 0.6 mm
(C) 0.9 to 1.0 mm
(D) 1.2 to 1.3 mm

21.17 The assessment of coronary endothelial function 6 months after SES implantation compared with BMS, assessed with bicycle exercise as a physiologic stimulus (Fig. Q21-17), revealed that an:

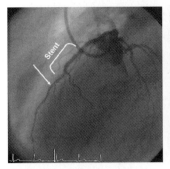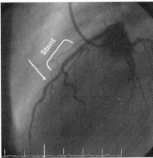

Figure Q21-17

(A) Implantation of a BMS does affect physiologic response to exercise proximal and distal to the stent

(B) Implantation of a BMS does not affect physiologic response to exercise proximal and distal to the stent

(C) Implantation of an SES does not affect physiologic response to exercise proximal and distal to the stent

(D) Implantation of an SES does affect physiologic response to exercise proximal and distal to the stent

  E) B and C

(F) B and D

21.18 What are possible pitfalls of biodegradable DESs using a pure polymer platform?

(A) Lack of radiopacity

(B) Reduced radial force in comparison with a stainless steel or a cobalt–chromium stent platform

(C) Hypersensitivity reactions to the polymer

(D) Reduced deformability of the stent

  E) A, B, and C

(F) A–D

21.19 The sirolimus- (Cypher), zotarolimus- (Endeavor), and the everolimus-eluting (Xience V) stent platform share the following characteristics:

(A) Stainless steel stent

(B) Release of drug within 28 days: ≥80%

(C) Strut thickness 130 to 140 μm

(D) Polymer thickness 12 to 16 μm

(E) A and B

(F) A and C

21.20 A 59-year-old patient is referred from another hospital due to an acute anterior ST-elevation myocardial infarction (STEMI) 7 years after SES implantation. The reangiography shows the following (Fig. Q21-20):

Based on the published data, which interventional treatment is supposed to be the most effective one for the treatment of this subtotal in-stent restenosis?

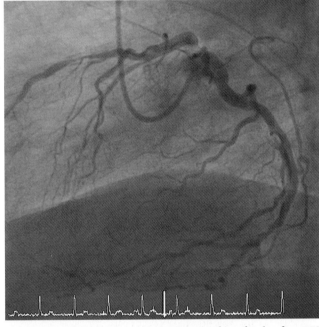

Figure Q21-20. Very late (>1 year) stent thrombosis after DES implantation.

(A) Balloon dilatation

(B) SES and PES implantation are equally effective

(C) SES is superior to PES implantation

(D) Second-generation DES implantation is always the therapy of choice

21.21 A 55-year-old patient presents with acute chest pain and 2-mm ST-elevation in the inferior leads. The ostial right coronary artery (RCA) is subtotally occluded due to a thrombus (Fig. Q21-21A). After aspiration of thrombus, balloon dilatation, and BMS implantation, the vessel is open with normal TIMI flow (Fig. Q21-21B). The left coronary system shows diffuse coronary artery disease with no significant stenosis. Six weeks later, the patient presents again with acute chest pain and ST elevation in the inferior leads. What is the most probable cause for the recurrent symptoms?

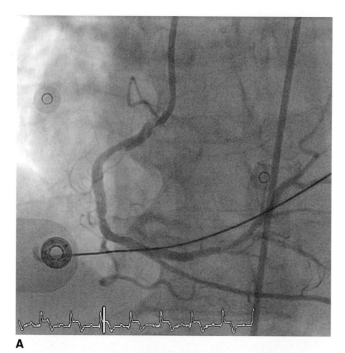

A

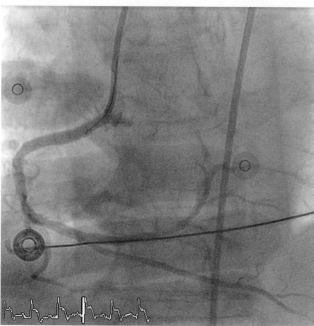

B

Figure Q21-21

(A) Severe in-stent restenosis
(B) Vasospasm of the RCA
(C) Allergic reaction to medication
(D) Stent thrombosis

21.22 The patient is brought to the catheterization laboratory and the invasive evaluation shows a thrombotic occlusion of the ostium of the RCA (Fig. Q21-22). What are the possible causes for stent thrombosis?

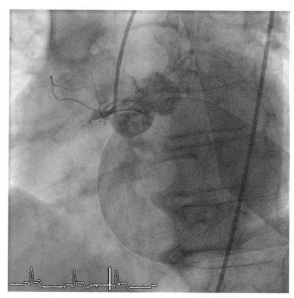

Figure Q21-22

(A) Stent fracture not recognized during the first intervention
(B) Hyporesponsiveness to dual antiplatelet treatment
(C) Rupture of the thin neointima
(D) Malcompliance to drug intake with discontinuation of dual antiplatelet treatment
(E) All of the above but A
(F) All of the above (A–D)

21.23 After passage of the occlusion with a wire, an evaluation of the occluded part of the artery is performed. An optical coherence tomography shows the image in Figure Q21-23. What is your interpretation?

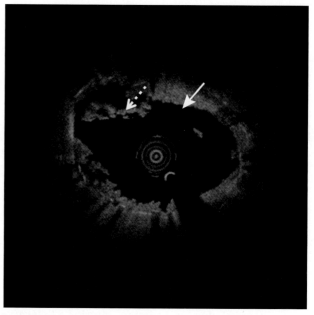

Figure Q21-23 (see color insert)

(A) Thrombotic stent occlusion with normal stent expansion
(B) Stent underexpansion due to fracture and thrombus formation
(C) Plaque rupture of the thin neointima
(D) Malapposition with thrombus formation
(E) All of the above

21.24 What is your strategy for the treatment of this patient with reinfarction of the RCA?

(A) Aspiration of thrombus and balloon dilatation
(B) Stent-in-stent implantation
(C) Emergency coronary artery bypass operation
(D) Platelet function testing
(E) A and B
(F) A, B, and D
(G) C and D

21.25 A 69-year-old female patient was successfully treated with acute PCI and single BMS implantation for an anterior myocardial infarction 6 months ago. Otherwise the coronaries were normal. An echocardiographic follow-up exam reveals an only mildly reduced left ventricular ejection fraction. A treadmill stress test demonstrates borderline ST-segment depression and mild chest discomfort after 6 MET. The patient is examined invasively including an optical coherence tomography. What is your interpretation of the image (Fig. Q21-25)?

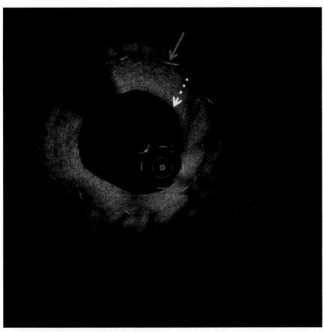

Figure Q21-25 (see color insert)

(A) Optimal result with a thin layer of neointima
(B) Borderline restenosis due to excessive formation of neointima
(C) Single stent fractures with formation of thrombus
(D) Stent underexpansion with thrombotic material in the vessel lumen

21.26 A randomized comparison of the everolimus-eluting Xience stent (EES) with the zotarolimus-eluting Resolute stent (ZES) has demonstrated in an all-comer patient population embracing 2,300 patients:

(A) Clinically indicated target lesion revascularization was below 10% in both groups
(B) Resolute ZES was found to be noninferior to EES with respect to the primary clinical end point of target lesion failure
(C) The mean in-stent diameter restenosis was significantly higher in the ZES than in the EES group
(D) The rate of overall stent thrombosis was higher in the EES than in the ZES group
(E) A and B
(F) C and D

21.27 DES with biodegradable polymers:

(A) May offer the antiretinoic effect of a standard DES
(B) Carry the risk of polymer breakdown and consecutive inflammatory reaction
(C) Have been shown to be as safe as DES with durable polymers in long-term clinical trials
(D) Are designed to become BMS after several months after implantation
(E) All of the above are correct
(F) All but C are correct
(G) All but B are correct

21.28 The endothelial progenitor cell (EPC) capture technology:

(A) Is able to build a very thin neointima resulting in a late lumen loss of <0.10 mm
(B) Aims to form rapidly a functional endothelial coverage of the stent struts
(C) Increases the risk of stent thrombosis due to irregular forming of a neointima
(D) Uses CD34+ markers specific for capturing endothelial progenitor cells

21.29 Poly-L-lactic acid (PLLA):

(A) Is metabolized via the Krebs cycle over a period of 12 to 18 months

(B) Is the most frequently used polymer for the current generation of biodegradable stents

(C) Is in use for restorable sutures and different implants

(D) Is radiopaque and provides as much radial force as a metallic stent

(E) Is phagocytosed by macrophages

(F) All but E are correct

(G) A, B, and C are correct

(H) All but D are correct

21.30 The bioresorbable vascular scaffold (BVS) stent technology:

(A) Uses poly-D,L-lactide acid for controlled release of everolimus

(B) Is associated with a late loss of 0.4 to 0.5 mm

(C) Represents the first biodegradable stent with CE mark

(D) Is associated with an increased risk of stent thrombosis and local inflammatory reaction

(E) A–C

(F) A, B, and D

21.1 **Answer C.** The main effect of the drugs is on the inhibition of smooth muscle cell proliferation and migration by interfering with the cell cycle (*Curr Pharm Des* 2010;16:4002–4011). The radial force of a stent inhibits a potential elastic recoil of the vessel (*Heart* 2000;83:481–490) (Fig. A21-1). As a side effect, positive arterial remodeling resulting in, for example, late malapposition of the stent might be induced by the implantation of a DES (*Minerva Cardioangiol* 2009;57:621–628).

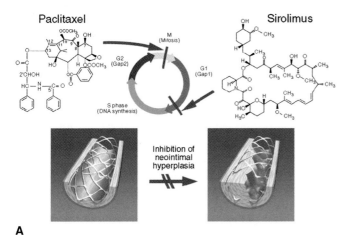

A

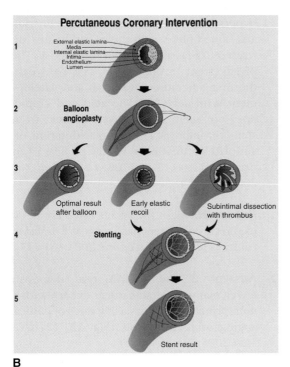

B

Figure A21-1

21.2 **Answer E.** Developed primarily as immunosuppressant inhibiting the expression of hypoxia-inducible factor (e.g., HIF-1) and reducing the expression of vascular endothelial growth factor, it was found to be useful in the prevention of coronary restenosis (*N Engl J Med* 2003;349:847–858).

21.3 **Answer C.** Paclitaxel promotes the polymerization of tubulin and does not induce the disassembly of microtubules like other antimicrotubule agents like vinca alkaloids (*N Engl J Med* 1995;332:1004–1014).

21.4 **Answer C.** The sirolimus-eluting Cypher stent was the first DES, tested in a randomized clinical trial (Fig. A21-4). For drug release, two nonerodable polymers were used: polyethylene-co-vinyl acetate (PEVA) and poly *n*-butyl methacrylate (PBMA). A drug-free coat of PBMA is also applied to the stent surface to control drug release. Only some specific drugs can be loaded directly onto metallic surfaces (e.g., biolimus, prostacyclin, paclitaxel) (*Circulation* 2003;107:2274–2279).

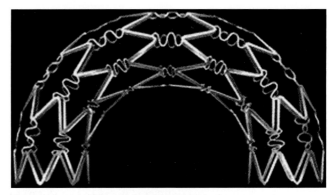

Figure A21-4. (www.cypherstent.com)

21.5 **Answer F.** A polymer is a natural or man-made high-molecular-weight organic compound, consisting of many repeating simpler chemical units or molecules called monomers (Fig. A21-5). Natural examples of polymers are proteins (polymer of amino acids) and cellulose (polymer of sugar molecules).

Polymers bind and release drugs from a coronary stent, serve therefore as a drug reservoir, and may induce inflammation in the vessel wall (hypersensitivity reaction) (*Pharmacology & Therapeutics* 2004;102:1–15).

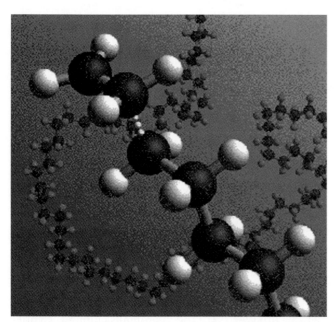

Figure A21-5. Example of synthetic polymer: PVC (a polymer of vinyl chloride).

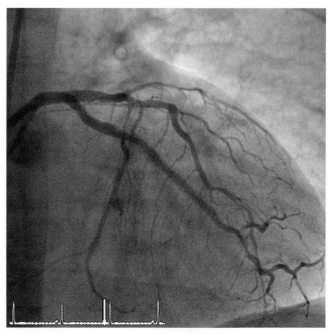

Figure A21-8. After PTCA and DES implantation.

21.6 Answer D. There is no predetermined correlation of effectiveness between the dose needed locally and the dose given systemically. Other statements are correct (*Pharmacology & Therapeutics* 2004;102:1–15).

21.7 Answer D. None of the patients in the sirolimus-stent group, as compared with 26.6% of those in the standard stent group, had restenosis of 50% or more of the luminal diameter (*p* < 0.001) (*N Engl J Med* 2002;346:1773–1780).

21.8 Answer D. A direct comparison of balloon angioplasty with a treatment with sirolimus- (Cypher) and paclitaxel-eluting (Taxus) stent showed a significantly lower restenosis rate with either stent (Fig. A21-8). SES implantation may be superior to PES for the treatment of BMS restenosis. β-Radiation significantly reduced in-stent restenosis in comparison with balloon angioplasty but is nowadays no longer used due to the high risk of late stent thrombosis and malapposition. A direct comparison of primary transluminal coronary angioplasty (PTCA) with paclitaxel-coated balloon vs. a PES implantation for the treatment of in-stent restenosis showed comparable results. (*J Am Coll Cardiol* 2010;56:1897–1907; *N Engl J Med* 2006;355:2113–2124; *JAMA* 2005;293:165–171; *Circulation* 2009;119:2986–2994).

21.9 Answer D. Complete re-endothelialization is usually achieved within 1 month after BMS implantation. After DES implantation, even for second-generation DES (e.g., everolimus-eluting stent), the healing process is prolonged (*EuroIntervention* 2010;6:630–637).

21.10 Answer D. Several factors have been associated with the risk of late stent thrombosis. Especially hypersensitivity to drug coating or polymer and incomplete endothelialization are device-related risk factors for stent thrombosis. The rate of late stent thrombosis is <1% per year with the first-generation DES. Dual antiplatelet treatment with acetylsalicylic acid and clopidogrel does not seem to effectively protect from late stent thrombosis. The optimal duration of dual antiplatelet treatment is still unclear (*Circulation* 2003;108:1701–1706; *J Am Coll Cardiol* 2008;52:1134–1140).

21.11 Answer H. All of the agents listed are in clinical use on coronary stent platforms (A–E) or have been clinically tested (F–G) (*Lancet* 2003;361:247–249).

21.12 Answer B. The SIRTAX trial demonstrated fewer major adverse cardiac events with sirolimus, primarily by decreasing rates of clinical and angiographic restenosis (Fig. A21-12) (*N Engl Med* 2005;353:653–662).

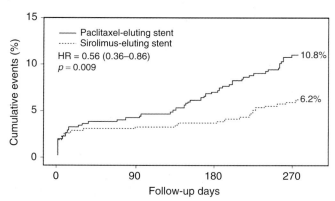

Figure A21-12.   Primary end point: composite of cardiac death, myocardial infarction, and target lesion revascularization.

21.13   Answer C. The meta-analysis by Kastrati et al. (*JAMA* 2005;294:819-825.) demonstrated that patients receiving SES had a significantly lower risk of restenosis and target vessel revascularization compared with those receiving PES. Rates of death, death or MI, and stent thrombosis were similar.

21.14   Answer F. Stent thrombosis is angiographically defined as reduced TIMI flow and visible thrombus. Clinically, stent thrombosis can be suspected if the patient presents with acute chest pain and dynamic ST changes in the leads of the previously treated target vessel. The treatment should follow the guidelines for the treatment of acute myocardial infarction (*Eur Heart J* 2008;29:2909-2945).

21.15   Answer D. The study by Kaiser et al. (*Lancet* 2005;366:921-929) suggested that in a real-world setting, use of DES in all patients is less cost-effective than in studies with selected patients. Use of these stents could be restricted to patients in high-risk groups.

21.16   Answer B. The late loss is minimal lumen diameter (MLD) at follow-up minus the postprocedural MLD at baseline. Current data suggest that a late loss of 0.5 to 0.6 mm triggers a target lesion revascularization (*J Am Coll Cardiol* 2005;45:1193-2000.).

21.17   Answer F. Implantation of a BMS does not affect physiologic response to exercise proximal and distal to the stent. However, SES or PES is associated with exercise-induced paradoxic coronary vasoconstriction of the adjacent vessel segments, although vasodilatory response to nitroglycerin is maintained (*J Am*

Coll Cardiol 2005;46:231-236; *Int J Cardiol* 2007;120:212-220).

21.18   Answer F. As there is no radiopacity of a polymer stent, radiopaque markers need to be added to the stent. The radial force of a pure polymer stent is clearly inferior to a stainless steel or a cobalt–chromium stent. It remains to be determined if certain polymers provoke hypersensitivity reactions. The reduced deformability of a polymer stent might be a disadvantage with respect to deliverability of the stent (*Lancet* 2008;371:873-874; *J Am Coll Cardiol* 2010;56:S43-S78).

21.19   Answer B. Cypher is a stainless steel stent with a strut thickness of 140 μm and a polymer thickness of 12.6 μm. The Endeavor and Xience V stents are cobalt–chromium stents with reduced strut and polymer thickness (91/81 μm as well as 4.1/7.6 μm, respectively) (*J Am Coll Cardiol* 2010;56:S43-S78).

21.20   Answer B. For the treatment of a sirolimus-eluting restenosis, both a new SES and PES implantation were associated with comparable degree of efficacy and safety in a comparative study. For the treatment with second-generation DES, no sufficient clinical data are available so far (*J Am Coll Cardiol* 2010;55:2710-2716).

21.21   Answer D. In-stent restenosis rarely induces an acute myocardial infarction. A restenosis after BMS implantation is usually not earlier than several months after the implantation observed. Vasospasm is unlikely as the patient suffers from diffuse coronary artery disease and the treated lesion was at the ostium of the RCA. Stent thrombosis is therefore the most likely diagnosis.

21.22   Answer F. All the mentioned answers are correct. The phenomenon of stent thrombosis is associated with a number of procedural, blood, and patient factors (*J Am Coll Cardiol* 2010;56:1357-1365).

21.23   Answer B. The optical coherence tomography images show an underexpanded stent (*solid arrow*) with thrombus formation (*dashed arrow*).

21.24   Answer F. The immediate percutaneous intervention with restoration of blood flow is the therapy of choice in the setting of an acute myocardial infarction and superior to an emergency CABG operation. The aspiration of thrombus reduces the risk of peripheral embolization and the risk of a no-reflow phenomenon with associated poor outcome. Therefore, aspiration is recommended in this setting. Stent-in-stent implantation is warranted to overcome the problem of stent fracture. A stent with high radial force or a stent with thick stent struts is considered the therapy of choice in order to apply maximal radial with underexpanded stents. Platelet function testing may be useful to rule out antiplatelet therapy resistance.

21.25 **Answer B.** The OCT image shows a "borderline" restenosis (50%) due to excessive formation of neointima. *Solid arrow*: stent strut and *dashed arrow*: neointima.

21.26 **Answer E.** This large randomized clinical trial including mainly off-label patients showed equal effectiveness of both stent types with no difference with respect to target lesion failure, overall rate of stent thrombosis, or in-stent diameter restenosis with a target lesion revascularization rate of 3.4% and 3.9%, respectively (Fig. A21-26) (*New Engl J Med* 2010;363:123–135).

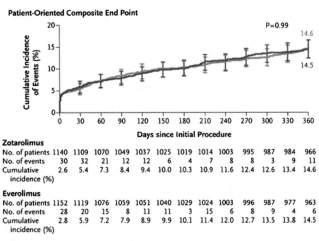

Patient-Oriented Composite End Point

Zotarolimus
No. of patients	1140	1109	1070	1049	1037	1025	1019	1014	1003	995	987	984	966
No. of events	30	32	21	12	6	4	7	8	8	3	9	11
Cumulative incidence (%)	2.6	5.4	7.3	8.4	9.4	10.0	10.3	10.9	11.6	12.4	12.6	13.4	14.6

Everolimus
No. of patients	1152	1119	1076	1059	1051	1040	1029	1024	1003	996	987	977	963
No. of events	28	20	15	8	11	11	3	15	6	8	9	4	6
Cumulative incidence (%)	2.8	5.9	7.2	7.9	8.9	9.9	10.1	11.4	12.0	12.7	13.5	13.8	14.5

Figure A21-26

21.27 **Answer G.** Despite all the benefits of DES, concerns have been raised over their long-term safety, with particular reference to stent thrombosis. In an effort to address these concerns, newer stents have been developed that include DES with biodegradable polymers, DES that are polymer free, stents with novel coatings, and completely biodegradable stents. Many of these stents are currently undergoing preclinical and clinical trials; however, early results seem promising (*J Am Coll Cardiol* 2010;56:S43–S78).

21.28 **Answer B.** This bare-metal stainless steel stent (OrbusNeich, Fort Lauderdale, Florida) is unique

in containing on its luminal surface immobile CD34 antibodies (Fig. A21-28). In preclinical studies, these antibodies were able to bind to EPCs, resulting in a rapidly formed, functional endothelial covering of the stent's struts, which ultimately has the potential to reduce ST and restenosis (*J Am Coll Cardiol* 2010;56:S43–S78).

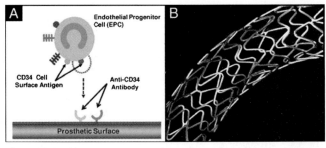

Figure A21-28

21.29 **Answer H.** The most frequently used polymers for bioresorbable stents are aliphatic polyesters, such as PLLA, poly(glycolic acid) (PGA), and poly(ε-caprolactone) (PCL) (*Circulation* 2010;122:2236–2238). PLLA is radiolucent.

21.30 **Answer E.** Bioabsorbable everolimus-eluting stent, or BVS, is made up of two layers of a biodegradable polymer: one that contains the immunosuppressant drug everolimus, the other forming a longer-lasting backbone. Over time, the body breaks down and absorbs the polymer, ultimately leaving nothing behind (Fig. A21-30). (*J Am Coll Cardiol* 2010;56:S43–S78; *Lancet* 2009;373:897–910).

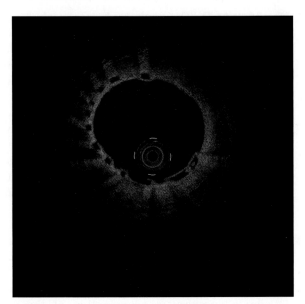

Figure A21-30. Example of 6 month follow-up OCT image of a BVS stent showing complete coverage of the stent struts. (see color insert)

22

Percutaneous Interventions in Aortocoronary Saphenous Vein Grafts

Stephane Noble and Marco Roffi

22.1 Which statement(s) about the historical background of surgical revascularization in humans is/are TRUE?

(A) Coronary artery bypass grafting (CABG) using saphenous vein grafts (SVGs) was first performed in the 1960s

(B) SVGs were used as bypass conduits earlier than the left internal mammary artery (LIMA)

(C) The first venous bypass grafting was performed in the 1950s

(D) The first conduit used was the LIMA

(E) A and D are true

22.2 Which statement(s) concerning patency rate of aortocoronary SVGs is/are TRUE?

(A) 95% of vein grafts are patent at 7 to 10 days

(B) 20% of vein grafts are patent at 10 years

(C) 40% of vein grafts are patent at 10 years

(D) 60% of vein grafts are patent at 10 years

(E) A and D are true

22.3 Which of the following morphologic features is the least representative for vein graft atherosclerosis (Fig. Q22-3)?

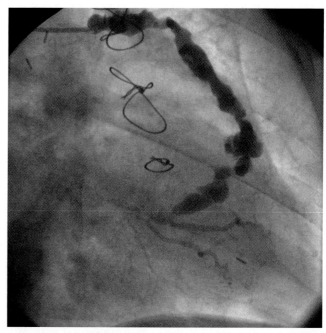

Figure Q22-3. Massively degenerated SVG to a marginal branch of the LCX. The extension of the disease is such that PCI does not appear to be a reasonable option.

(A) Neointimal hyperplasia

(B) Atherosclerotic plaque with highly developed fibrous cap

(C) Thrombosis

(D) Absence of calcification

(E) Diffuse involvement

22.4 A 75-year-old woman presents with an acute coronary syndrome (ACS) and dynamic ST-segment depression in the lateral leads. She underwent CABG 4 months earlier (LIMA to LAD, right

251

internal mammary artery [RIMA] to the right coronary artery [RCA], SVG to the first diagonal branch and jump graft to the first obtuse marginal branch of the LCX). Her preoperative left ventricular ejection fraction (LVEF) was 30%. Coronary angiography demonstrated an occlusion of the SVG to the diagonal branch and marginal branch. Which statement(s) about SVG occlusion within the first 6 months after surgery is/are TRUE?

(A) Female gender is a significant predictor of early SVG graft occlusion
(B) Dyslipidemia reduces 6-month vein graft patency
(C) Optimal graft flow at the end of surgery has a protective effect against graft occlusion
(D) Preoperative congestive heart failure is a significant predictor of early SVG occlusion
(E) C and D are correct

22.5 A 74-year-old gentleman presents with angina CCS III 1 year following CABG. Which of the following statements is NOT correct?

(A) Vein graft thrombosis is the principal underlying mechanism of early vein graft occlusion
(B) Compared with aspirin monotherapy, the combination of aspirin plus clopidogrel significantly reduces the probability of SVG neointimal hyperplasia one year after CABG according to intravascular ultrasound (IVUS) assessment
(C) Reduction of graft flow due to anastomosis proximal to an atherosclerotic segment or to a stricture at the anastomosis site predisposes to graft thrombotic occlusions
(D) Oral anticoagulants are not superior to aspirin in preventing SVG thrombosis
(E) The combination of aspirin and oral anticoagulants is not routinely recommended following CABG

22.6 A 68-year-old diabetic man presented with ACS and dynamic ST depression in leads V4–V6. Eight months earlier, he underwent CABG (LIMA to LAD, vein to diagonal branch and jump graft to LCX, vein to RCA). The likely cause(s) of ischemia is/are:

(A) A stenosis at one distal anastomosis site
(B) A midgraft stenosis of an SVG conduit due to neointimal hyperplasia
(C) A subacute thrombotic SVG occlusion
(D) A stenosis at the proximal anastomosis due to aorto-ostial disease
(E) A and B

22.7 Which statement about SVG atherosclerosis is CORRECT?

(A) Lipid handling of SVG endothelium is characterized by fast lipolysis, less active lipid synthesis, and low lipid uptake
(B) Late thrombotic occlusion occurs rarely in old degenerated SVG with advanced atherosclerotic plaque formation
(C) SVG atherosclerosis tends to be diffuse with plaque having a highly developed fibrous cap and little evidence of calcification
(D) Compared to the native vessel atherosclerotic process, SVG atherosclerosis is more rapidly progressive
(E) From a histologic perspective, SVG atherosclerosis has fewer foam cells and inflammatory cells than the native coronary one

22.8 Which of the following factors influence long-term SVG patency?

(A) Native vessel diameter distal to the anastomotic site
(B) Cigarette smoking
(C) Hyperlipidemia
(D) Severity of native vessel atherosclerosis proximal to the anastomotic site
(E) All of them

22.9 One of your referring general practitioners is asking you which of the following strategies is not associated with improved outcomes among patients post-CABG.

(A) Antiplatelet therapy
(B) Routine coronary angiogram 1 year postsurgery
(C) Lipid-lowering therapy
(D) The use of arterial grafts
(E) Smoking cessation

22.10 The same general practitioner challenges you on the antithrombotic therapy in patients who have undergone CABG. Which one of his statements is NOT correct?

(A) Clopidogrel or dipyridamole in addition to aspirin are more effective than aspirin alone to improve SVG patency
(B) Clopidogrel 300 mg as a loading dose 6 hours after surgery followed by 75 mg/d is a safe alternative for patients undergoing CABG who are aspirin intolerant
(C) In patients who undergo CABG for non–ST-segment elevation ACS, clopidogrel 75 mg per day for 9 to 12 months following the procedure in addition to aspirin is recommended
(D) For patients undergoing CABG and mechanical valve replacement, aspirin is recommended on top of Coumadin

22.11 You are starting an elective percutaneous coronary intervention (PCI) of an aorto-ostial long-segment stenosis in a patient with a 7-year-old vein graft (Fig. Q22-11). Which of the following complications should be of LEAST concern in this setting?

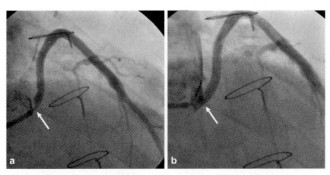

Figure Q22-11. An aorto-ostial lesion (*arrow*) of an SVG to the LAD is demonstrated in panel A. Panel B shows the result following stenting.

(A) Dissection
(B) Distal embolization
(C) No-reflow
(D) Abrupt closure
(E) Proximal anastomosis rupture

22.12 A 77-year-old man underwent stent implantation without emboli protection of a long segment involving the proximal portion of the SVG in a 15-year-old vein conduit (Fig. Q22-12) and suffered a periprocedural MI following prolonged no-reflow after stenting. The antithrombotic regimen included aspirin, clopidogrel, and unfractionated heparin. What should have been done differently?

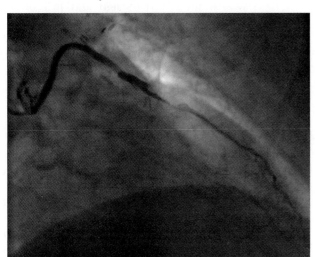

Figure Q22-12. Long stenosis involving the mid and distal portion of the SVG to the diagonal branch (15-year-old vein conduit).

(A) The use of a mechanical emboli protection device would have reduced the risk of periprocedural MI
(B) The use of glycoprotein IIb/IIIa inhibitors would have reduced the risk of periprocedural MI
(C) A distal balloon occlusion emboli protection device should have been used since it has been demonstrated to be superior to filter devices in SVG PCI
(D) It was correct not to use mechanical emboli protection devices since safety and efficacy data for those devices are currently insufficient
(E) Randomized data support the notion that bivalirudin should have been used instead of unfractionated heparin to significantly decrease the periprocedural MI risk

22.13 A 62-year-old gentleman underwent CABG ×4 (LIMA to LAD and first diagonal branch, SVG to the second obtuse marginal branch and SVG to the posterolateral branch of the RCA). At postoperative day 2, he developed ST-elevation myocardial infarction (STEMI) in the lateral leads. The coronary angiogram (Fig. Q22-13) shows an ostial lesion (arrow) associated with a suspected thrombus in the SVG. You plan to perform a PCI of the SVG. Which answer is NOT correct?

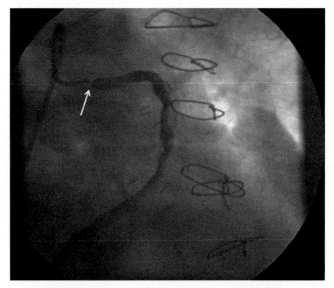

Figure Q22-13. Aorto-ostial SVG lesion (*arrow*) associated with a suspected thrombus in a 2-day-old SVG to the posterolateral branch of the RCA.

(A) Disruption of fresh thrombus may lead to no-reflow

(B) Use of distal embolic protection device offers up to 40% reduction in 30-day MACE (major adverse cardiac event)

(C) In addition to distal embolization, suture rupture at the aortic anastomosis site is a concern and the intervention should be done after agreement with the surgical colleague

(D) Direct stenting may be associated with a reduction in the volume of atheroembolic debris

(E) None of the above

22.14 A 78-year-old lady experienced a malaise. She presented 6 hours later to the emergency room because of ongoing chest pain and shortness of breath. She had previous pacemaker implantation, and the ECG showed a left bundle branch block. She underwent CABG × 2 10 years earlier (SVG to LAD and SVG to RCA). Which of the following statements is NOT correct?

(A) Further revascularization is required in approximately 20% at 10 years after SVG

(B) SVG to the LAD has worse patency rate than that to the RCA or LCX

(C) Smoking is a risk factor for early and late graft thrombosis

(D) Diameter of the recipient artery by angiography is highly predictive of SVG patency

22.15 In the patient detailed in Question 22.14, two drug-eluting stent (DES) were implanted in the SVG to the LAD 2 years ago. Clopidogrel was stopped 15 days prior to this event. At the time of angiography (Fig. Q22-15), 8 hours after symptom onset, the patient still had chest pain. SVG to RCA is patent, and the native LCX shows only nonsignificant lesions. LVEF is not known. Proximal native LAD is chronically occluded with heavy calcification. What is your strategy?

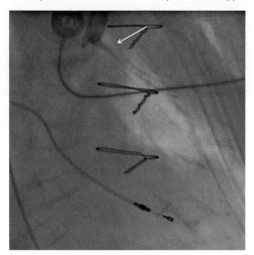

Figure Q22-15.   Proximal SVG to LAD occlusion 2 years after DES implantation.

(A) Acute anterior MI following SVG to LAD occlusion, medical management

(B) Acute anterior MI following SVG to LAD occlusion, SVG PCI attempted

(C) Acute anterior MI following SVG to LAD occlusion, native LAD recanalization attempted

(D) Chronic SVG to LAD occlusion, medical management

(E) B or C

22.16 A 71-year-old diabetic man underwent surgical revascularization 13 years before with SVG × 2 to the LCX and RCA (LAD was free of significant lesions). Two years prior to current presentation, PCI of the proximal portion of the SVG to the RCA was performed with implantation of a DES. At that time, LVEF was 45%. The patient is now admitted for progressive shortness of breath, pulmonary edema, mild upper abdominal pain, and diffuse ST depression in the anterior leads. Troponin I was 10 UI/L (100 times of the upper limit of normal) at presentation but declined 4 hours later. LVEF was 35%. At day 2, coronary angiography showed occlusion of the SVG to the RCA, a severely diffused disease SVG to the LCX and a diffusely infiltrated left main stem (degree of stenosis estimated at 70%) involving the bifurcation, and a long proximal LAD lesion. The native RCA was occluded, on the ECG there were Q waves in the inferior leads, the inferior territory was akinetic on echocardiography, and nuclear imaging shows no viability in the same territory. What is your attitude?

(A) Deobstruction of the SVG to the RCA that was stented 2 years ago and PCI of the stenosis on the SVG to the LCX

(B) PCI of the left main stem and LAD with DES

(C) Optimal medical treatment with ICD implantation

(D) Redo surgery

(E) A and B

22.17 Which of the following statement(s) about redo CABG is/are NOT correct?

(A) Redo surgery carries a higher mortality rate than the first CABG

(B) Redo surgery carries a higher morbidity rate than the first CABG

(C) Redo surgery is associated with reduction of SVG patency as compared with initial surgery

(D) Redo surgery conveys less relief from angina than the first CABG

(E) Redo surgery conveys the same degree of relief from angina as the first CABG

22.18 A 70-year-old man underwent surgical revascularization 10 years previously (LIMA to the LAD, SVG to the RCA, and SVG to the second obtuse marginal of the LCX) and presented with angina CCS II. Coronary angiography (Fig. Q22-18) showed an ostial lesion on the SVG to obtuse marginal. Which one of the following statements is CORRECT?

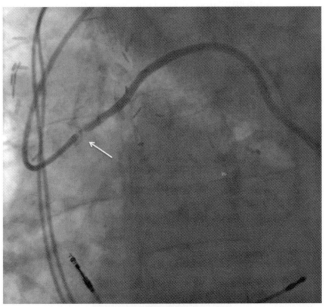

Figure Q22-18. Coronary angiography 10 years postsurgical revascularization showing an ostial lesion on an SVG to the marginal branch of the LCX (*arrow*).

(A) PCI of this ostial SVG lesion carries a high risk of vessel rupture

(B) Distal embolization during this type of PCI is too low to consider distal embolic protection

(C) Rate of DES in-stent restenosis is not higher in SVG than in native coronary arteries

(D) Glycoprotein IIb/IIIa inhibitors are associated with improved outcome in PCI of SVG

(E) Primary stenting is contraindicated in SVG PCI

22.19 A 67-year-old man treated for hypertension and dyslipidemia underwent surgical revascularization (LIMA to LAD, SVG to RCA, SVG to an obtuse marginal branch of the LCX) for three-vessel coronary artery disease with focal proximal RCA stenosis, an ostial lesion of the left main stem, and normal LVEF. At postoperative day 2, the patient became dependent to inotropic agents, and developed diffuse ST-segment depression on ECG as well as a mild rise of cardiac biomarkers beyond what expected following CABG. Urgent coronary angiography was performed and the SVG to the marginal branch and to the RCA are demonstrated in Figure Q22-19. Injection of the native coronary arteries demonstrated, in addition to the preoperative findings, a diffuse luminal narrowing of all three vessels. What statement regarding this case is NOT correct?

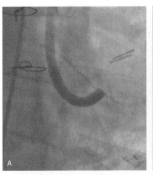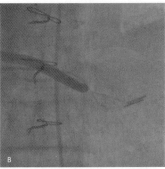

Figure Q22-19. Two SVGs anastomosed to a spastic marginal branch of the LCX (Panel A) and a spastic distal RCA (Panel B).

(A) In patients undergoing CABG, urgent coronary angiography should be performed when medium-size or large perioperative MI is suspected

(B) Perioperative MI is not associated with increased risk of subsequent congestive heart failure and adverse long-term outcomes

(C) In this case, inotropic support should be discontinued—if needed following insertion of an intraaortic balloon pump—and whenever possible nitroglycerine perfusion should be started

(D) None of the above

22.20 An 84-year-old man underwent surgical revascularization (SVG to the LAD, SVG to the obtuse marginal branch of the LCX) for two-vessel coronary disease 8 years ago. He presents now with angina on exertion (CCS II) despite optimal medical therapy. Coronary angiography shows a stenosis on the proximal portion of the SVG to the obtuse marginal branch (Fig. Q22-20). Which statement is TRUE?

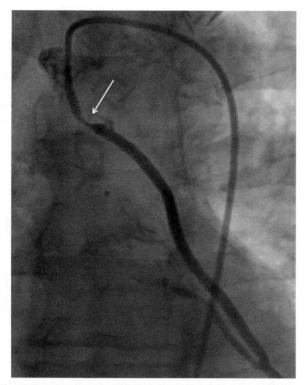

Figure Q22-20. Proximal lesion (*arrow*) on an 8-year-old SVG to the obtuse marginal branch in a patient presenting with angina CCS 2.

(A) PCI of SVG is associated with worse outcome than native coronary artery disease

(B) In-stent restenosis rate after BMS implantation in an SVG is over 20%

(C) Covered stents do not reduce periprocedural complications

(D) Incidence of clinical events after SVG stenting approaches 50% by 5 years

(E) All of the above

22.21 A 64-year-old patient presented with angina on exertion 5 years after having undergone CABG (LIMA to LAD and SVG to RCA). The coronary angiogram showed a significant lesion in the midportion of the SVG, and PCI was performed using a DES. Which statement about DES use in SVG PCI is NOT correct?

(A) Compared to BMS, DES use is associated with reduced target lesion revascularization (TLR) and TVR rates up to 30 months

(B) Strong evidence suggests increased rates of mortality with DES vs. BMS

(C) No evidence to date suggests increased rates of MI or stent thrombosis with DES vs. BMS

(D) A randomized study comparing DES and BMS observed higher mortality was associated with DES use at 32 months

(E) B and C

22.22 A 71-year-old patient anticoagulated for chronic atrial fibrillation presented with angina on exertion 12 years post-CABG (SVG to LAD, SVG to the obtuse marginal branch of the LCX). Coronary angiogram showed a distal anastomosis stenosis on the SVG to the obtuse marginal branch (Fig. Q22-22A). Direct stenting was performed with a 2.5- × 12-mm BMS with a good angiographic result (Fig. Q22-22B). Six months later, the patient experienced recurrent typical angina and in-stent restenosis was demonstrated on repeat coronary angiography (Fig. Q22-22C). All the factors listed below should be considered predictors of BMS in-stent restenosis following SVG interventions, EXCEPT:

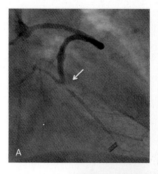
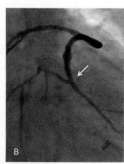
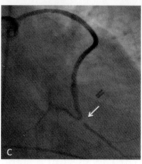

Figure Q22-22. **A:** Twelve years post-SVG to the obtuse marginal branch, presence of a severe lesion involving the distal anastomosis (*arrow*). **B:** result post-PCI with a 2.5- × 12-mm BMS. **C:** Angiographic control at 6 months because of recurrent angina showing severe in-stent restenosis.

(A) Diabetes mellitus

(B) Small posttreatment stent diameter

(C) Small reference diameter (<3mm)

(D) Lesion already stented (in-stent restenosis)

(E) Presentation with ACSs

22.23 A 70-year-old diabetic lady underwent surgery for a three-vessel disease (LIMA to LAD, SVG to LCX and RCA). Four years later, coronary angiography was performed because of worsening dyspnea on exertion and showed an ostial lesion on the SVG to the LCX that was treated by PCI using a filter emboli protection device

(Fig. Q22-23). What statement is NOT correct concerning the use of embolic protection device in SVG interventions?

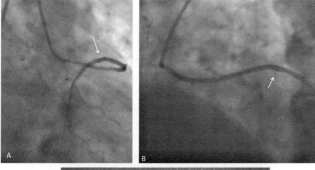

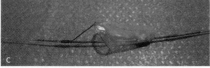

Figure Q22-23. Angiography showing (*arrow*) a deployed FilterWire EX (Boston Scientific, Natick, MA, USA) (*arrow*) in RAO 30 (A) and LAO 30 cranial 10 (B). FilterWire EX with SVG debris trapped in the basket (C). Note the ostial SVG lesion at the tip of the catheter.

(A) In the SAFER trial, a study comparing the use of distal occlusion balloon vs. no protection device, primary composite end point (death, MI, emergency CABG, and TLR) was reduced by 42% at 30 days

(B) In the SAFER trial, the primary composite end point reduction was driven by lower incidence of MI

(C) Proximal protection device was associated with significantly lower 30-day MACE compared to distal protection device in the PROXIMAL trial (randomized comparison between proximal and distal protection device)

(D) Postprocedural measures of epicardial blood flow and angiographic complication rates were similar between two different distal protection devices (filter vs. distal balloon occlusion) tested in the randomized FIRE Trial

22.24 A 63-year-old obese woman underwent CABG (LIMA to LAD, SVG to RCA and to the first obtuse marginal of the LCX) for a three-vessel disease. Fourteen days postsurgery, she developed transient ST-segment elevation in the lateral leads and cardiac enzyme elevation. The angiogram is shown in Figure Q22-24. Which statements apply for early SVG failure?

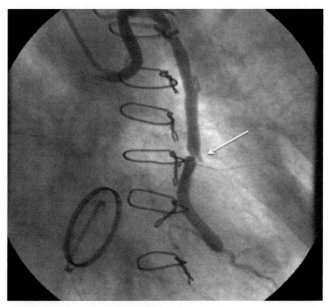

Figure Q22-24. Early SVG failure resulting from clips (*arrow*) compromising flow in the SVG.

(A) It results from surgical technical issue

(B) It results from nonlaminar flow patterns secondary to SVG–coronary artery mismatch

(C) It results from venous varicosities

(D) It results from compromised outflow from distal coronary artery disease

(E) All of the above

22.25 Major breakthrough(s) in SVG-PCI has/have been:

(A) Glycoprotein IIb/IIIa receptor antagonist

(B) Mechanical distal emboli protection

(C) Covered stent

(D) Atherectomy device

(E) All of the above

ANSWERS AND EXPLANATIONS

22.1   Answer E. The first aortocoronary SVG was implanted by Garrett and colleagues in May 1967 (*JAMA* 1973;223:792–794), and the technique was subsequently refined and brought to success by René Favaloro, an Argentinean cardiac surgeon working at the Cleveland Clinic Foundation, Cleveland, Ohio. The LIMA was the first conduit used as a coronary bypass graft in humans. A sutured end-to-end anastomosis between the LIMA and a marginal branch of the left circumflex coronary artery (LCX) was first performed in February 1964 in Leningrad (*J Thorac Cardiovasc Surg* 1967;54:535–544).

22.2   Answer C. A major limitation of SVG as conduits for CABG is the atherosclerosis developing in the vein grafts. Historically, the perioperative and 10-year SVG occlusion rates were 10% and 50%, respectively (*J Am Coll Cardiol* 2002; 40(11):1951–1954). More recent data from a multicentric cohort of 1,074 patients reported that 95% of SVGs were patent by angiography at 7 to 10 days. One-week patency or early patency was associated with a 76% 6-year patency rate and 68% 10-year patency. The overall 10-year SVG patency rate was 61%. The strongest long-term predictors of SVG graft patency are grafting into the left anterior descending coronary artery (LAD) and grafting into a vessel that is at least 2.0 mm in diameter (*J Am Coll Cardiol* 2004;44:2149–2156).

22.3   Answer B. Three distinct and temporally separated pathophysiologic processes are observed in SVG disease: subacute thrombosis (usually occurring within <1 month of surgery), neointimal hyperplasia (between 1 month and 1 year post-CABG) and vein graft atherosclerosis (usually clinically relevant >3 years after surgery). Morphologically, vein graft lesions tend to be diffuse, concentric, and friable with a poorly developed or absent fibrous cap. SVG atherosclerosis is often rapidly progressive and associated with greater numbers of foam and inflammatory cells. Severe calcifications are rare (*Circulation* 1998;97:916–931).

22.4   Answer E. Optimal graft flow as assessed at the end of surgery has a protective effect against graft occlusion. Good flow conditions are observed in patients with larger target vessels, lack of significant native disease distal to the anastomosis, and several run-off branches. Since SVG lack side branches, any process resulting in decreased flow may precipitate thrombosis. Significant predictors of SVG attrition or occlusion at 6 months after surgery in a study on 200 patients (*J Thorac Cardiovasc Surg* 2005;129:496–503) included congestive heart failure, grafting to diagonal arteries, larger vein graft size, and poor run-off. Hypertension, gender, dyslipidemia, and previous myocardial infarction (MI) did not affect early graft patency (*Circulation* 1993;88(5 Pt 2):II93–II98). Accordingly, graft attrition during the first postoperative year results principally from early thrombotic occlusion related to rheologic and technical issues rather than from vein graft atherosclerosis.

22.5   Answer B. Vein graft thrombosis is the principal underlying mechanism of early vein graft occlusion. The reduction of graft flow due to graft anastomosis proximal to a diseased coronary segment or a stricture at the anastomosis site is a predisposing factor for graft thrombosis. Several comparative antithrombotic trials have shown that oral anticoagulants are equivalent to aspirin in terms of 1-year vein graft patency rates (*Circulation* 1998;97:916–931) and there is no data to support the combination of aspirin and oral anticoagulants. Similarly, the combination of aspirin plus clopidogrel compared to aspirin alone did not significantly reduce the process of SVG intimal hyperplasia or the graft patency rate at 1 year post-CABG in a randomized study including 113 patients and performing angiography and IVUS assessment at 1 year (*Circulation* 2010;122(25):2680–2687). Similar to this study, Gao et al. showed that the 1-year SVG patency did not differ between two randomized groups (93.5% vs. 96.3% for clopidogrel [*n* = 102] alone vs. clopidogrel plus aspirin [*n* = 95]), *p* = 0.25) as assessed by computed tomography angiography (*Ann Thorac Surg* 2009;88:59–62).

22.6   Answer E. While within the first month after surgery, thrombosis is the main mechanism of vein graft disease. From 1 month to 1 year, ischemia in the territory supplied by an SVG is most often due to lesions at the distal perianastomotic site or midgraft stenosis caused by neointimal hyperplasia. Neointimal hyperplasia, defined as proliferation of smooth muscle cells and accumulation of extracellular matrix in the intimal compartment, is the characteristic adaptive mechanism of venous conduits to systemic blood pressure. This process represents the foundation for later development of graft atherosclerosis. Graft occlusion due to subacute thrombosis and problems at the proximal anastomotic site less frequently cause ischemia between 1 month and 1 year after CABG.

22.7 **Answer D.** Although the fundamental processes of atherosclerosis in native coronary vessels and in vein grafts are similar, there are several temporal, histologic, and metabolic differences between the two pathologies. Lipid handling by SVG endothelium is characterized by slower lipolysis, more active lipid synthesis, and higher lipid uptake than in the native coronary arteries. In addition, SVG atherosclerosis is more rapidly progressive. From a histologic point of view, SVG atherosclerosis is characterized by the presence of a larger number of foam and inflammatory cells. SVG atherosclerotic involvement is diffuse, and lesions are friable with a poorly developed fibrous cap and little evidence of calcification (*Circulation* 1998;97:916–931).

22.8 **Answer E.** A number of morphologic factors have been associated with reduced vein graft patency. It has been observed that 1-year vein graft patency was significantly lower if the native grafted vessel was <1.5 mm compared to grafted vessels with a diameter >1.5 mm (*Ann Thorac Surg* 1979;28:176–183). More recently, Goldman et al. confirmed that the diameter of the recipient artery by angiography is highly predictive of SVG patency (grafting of a vessel > 2 mm in diameter has an 88% 10-year patency rate compared with an artery ≤2 mm which has 55% 10-year patency rate (*p* < 0.001) (*J Am Coll Cardiol* 2004;44(11):2149–2156). The severity of native vessel atherosclerosis proximal to the anastomotic site influences the flow in the vein graft. Sustained competitive flow through mild stenotic native vessels has been described as a predisposing factor for vein graft occlusion. However, this mechanistic view remains a source of debate since the available data are conflicting (*Ann Thorac Surg* 1979;28:176–183; *J Thorac Cardiovasc Surg* 1981;82:520–530). Cigarette smoking is an important predictor of recurrent angina during the first year after surgery and of poor long-term clinical outcome. The evidence implicating hyperlipidemia as a key risk factor in the development of vein graft atherosclerosis is as consistent and strong as it is for native coronary disease.

22.9 **Answer B.** Aspirin has been shown to increase short- and mid-term vein graft patency. Cessation of smoking is a highly effective strategy in preventing atherosclerosis. Accordingly, it has been shown that persistent smokers had more than twice the risk of suffering MI or requiring redo surgery at one year following CABG compared with patients who quit smoking at the time of surgery (*Circulation* 1996;93:42–47). Several trials have shown a clear-cut benefit for aggressive lipid-lowering therapy in the post-CABG setting. Similarly, the use of arterial grafts has been a major breakthrough in bypass surgery due to the better long-term patency compared with SVG. Routine follow-up angiography post-CABG is not recommended because it has never been shown to improve long-term patency rates.

22.10 **Answer A.** For patients undergoing CABG, addition of dipyridamole to aspirin therapy is not recommended (*BMJ* 1994;308:159–168). According to the American College of Chest Physicians guidelines, for patients intolerant to aspirin an oral loading dose of 300-mg clopidogrel 6 hours after surgery followed by 75 mg/d is recommended (*Chest* 2004;126:600S–608S). According to the same guidelines, patients undergoing CABG who require at the same time oral anticoagulation (e.g., for atrial fibrillation or mechanical valve prosthesis) qualify also for aspirin. In patients who undergo CABG for non–ST-segment elevation ACS, the CURE study has demonstrated that the combination of aspirin and clopidogrel, 75 mg/d for 9 to 12 months, is superior to aspirin alone (*Circulation* 2004;110:1202–1208). Nevertheless, that benefit was only observed in the preoperative phase, while no additional benefit for clopidogrel was demonstrated after CABG.

22.11 **Answer E.** Suture line rupture is of concern only in the early phase after surgery. Characteristic complications of PCI in degenerated SVG include distal embolization, no-reflow, dissection, and abrupt closure. Overall SVG PCI is associated with significantly worse outcomes compared to interventions in the native coronary circulation (Table A22-11) (*Circulation* 2002;106:3063–3067).

Table A22-11. Event Rates in SVG PCI (Compared to PCI in Native Vessels)

	Grafts PCI (N = 627)	Native PCI (N = 13158)	*p*
30-day events (%)			
Death	2.1	1.0	0.006
MI	13.1	7.7	<0.001
Urgent revascularization	2.6	3.6	0.15
Death/MI	14.0	8.2	<0.001
Death/MI/urgent revascularization	15.2	10.0	<0.001
6-mo events (%)			
Death	4.7	2.0	<0.001
MI	18.3	9.4	<0.001
Revascularization	24.5	19.1	0.003
Death/MI	20.4	10.6	<0.001
Death/MI/ revascularization	37.1	25.4	<0.001

PCI, percutaneous coronary intervention; MI, myocardial infarction.

22.12   Answer A. Mechanical emboli protection is based on the concept of either interposing a filter device between the lesion treated and the distal vasculature supplied by the graft or interrupting the flow—by either proximal or distal balloon occlusion—and then aspirating the blood column with the debris as a prevention of distal embolization. Filter-based emboli protection allows blood flow throughout the procedure, but particles smaller than the pore size (usually 100 μm) may reach the distal vasculature. Flow occlusive devices allow for more complete retrieval of small particles suspended in the blood column at the time of intervention, but they have the disadvantages of inducing ischemia and of poor visualization of the lesion. The use of a filter device was proved to be equivalent to distal balloon occlusion for reducing periprocedural MI in a randomized trial involving 651 patients (Fig. A22-12) (*Circulation* 2003;108:548–553). Distal balloon

occlusive devices should not be used for aorto-ostial vein graft lesions since a lack of antegrade flow during distal occlusion may lead to debris embolization into the ascending aorta and the brain. The use of glycoprotein IIb/IIIa inhibitors in SVG interventions is not useful (see answer to Question 22.18). No randomized data on bivalirudin in SVG PCI are available. In a retrospective study, administration of bivalirudin as single antithrombotic agent (54 patients) vs. heparin alone (60 patients) in the context of SVG PCI with a distal protection device was described as clinically safe and associated with a trend toward fewer in-hospital non–Q-wave MI, repeat revascularization, overall vascular complications, and significantly fewer major creatine kinase-MB increases compared with heparin. The bivalirudin group also showed a trend towards fewer major adverse cardiac events at 1-month clinical follow-up (*Am J Cardiol* 2005;96:67–70).

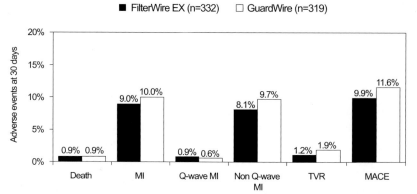

Figure A22-12.   Major adverse cardiac events (death, MI, TVR) at 30 days among 651 patients undergoing SVG PCI randomized to a filter emboli protection (FilterWire EX, Boston Scientific, Natick, MA) or to distal balloon occlusion (Percusurge GuardWire, Medtronic, Minneapolis, MN). For all end points, no statistically significant difference was observed.

22.13 **Answer E.** Recurrent ischemia early after surgical revascularization with SVG is usually caused by acute SVG thrombosis. Stenosis at proximal or distal anastomosis may exist. Disruption of fresh thrombus at the time of PCI may lead to no-reflow from embolization of platelet aggregates, intense microvascular constriction following the release of soluble mediators of vasoconstrictions (serotonin, thromboxane A2). Risk factors for distal embolization include angiographically visible thrombus, intervention in ACS, plaque ulceration, and SVG degeneration. Inability to restore TIMI 3 flow is associated with a 32% incidence of Q-wave or large non–Q-wave MI (CKMB > 50 IU/L) and 8% of in-hospital mortality (*Circulation* 1994;89(6):2514–2518). There is some nonrandomized evidence that direct stenting of SVG (i.e., without predilatation) may be associated with a reduction in the volume of atheroembolic debris.

22.14 **Answer B.** Additional revascularization (redo CABG or PCI) is required in approximately 5% of patients at 5 years and 20% at 10 years (*Am J Cardiol* 1994;73:103–112). In a series of 1,074 patients, it has been suggested that the location of SVG anastomosis predicted 10-year SVG patency: 69%, 58%, and 56% for LAD, LCX, and RCA, respectively (*J Am Coll Cardiol* 2004;44:2149–2156). The diameter of the recipient artery is highly predictive of SVG patency (grafting of vessel > 2 mm in diameter has an 88% 10-year patency rate compared with only 55% for a recipient or target vessel ≤2 mm (*p* < 0.001) (*J Am Coll Cardiol* 2004;44(11): 2149–2156) (see also answer to Question 22.8).

22.15 **Answer B.** Two weeks after clopidogrel cessation and according to the clinical presentation and coronary angiography, a very late DES thrombosis in the SVG to the LAD is the most likely diagnosis. Native LAD is occluded in its midportion and not suitable for PCI (chronically occluded and heavily calcified). Medical management was not selected in the context of ongoing chest pain. PCI of SVG was successfully performed. A BMW wire was easily advanced across the thrombus burden, and thromboaspiration brought large volume of atheroembolic debris. Intragraft administration of verapamil was performed before balloon dilatation to improve flow in this SVG with no-reflow. Flow then increased from TIMI 1 to TIMI 3 (Fig. A22-15). However, it is important to underscore that, with the exception of an acute MI in the presence

of a native circulation nonaccessible to revascularization, recanalization of an occluded SVG is generally not recommended.

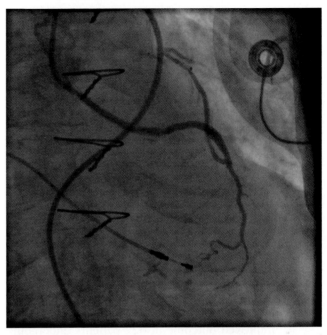

Figure A22-15. **SVG to LAD postcatheter thromboaspiration and balloon angioplasty.**

22.16 **Answer D.** PCI of the native vessels or of the grafts is a viable option if the lesions are suitable. In this patient, based on the fact that he is diabetic, has a moderately depressed LV function, has advanced SVG disease to the LCX, and has a complex left main-LAD lesion, redo CABG should be considered, particularly because no IMA grafting was previously performed. The use of LIMA has been associated with improved long-term graft patency and survival. In addition, in the SYNTAX (SYNergy between percutaneous coronary intervention with TAXus and cardiac surgery) trial (*J Am Coll Cardiol* 2010; 55(11):1067–1075), diabetic patients with high SYNTAX score (i.e., complex anatomy like in this case) randomized to surgery had a survival benefit compared to those allocated to DES. However, these data should be interpreted cautiously with respect to our patient because the SYNTAX trial excluded patients with previous cardiac surgery.

22.17 **Answer E.** As compared with the first surgery, redo CABG is associated with higher mortality rate (3% vs. 7%) and higher rate of perioperative MI (4% vs. 11.5%). In addition, redo surgery is less efficacious in relieving angina, and the patency rate of venous conduits is decreased (*Circulation* 1998;97:916–931).

22.18 **Answer C.** PCI of ostial SVG lesions can be safely performed a few months after CABG. Early following surgery, the risk of suture-line disruption and severe hemorrhagic complications is higher, and balloon sizing should be conservative. The SAFER (*Circulation* 2002;105:1285–1290)—randomizing patients undergoing SVG PCI to emboli protection with distal balloon occlusion or no protection—and FIRE (*Am Heart J* 2006;151:915.e1–917.e1)—randomization to emboli protection with filter vs. distal balloon occlusion in the same patient population—trials showed a dramatic reduction in no-reflow and its clinical sequelae with the use of embolic protection devices but no difference between different emboli protection strategies. Administration of glycoprotein IIb/IIIa receptor antagonists in nonrandomized trials has been associated with increased MACE risk in patients undergoing SVG PCI, potentially because of biased patient selection (*Circulation* 2008;117:790–797). A meta-analysis of five randomized trials of glycoprotein IIb/IIIa inhibitors also failed to show improved outcome in 627 patients undergoing SVG PCI (*Circulation* 2002;106:3063–3067). At 30 days, MI or target vessel revascularization (TVR) occurred in 16.5% of patients treated with glycoprotein IIb/IIIa inhibitors vs. 12.6% in the placebo group. Given the propensity of SVG atheroma to embolize, primary stenting without predilatation should be the preferred option whenever possible. Most of the time, postdilatation can be avoided when the correct stent size is used and implantation is performed at high pressure. When high-pressure postdilatation is required because of insufficient stent expansion, it should be performed with an embolic protection device in place, as this step carries the highest risk of all for distal embolization. Similarly to what is observed for BMS, the restenosis rate following DES implantation is higher for SVG PCI than for native vessel interventions and, overall, DES-based PCI of SVG carry a higher risk of restenosis than native vessel interventions.

22.19 **Answer B.** Repeat coronary angiography should be performed urgently when a sizable perioperative MI is suspected. This allows for a discrimination between graft-related ischemic events from other causes of myocardial damage such as prolonged extracorporeal circulation and for a minimization of the ischemic time. In the presence of acute ST-segment elevation in a coronary territory, rise of cardiac biomarkers, and

hemodynamic instability or sustained ventricular arrhythmia, a sudden graft occlusion should be suspected. Perioperative MI is associated with increased risk of subsequent congestive heart failure and short- and long-term adverse outcomes (*Eur Heart J* 2002;23:1219–1227). Emergency PCI—either by treating the graft (e.g., in the presence of an anastomosis stenosis) or by approaching the native vessel supplied by the occluded graft—is an alternative to redo surgery for acute graft occlusion. The choice between percutaneous and surgical revascularization should be made on a case-by-case basis based on the nature of the graft dysfunction, the territory affected, and the patency of the corresponding native vessel. In the case presented, ischemia was secondary to diffuse spasm of the native coronary vessel, likely induced by inotropes. A conservative treatment with hemodynamic support by intraaortic balloon pump was the preferred option, allowing for a discontinuation of inotrope agents and subsequent introduction of vasodilators. The clinical course was uneventful.

22.20 **Answer E.** Although partially explained by the increased prevalence of high-risk characteristics among the patients undergoing graft intervention, it has been demonstrated that SVG PCI per se is associated with worse outcomes compared with interventions of the native circulation (*Circulation* 2002;106:3063–3067). In-stent restenosis rate after BMS implantation in an SVG is over 20%. The Symbiot trial (*Catheter Cardiovasc Interv* 2006;68:379–388) showed that covered stents have a higher binary in-stent restenosis than BMS with no difference in MACE. Therefore the hypothesis that covered stents may reduce periprocedural complications by potentially preventing distal embolization and reduce restenosis by serving as a possible barrier to cell migration has been invalidated. The incidence of clinically adverse events in patients following SVG stenting approaches 50%, mainly because of disease progression at non–target sites within the treated SVG, the attrition of other SVGs, and the progression of native coronary artery disease (*J Am Coll Cardiol* 1997;30:1277–1283).

22.21 **Answer B.** The DELAYED RRISC (*J Am Coll Cardiol* 2007;50:261–267) study (prospective, randomized trial of DES vs. BMS in SVG lesions) showed at a median follow-up of 32 months that DES use was not associated with a reduction in repeat revascularization procedures.

Moreover, higher mortality was observed with DES implantation. However, the study was small, and this observation was not replicated in two recent meta-analyses. Accordingly, the DELAYED RRISC study included only 75 patients and obviously did not provide sufficient power to detect true effects in terms of repeat revascularization, morbidity, or mortality. In addition, most fatal adverse outcomes were neither cardiac nor procedure related. The first meta-analysis (*Circ Cardiovasc Interv* 2010;3:565–576) using Bayesian methods addressing DES and BMS use in SVG PCI included 25 studies (3 randomized studies and 22 nonrandomized studies, for a total of 5,755 patients) and concluded that DES use in SVG PCI was associated with improved TLR and TVR rates up to 30 months in the absence of increased rates of mortality, MI, or stent thrombosis. The second meta-analysis published thus far (*JACC Cardiovasc Interv* 2010;3:1262–1273) included 23 studies (4 randomized and 19 nonrandomized studies), and the median follow-up was 18 months. DES use was associated with improved mortality, MACE, TLR, and TVR, and there was no evidence of increased risk of MI or stent thrombosis.

22.22 **Answer E.** In multivariate analysis in a population of 589 patients undergoing BMS-PCI of SVG (*J Am Coll Cardiol* 1995;26:704–712), in-stent restenosis predictors included diabetes mellitus, small posttreatment stent diameter, small reference diameter (<3 mm), and treatment of an in-stent restenosis. Conversely, presentation with an ACS did not predict in-stent restenosis.

22.23 **Answer C.** Different types of embolic protection device exist: (1) distal occlusion balloon (GuardWire, Medtronic, Santa Rosa, CA), (2) distal filter (such as the FilterWire EX, Boston Scientific, Natick, MA [see Fig. Q22-23]; or Spider, EV3 Inc, Plymouth, MN; or Emboshield, Abbott Vascular, Abbott Park, IL) and (3) proximal occlusion device (Proxis, St. Jude Medical, St. Paul, MN). The SAFER trial (*Circulation* 2002;105:1285–1290) randomized patients undergoing SAVG PCI to emboli protection with the distal occlusion balloon GuardWire vs. no protection and was the first to show a dramatic improvement of the outcomes and a clear cost-effectiveness. The use of a filter device (FilterWire EX) was proved to be equivalent to distal balloon occlusion (GuardWire) in terms of periprocedural MI in the FIRE trial, a randomized study involving 651 patients undergoing SVG PCI (*Circulation* 2003;108:548–553). At 6-month follow-up (*Am Heart J* 2006;151:915.e1–917.e1), the use of FilterWire EX or GuardWire devices also resulted in similar outcomes although the clinical course after hospital discharge was not benign, with significant rates of death (3.0% and 4.1%, respectively) and repeat interventions (8.2% and 10.0%, respectively). The PROXIMAL trial (*J Am Coll Cardiol* 2007;50:1442–1449) was a multicenter, prospective randomized trial comparing proximal balloon occlusion vs. distal protection with either a balloon occlusion or a filter wire. The primary composite end point (death, MI, TVR) at 30 days by intention-to-treat analysis occurred in 9.2% of the proximal protection group and 10% of the distal protection group ($p = 0.0061$ for noninferiority). In patients amenable to both protection methods, 30-day MACE was numerically lower (although not statistically significant) with the proximal protection.

22.24 **Answer E.** Early SVG failure may result from any process that contributes to flow reduction or thrombosis such as prothombotic states, surgical issues—such as constrictive sutures or clips (as in this case), severe stenosis at the distal anastomosis site, graft kinking or overstretching—nonlaminar flow patterns secondary to SVG coronary artery mismatch, compromised outflow from distal coronary artery disease, and venous varicosities (*Eur J Cardiothorac Surg* 2006;30:117–125. Epub 2006 May 24). The diameter of the recipient artery is highly predictive of the 10-year patency rate of the corresponding vein graft (*J Am Coll Cardiol* 2004;44:2149–2156).

22.25 **Answer B.** A summary of the efficacy of different strategies for SVG interventions is demonstrated in Table A22.25. GP IIb/IIIa inhibitors showed no benefit in SVG interventions (*Circulation* 2002;106:3063–3067) (see Answer 22.18). Mechanical emboli protection is based on the concept of interposing a device between the lesion treated and the distal vasculature supplied by the graft as a prevention of distal embolization. The use of mechanical emboli protection devices has been a major breakthrough in SVG PCI (see answers to Questions 22.18 and 22.23 and Figs. Q22-24 and A22-25A,B). Symbiot trial (*Catheter Cardiovasc Interv* 2006;68:379–388) showed that covered stents have a higher binary in-stent restenosis than BMS with no difference in MACE.

Table A22-25.   Efficacy of Different Treatment Strategies in PCI of SVG

Therapy	Efficacy	Comments
Stents	Likely	Not prospectively addressed in large-scale randomized trials
		Majority of SVG PCIs performed are stent based
Covered stents	Failed	Lack of efficacy demonstrated in a randomized trial
		Preliminary data on new generation covered stents promising
Drug-eluting stents (DESs)	Effective	Two meta-analyses comparing DES vs. BMS showed improved TLR and TVR in the absence of increased risk of MI or stent thrombosis associated with the use of DES. One of the two meta-analyses showed a reduced mortality rate with the use of DES.
Glycoprotein IIb/IIIa inhibitors	Failed	Not recommended
Emboli protection devices	Highly effective	Efficacy in terms of MACE reduction demonstrated in randomized trials
		Distal balloon occlusion and filter devices equally effective
Ultrasound thrombolysis	Failed	Tested in a randomized trial
Atherectomy devices	Unknown	Insufficient safety and/or efficacy data

PCI, percutaneous coronary intervention; TLR, target lesion revascularization; TVR, target vessel revascularization; MACE, major adverse cardiac events; DES, drug-eluting stent; BMS, bare-metal stent

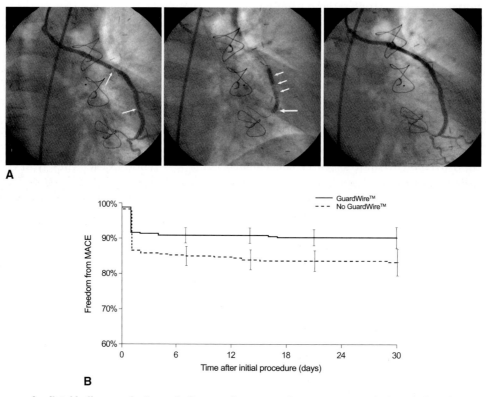

Figure A22-25.   A: The use of a distal balloon occlusive emboli protection system (Percusurge GuardWire, Medtronic, Minneapolis, MN) is demonstrated. Panel A shows two significant lesions (*arrows*) in the mid to distal portion of an SVG to the marginal branch of the LCX. In Panel B, the distal balloon is inflated (*large arrow*) and the graft occluded. The no-flow state is documented by the stagnant column of contrast media (*small arrows*). Panel C demonstrates final result following stent and retrieval of the distal protection. B: Freedom from major adverse cardiac events (i.e., death, MI, emergent bypass surgery, or TVR) at 1 month among 800 patients undergoing SVG PCI randomized to distal balloon occlusion (Percusurge GuardWire, Medtronic, Minneapolis, MN) vs. conventional guidewire. The event rate was 9.6% in the GuardWire group and 16.5% in the control group, and the difference was statistically significant (*p* = 0.004).

23 Closure Devices

Robert J. Applegate

23.1 The proven benefits of vascular closure devices include all of the following, EXCEPT:

(A) Lower incidence of pseudoaneurysm and hematoma
(B) Earlier ambulation of patients
(C) Reduction in time to hemostasis
(D) Earlier discharge for some patients

23.2 Match the mechanism of closure with a device:

(A) Utilizes a nitinol clip to close the arteriotomy site Angio-Seal
(B) Suture-mediated closure Duett
(C) Mechanical seal by sandwiching the arteriotomy between a bioabsorbable anchor and the collagen sponge Mynx
(D) Balloon catheter that initiates hemostasis and ensures the precise placement of procoagulant (a flowable mixture of thrombin, collagen, and diluent) at the puncture site in the entire tissue tract Perclose
(E) Polyethylglycol sealant delivered to the surface of the arteriotomy Devices: Angio-Seal, Duett, Mynx, Perclose, StarClose

23.3 Which of the following is not bioresorbable?

(A) Angio-Seal
(B) Duett
(C) Mynx
(D) Perclose
(E) VasoSeal

23.4 Match the image of the closure device with the device (Fig. Q23-4 (1-5)):

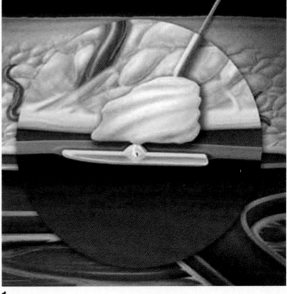

1

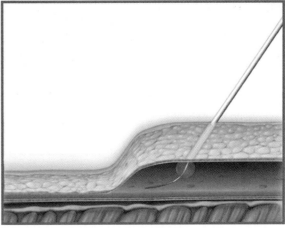

2

265

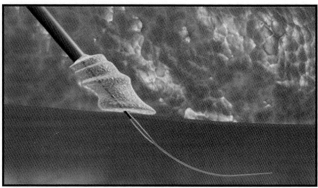

3

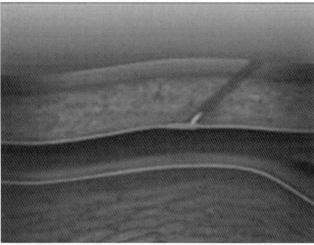

4

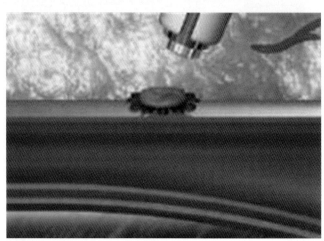

5

Figure Q23-4(1-5)

(A) Angio-Seal
(B) Duett
(C) Mynx
(D) Perclose
(E) StarClose

23.5 Which of the following does not achieve active approximation or result in immediate closure of the access site?

(A) Angio-Seal
(B) StarClose
(C) Perclose
(D) Mynx

23.6 Which of the following is made of a soft, white, sterile, nonwoven pad of cellulosic polymer and poly-*N*-acetyl glucosamine isolated from a microalgae?

(A) Angio-Seal
(B) Duett
(C) Syvek
(D) Perclose
(E) StarClose
(F) Mynx

23.7 Clinical studies have suggested increased vascular complications with which of the following devices?

(A) Angio-Seal
(B) VasoSeal
(C) Duett
(D) Perclose
(E) StarClose
(F) Mynx

23.8 A 68-year-old diabetic man underwent percutaneous coronary intervention (PCI) and uneventful closure of his femoral access site with a Perclose device. Two weeks later, he noted redness and swelling at the access site with drainage of serosanguineous material. Figure Q23-8 was taken at the time of exploration of his groin and most likely represents which of the following?

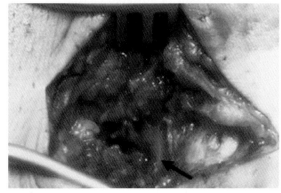

Figure Q23-8

(A) Generalized sepsis

(B) Mycotic pseudoaneurysm

(C) Carbuncle

(D) Infective endocarditis

(E) Femoral endarteritis

23.9 A 55-year-old man undergoes uncomplicated cardiac catheterization and PCI of the right coronary artery (RCA). Aspirin, clopidogrel, and bivalirudin were administered during the case. A femoral angiogram is obtained through the procedural sheath in anticipation of use of a closure device (Fig. Q23-9). What is the most optimal next step?

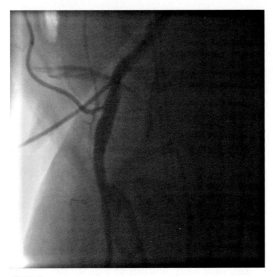

Figure Q23-9

(A) Place a FemoStop and pull the sheath

(B) Obtain an abdominal CT scan and call vascular surgery

(C) Place an Angio-Seal device

(D) Wait 2 hours, and then pull the sheath and apply manual compression

23.10 A 65-year-old woman undergoes elective uncomplicated cardiac catheterization and PCI of the left anterior descending (LAD). Aspirin, clopidogrel, and heparin were administered during the case. A femoral angiogram is obtained through the procedural sheath in anticipation of use of a closure device (Fig. Q23-10). What closure device should be chosen in this case?

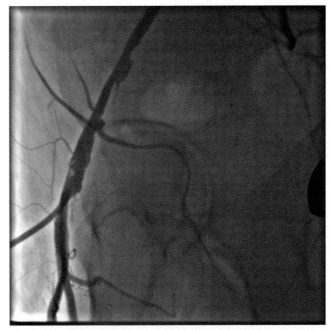

Figure Q23-10

(A) Angio-Seal

(B) Perclose

(C) Mynx

(D) StarClose

(E) None of the above

23.11 A 48-year-old man undergoes uncomplicated cardiac catheterization and PCI of the LAD after a non–ST elevation myocardial infarction (NSTEMI). Aspirin, prasugrel, and bivalirudin were administered during the case. Since the initial femoral access was achieved with a single anterior wall stick, the operator placed a closure device without apparent complication. Throughout the night, the patient complained of pain and swelling at the access site. A pulsatile mass was found in the groin the following morning. Which of the following likely corresponds to this case?

(A) Arteriovenous fistulae

(B) Occlusion

(C) Pseudoaneurysm

(D) High stick

23.12 A 45-year-old woman undergoes a diagnostic catheterization after having a positive stress test for atypical chest pain. She is found to have mild luminal irregularities, and the cardiologist decides to close her groin. The patient is very obese, so he elects to place a buddy wire in the event he does not get complete closure with an Angio-Seal device. She complains of immediate leg pain and is found to be pulseless and have pain, pallor, and paresthesia of her right leg. A sheath is inserted over the buddy wire, and the following angiogram is obtained (Fig. Q23-12). What should you do next?

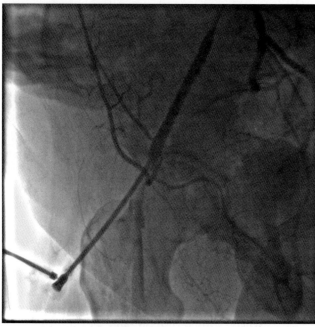

Figure Q23-12

  (A) Urgent surgery consult or urgent percutaneous peripheral vascular intervention

  (B) IV heparin and glycoprotein (GP) IIb/IIIa inhibitor

  (C) IV fibrinolytic therapy

  (D) Give pain pills for relief

23.13 A 67-year-old woman is admitted to the hospital with an acute coronary syndrome and suffers an NSTEMI. Cardiac catheterization is performed revealing diffuse three-vessel CAD. At the end of the procedure, she appears to be uncomfortable and complains of vague abdominal discomfort. The angiogram in Figure Q23-13 is obtained. What should be the next step?

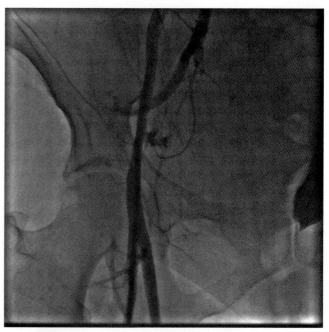

Figure Q23-13

  (A) Place a closure device

  (B) Pull the sheath in the lab and apply manual compression

  (C) Gain contralateral access and perform balloon angioplasty

  (D) Continue anticoagulation in preparation for coronary artery bypass graft

23.14 What are the distinguishing features on the physical examination of a groin hematoma from femoral artery pseudoaneurysm?

  (A) Pulsatile groin mass and bruit

  (B) Pain and audible bruit

  (C) Groin mass

  (D) Continuous groin pain and neuralgia

23.15 An 81-year-old patient undergoes an urgent catheterization for acute myocardial infarction. She is found on angiogram to have 100% occlusion of LAD artery. She has a successful PCI to LAD with 3.0/33 mm drug-eluting stent and 3.0/28 mm drug-eluting stent with heparin and GP IIb/IIIa inhibitor, abciximab. She is allergic to latex. She is unable to keep her leg still. Can you use Angio-Seal?

  (A) Yes, Angio-Seal can be used in patients with latex allergy

  (B) No, Angio-Seal cannot be used in patients with latex allergy

  (C) Only manual pressure should be applied to patients with latex allergy

  (D) No, only Perclose can be used in patients with latex allergy

23.16 A 78-year-old man undergoes PCI to the RCA with bivalirudin. He responds well and is sealed with Angio-Seal without any complication. He is discharged home. He returns to your office within a month, complaining of severe chest pain with minimal exertion. You examine him, and he is found to have slightly decreased right lower extremity pulse but is otherwise unremarkable and denies claudication. You elect to proceed with catheterization from the right leg, and the angiogram in Figure Q23-16 is obtained. What is the optimal next step?

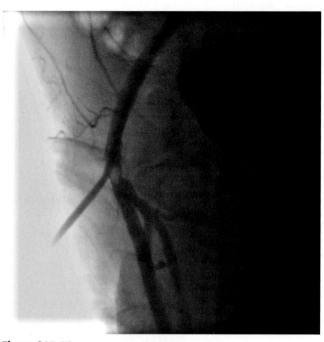

Figure Q23-16

(A) Manual compression, and obtain ABIs
(B) There is no such thing as subacute limb ischemia from vascular closure device; therefore, he has peripheral arterial diseases
(C) Access from contralateral femoral artery and balloon angioplasty of the affected side
(D) Surgical intervention

23.17 An 80-year-old woman undergoes an elective PCI to a dominant left circumflex (LCX). Her right femoral artery is sealed with new generation Angio-Seal. Three days later she presents with chest pain, ST elevation, and hypotension in the emergency room. She is taken back to the catheterization laboratory. Can you reaccess the same site?

(A) No, the same site cannot be accessed for 7 days
(B) No, right femoral artery cannot be accessed for 90 days
(C) No, the same site cannot be accessed for 30 days
(D) Yes, as long as it is 1 cm proximal to the previously accessed site

23.18 The following devices are approved for use outside of the common femoral artery:

(A) Angio-Seal
(B) StarClose
(C) Perclose
(D) Mynx
(E) None of the above

23.19 Which of the following has been associated with acute vessel closure at the time of device deployment?

(A) Angio-Seal
(B) StarClose
(C) Perclose
(D) Mynx
(D) All of the above

23.20 The femoral angiogram was taken after placement of the arterial sheath (Fig. Q23-20). The arrow points to which artery?

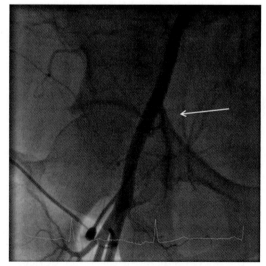

Figure Q23-20

(A) The superficial femoral artery
(B) The inferior epigastric artery
(C) The pudendal artery
(D) The lateral CX artery

23.1 **Answer A.** Vascular closure devices have some obvious advantages. The time spent by catheterization laboratory staff in manually compressing the puncture site is reduced, which in turn improves the patient flow throughput in busy catheterization laboratories. Other proven benefits include the reduction in time to hemostasis, and earlier ambulation of patients and earlier discharge for some patients. Small studies comparing patient satisfaction after management of the access site indicate that closure devices enhance patient comfort. A rigorously performed systematic review and meta-analysis of first-generation devices suggested that vascular closure devices may actually increase the risk of hematoma and pseudoaneurysm (*JAMA* 2004;291:350–357).

23.2 **Answers.** **A**-StarClose. **B**-Perclose. **C**-Angio-Seal. **D**-Duett. **E**-Mynx.

23.3 **Answer D.** All of the devices listed except for Perclose undergo breakdown and eventually resorption by the body. Perclose utilizes a nonbiodegradable suture, similar to the suture that is used to directly close the artery by surgeons. Perclose did offer a biodegradable suture at one point, but the product was withdrawn from the market because of issues with suture breakage.

23.4 **Answer.** A-1; B-2; C-3; D-4; E-5

23.5 **Answer D.** The Mynx device utilizes an extravascular polyethylene glycol sealant to tamponade the access site at the base of the tissue tract. There is no permanent intra-arterial component to the device, but rather a balloon inflated in the vessel is used during activation of the sealant to achieve temporary mechanical hemostasis. After a brief period of manual compression, longer for PCI procedures, the balloon is deflated and removed, leaving the sealant to tamponade the access site. All of the other devices utilize active approximation of the access site either with an intra-arterial component (Angio-Seal) or by direct closure of the arteriotomy (Perclose, StarClose).

23.6 **Answer C.** The Syvek patch is made of a soft, white, sterile, nonwoven pad of cellulosic

polymer and poly-*N*-acetyl glucosamine isolated from a microalgae (Fig. A23-6). It leaves no subcutaneous foreign matter, is nonallergenic, and does not restrict immediate same site reentry. Although there are no known contraindications, it does not eliminate manual compression, but may shorten the duration of compression needed.

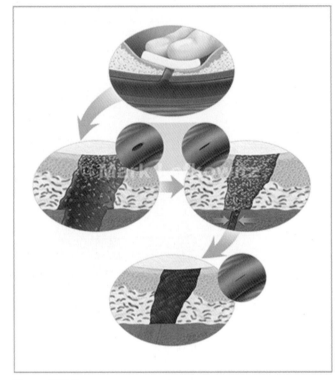

Figure A23-6

23.7 **Answer B.** The pooled analyses by Vaitkus et al. (*J Invasive Cardiol* 2004;16:243–246) demonstrated that the Angio-Seal and Perclose devices might be superior to or at least equivalent to manual compression for both interventional and diagnostic cases. The results of controlled clinical trials with VasoSeal, however, indicated a potentially increased risk of complications. Another analysis by Nikolsky et al. (*J Am Coll Cardiol* 2004;44:1200–1209) showed that in interventional cases, the rate of complications was also higher with VasoSeal. VasoSeal is no longer commercially available, although this appeared to stem from withdrawal from the market due to lack of utilization rather than for regulatory reasons.

23.8 **Answer B.** Sohail et al. reviewed all cases of closure device–related infection seen in their institution and searched the English language medical literature for all previously published reports (*Mayo Clin Proc* 2005;80:1011–1015). They identified 46 cases from the medical literature and 6 cases from their institutional database. Diabetes mellitus and obesity were the most common comorbidities. The median incubation period from device insertion to presentation with access-site infection was 8 days (with a range of 2 to 29 days). The most common presenting symptoms were pain, erythema, fever, swelling, and purulent drainage at the access site. Mycotic pseudoaneurysm was the most common complication (22 cases). *Staphylococcus aureus* was responsible for most of the infections (75%). The mortality rate was 6% (3 patients). This suggests that infection associated with closure device placement is uncommon but is an extremely serious complication. Morbidity is high, and aggressive medical and surgical interventions are required to achieve cure.

23.9 **Answer D.** The femoral angiogram indicates that the access site is above the inferior epigastric artery, and likely within the external iliac artery. Several recent retrospective observational studies have identified a "high stick" such as this as associated with an increase in the incidence of retroperitoneal hemorrhage. Moreover, these studies found an association with closure device use and an increase in the likelihood of a retroperitoneal hemorrhage, although there was not complete consensus on this point. However, in the study of Tiroch et al., the absolute rate of a retroperitoneal hemorrhage after a "high stick" was only about 4%. At this point in time, watchful waiting would be indicated, unless there was active concern about retroperitoneal hemorrhage, and avoidance of a closure device. Pulling the sheath in an actively anticoagulated patient in the absence of a complication may not be the wisest course of action even if a FemoStop is applied.

23.10 **Answer E.** Appropriate use of all of the commercially available closure devices rely on review of a femoral angiogram prior to use of a closure device. Each of the information for use instructions indicate that the device can be used for closure of access within the common femoral artery, of an appropriately sized vessel (4 to 6 mm depending on the device), and the absence of significant atherosclerotic disease at the access site. This patient has evidence of severe atherosclerosis at the access site with a vessel diameter at the access site of only 2 mm. Thus, none of the currently available devices, including the extravascular closure devices, are approved for use in this patient.

23.11 **Answer C.** The patient's symptoms and findings are consistent with a pseudoaneurysm. The angiogram not only reveals a pseudoaneurysm (Fig. A23-11) but indicates that the access site was likely in the femoral bifurcation. A "low stick" is associated with an increase in the risk of both pseudoaneurysm and arteriovenous fistulae. Moreover, there is no evidence that closure device use decreases this risk (as noted elsewhere, they have been associated with an increase in the risk of these two local access complications). The operators' failure to obtain a femoral angiogram prior to placement of a closure device, in spite of a single anterior wall stick, may have contributed to the development of the pseudoaneurysm, although a "low stick" itself is also associated with an increase in the incidence of this complication.

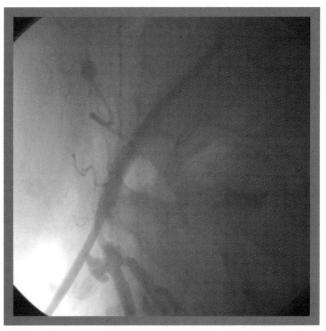

Figure A23-11

23.12 **Answer A.** She has acute femoral artery thrombosis. There is approximately 1% to 2% risk of major complication from vascular closure device. Acute femoral artery thrombosis requires urgent intervention (*JAMA* 2004;291:350–357).

23.13 **Answer C.** This patient has developed a retro-peritoneal hemorrhage with extravasation of contrast from the access site in the external iliac artery. Closure devices have been associated with a higher rate of retroperitoneal bleeding in cases of "high sticks" and are not recommended for use in this situation. Manual compression is unlikely to achieve hemostasis this deep into the pelvis, and pulling the sheath may exacerbate the situation. Given the compression of the bladder, this patient has an active retroperitoneal bleed and needs to be urgently treated with endovascular rescue using contralateral access to tamponade the bleeding and potentially place a covered stent, or taken for urgent surgery.

23.14 **Answer A.** A hematoma is associated with a groin mass, but there should not be an audible bruit. Patients with preexisting atherosclerotic disease may have a preexisting bruit, which can make the specificity of this combination reduced. A pseudoaneurysm can be diagnosed on physical examination by pulsatile mass and audible bruit. Most are asymptomatic. In this era, a groin mass and bruit would signal the need to obtain a groin ultrasound to more specifically diagnose the underlying complication.

23.15 **Answer A.** Angio-Seal is comprised of a poly lactic-glycolic acid anchor, bioresorbable collagen suture, and bovine collagen extravascular sponge. Although patients with a beef allergy may experience a mild inflammatory reaction to the collagen in Angio-Seal, this device can be used safely in patients with latex allergy.

23.16 **Answer A.** This patient has a filling defect at the site of the previous Angio-Seal deployment. This may represent thrombus formation at the site, inflammation, and/or neointimal proliferation in response to the device. In the absence of obstruction and accompanying symptoms and findings consistent with limb ischemia, this may resolve. All of the commercially available closure devices may potentially cause limb ischemia, although the incidence is exceedingly low. While a simple surgical patch angioplasty can

be performed with low morbidity, and this may also be treated with balloon angioplasty from contralateral access and would be preferred by many patients (*Catheter Cardiovasc Interv* 2002;57:12–23), neither of these may be required in the absence of claudication.

23.17 **Answer D.** Applegate RJ et al. studied the restick issue with Angio-Seal and found that restick can occur safely within 1 to 7 days of Angio-Seal (*Catheter Cardiovasc Interv* 2003;58:181–184). In this study, the femoral angiogram taken at the time of the initial Angio-Seal deployment was reviewed, and the second access was attempted 1 cm above or below the initial access site (but trying to stay within the common femoral artery).

23.18 **Answer E.** While each of the devices listed have been used in access sites outside of the common femoral artery, none of these devices are approved for use in this location. This would be considered an "off-label" use of a closure device and should be monitored closely at each institution until definitive studies confirm the safety of this strategy.

23.19 **Answer E.** All of the closure devices listed have been reported to be associated with acute vessel closure at the time of device deployment. Fortunately, the incidence of this potentially devastating complication has decreased dramatically since the introduction of closure devices in 1994, occurring in <0.1% of cases in most series.

23.20 **Answer B.** The point of the most caudal position of the inferior epigastric artery demarcates the thigh compartment from the retroperitoneal space. As such, it is a useful landmark to determine if the access site is within the common femoral artery. If the access site is above the lowest portion of the inferior epigastric artery, then it is likely that the sheath entered the external iliac artery and is located within the retroperitoneal space. This has also been termed a "high stick" to demarcate its position outside of the common femoral artery.

24

Management of Intraprocedural and Postprocedural Complications

Ferdinand Leya

QUESTIONS

24.1 A 35-year-old otherwise healthy woman was found to have a diastolic murmur during routine physical exam. The patient underwent noninvasive testing that was inconclusive and the pressure wave forms in Figure Q24-1 were found upon hemodynamic evaluation.

What is the best treatment plan (assuming that this patient has no contraindication for the therapy listed) based on Figure Q24-1?

(A) Refer for mitral valve surgery
(B) Holter monitoring with medical management with β-blockade
(C) Percutaneous balloon valvotomy
(D) Annual transthoracic echocardiography and watchful waiting for disease progression

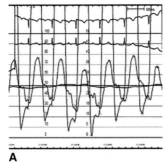

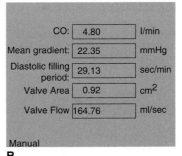

CO:	4.80	l/min
Mean gradient:	22.35	mmHg
Diastolic filling period:	29.13	sec/min
Valve Area	0.92	cm²
Valve Flow	164.76	ml/sec

Manual

A   B

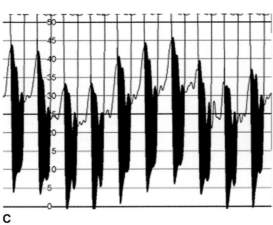

C

Figure Q24-1

24.2 A 38-year-old previously healthy woman presents to the emergency room (ER) with severe chest pain and an ECG showing ST-segment elevation. An emergent coronary angiogram was performed and revealed moderate diffuse stenosis in the left anterior descending (LAD) and thrombolysis in myocardial infarction (TIMI) III flow with no significant coronary artery disease (CAD) noted in the other epicardial coronary arteries. Intravascular ultrasound (IVUS) of the LAD was performed (Fig. Q24-2):

What is the diagnosis based on Figure Q24-2?

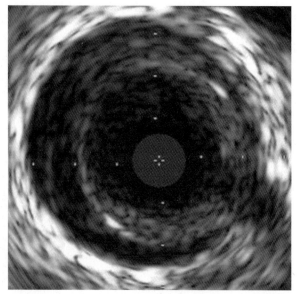

Figure Q24-2

(A) Pericarditis
(B) Plaque rupture leading to ST elevation myocardial infarction (MI)
(C) Coronary artery dissection
(D) Moderate nonobstructive CAD

24.3 Based on recently presented CLOSURE 1 trial, what would you recommend in this 58-year-old patient with history of cryptogenic stroke (Fig. Q24-3)?

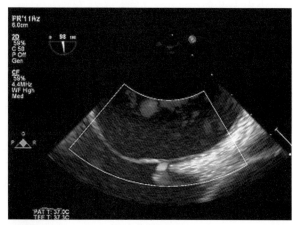

Figure Q24-3 (see color insert)

(A) Medical therapy
(B) Percutaneous closure with STARflex device and stop medical therapy
(C) Percutaneous closure with STARflex device and medical therapy
(D) Surgical closure

24.4 An 86-year-old patient with hypertension (HTN), diabetes mellitus (DM), hyperlipidemia, chronic renal insufficiency, and previous coronary artery bypass grafting (CABG) in 2000 with saphenous vein graft (SVG) to LAD, SVG to posterior descending artery (PDA), and SVG to circumflex (CX) presents to your office with 4 weeks of exertional chest pain. He undergoes stress thallium, which shows left ventricular (LV) dilatation and possible anterior ischemia. His ejection fraction (EF) is 55% on the stress test.

He is taken to catheterization laboratory. His native arteries are occluded and his SVG to PDA and SVG to CX are also occluded. His SVG to LAD has severe 95% hazy lesion. SVG to LAD provides collateral flow to the right coronary artery (RCA) as well as to the CX. He is evaluated by the surgeons and turned down for surgery. You decide to proceed with percutaneous coronary intervention (PCI) to SVG to LAD. Given the high-risk nature of his lesions, you decide to use the device that is shown in Figure Q24-4. How much blood is pumped from the LV to aorta by the system above?

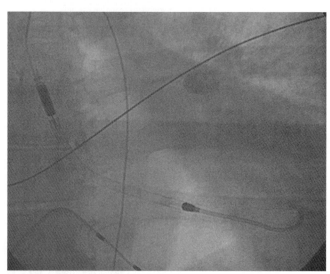

Figure Q24-4

(A) 2.0 L/min
(B) 2.5 L/min
(C) 3.0 L/min
(D) 3.5 L/min

24.5 During the procedure of SVG to LAD, he has no reflow and he goes into ventricular fibrillation and cardiac arrest. He is resuscitated with defibrillation. Then after repeated pharmacologic intervention, his SVG to LAD has TIMI 2 flow and he is taken to the intensive care unit (ICU), intubated, and on 2 pressors. He recovers after several days and his EF is now 15% to 20%. He and his family are upset that this happened and are threatening to sue you. They claim that it was the device that made him have complications. Based on trial data, what is known about the device in Figure Q24-4?

(A) There has not been a study of nonemergent high-risk PCI patients using Impella device

(B) There was a study of nonemergent high-risk PCI patients using Impella and it showed significant reduction of major adverse cardiac event with the Impella device

(C) There was a study of nonemergent high-risk PCI patients using Impella and it showed higher risk of complications and major adverse cardiac event with the Impella device

(D) There was a study of nonemergent high-risk PCI patients using Impella and there was no difference between intraaortic balloon pump (IABP) and Impella

24.6 A 69-year-old man with HTN and renal insufficiency (glomerular filtration rate 65) presents to your office for consult from an internist. He has been experiencing chest pain with exertion and underwent stress thallium, which showed anterior defect. He then had cardiac catheterization that showed severe three-vessel disease with EF of 45%. He refused CABG and presents to your office for multivessel PCI. He is concerned about his risk. What is his risk of emergent CABG with contemporary percutaneous revascularization with use of stents?

(A) 0.4%

(B) 1.5%

(C) 3.7%

(D) 5.0%

24.7 During the selective cannulation of the left main coronary ostium, the blood pressure (BP) waveform, as seen in Figure Q24-7, was recorded. Which of the following is the most likely explanation for the waveform?

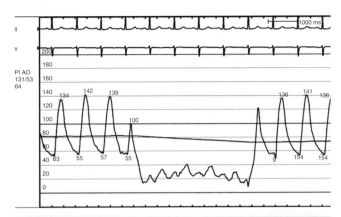

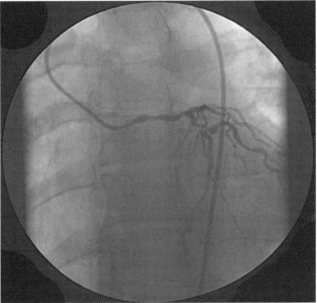

Figure Q24-7

(A) The pressure waveform indicates that the catheter tip prolapsed into the left ventricle

(B) The pressure transducer contains air

(C) There is catheter kink

(D) The catheter is up against the wall

(E) The catheter is engaged into a diseased left main artery

24.8 A 67-year-old retired lawyer with DM, hyperlipidemia, and HTN presents to you for a second opinion. He underwent cardiac catheterization for increasing exertional chest pain and was found to have chronically occluded moderate-size RCA, 50% LAD artery, and CX lesions. He underwent PCI to RCA and had 2.5/28, 2.5/33, and 2.25/28 bare-metal stent. Drug-eluting stents were not used because of the patient's history of ulcers. Immediately after the intervention, the patient started complaining of chest pain and had inferior ST elevation. He underwent immediate catheterization and was found to have an occluded RCA. However, the artery could not be successfully opened. In the stent era, all factors have been correlated with abrupt vessel closure, EXCEPT:

(A) Stent length
(B) Small vessel diameter
(C) Poor distal runoff
(D) Excessive tortuosity
(E) Unstable angina

24.9 A 51-year-old woman presents to you for second opinion. She underwent successful elective PCI to CX for exertional chest pain. Her hospitalization was uneventful until the time of discharge when she was told that her creatine kinase-MB (CK-MB) isoform was three times the normal limit. She was discharged home and has been doing well but cannot stop worrying. Which of the following statements is TRUE regarding procedure-related enzyme release?

(A) CK-MB elevation does not occur after angiographically successful uncomplicated coronary interventions
(B) Routine monitoring of cardiac enzymes is not necessary to detect patients who suffer from myocardial injury after coronary intervention
(C) The incidence of CK-MB enzyme elevation after angiographically successful percutaneous intervention is >50%
(D) Elevation of CK-MB after PCI predicts increased long-term cardiac mortality and morbidity

24.10 A 45-year-old patient with diabetes who was hypercholesterolemic, hypertensive, and a heavy (two-packs-a-day) smoker underwent a successful angioplasty and stent placement to mid-LAD lesion. Before angioplasty, the patient received acetylsalicylic acid (ASA) 325 and glycoprotein (GP) IIb/IIIa inhibitor treatment. The angioplasty procedure was uneventful. The Cypher 3.0- × 28-mm stent was deployed at 16 atm. The final angiogram showed a well-expanded vessel with TIMI 3 flow. The following morning, a routine troponin was 1.5 ng/mL. The patient remained asymptomatic and his cardiac examination was normal. His electrocardiogram (ECG) showed nonspecific ST–T-wave changes, which were unchanged from the admitting ECG. The best course of action for this patient now is as follows:

(A) Discharge the patient immediately with β-blockers, nitrates, statin, ASA, Plavix, and an angiotensin-converting enzyme (ACE) inhibitor
(B) Bring the patient back to the catheterization laboratory for a repeat angiogram

(C) Transfer the patient to a coronary care unit (CCU)
(D) Continue to monitor the patient in telemetry for 48 hours
(E) Check another set of troponin in 8 hours. If the trend is down then discharge him on Plavix, ASA, β-blockers, statins, and an ACE inhibitor

24.11 A 75-year-old patient traveled 4 hours by car to get to the hospital for a 7:00 AM, first case, elective, complex, multilesion, multivessel coronary intervention. Although the angioplasty procedure was difficult to perform because of lack of adequate guide support, finally after trying several guide catheters, an Amplatz no. 3 guide catheter was found to give a good guide support to deliver three long Taxus stents. At the end of the procedure, the operator informed the patient that he was successful in opening all the blockages. The catheterization laboratory staff moved the patient to the recovery room. The patient was asymptomatic without any complaint and had normal vital signs. Later, the recovery room registered nurse (RN) noticed that the patient became progressively lethargic and less responsive to her. The physician in charge was notified. After obtaining the vital signs, which were noted to be unchanged, the most appropriate action at this time should be:

(A) Have the RN check the patient's ECG and his vital signs again
(B) Give the patient naloxone (Narcan)
(C) Perform a screening neurologic examination or obtain an urgent neurology consult
(D) Check the patient's complete blood count (CBC), blood sugar, blood urea nitrogen, and creatinine level

24.12 The patient mentioned in the preceding text recovers and is discharged without any residual deficits. He has filed a formal complaint against you to the hospital. The Chief of Staff's office would like to know about periprocedural stroke during coronary interventions. Which of the following statements is correct?

(A) Periprocedural stroke occurs approximately 0.5%
(B) Patients who suffer a stroke have an increased in-hospital mortality of 37%
(C) Patients who suffer a stroke have an increased 1-year mortality of 56%
(D) It is mostly embolic and not hemorrhagic stroke

(E) A, B, and C are true

(F) B, C, and D are true

(G) C and D are true

(H) A, B, C, and D are true

24.13 You are asked to examine a 65-year-old heavy smoker with a strong family history of CAD and history of multivessel PCI with left-sided stroke for cardiology evaluation. His past medical history is notable for PCI to heavily calcified ostial LAD and mid-CX 8 months ago. Recently, he has been under treatment for methicillin-resistant *Staphylococcus aureus* bacteremia following his right below-knee amputation for gangrene. At baseline, he has an abnormal ECG with nonspecific ST changes in the precordial leads. The two-dimensional (2D) echo demonstrated moderate aortic insufficiency with multiple large vegetations on the aortic valve. He is examined by the cardiothoracic surgeons who would like to operate on him. They would like to visualize his coronary anatomy first and then ask for your opinion. The most appropriate action at this time is:

(A) Because of high risk of embolization with left heart catheterization, he should undergo cardiac computed tomography (CT) to assess patency of ostial LAD and mid-CX stents

(B) Send the patient for emergency heart surgery without cardiac angiogram

(C) Perform left-sided cardiac catheterization to visualize coronary anatomy

(D) Transfer the patient to neuro-ICU for stroke management and treat endocarditis medically

24.14 A 75-year-old morbidly obese patient (378 lb, 5 ft. 5 in. tall) is referred from an outside hospital for angioplasty and stenting of a large proximal dominant RCA lesion. She has an infected skin lesion in the right groin beneath a large abdominal pannus. The operator decides to cannulate the left groin instead, and after multiple sticks, he is finally able to cannulate the left leg artery and to place a 7-F arterial introducer. The angioplasty procedure is successful using a 3.5-/33-mm Cypher stent to RCA with heparin and GP IIb/IIIa inhibitor eptifibatide (Integrilin). Following the angioplasty procedure, all equipment is removed from the patient's heart. At the end of the procedure, the activated clotting time is measured at 287 seconds. The operator decides to close the left groin artery entry site with an 8-F Angio-Seal device. Before doing so, he performs a peripheral angiogram using the introducing sheath to inject dye. The angiogram shows that the introducer was placed in the proximal

profunda femoris artery too close to its bifurcation. The operator elects to place the Fem Stop instead. The Fem Stop is successfully applied and the patient is moved to the recovery room. In the recovery room, the RN notices that the patient's BP has dropped from 130/90 to 96/70, and her pulse has increased from 68 to 78 bpm. The physician is notified, and he orders an increase in intravenous fluids to 200 mL/hour for 1 hour. The patient's BP normalizes, but an hour later, it drops again. This time it measures 90/68, with a pulse of 90 bpm. Soon after that, the patient starts to complain that the Fem Stop causes her to have left groin pain. The physician comes and adjusts the Fem Stop. He examines the groin and it appears normal. The intravenous fluids are increased and the systolic BP returns to 102/70 mm Hg. After a while, the patient again starts complaining of being uncomfortable in bed with the Fem Stop compressing her groin, and she becomes diaphoretic, her BP drops to 75/50, and her heart rate (HR) slows down to 45 bpm. The physician is notified. The most appropriate initial response at this time should be:

(A) Loosen or reposition the Fem Stop and give the patient a pain medication with sedation for comfort

(B) Send the patient for CT scan

(C) Send the patient to vascular laboratory for ultrasound

(D) Order patient's CBC, and type and cross

(E) Remove Fem Stop and apply direct manual pressure on the artery entry site

(F) Continue rapid fluid infusion to expand the volume

(G) Stop GP IIb/IIIa inhibitors

(H) Consult a vascular surgeon to consider surgery

(I) A, B, and C are correct

(J) D, E, F, and G are correct

(K) A–H are correct

24.15 The patient mentioned in the preceding text does well with manual pressure and goes upstairs to the telemetry floor. In 3 hours, you are called to see the patient because she has developed pulselessness, pain, pallor, and paresthesia of her left leg. What is the best way to treat this patient at this time?

(A) Start intravenous heparin and careful clinical monitoring

(B) Start intravenous heparin, GP IIb/IIIa inhibitor, and careful monitoring

(C) Intravenous fibrinolytic therapy

(D) Urgent peripheral vascular (PV) surgery consultation or urgent percutaneous PV intervention

24.16 Complication of groin hematoma may lead to sensory or motor neurologic deficit by compressing the surrounding nerves. Which nerves are most commonly affected by groin hematoma?

(A) Femoral and sciatic nerves
(B) Sciatic, femoral, and lateral cutaneous nerves
(C) Femoral and lateral cutaneous nerves

24.17 The most common cause of procedurally related retroperitoneal (RP) hematoma includes:

(A) Spontaneous RP venous bleeding triggered by aggressive anticoagulant therapy
(B) Arterial bleed caused by a back wall puncture of the femoral artery distal to the origin of the superficial CX iliac artery
(C) Arterial bleeding caused by a back wall puncture of the femoral artery proximal to the origin of the deep CX iliac artery

24.18 A 54-year-old woman is transferred to the medical center from an outside hospital for an elective angioplasty of the RCA artery lesion. Three days before admission, the patient suffered an acute inferior wall MI, which was successfully treated with IV tPA. On the day of the procedure, the patient was asymptomatic, but she was quite anxious about the upcoming coronary angioplasty. The 80% lesion in the proximal RCA was opened with a 3.5- × 23-mm Cypher stent. The final angiogram showed a widely patent RCA, normal left coronary system, and EF of 50% with moderate inferior wall hypokinesia. The right groin entry site was successfully closed with a Perclose device after angiogram was taken (Fig. Q24-18).

The patient was transferred to the recovery unit, and within 45 minutes, she began to complain of right groin and right flank pain, which improved when she adjusted her position. Thirty minutes later, her BP and pulse, which previously read 130/70 and 70, respectively, measured 100/60 and 80. Fluids were administered, and her BP improved, but she continued to complain about the right lower abdominal quadrant pain. The physician was called. He examined the groin and found no evidence of bleeding and hematoma. Bowel sounds were weak but present. He reassured the patient and returned to the catheterization laboratory. Fifteen minutes later, her BP dropped again to 76 mm Hg with a pulse of 60 bpm. The patient became slightly diaphoretic and restless, complaining of increasing abdominal discomfort. Soon thereafter, her BP dropped to 60/40, HR was 45 bpm, and the patient began to retch but could not vomit. The most likely diagnostic explanation of this patient's problem is:

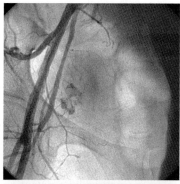

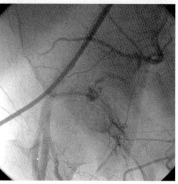

Figure Q24-18

(A) The patient is allergic to intravenous pyelogram dye
(B) The patient has femoral artery dissection
(C) The patient has spontaneous RP bleed
(D) The patient has adverse reaction to midazolam (Versed) and fentanyl
(E) The patient has arterial external iliac artery perforation with RP dye extravasation

24.19 The best treatment for a patient who, during the percutaneous intervention, suffers an accidental large right iliac artery laceration is:

(A) Aggressive fluid and blood replacement therapy
(B) Emergency consultation from vascular
(C) Immediate percutaneous intervention using contralateral approach to block bleeding from the iliac artery by inflating properly sized angioplasty balloon followed by placing covered stent to seal the vessel wall
(D) Manual pressure

24.20 Match each of the following figures to a diagnosis (Fig. Q24-20 (1-6)):

(A) RP hematoma
(B) Thigh hematoma
(C) Rectus muscle hematoma
(D) Aortic dissection
(E) Coronary atrioventricular (AV) malformation
(F) Coronary perforation

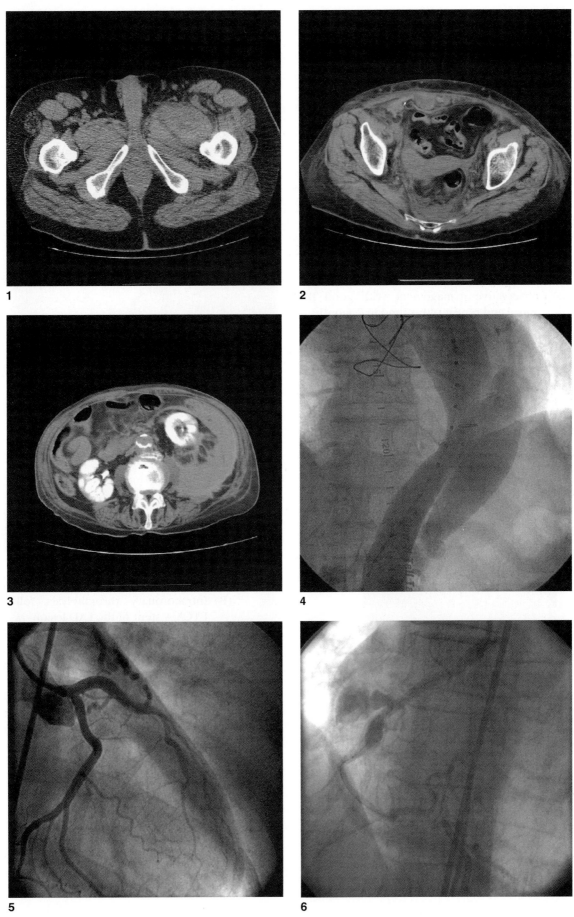

Figure Q24-20 (1-6)

24.21 A 63-year-old morbidly obese woman presents to your office for follow-up. She underwent successful uneventful PCI to RCA, which was complicated by the development of pseudoaneurysm. On initial duplex, it was measured at 2.5 cm. It was treated with ultrasound-guided thrombin injection. She underwent a repeat duplex study 2 months later, and the aneurysm has remained unchanged. However, she is asymptomatic. What are the appropriate therapeutic options at this time?

(A) Ultrasound-guided compression of the neck of the pseudoaneurysm
(B) Injection of the cavity of the pseudoaneurysm with procoagulant or embolization coils
(C) Surgery
(D) Conservative management with good BP control and repeat ultrasound in 2 months

24.22 The angiogram in Figure Q24-22 demonstrates which of the following abnormalities?

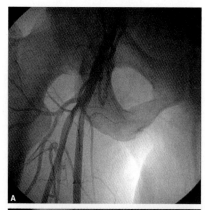

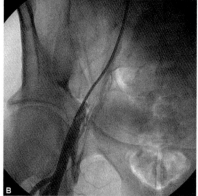

Figure Q24-22

(A) Iliac artery lesion
(B) Femoral artery dissection
(C) Postprocedural AV fistula
(D) Right groin mass
(E) Congenital AV malformation

24.23 A 75-year-old woman with HTN and hyperlipidemia was admitted to an outside hospital for an anterior wall MI 4 days ago. She was given thrombolytic therapy and was doing well until this morning when she developed shortness of breath (SOB). She has been transferred to your hospital, and a diagnostic angiogram was performed. The coronary angiogram showed TIMI 3 flow in LAD with 85% proximal lesion and small residual clots. The LV angiogram was performed, demonstrating an EF of 65% and no mitral regurgitation (Fig. Q24-23). The best course of action for the patient is to have:

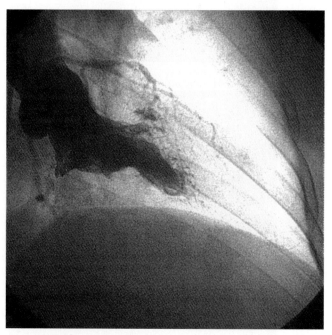

Figure Q24-23

(A) PTCA + stent of the residual LAD lesion
(B) Intracoronary thrombolysis, followed by PTCA + stent of the LAD lesion
(C) AngioJet procedure, followed by PTCA + stent of the LAD lesion
(D) Immediate Doppler echocardiogram and open heart surgery

24.24 The incidence of coronary perforation during coronary intervention is low. These preprocedural and postprocedural angiograms (Fig. Q24-24) demonstrate:

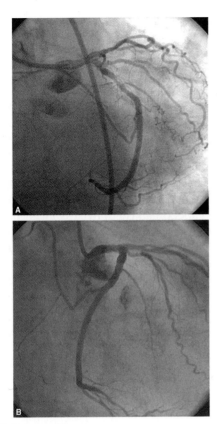

Figure Q24-24

(A) Type I coronary perforation

(B) Type II coronary perforation

(C) Type III coronary perforation

24.25 Which of the following options is NOT a correct choice to treat coronary perforation?

(A) Prolonged inflation of the balloon across the perforation

(B) Reverse anticoagulation, giving protamine 1 mg for each 100 units of heparin

(C) Reverse anticoagulation, giving protamine 0.1 mg for each 1,000 units of heparin

(D) Use of covered stent

(E) Use of coils to embolize leaking branch

(F) Pericardiocentesis

24.26 If a severe reaction to dye occurs, with which of the initial concentration of IV epinephrine can it be reversed before it is diluted further?

(A) 1 mL of 1:1,000 epinephrine

(B) 1 mL of 1:100,000 epinephrine

(C) 1 mL of 1:10,000 epinephrine

24.27 A 68-year-old man with history of CABG 10 years ago presents with chest pain. He is noted to have nonspecific ST changes, but his initial troponin is 2.0 ng/mL. He is brought to the cardiac catheterization laboratory. His angiograms are given in Figure Q24-27. He undergoes PCI to a diseased

SVG with embolic protection device. During the procedure after stent deployment, he has severe chest pain with ST elevation. An angiogram at that time is shown in Figure Q24-27. What would you do next?

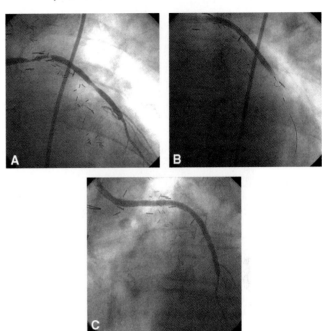

Figure Q24-27

(A) Capture and remove the filter device because it did not adequately capture the debris

(B) Capture and remove the filter device because it is full of debris

(C) Give intracoronary nitroglycerin (IC NTG)

(D) IVUS of the stent site because there might be a dissection

24.28 What is the most common cause of no reflow and CK elevation during SVG PCI?

(A) No reflow is primarily caused by intense vasospasm

(B) No reflow is caused by acute platelet aggregation

(C) No reflow is caused by particulate matter embolization from friable plaque and thrombus

(D) No reflow is completely preventable by using emboli protection device

24.29 A 24-year-old patient was admitted to the ER with severe chest pain and anterior wall ST elevation. The patient was "partying" and drinking alcohol and using cocaine all night long. The patient was taken to the catheterization laboratory, and the selective coronary angiogram showed severe mid-LAD lesion (Fig. Q24-29). What would you do next?

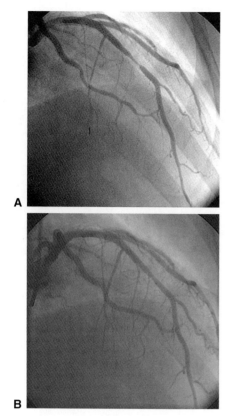

Figure Q24-29

(A) Heparin and GP IIb/IIIa inhibitor
(B) Angioplasty and stent
(C) IC NTG and repeat angiogram
(D) IV β-blockers

24.30 A 51-year-old man comes to your ER with severe chest pain for 2 hours. His past medical history is unremarkable except for hyperlipidemia. He is found to have ST elevation in the anterior leads and is taken to the catheterization laboratory, where he undergoes successful PCI to mid/distal LAD with 3.0/28 drug-eluting stent, heparin, and abciximab (ReoPro). His EF is 50%. He does well and is transferred to CCU. Two hours later, he becomes very short of breath and hypoxemic. He has hemoptysis, goes into respiratory distress, and is intubated. His chest x-ray shows alveolar infiltrates. What is the most likely cause of his SOB?

(A) Pulmonary hemorrhage from ReoPro
(B) Congestive heart failure
(C) LV rupture
(D) Papillary muscle rupture
(E) Aortic dissection

24.1 Answer C. The patient has mitral stenosis. For patients who have symptomatic mitral stenosis without contraindications, percutaneous balloon valvuloplasty is the treatment of choice. Watchful waiting and putting her on Holter monitoring with medical management would not help her.

24.2 Answer C. IVUS shows a dissection of the LAD. This was a spiral dissection that started in the proximal LAD and extended down to the distal portion.

24.3 Answer A. The result of the CLOSURE 1 trial, the first randomized controlled trial of patent foramen ovale (PFO) closure for stroke/transient ischemic attack (TIA) to reach completion, found no differences in the primary end point of stroke or TIA at 2 years, all-cause mortality at 30 days, and neurologic mortality between 31 days and 2 years.

24.4 Answer B. The figure is that of an Impella device that is placed across the aortic valve through a femoral artery site to pump blood from the left ventricle into the ascending aorta at 2.5 L/min.

24.5 Answer D. PROTECT II was a randomized, multicenter trial comparing the Impella system with an IABP in patients undergoing nonemergent high-risk PCIs. The primary end points were the composite rate of 10 major adverse events, including death, MI, stroke, or repeat revascularization within 20 to 40 days after the procedure; secondary end points were maximum chronic left ventricular pressure overload (CPO) decrease from baseline and the rate of in-hospital major events between the Impella and IABP. The company stopped the trial on December 6 after the data safety and monitoring committee reviewed halfway data because they felt that the study could not reach primary end point. However, the preliminary study shows no difference between IABP and Impella.

24.6 Answer C. Typically, CABG is performed as a rescue revascularization procedure to treat acute ischemia or infarction resulting from PCI-induced acute coronary occlusion. In the balloon angioplasty era, the rate of emergent CABG was 3.7%. However, in the stent era, the reported rate has been 0.45% (*Circulation* 2000;102:2945–2951).

24.7 Answer E. There is ostial left main coronary trunk stenosis with no reflux of dye.

24.8 Answer D. In the stent era, unstable angina, bailout stenting, small vessel diameter, long lesions, large plaque volume, residual uncovered dissection, slow flow or poor distal runoff, and suboptimal final procedural lumen have all been associated with abrupt vessel closure. Excessive tortuosity is a risk factor for abrupt vessel closure during balloon angioplasty but not stent thrombosis (*Textbook of interventional cardiology*, Chapter 13).

24.9 Answer D. Elevation of CK-MB over five times the normal baseline carries the same adverse impact on long-term prognosis as a Q-wave infarction (*Circulation* 1996;94:3369–3375; *Catheter Cardiovasc Interv* 2004;63:31–41; *J Am Coll Cardiol* 1999;34:672–673).

24.10 Answer E. The long-term prognostic significance of smaller postprocedural troponin T elevations is unknown. Therefore, there is no need to prolong hospitalization beyond what is necessary to document that troponin has peaked and has begun to fall. It is of note that one study suggests a postprocedural increase in troponin T of five times normal is predictive for adverse events at 6 years (*ACC/AHA 2005 Guideline Update*, 2006).

24.11 Answer C. Strokes are rare but devastating complications of cardiac interventions. The interventionalist should be familiar with potential etiologies, preventive strategies, and treatments for catheterization-related stroke and should develop the routine habit of speaking with the patient directly at the end of the procedure. If the patient is less alert, has slurred speech, and has visual, sensory, or motor symptoms, there should be a low threshold for performing a screening neurologic examination or obtaining an urgent stroke neurology consult. For most hemispheric events, an urgent carotid angiogram and neurovascular rescue should be considered (*Cathet Cardiovasc Diagn* 1998;44:412–414).

24.12 **Answer H.** Stroke related to contemporary PCI is associated with substantial increased mortality. Patients who suffer procedural stroke tend to be older, have lower LV EF and more diabetes, and experience a higher rate of intraprocedural complications necessitating emergency use of IABP. The in-hospital mortality and 1-year mortality are substantially higher in patients with stroke (*Circulation* 2002;106:86–91).

24.13 **Answer C.** The question of central nervous system embolic risk arises when it is necessary to perform catheterization on a patient with endocarditis of left-sided (aortic or mitral) heart valves. Although echo appearance of these vegetations looks friable and they can embolize spontaneously, left heart catheterization can be done safely in these patients. In a series of 35 patients with active endocarditis who had left heart catheterization, none had catheterization-induced embolic events. Patency is difficult to visualize with heavily calcified arteries with cardiac CT (*Am J Cardiol* 1979;44:1306–1310).

24.14 **Answer J.** Occult bleeding at the arterial entry site is the cause of this patient's hypotension. The patient needs to be stabilized first before being sent to CT scan or vascular laboratory (*J Am Coll Cardiol* 2005;45:363–368).

24.15 **Answer D.** This patient has acute femoral artery thrombosis. This is an emergency case that needs immediate surgery or PV intervention.

24.16 **Answer C.** Nerve complications following cardiac catheterization through the femoral route are rare. Although femoral nerve is most likely to be affected, lateral cutaneous nerve can also be affected (*Catheter Cardiovasc Interv* 2002;56:69–71).

24.17 **Answer C.** Arterial back wall puncture is the most common cause of RP hematoma (*Eur J Vasc Endovasc Surg* 1999;18:364–365).

24.18 **Answer E.** The angiogram shows external iliac artery perforation with dye extravasation.

24.19 **Answer C.** Bleeding from lacerated iliac artery could be fatal within a matter of minutes without catheter-based control of large bleeding. Therefore, immediate posterior tibial artery using contralateral approach is appropriate.

24.20 **Answer.** A-2, B-3, C-1, D-4, E-5, F-6.

24.21 **Answer C.** This aneurysm has been treated in the past and still persists after 2 months. Therefore, it should be operated (*J Vasc Surg* 1993;17:125–131, discussion 131–133; *Catheter Cardiovasc Interv* 2001;53:259–263; *J Vasc Surg* 1999;30:1052–1059).

24.22 **Answer C.** AV fistula is noted in the figure. Small AV fistulas are often monitored with ultrasound imaging. Indications for intervention are lack of spontaneous closure, increase in fistula size, and/or the development of symptoms.

24.23 **Answer D.** The LV angiogram demonstrates impending LV rupture (high anterior wall) with dye staining the fistula track in the LV wall. Echocardiography showed moderate pericardial effusion. The patient had an emergency surgery.

24.24 **Answer B.** The angiographic appearance of coronary perforations could be classified as: Type I—Extraluminal crater without extravasation, Type II—Pericardial and myocardial blush, and Type III—Dye extravasation (*Circulation* 1994;90:2725–2730).

24.25 **Answer C.** The current dose of protamine is 1 mg for each 100 units of heparin (*Am J Cardiol* 2002;90:1183–1186).

24.26 **Answer C.** Epinephrine of 0.5 to 1.0 mL of 1:10,000 administered intravenously over several minutes should be considered. This may be repeated at intervals of 5 to 10 minutes, preferably with cardiac monitoring because adverse effects of intravenous epinephrine may occur. In the setting of profound hypotension, a continuous infusion of epinephrine (5 to 15 μg/min) titrated to effect may be administered. If intravenous access cannot be obtained immediately, epinephrine (3 to 5 mL of 1:10,000 dilution of epinephrine) can be delivered through the endotracheal tube.

24.27 **Answer B.** The filter device is full of debris. Although it is possible that distal embolization occurred, if there was good apposition of the filter to the vessel wall throughout the case, it is less likely. Therefore, at this point, you can wire with another wire and capture and remove the emboli filter device. After the removal of filter wire, the angiogram shown in the figure was taken.

24.28 **Answer C.** The Saphenous Vein Graft Angioplasty Free of Emboli Randomized (SAFER) trial compared emboli protection device vs. conventional therapy in SVG PCI. The primary end point (a composite of death, MI, emergency bypass, or target lesion revascularization by 30 days) was observed in 16.5% assigned to the control group and 9.6% assigned to the embolic protection device ($p = 0.004$). This 42% relative reduction in major adverse cardiac events was driven by lower MI and no-reflow phenomenon in the emboli filter arm. This study demonstrated the importance of distal embolization in causing major adverse cardiac events and the value of embolic protection devices in preventing such complications (*Circulation* 2002;105:1285–1290; *J Am Coll Cardiol* 2002;40:1882–1888).

24.29 **Answer C.** The follow-up angiogram demonstrates the normal LAD lumen size, indicating the presence of cocaine-induced coronary spasm. An IV β-blocker would not be appropriate and may cause more spasm. Calcium channel blockers would be more appropriate.

24.30 **Answer A.** Pulmonary alveolar hemorrhage has been rarely reported during use of abciximab. This can present with any or all of the following in close association with ReoPro administration: Hypoxemia, alveolar infiltrates on chest x-ray, hemoptysis, or an unexplained drop in hemoglobin.

25

Qualitative and Quantitative Angiography

Raúl A. Schwartzman and Sorin J. Brener

QUESTIONS

25.1 Characteristics of type *non*-C lesions, as defined by ACC/AHA criteria, include all of the following, EXCEPT:

(A) Length > 20 mm
(B) Ostial location
(C) Moderate calcification
(D) Eccentric localization

25.2 Which of the following statements related to saphenous vein grafts (SVGs) is FALSE?

(A) The rate of embolic complications is related to both the degree of overall SVG degeneration as well as the length of the lesion
(B) Fifty percent of SVGs are occluded within 1 year after coronary bypass surgery
(C) Embolic protection devices may not be necessary for the treatment of in-stent restenosis
(D) Compared with balloon angioplasty, stents reduce restenosis rate

25.3 Predictive factors for stent thrombosis include all of the following, EXCEPT:

(A) Longer stent length
(B) Chronic kidney disease
(C) Reduced ejection fraction
(D) Greater final minimal lumen diameter (MLD) within the stent

25.4 Which of the following cases is expected to have the highest complication rate?

(A) Coronary perforation type II
(B) Coronary perforation type I
(C) Coronary perforation type III
(D) Coronary aneurysm

25.5 Stent thrombosis that occurs between 6 and 12 hours after the procedure is defined as:

(A) Hyperacute
(B) Acute
(C) Late
(D) Subacute

25.6 Restenosis after drug-eluting stent (DES) implantation is:

(A) More diffuse than after bare-metal stent (BMS) placement
(B) Equally distributed as after BMS implantation
(C) Less commonly seen at the margin of the stent
(D) Generally more focal than after BMS placement

25.7 All of the following are limitations of the TIMI flow classification, EXCEPT:

(A) Good correlation with mortality for STEMI patients
(B) Flow in reference artery(ies) may not be totally normal
(C) Categorical nature
(D) It does not evaluate myocardial perfusion

25.8 Which of the following describe the correct landmarks for TIMI frame count (TFC) assessment in the left anterior descending (LAD) and left circumflex (LCX) arteries respectively?

(A) LAD—"moustache" or fork at the apex

(B) LAD—last diagonal branch

(C) LCX—the most distal bifurcation of the segment with the longest total distance that includes the culprit lesion for the LCX

(D) LCX—end of most distal obtuse marginal branch

25.9 Advantages of corrected TFC (CTFC) over TIMI flow grades include:

(A) Lower interobserver variability

(B) Continuous nature

(C) Relationship with clinical outcomes

(D) All of the above

25.10 Choose the combination of values associated with the lowest risk for mortality after STEMI:

	TIMI Flow Grade	TIMI Myocardial Perfusion Grade (TMPG)
A	3	2
B	2	2
C	3	3
D	3	0/1

(A) A

(B) B

(C) C

(D) D

25.11 Which of the following can lead to erroneous quantitative coronary angiography (QCA) evaluation of coronary stenoses?

(A) Analyzing systolic frames

(B) Analyzing end-diastolic frames

(C) Analyzing two orthogonal views

(D) None of the above

25.12 Late luminal loss after DES implantation:

(A) Is defined as the difference in minimal luminal diameter between post-PCI and follow-up angiograms, and shows the distribution depicted in Figure Q25-12A)

(B) Does not differ from the distribution observed for BMS

(C) Is defined as the difference in luminal diameter between baseline and follow-up angiograms, and shows the distribution depicted in Figure 25-12B)

(D) Is defined as the change in minimal luminal diameter that occurs immediately after PCI

25.13 Choose the correct QCA-based statement regarding angiographic results after stent-based PCI compared with balloon angioplasty alone:

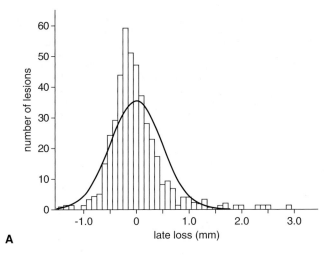

A

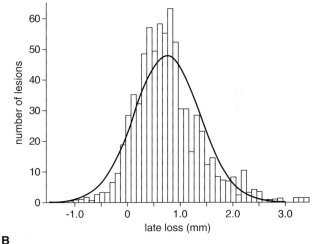

B

Figure Q25-12

(A) Residual lumen is smaller after stenting

(B) Stent placement leads to smaller amount of intimal hyperplasia and of late lumen loss

(C) Stents provide a net larger late lumen gain than balloon angioplasty

(D) Although residual lumen is larger after stenting, stents lead to a greater degree of late luminal loss

25.14 The TIMI myocardial perfusion (TMP) grade evaluates the quality of:

(A) Epicardial flow

(B) Myocardial flow

(C) Epicardial and myocardial flow

(D) Neither

25.15 Determination of the reference diameter (RD) in this right coronary artery (RCA) lesion (Fig. Q25-15) is best done at:

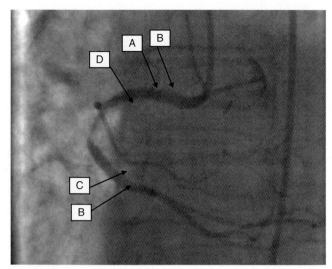

Figure Q25-15

(A) Point A (10 mm proximal to lesion)
(B) Points B (Two 10-mm segments without irregularities proximal and distal to lesion)
(C) C (10 mm distal to lesion)
(D) D (proximal shoulder of the lesion)

25.16 As compared with quantitative methods, visual estimation of diameter stenosis before PCI is:

(A) Greater
(B) Similar
(C) Lower
(D) Unpredictable

25.17 Compared with patients without progression of CAD, those who show angiographic progression by quantitative coronary analysis (QCA) have:

(A) Smaller plaque volume at baseline IVUS examination but significantly increased plaque volume over time
(B) Larger plaque volume at baseline IVUS examination without a significant increase in plaque volume over time
(C) Both greater plaque volume at baseline IVUS and significantly higher increases in plaque volume over time
(D) None of above

25.18 The Medina classification of bifurcation lesions is based on the severity and location of lesion in the proximal and distal segments of the parent vessel and the ostium of the side branch. Which of the bifurcations represented in Figure Q25-18 is (are) "true bifurcation lesions"?

(A)

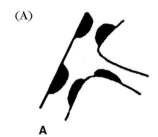

A

Figure Q25-18A

(B)

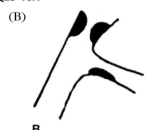

B

Figure Q25-18B

(C)

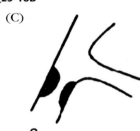

C

Figure Q25-18C

(D)

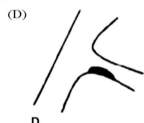

D

Figure Q25-18D

25.19 Which of the following pair of values is typical of TFCs in noninfarct arteries after reperfusion and in arteries examined during elective angiography?

(A) 45 and 28
(B) 35 and 28
(C) 21 and 21
(D) 31 and 21

25.20 All the definitions below describe restenosis after PCI, EXCEPT:

(A) Late loss ≥ 0.72 mm
(B) Loss of >50% of acute gain at follow-up
(C) Diameter stenosis >70% at follow-up
(D) Diameter stenosis >50% at follow-up

25.1 **Answer A.** The relation of lesion morphology to angioplasty outcome has been known for many years. The more complex the morphology, the less favorable the initial (and later) results of coronary angioplasty. Diffuse (>20-mm length), excessive tortuosity of proximal segment, extremely angulated segments (>90 degrees), total occlusion >3 months duration, inability to protect major side branches, and degenerated vein grafts with friable lesions are all characteristics of type C lesions (*J Am Coll Cardiol* 1988;12:529–545; *J Am Coll Cardiol* 1992;19:1641–1652).

25.2 **Answer B.** Despite the widespread use of aspirin, clopidogrel, and statins, graft failure after bypass surgery continues to be a major problem. The rate of SVG occlusion within a year after surgery is around 30%. In comparison, ITA graft failure is much lower than for vein grafts (around 8% at 1 year) (*JAMA* 2005;294:2446–2454). It is well established that the risk of 30-day MACE after percutaneous intervention in aortocoronary SVGs is increased in more diffusely diseased grafts and in bulkier lesions (*Am J Cardiol* 2005;95:173–177). As demonstrated in randomized clinical trials, the use of distal protection devices during stenting of stenotic SVGs has shown to significantly reduce major adverse events compared with stenting over a conventional angioplasty guidewire (*Circulation* 2002; 105:1285–1290; *J Am Coll Cardiol* 2002;40: 1882i–1888i). For patients who require SVG revascularization, bare-metal stenting reduces restenosis compared with balloon angioplasty. In one study of 454 patients, procedural success achieved by plain old balloon angioplasty (POBA) was 90% with a 5-year MACE-free survival of just 26%. In comparison, in a higher-risk, unselected population, utilizing DESs for percutaneous intervention of degenerate SVGs, MACE-free rate was 84% and TLR rate 5% at just over 1 year of follow-up (*J Invasive Cardiol* 2004;16: 230–233).

25.3 **Answer D.** Thrombotic events remain the primary cause of death after percutaneous coronary interventions. In a large cohort of consecutive patients undergoing DES implantation, premature discontinuation of antiplatelet therapy was the most important predictor of stent thrombosis after implantation. In addition, other key predictors of stent thrombosis were renal failure, bifurcation lesions, diabetes, low ejection fraction, and, for subacute thrombosis, stent length (*JAMA* 2005;293:2126–2130). In a pooled analysis of six multicenter RCTs and associated registries (6,186 patients treated with at least one coronary stent followed by dual antiplatelet therapy) the variables most significantly associated with the probability of stent thrombosis were persistent dissection NHLBI grade B or higher after stenting, total stent length, and a smaller final MLD within the stent (*Circulation* 2001;103:1967–1971).

25.4 **Answer C.** Coronary perforation during PCI occurs very infrequently. In contrast with type I (fully contained) and type II (limited extravasation), that rarely develop tamponade or result in ischemia, type III perforations (brisk extravasation) are associated with a high incidence of dramatic complications including abrupt tamponade, need for urgent bypass surgery, and a high mortality (up to 19% in the original multicenter report who evaluated this complication) (*Circulation* 1994;90:2725–2730).

25.5 **Answer B.** The Academic Research Consortium recommends temporal categories of acute stent thrombosis (0 to 24 hours after implantation), subacute stent thrombosis (>24 hours to 30 days after implantation), late (31 days to 1 year), and very late (>1 year) stent thrombosis. The purpose of this classification was to create consensus definitions for DES study end points to distinguish likely differences in the contribution of the various pathophysiological processes during each of these intervals. Acute or subacute (0 to 30 days) are frequently replaced by the term early stent thrombosis in numerous clinical trials (*Circulation* 2007;115:2344–2351).

25.6 **Answer D.** Compared with treatment using a BMS, treatment with DES reduces all angiographic parameters of restenosis in patients with complex native vessel disease. In a substudy of the SIRIUS trial, which used QCA to assess restenosis after sirolimus-eluting stent (SES) implantation in native coronaries, the authors reported that restenosis occurred at the stent margins in 64.5% of the cases, and that in 87% of the cases, restenosis was focal (*Circulation* 2004;110:3773–3780). An elegant study from the Netherlands that employed IVUS to analyze morphological patterns of restenosis after SES showed that in the vast majority of patients with in-stent restenosis, the lesion was very localized and bordered by segments with no evidence of neointima. IVUS identified stent discontinuity in 36% of cases suggesting that a decrease in local drug availability may have contributed to the development of restenosis in these cases (*Circulation* 2003;108:257–260).

25.7 **Answer A.** Almost two decades ago, the GUSTO trial demonstrated that the more rapid the restoration of flow through the infarct-related artery, the better the preservation of left ventricular systolic function and the survival (*N Engl J Med* 1993;329:1615–1622). Using the CTFC, in which the number of frames required for contrast material to reach standardized distal landmarks is counted. The TIMI group investigators demonstrated that AMI slows flow not only in the culprit artery, but also in the nonculprit ones by up to 45%. Although improved post-PTCA, both culprit and nonculprit artery flows were still 45% slower than normal (*J Am Coll Cardiol* 1999;34:974–982). The categorical, rather than continuous nature of the TIMI flow classification clearly limits its statistical power in clinical trials. The TMP grade is used to characterize the filling and clearance of the microcirculation, serving as an index of myocardial reperfusion (*Circulation* 2000;101:125–130).

25.8 **Answers A and C.** Two of the limitations of the TIMI flow grade are its subjective and categorical nature. The TFC was created to overcome those deficiencies and standardize the assessment of coronary flow. It consists of a simple, continuous measure of coronary flow in which the number of cine frames required for contrast material to reach standard distal coronary landmarks is determined. The first frame used for TIMI frame counting is the first frame in which dye fully enters the artery. This occurs when three criteria are met: (1) A column of nearly full or fully concentrated dye must extend across the entire width of the origin of the artery; (2) Dye must touch both borders of the origin of the artery; and (3) There must be antegrade motion to the dye. If the LAD is subselectively engaged and the LCX is the culprit vessel, the TFC begins

when the dye first touches both borders at the origin of the LCX. The same rule holds for subselective engagement of the LCX. The last frame is counted or included as one of the frames and is defined as the frame when dye first enters the distal landmark point. The standard distal landmarks are the first branch of the posterolateral artery for the RCA; the most distal bifurcation of the segment with the longest total distance that includes the culprit lesion for the LCX; and the distal bifurcation ("moustache' or "fork") in the LAD. Proper planning is essential for counting the number of cineframes required to first opacify the distal artery, particularly the LAD. The TFC of the LAD and circumflex arteries is often assessed best in either the right or left anterior oblique views with caudal angulation, and the RCA often is assessed best in the left anterior oblique projection with steep cranial angulation. Since the LAD is a longer artery, its frame counts are divided by 1.7 to derive the CTFC (*Circulation* 1996;93:879–888).

25.9 **Answer D.** There is a modest rate of agreement between an angiographic core laboratory and clinical centers in the assessment of TIMI grade 2 flow, which may limit the broad clinical applicability of this measure. In addition, a categorical variable such as TIMI flow grade limits its statistical power and sensitivity. For example, if new interventions achieve a higher incidence of TIMI grade 3 flow, a categorical scale may fail to distinguish their efficacies, because there is a range of dye velocities that constitute TIMI grade 3 flow. Therefore, even if two interventions result in the same proportion of TIMI grade 3 flow, there may be a difference in dye velocity between the two agents when analyzed as a continuous variable with the CTFC. Despite high rates of TIMI grade 3 flow reported in the literature, only a third of patients with an open artery actually achieve flow that is truly within the normal range (CTFC $\leq$ 27). In contrast to the conventional TIMI flow-grade system, it has been shown that the CTFC is a simple, reproducible, objective, and quantitative index of coronary flow that allows standardization of TIMI flow grades and facilitates comparisons of angiographic end points between trials (*Circulation* 1996;93:879–888).

25.10 **Answer C.** It has been demonstrated that impaired myocardial perfusion, graded with the TMP grade is related to a higher mortality after administration of thrombolytic drugs, independent of flow in the epicardial artery. Gibson et al. reported a mortality gradient across the TMP grades, with mortality being the lowest in those patients with TMP grade 3 (2.0%), intermediate in TMP grade 2 (4.4%), and highest in TMP grades 0 and 1 (6.0%; 3-way $p < 0.05$). Even among patients with TIMI grade 3 flow in the epicardial artery, the TMP grades allowed further risk stratification of 30-day mortality: 0.73% for TMP grade 3; 2.9% for TMP grade 2; 5.0% for TMP grade 0 or 1. Patients with both normal epicardial flow (TIMI grade 3 flow) and normal tissue level perfusion (TMP grade 3) have an extremely low risk of mortality (*Circulation* 2000;101:125–130).

25.11 Answer A. There are many potential sources for error in the quantitative assessment of the coronary arteries. Among others, frame selection is associated with substantial interobserver variability: the end-diastolic frame showing the sharpest and tightest view of the stenosis should be used (*Cathet Cardiovasc Diagn* 1993;29:314–321).

25.12 Answer A. The pattern of late lumen loss after DES implantation follows a peculiar behavior that differs from lesions treated with conventional stents. The distribution of late loss of DES is largely skewed to the left (i.e., most patients exhibit small amounts of late loss). In contrast, the pattern of late angiographic observed after bare stent implantation follows an almost-Gaussian distribution (*Circulation* 2004;110:3199–3205).

25.13 Answer C. Compared with POBA, coronary stents provide a superior residual lumen. Since stents may result in higher degree of late intimal hyperplasia and late luminal loss, the net balance is that stents lead to a net larger late lumen size (*J Am Coll Cardiol* 1993;21:15–25).

25.14 Answer B. There are two important methods for the determination of TMPG: the densitometric method (evaluates maximal density of contrast in region of interest) and the kinetic method (evaluates the speed of entry and exit of contrast in the area of interest). While epicardial flow is necessary for myocardial perfusion, it is not sufficient. Patients may experience TIMI 3 flow in the infarct-artery with poor myocardial perfusion due to destruction of the microcirculation or distal embolization of plaque and thrombus after reperfusion. Conversely, patients may have suboptimal TIMI flow (usually TIMI 2) in the infarct-artery with excellent myocardial perfusion. Rarely, even collateral flow may be sufficient to provide adequate myocardial perfusion (TMPG 2 or 3) (*Circulation* 1996;93:223–228; *Circulation* 2002;105:1909–1913; *Circulation* 1998;97:2302–2306).

25.15 Answer B. There are two methods to estimate RD at the point of maximal stenosis. The interpolation method uses a second-order polynomial equation to estimate the RD by tracking the arterial contour proximal and distal to the lesion. A second method uses an arithmetic average of the diameter of two 10-mm segments without obvious irregularities located equidistantly from the maximal stenosis (*Cathet Cardiovasc Diagn* 1992;25:110–131; *Cathet Cardiovasc Diagn* 1997;40:343–347).

25.16 Answer A. The degree of discrepancy between visual and quantitative evaluation of coronary lesions' severity should not be overlooked. For example, Fleming et al. have reported that for "moderately" severe lesions ranging from 40% to 60% stenosis, visual estimates were 30% higher than the measured percent diameter stenosis, with individual visual errors ranging up to 60% and unrelated to observer experience. When stenosis severity by visual and quantitative estimates from coronary angiograms were obtained before and after angioplasty, these authors demonstrated visual overestimation of lesions with ≥50% diameter stenosis, and underestimation of lesions with <50% diameter stenosis (*J Am Coll Cardiol* 1991;18:945–951).

25.17 Answer C. The relationships between atherosclerosis progression (or regression) as assessed by QCA and IVUS were evaluated in a substudy of the *Avasimibe and Progression of Coronary Lesions Assessed by Intravascular Ultrasound (A-PLUS)* trial, a multicenter placebo-controlled study of the acyl coenzyme A: cholesterol acyltransferase enzyme inhibitor avasimibe. The authors concluded that, although there is no correlation between changes in QCA measures and changes in plaque volume on IVUS as continuous variables, patients with angiographic progression have both greater plaque volume at baseline on IVUS and significantly higher increases in plaque volume over time compared with patients without angiographic progression (*Circulation* 2007;115:1851–1857).

25.18 **Answer A.** Type 1,1,1 is the most common cause of bifurcation lesions (45%) and is associated with the highest rate of branch compromise during PCI (15% to 20%) (*Rev Esp Cardiol* 2006;59:183).

25.19 **Answer D.** During the analysis of infarct-artery flow in reperfusion studies with fibrinolytic agents, it was observed that the flow in noninfarct arteries is slower (higher TFC) than the flow observed in patients undergoing elective angiography. This important observation strengthens the current paradigm claiming that during an acute coronary syndrome, systemic activation of platelets occurs and marked secretion of vasoactive substances leads to diffuse slowing of coronary flow (*Circulation* 1996;93:879–888; *J Am Coll Cardiol* 1999;34:974–982).

25.20 **Answer C.** Numerous definitions have been used to describe the response to arterial injury during PCI. Classically, binary restenosis has been defined as >50% stenosis at follow-up. The 0.72-mm cut-off point is derived from doubling the expected variability in serial angiographic studies. The 70% cut-off is better associated with recurrent angina, positive stress tests, or ischemia-driven revascularization (*J Am Coll Cardiol* 1992;19:258–266; *Circulation* 1985;71:280–288; *J Am Coll Cardiol* 1992;19:939–945).

26

Interventional Doppler and Pressure Monitoring

Morton J. Kern

QUESTIONS

26.1 A 65-year-old man presents with stable yet troublesome angina pectoris and anterior T-wave inversions without cardiac biomarker elevations. He has been treated with β-blockers, aspirin, and angiotensin converting enzyme inhibitors. He does not have diabetes mellitus. His angiogram shows severe left anterior descending (LAD) disease and intermediate and serial OM1 disease (Fig. Q26-1). The right coronary artery (RCA) has only luminal irregularities. Which of the following percutaneous coronary intervention (PCI) approaches is best supported by available studies?

(A) Proceed with PCI of all visible lesions
(B) Drug-eluting stent (DES) to LAD and bare-metal stent (BMS) to OM1
(C) DES to both LAD and OM1
(D) DES to LAD and fractional flow reserve (FFR) of OM1—proceed with stent if FFR < 0.80
(E) DES to LAD and intravascular ultrasound (IVUS) of OM1—proceed with stent if IVUS minimum lumen area (MLA) < 4.2 mm²

26.2 In assessing the physiology of a coronary artery narrowing, in which of the following relationships is the flow related to the pressure?

(A) Directly and linearly
(B) Directly and exponentially
(C) Inversely and linearly
(D) Indirectly and exponentially
(E) Indirectly and linearly

26.3 After stenting a proximal LAD in a 67-year-old diabetic woman as shown in Figure Q26-3, the distal FFR is still abnormal (FFR = 0.41). What is the best way to assess the final result of stenting in this patient?

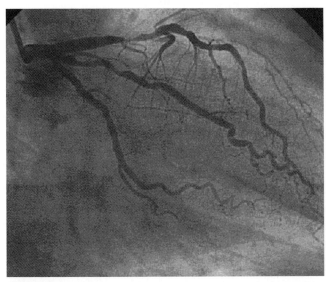

Figure Q26-1

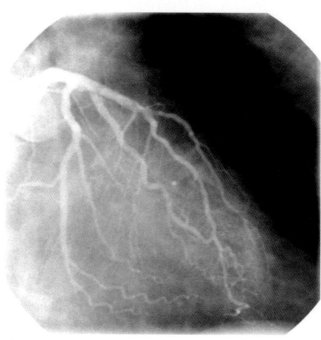

Figure Q26-3

(A) IVUS
(B) CFR
(C) FFR during pullback
(D) SPECT scanning
(E) RCFR

26.4 A 65-year-old woman has a RCA stent placed for acute inferior ST-elevation myocardial infarction (STEMI). She has an LAD lesion of 65% on angiography. She returns 4 weeks later for evaluation of the LAD and on stress testing demonstrates hypertension (200/105), dyspnea, nonsustained ventricular tachycardia (4 to 6 beats), and 2-mm ST-segment depression (left ventricular hypertrophy [LVH] on ECG at rest). The referring physician sends the patient to the catheterization laboratory before the radionuclide perfusion study result is available. Angiography shows the RCA stent to be patent, normal left ventricular (LV) function, and a 60% LAD lesion in only one view. The radionuclide perfusion images are normal. What is the best way to approach this patient?

(A) Place LAD stent
(B) Obtain true lateral image of LAD lesion then stent
(C) Stop procedure and repeat stress test
(D) FFR and place stent if abnormal
(E) IVUS and place LAD stent if cross-sectional area (CSA) < 4 mm²

26.5 A 42-year-old man returns to your catheterization laboratory for follow-up 3 years after cardiac transplantation. He is asymptomatic. Routine angiography is normal. The attending physician wants to evaluate his microcirculatory responses to a new antirejection drug. What is the best method to evaluate this agent?

(A) FFR
(B) RCFR
(C) CFR
(D) IVUS
(E) MRI

26.6 A 75-year-old man with progressive angina and positive stress testing undergoes catheterization and is found to have multivessel coronary artery disease (CAD): LAD 60%, circumflex (CFX) 80%, and RCA 90% with normal LV systolic function. Which of the following correctly states the case for the use of coronary physiology in this setting?

(A) FFR of the LAD alone is sufficient to assist in revascularization by PCI or coronary artery bypass grafting (CABG)
(B) FFR of all vessels provides information useful to the surgeon alone
(C) FFR of all vessels is unnecessary, proceed to CABG
(D) FFR of the LAD is not reliable in 3V CAD
(E) IVUS is preferable to FFR in patients with 3V CAD

26.7 A 60-year-old woman with diabetes mellitus has atypical chest pain and an equivocal stress echocardiographic examination. She smokes 1 pack/day. Her ECG is normal. Her weight is 285 lb. She is 5' 2". On angiography she has an intermediate stenosis shown in Figure Q26-7. Which is the best way to treat this lesion?

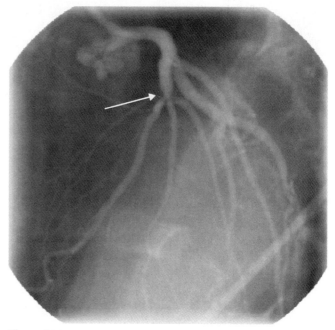

Figure Q26-7

(A) Rotablator

(B) Crush stenting

(C) Plain old balloon angioplasty

(D) Determine CFR for individual branches

(E) Determine FFR for individual branches

(F) CABG

26.8 A 69-year-old man had a STEMI 2 weeks ago and now comes to the catheterization laboratory with atypical chest pain. No risk stratification testing has been performed. The ECG shows evolutionary changes with small inferior Q waves and no dynamic or acute ECG changes. His physical examination is unremarkable with normal and stable BP and HR. In the catheterization laboratory, the LAD has a 65% narrowing, the CFX is nondominant and unobstructed, and the RCA has a 50% hazy-appearing lesion. Which of the following is an appropriate use of FFR?

(A) FFR of the RCA to determine necessity to stent

(B) FFR of the LAD only to determine necessity to stent at this sitting

(C) FFR of both the RCA and LAD to determine necessity to stent both in this sitting

(D) FFR of the LAD only to determine necessity to stent at another time

(E) FFR of both the RCA and LAD to determine necessity to stent both at another time

26.9 You have performed both FFR and CFR on an intermediate (60%) diameter narrowing in the LAD of a patient with hyperlipidemia. CFR was 1.7 and FFR was 0.88. What is the most likely explanation?

(A) The FFR overestimated lesion severity

(B) The FFR underestimated lesion severity

(C) There is a hyperdynamic response to pharmacologic hyperemia

(D) There is an impairment of the microcirculation

(E) The lesion is physiologically significant

26.10 A 49-year-old woman who received radiation therapy to the chest for Hodgkin's lymphoma >15 years ago complains of atypical chest pain. Her ECG shows normal sinus rhythm with nonspecific STT changes. The physical examination is normal; laboratory work is normal; and echocardiogram is normal. An exercise stress test shows equivocal small area of reperfusion. Coronary angiography shows a 40% to 50% left main in one projection only. Catheter damping is inconsistent during several angiograms. What is the preferred method of using FFR to assess the ostial LM lesion?

(A) Intracoronary (IC) bolus adenosine through the engaged guide catheter

(B) IV infusion adenosine, guide catheter engaged, with side holes

(C) IV infusion adenosine, guide catheter engaged, no side holes

(D) IV infusion adenosine, guide catheter disengaged

(E) IV bolus adenosine, guide catheter disengaged

26.11 Which of the following is the correct FFR calculation?

(A) P_a/P_d

(B) $P_a - P_{pcw}/P_d - P_{pcw}$

(C) P_a/P_v

(D) P_d/P_a

(E) $P_d - P_a$

26.12 Identify the following tracings labeled A, B, C, and D correctly (Fig. Q26-12):

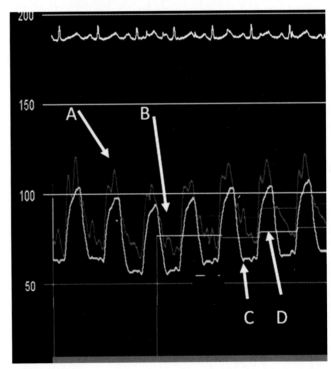

Figure Q26-12

(A) A = distal coronary systolic, B = distal diastolic, C = aortic systolic, D = mean diastolic pressure

(B) A = aortic systolic, B = mean aortic, C = distal coronary diastolic pressure, D = mean distal coronary pressure

(C) A = aortic mean, B = coronary mean, C = distal diastole, D = aortic diastole

(D) A = coronary mean, B = aortic mean, C = aortic diastole, D = coronary diastole

(E) A = aortic diastole, B = aortic mean, C = coronary diastolic, D = coronary mean

26.13 A 71-year-old man presents with STEMI involving the anterior leads. The ST segments normalize after initiation of heparin, aspirin, and eptifibatide. Urgent cardiac catheterization is refused, and the patient is treated medically for 4 days and then discharged. He returns with atypical chest complaints 2 weeks later and is taken to the catheterization lab where a 50% LAD lesion with thrombolysis in myocardial infarction 3 flow is seen and a small right ventricular marginal branch with a 95% narrowing. What is the next most appropriate step?

(A) Treat both lesions
(B) Complete angiography, discharge, obtain perfusion imaging, and treat later
(C) Defer PCI and treat with clopidogrel alone
(D) Defer PCI if FFR > 0.80
(E) Treat LAD empirically with PCI since it is too soon to use FFR after myocardial infarction (MI)

26.14 A 79-year-old man has atypical chest pain with exertional dyspnea. He has no CAD risk factors. No other medical problems or significant past surgical or medical history exists. A maximal exercise Cardiolite perfusion study is negative. Because of persistent chest pain at rest without ECG abnormalities, coronary angiography was performed and demonstrated a 50% LAD lesion and no other evidence of CAD. FFR is 0.88. Treatment with PCI is deferred. Aspirin, β-blockers, ACE, and statins are prescribed. What is the expected major adverse cardiovascular event (MACE) rate for this patient over the next 2 years?

(A) Unpredictable because CAD is highly variable
(B) Acute MI can be expected because this is an intermediate lesion
(C) Greater than 15% at 1 year
(D) 4%, the same as any patient with CAD
(E) 10%, twice the rate as patients with CAD

26.15 A 49-year-old woman presents with acute coronary syndrome (ACS) and is found to have a severe RCA lesion and mild disease in the LAD and CFX. She has insulin-requiring diabetes mellitus and hypertension that is controlled with lisinopril. She receives a 3.0- × 18-mm sirolimus-eluting stent, but the operator is not confident that the stent is adequately deployed by angiography. What is the best method to assure adequate deployment and reduce chances of subacute thrombosis?

(A) Quantitative coronary analysis (QCA) in multiple projections visualizing step up and step down
(B) CFR
(C) FFR
(D) IVUS
(E) None of the above

26.16 Your patient undergoes CABG surgery for three-vessel CAD. The LAD had a 65% narrowing with FFR 0.86, the CFX an 80%, FFR 0.72 and the RCA 95%, FFR 0.70. LV wall motion was severely hypokinetic inferiorly. Which of the grafts has a 25% likelihood of being occluded at the end of 1 year?

(A) LAD alone
(B) CFX alone
(C) RCA alone
(D) RCA and CFX
(E) RCA, CFX, and LAD

26.17 CFR by Doppler is no longer used as a reliable indicator of lesion significance. Which of the following explains this?

(A) The wire was too stiff
(B) An abnormal CVR did not necessarily mean that the lesion was flow limiting
(C) Doppler intervention was too difficult to use by the average interventionalist
(D) Pharmacologic hyperemia was unreliable compared to exercise
(E) The Doppler signal did not reflect volumetric flow

26.18 A 42-year-old woman has a chest pain syndrome and is evaluated for CAD and microvascular angina. This patient has a family history of CAD, migraine headaches, and treated hyperlipidemia. Coronary angiography shows a 40% eccentric RCA stenosis. The results of her physiologic studies are shown in Figure Q26-18. Based on these findings, what can be concluded?

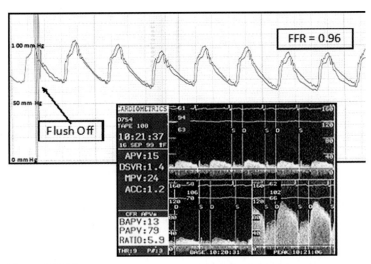

Figure Q26-18

(A) This patient has significant microvascular disease accounting for chest pain
(B) This patient has significant epicardial coronary disease accounting for chest pain
(C) This patient has impaired coronary flow reserve and normal FFR
(D) This patient has combined abnormalities of CFR and FFR
(E) This patient has a noncardiac cause of chest pain

26.19 A 73-year-old man has atypical chest pain and undergoes coronary angiography. He is treated for hypertension, hyperlipidemia, and diabetes mellitus. The left coronary angiogram shows mild irregularities with no diameter narrowing >40%. The RCA angiogram is shown in Figure Q26-19A. The cardiologist performs an FFR which is shown in Figure Q26-19B. What would be the appropriate approach?

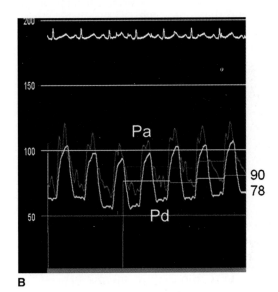

B
Figure Q26-19B

(A) Stent the RCA because the angiogram underestimates the severity of the lesion in a symptomatic patient with an erroneous FFR in a patient with diabetes
(B) Stent the RCA because the FFR is abnormal
(C) Treat medically because this is severe single-vessel disease without ischemia
(D) Treat medically because this patient has diabetes and the symptom presentation is not reliable. Furthermore, the FFR is in the nonischemic range
(E) Stent this RCA to prevent future MIs because this is a vulnerable plaque

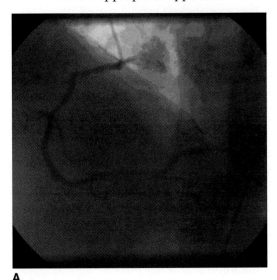

A
Figure Q26-19A

26.20 Which of the following BEST states the rationale for use of in-laboratory coronary physiology to assess stenoses?

(A) Chest pain is an unreliable indication of ischemia

(B) The use of stress testing has a low specificity and sensitivity

(C) The angiogram cannot provide enough information to determine flow for diameter stenosis in the 40% to 70% range

(D) CAD is often diffuse, obscuring the degree of focal atherosclerosis

(E) IVUS imaging shows plaque distribution and flow limitations

26.21 A 61-year-old man has intermediately severe LAD disease, and the FFR is measured. During pullback across the lesion, the FFR changes from abnormal to normal as shown in Figure Q26-21. What would you do to ensure this is a CORRECT value?

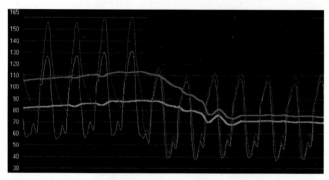

Figure Q26-21

(A) Repeat pullback with higher adenosine dose

(B) Check IV infusion pump for delivery of adenosine

(C) Use side hole guide catheter and repeat pullback

(D) Change to 8-F guide catheter for better signal fidelity

(E) Continue IV adenosine and remove guide catheter from ostium

26.22 A 59-year-old man presents with chest pain at rest and LVH with nonspecific ST-T wave changes. Troponins are negative. Coronary angiography demonstrates a 50% to 60% narrowing of the LAD. What is the role of FFR/CVR in this setting?

(A) FFR with pullback is most accurate to define the lesion

(B) IVUS will better define the need to intervene

(C) FFR will indicate whether to proceed with intervention

(D) CVR is better than FFR to assess a lesion in the ACS

(E) Neither FFR nor CVR is indicated in ACS

26.23 Coronary blood flow across a stenosis is reduced because of resistance. Factors producing resistance to flow are shown in Figure Q26-23. Which of the following factors is used to assess lesion significance by IVUS?

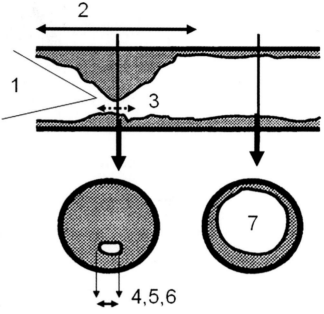

Figure Q26-23

(A) Entrance Angle (1) and disease length (2)

(B) Eccentricity (4) and reference diameter (7)

(C) Minimal lumen area (5) and minimal lumen diameter (6)

(D) Lesion length (3)

(E) Lesion length (3) and minimal lumen diameter (6)

26.24 Based on Figure Q26-23, what factors BEST explain the discrepancy between IVUS findings and FFR for determination of lesion significance?

(A) Entrance angle (1) and disease length (2)

(B) Lesion length (3), eccentricity (4), and reference diameter (7)

(C) Minimal lumen area (5) and minimal lumen diameter (6)

(D) Lesion length (3) and minimal lumen diameter (6)

26.25 Myocardial oxygen demand is balanced by oxygen supply. Which of the following is NOT involved in increasing myocardial oxygen demand?

(A) Myocardial contractility

(B) Systolic pressure

(C) LV end diastolic dimension

(D) Diastolic relaxation

(E) R-R interval

26.1 **Answer D.** The LAD lesion is severe and associated with angina and ECG changes. Stenting the LAD is Class I indication to treat without ancillary assessment. The OM1 has serial intermediate lesions and does not justify treatment without evidence of ischemia (IIa recommendation). FFR should be performed, and if <0.80, proceed to treat according to FAME and DEFER studies. IVUS cannot fully assess lesion for flow limitation, and according to FFR/IVUS comparison study (Takagi A, Tsurumi Y, Ishii Y, et al. *Circulation* 1999;100:250–255), lesions with >4.0 mm² MLA had negative FFR values.

26.2 **Answer E.** Flow is related to pressure directly in relationship to viscous friction and exponentially in terms of the separation coefficient. Overall the pressure–flow relationship is curvilinear and approximately exponential.

26.3 **Answer C.** FFR during pullback will show the physiologic impact of the entire artery and any focal lesions as well as the effect of flow immediately distal to stent (Fig. A26-3). CFR will be abnormal in diffuse disease and diabetics with microvascular impairment. IVUS will show diffuse disease but not specific lesions in a diffuse disease vessel. SPECT scanning will likely be abnormal but not helpful in diffuse disease. RCFR may be helpful but not for diffuse disease.

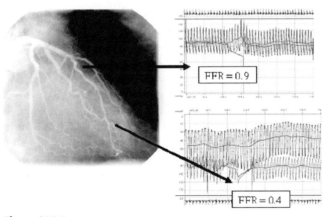

Figure A26-3

26.4 **Answer D.** FFR and stent if abnormal. The FFR turned out to be 0.89 × 2 with 50, 60 μg IC adenosine. The correspondence between radionuclide stress and FFR is good. ST-segment changes on exercise tolerance test with an abnormal resting ECG are unreliable. VT is not specific in this setting, and symptoms of dyspnea with uncontrolled hypertension are likewise not specific for ischemia.

26.5 **Answer C.** CFR measures both conduit and microvascular bed flow. FFR is only useful when there is a lesion in a vessel. RCFR would also give information about the bed but only relative comparison. IVUS is an anatomic tool without physiologic information. MRI is not yet widely available to test coronary flow and reserve.

26.6 **Answer A.** FFR is useful to identify which vessels have hemodynamically significant lesions. If FFR of the LAD is abnormal, CABG > PCI for revascularization strategies is suggested, whereas if FFR of the LAD is normal, PCI of the CFX and RCA is preferred. FFR can be used in multivessel disease, and it is superior to IVUS for physiologic decisions. IVUS is mainly indicated for anatomic information.

26.7 **Answer E.** Because of the high risk and complex lesion characteristics, determination of ischemic potential is needed. No percutaneous intervention is optimal for trifurcation lesions. CFR is not lesion specific. FFR for each branch will identify which, if any, narrowing needs to be treated. FFR for each branch in this patient was 0.90, 0.91, and 0.90. No intervention was performed. GERD was treated successfully.

26.8 **Answer C.** This patient is stable after his infarction and several weeks away from the acute event. DeBruyne et al. found that the correlation between FFR and SPECT 2-methoxyisobutylisonitrile scanning for ischemia was high with a threshold value of approximately 0.80. In this patient, FFR can be used for both the RCA and LAD to identify the correlation to ischemia and for selection of revascularization on that basis. One might also stage the procedure and do only one of the two lesions, but at this time after the acute event, most operators would intervene on both lesions in one setting.

26.9 **Answer D.** Assuming that the technique of FFR and CFR was correctly performed, the FFR

299

accurately reflects the ischemic potential of the epicardial narrowing. The CFR reflects the status of both the epicardial conduit and the microvascular bed. Thus, the CFR is not a lesion-specific measurement, and in the presence of a near-normal FFR, it is a measure of microvascular disease.

26.10 **Answer D.** IV infusion adenosine, guide catheter disengaged. Obstruction of the presumed ostial lesion by the guide catheter will give a false high-pressure gradient and low FFR. Disengaging the guide is a key maneuver. Side holes may produce some relief of the obstruction but may create a stenosis of lesser magnitude. IC bolus and quick withdrawal of the guide catheter have been used but are more difficult and less reliable than an IV adenosine infusion of 140 μg/kg/min. IV bolus adenosine is not used for FFR.

26.11 **Answer D.** The full correct calculation of FFR is P_d-P_v/P_a-P_v, but for most clinical settings, P_v is negligible compared to P_a. Pcw is pulmonary capillary wedge pressure and has no role in the FFR calculation.

26.12 **Answer B.** The phasic tracings of aortic pressure on top of coronary pressure below are labeled with the aortic systolic peak and mean A and B and distal coronary diastolic and mean C and D. FFR = D/B = P_d/P_a (Fig. A26-12).

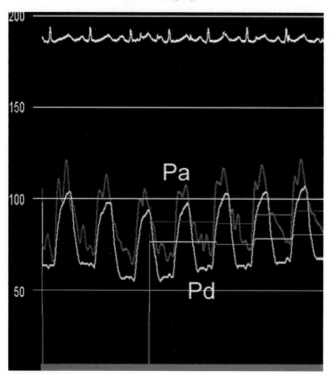

Figure A26-12

26.13 **Answer D.** A normal fractional flow reserve is indicative of reversal of myocardial perfusion defects in patients with prior MI. De Bruyne et al. examined FFR in 57 patients who had sustained an MI more than 6 days prior to investigation (*Circulation* 2001;104:157–162). Sensitivity and specificity of an FFR of 0.75 to detect abnormal scintigraphic imaging were 82 and 87 percent, respectively; the concordance between FFR and scintigraphy was 85 percent ($p < 0.001$). Excluding false-positive and negative studies, the corresponding values increased to 87, 100, and 94 percent respectively ($p < 0.001$). Patients with positive scintigraphic imaging before PCI had lower FFRs than patients with negative imaging (0.52 ± 0.18 vs. 0.67 ± 0.16, $p < 0.008$) and had significantly higher ejection fraction (63 ± 10 percent vs. 52 ± 10 percent, $p < 0.0009$). An FFR > 0.75 distinguished patients after MI with negative scintigraphic imaging. Similar findings relating FFR of infarct-related arteries in patients early after MI to reversible perfusion defects by SPECT scanning and myocardial contrast echocardiography has been reported by Samady H et al. (*J Am Coll Cardiol* 2006;47;2187–2193).

26.14 **Answer D.** Deferring PCI in patients with stable angina or atypical chest pain with normal FFR yields an excellent, low 2-year MACE. Patients with stable CAD have an event rate of 4% per year. MI has not been demonstrated in stable lesions undergoing FFR and is being followed up. CAD is highly variable but should be controllable with treatment and is associated with a low event rate.

26.15 **Answer D.** The question raised by the adequacy of stent deployment is anatomic. Are the struts fully apposed to the vessel wall? This question can only be answered by IVUS or OCT. QCA failed to define the stent and wall interface. FFR provides information that flow is normalized but not how much the lumen is open— only that it is open to permit good flow. There is no information on full strut deployment by FFR. CFR after stenting may be impaired despite full apposition due to the variability of factors producing CFR.

26.16 **Answer A.** Coronary stenoses with <50% narrowing by angiography or an FFR > 0.80 have a 20% to 25% chance of graft occlusion at 1-year follow-up (Fig. A26-16) (*Ann Thorac Surg* 2007;83:2093–2097).

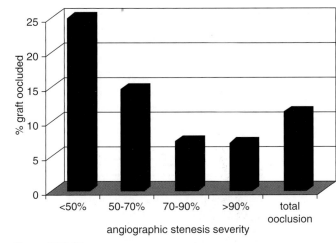

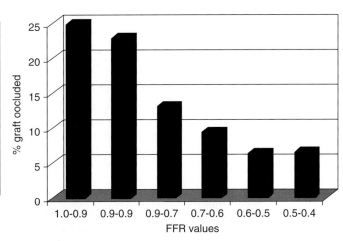

Figure A26-16

26.17 **Answer B.** CVR, although difficult at times to some operators and laboratories, was only useful if normal. If abnormal, CVR did not differentiate between flow impairment due to a stenosis or abnormal microvascular circulation. The technical aspects of the Doppler wire could easily be overcome, and pharmacologic hyperemia is as reliable as exercise for ischemic induction. CFR is a combined measure of the capacity of the major resistance components (the epicardial coronary artery and supplied vascular bed), to achieve maximal blood flow in response to hyperemic stimulation. A normal CFR implies that both the epicardial and minimally achievable microvascular bed resistances are low and normal. However, when abnormal, CFR does not indicate which component is affected, a fact limiting the clinical applicability of this measurement.

26.18 **Answer E.** The chest pain complaint is associated with a completely normal FFR (0.96, top panel) and normal CFR (Ratio 5.9, shown on lower IC Doppler tracing. The Doppler panel shows continuous flow at top half of signals and the bottom 2 panels show basal flow on left and peak hyperemic flow on right. The ratio of average peak velocity (APV) at base (BAPV = 13 cm/s) to peak (PAPV = 79 cm/s) produces the CFR ratio (Ratio = 5.9). This patient has no epicardial obstruction and no abnormalities of the coronary microvasculature.

26.19 **Answer D.** This patient has CAD with three risk factors. The angiographic appearance of the RCA is not severe, and treatment decision for stent should include assessment of ischemia by stress testing or other objective evidence of ischemia (e.g., FFR). Stenting with ischemia is class I recommendation for appropriateness. The FFR is

0.86 (78/90) and therefore nonischemic. The FFR is not influenced by diabetes or changing hemodynamics. Single-vessel CAD can be treated medically, but if ischemia is present, outcomes regarding symptoms and medication use are better with PCI (Courage Trial). Typical angina symptoms may not occur in patients with diabetes. Stenting for presumed vulnerable plaques is not justified at this time based on available data.

26.20 **Answer C.** While it is true that stress testing has a highly variable sensitivity and specificity depending on the test, the study population, and incidence of CAD, the rationale for in-laboratory physiology is that the angiogram for intermediate lesions cannot predict which lesions will or will not produce ischemia by whatever measures are used for testing. It is also true that chest pain syndromes are not specific, but the patient still has to have a coronary narrowing to require further testing. IVUS shows diffuse disease and its distribution but does not directly give a picture of flow responses in a single cross-sectional image. Coronary angiography produces a silhouette image and can neither identify intraluminal detail nor provide the angiographer with information about the characteristics of the vessel wall. Furthermore, the accurate identification of both the normal and diseased vessel segments is complicated by diffuse disease as well as angiographic artifacts of contrast streaming, image foreshortening, or calcification. Bifurcation or ostial lesion locations may be obscured by overlapping branch segments. Even with numerous angiographic angulations to reveal the lesion in its best view, the physiologic significance of a coronary stenosis, especially for an intermediately severe luminal narrowing (approximately 40% to 70% diameter narrowing), cannot be accurately determined.

26.21   **Answer E.** This tracing shows that the guide catheter was pulled into the ostium and obstructed the opening, producing a damped (ventricularized) pressure wave. This is not related to adenosine and should be repeated with the guide unseated. Side hole guide catheters also result in suboptimal signal because of pseudo gradient through the side hole into the ostium. The doses of adenosine are shown in Figure A26-21.

	Adenosine	Adenosine	Papaverine
Route	IV	IC	IC
Dosage	140 mcg/kg/min	30-60 mcg LCA 20-30 mcg RCA	15 mg LCA 10 mg RCA
T 1/2	1 – 2 min	30-60 sec	2 min
Time to max	≤1 – 2 min	5-10 sec	30 - 60 sec
Advantage	Gold Standard	Short action	Short action
Disadvantage	↓BP by 10-15%, Chest burning	AV delay, ↓BP	Torsades, severe ↓BP

Figure A26-21

26.22   **Answer E.** Neither FFR nor CVR is indicated in ACS. The dynamic and rapidly changing status of the artery, microcirculation, and the patient precludes accurate use of FFR/CVR. This dynamic variability holds for the acute MI as well. No data exists for the ACS within the first 24 hours or for the acute MI before 6 days of the event.

26.23   **Answer C.** IVUS only uses one parameter of the stenosis morphology to produce a minimal cross-sectional area, which is correlated to functional significance by FFR. The CSA of 4 mm² was the cut-point for FFR < 0.75, but the scatter around this point was large.

26.24   **Answer B.** The pressure gradient across a stenosis is determined principally by the area of the stenosis(A_s), the length of the stenosis (l), the area of the normal reference vessel segment (A_n) by the following relationship (Fig. A26-24). (Q = flow, f1 and f2 are the coefficients of friction and separation derived from Poiseuille and Bernoulli equations.)

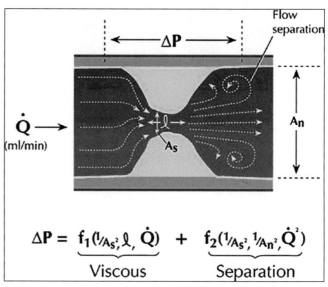

Figure A26-24

26.25   **Answer D.** Myocardial oxygen consumption (MVO_2) is directly related to contractility, LV wall stress, and frequency of contraction (HR or RR interval). LV wall stress is related to LV diameter and generated systolic pressure. Although diastolic function is energy consuming, it is not one of the major determinants of MVO_2. Myocardial ischemia results from an imbalance between the myocardial oxygen supply and demand. Coronary blood flow provides the needed oxygen supply for any given myocardial oxygen demand, and normally increases automatically from a resting level to a maximum level in response to increases in myocardial oxygen demand from exercise, neurohumoral, or pharmacologic hyperemic stimuli.

27 Intravascular Ultrasound

Khaled M. Ziada

QUESTIONS

27.1 Following an intravascular ultrasound (IVUS) imaging of a moderately diseased coronary artery (Fig. Q27-1A), offline measurements are performed (Fig. Q27-1B). All of the following statements about these measurements are true, EXCEPT:

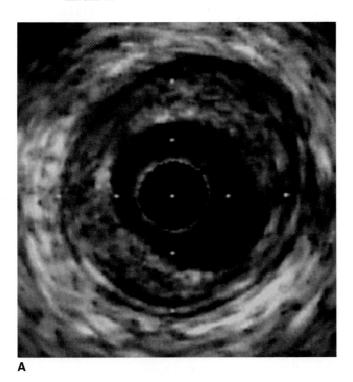

A

B

Figure Q27-1

(A) Line A traces the leading edge of the intima, defining the lumen area
(B) Line B traces the leading edge of the media, defining the vessel area
(C) Line C is the minimal luminal diameter in this cross section
(D) The difference between areas A and B represents the atheroma area
(E) Line D represents the minimal atheroma thickness

27.2 Following a difficult engagement of a large and mildly diseased right coronary artery (RCA), a subsequent angiogram reveals an extensive dissection (Fig. Q27-2A). Emergent bailout stenting is planned, and a guiding catheter is advanced to engage the RCA. The angioplasty wire is passed to the distal vessel with some difficulty. An IVUS catheter is then advanced over the wire to confirm its position. Figure Q27-2B is obtained from the mid and proximal RCA. The next best course of action is as follows:

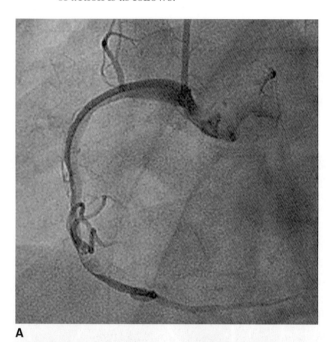

A

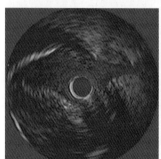 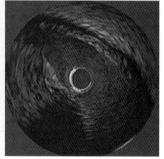

B

Figure Q27-2

(A) The wire should be removed and the procedure terminated
(B) The wire should remain in place; percutaneous transluminal coronary angioplasty (PTCA) and/or stenting should follow
(C) The wire should be removed, and another attempt at passing it in the true lumen should be performed
(D) The wire should remain in place, but another wire should be used to access the true lumen

27.3 Virtual histology (VH) is a technical advancement that allows for better characterization of coronary plaque morphology compared to standard grayscale IVUS imaging. Which of the following statements is NOT true regarding IVUS-derived virtual VH?

(A) VH technology is based on advanced frequency domain analysis of the radiofrequency backscatter of the ultrasound signals
(B) The color-coded display of the VH information allows for easier and faster interpretation of the information by operators
(C) Radiofrequency analysis is not reliable in distinguishing between lipid-laden plaque material and organizing thrombus
(D) The VH data superimposed on the cross-sectional image obtained by grayscale IVUS result in higher axial and lateral resolution

27.4 A physically active 66-year-old hypertensive patient is referred for coronary angiography because of typical angina precipitated by moderate exertion. In the catheterization laboratory, there is fluoroscopic evidence of calcification in the left main trunk. Right coronary angiography showed a severe focal lesion in the midsegment. Left coronary angiography revealed not only moderate disease in a marginal branch of the circumflex artery, but more importantly it also revealed ostial left main disease (Fig. Q27-4A). An IVUS imaging is then performed to better define the left main trunk disease. The minimal lumen area in the left main trunk was measured to be 7.4 mm² (Fig. Q27-4B). What is the most appropriate next step?

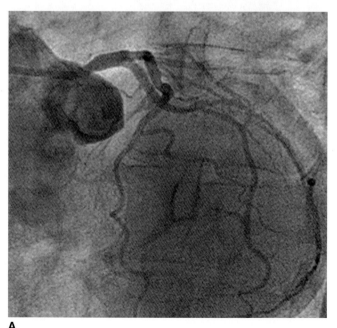

A

Figure Q27-4A

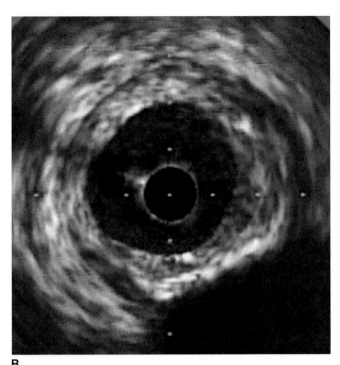

B

Figure Q27-4B

(A) Measure fractional flow reserve (FFR) distal to the left main stenosis

(B) Place an intraaortic balloon pump and arrange for three-vessel bypass surgery

(C) Consider right coronary angioplasty for symptom relief

(D) Reevaluate the patient with a pharmacologic nuclear stress test

27.5 Comparing an IVUS-guided with an angiography-guided bare-metal stent implantation strategy, which of the following statements is TRUE?

(A) In aggregate, the randomized trials comparing the two strategies demonstrated an advantage of IVUS guidance in reducing the rate of repeat revascularization

(B) The significantly higher acute gain seen in the angiography-guided stent implantation strategy was neutralized by the higher late loss seen at follow-up

(C) An angiography-guided strategy to stenting was associated with an increased number of balloons used per case

(D) The risk of subsequent myocardial infarction is significantly reduced with the use of an IVUS-guided strategy for stent implantation

(E) At 6 months, percent diameter stenosis is significantly smaller in the IVUS-guided strategy

27.6 A 70-year-old male patient with hypertension and hyperlipidemia presents with recurrent episodes of chest burning for several days. His electrocardiogram reveals T-wave inversion in leads V_3 through V_6 that resolve with the resolution of chest pain. His troponin I is 3.0, but the creatine kinase-MB is not elevated. Coronary angiography is performed: the right coronary angiogram is unremarkable, and the left coronary angiogram is seen in Figure Q27-6A. An IVUS imaging was then performed to better define the mid left anterior descending (LAD) segment. Figure Q27-6B and C demonstrate the representative images from the LAD at the level of the diagonal bifurcation and just proximal to the bifurcation, respectively. On a review of the angiograms and the IVUS images, which of the following statements would be considered as correct?

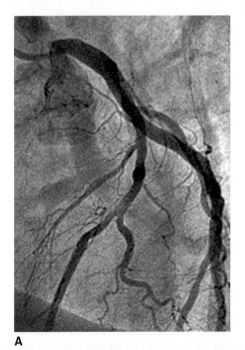

A

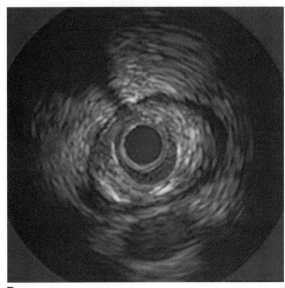

B

Figure Q27-6

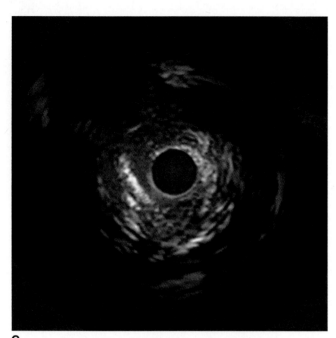

C

Figure Q27-6

- (A) The haziness of the mid LAD is caused by heavy calcification
- (B) An IVUS imaging did not provide an explanation for the angiographic haziness in the mid LAD
- (C) The clinical management of the patient will be influenced by the IVUS findings
- (D) FFR in the distal LAD will be ≥0.85
- (E) The patient is unlikely to develop more chest pain

27.7 IVUS imaging has been the primary imaging modality used in coronary atherosclerosis progression–regression trials of statin therapy in the last decade. All of the following statements regarding these trials are true, EXCEPT:

- (A) IVUS measures of atheroma volume (total or percent atheroma volume [TAV or PAV]) were the primary efficacy end points of these studies
- (B) The change in TAV or PAV was proportionate to the change in the low density lipoprotein (LDL) cholesterol level
- (C) These studies demonstrated an association between regression of disease and reduced adverse cardiac events
- (D) There was a significant reduction in the IVUS measures of atheroma volume with intensive or very intensive lipid lowering
- (E) There was evidence of progression in the IVUS measures of atheroma volume with moderate lipid lowering

27.8 Serial IVUS imaging of coronary lesions following the balloon angioplasty and atherectomy improved our understanding of the mechanisms of acute lumen gain and subsequent restenosis. Regarding these mechanisms, the following statement is TRUE:

- (A) At 6 months, the change in lumen area correlates more strongly with the change in the plaque area than with the change in the vessel area
- (B) The serial changes in the minimal luminal diameter seen by angiography correlate with the changes seen by IVUS imaging
- (C) At 1 month, the increase in vessel area is more significant in the nonrestenotic lesions compared with the restenotic lesions
- (D) Between 24 hours and 1 month after balloon angioplasty, there is significant adaptive remodeling
- (E) Between 1 month and 6 months, constrictive remodeling was less significant in restenotic lesions than in nonrestenotic lesions

27.9 Figure Q27-9 represents a longitudinal section of a severe focal coronary stenosis. Which of the following measurements are needed to calculate the remodeling index?

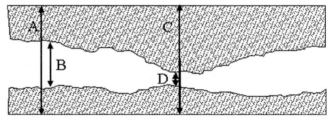

Figure Q27-9

- (A) A and B
- (B) C and D
- (C) A and C
- (D) B and D
- (E) A to D

27.10 A 52-year-old patient presented with angina on moderate exertion. On the treadmill, he stopped after 5.5 minutes because of chest pressure and 2-mm ST depression. A diagnostic angiogram of the left coronary system (Fig. Q27-10A) revealed a tight lesion in the major obtuse marginal branch of the circumflex artery. After deciding to proceed with percutaneous coronary intervention (PCI), a 6-F extra backup guiding catheter was selected. The catheter engagement was difficult, and the patient developed chest discomfort. Another angiogram was obtained just before passing the angioplasty wire (Fig. Q27-10B). IVUS imaging of the left main trunk was performed (Fig. Q27-10C). What is the most appropriate next step?

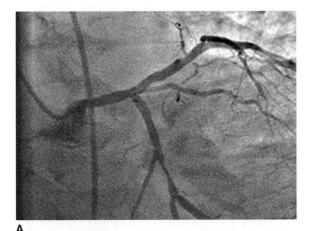

A

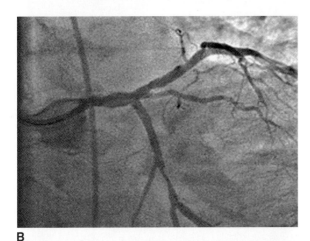

B

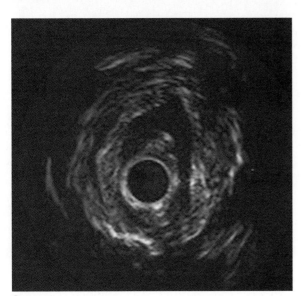

C

Figure Q27-10

(A) Abort the planned PCI, and schedule the patient to see a cardiac surgeon
(B) Abort the planned PCI, and consult with the cardiac surgeon in the laboratory
(C) Proceed with the planned PCI of the left circumflex artery
(D) Proceed with the planned PCI after inserting an intraaortic balloon pump

27.11 All of the following applications of IVUS imaging are appropriate, EXCEPT:

(A) Assessment of an angiographically hazy segment in the marginal branch of the circumflex artery after PTCA
(B) Measurement of the minimum lumen area and the adequacy of strut apposition after stenting the mid RCA
(C) Evaluation of an ostial LAD lesion considered for directional atherectomy
(D) Confirmation of the presence of atherosclerotic coronary disease in a patient with atypical symptoms whose angiograms reveal minimal disease
(E) Evaluation of a 40% to 50% ostial left main coronary artery lesion in a patient with class 2 to 3 angina

27.12 Which of the following images (Fig. Q27-12A–D) is obtained from the saphenous vein graft of a patient presenting with chest pain for the first time, 5 years after his bypass surgery?

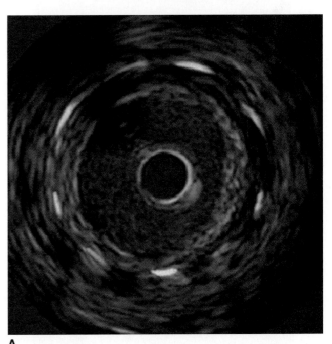

A

Figure Q27-12A

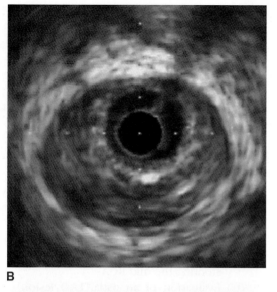

B

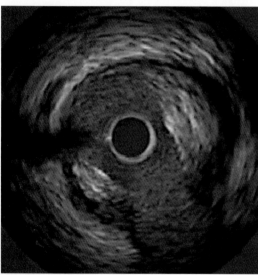

C

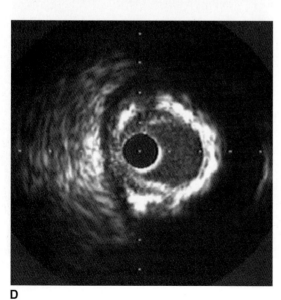

D

Figure Q27-12 (B-D)

27.13 A patient with typical angina is referred for coronary angiography after a nuclear stress test reveals an anterior reversible perfusion defect. The LAD angiograms reveal a 50% to 60% diameter stenosis in the midsegment (Fig. Q27-13A,B), though the other vessels contain only mild irregularities. An IVUS examination of the LAD is performed. The bottom left figure shows the section with the narrowest lumen (Fig. Q27-13C). The middle and right IVUS images represent more proximal LAD (Fig. Q27-13C). Which of the following conclusions about this patient is TRUE?

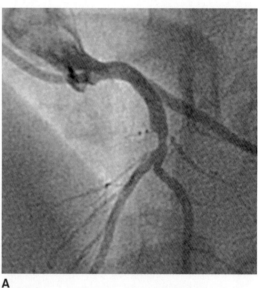

A

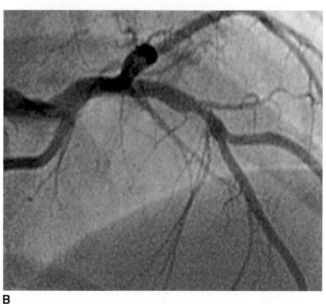

B

Figure Q27-13

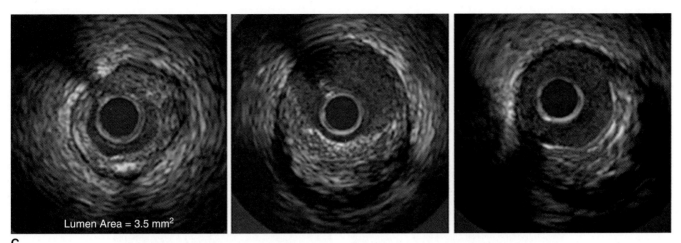

Lumen Area = 3.5 mm²

C

Figure Q27-13

(A) IVUS imaging did not explain the discrepancy between the angiogram and the result of the stress test
(B) The IVUS images explain why the stress test result was false positive
(C) An FFR of 0.70 would confirm the findings of the IVUS images
(D) The IVUS images are inconclusive because of the proximity of the diagonal branch

27.14 A patient is referred for PCI to a severe proximal LAD lesion. IVUS imaging is performed to evaluate the lesion and plan the intervention. A representative image from the diseased segment is shown in Figure Q27-14. On evaluating this lesion, which of the following statements would be considered TRUE?

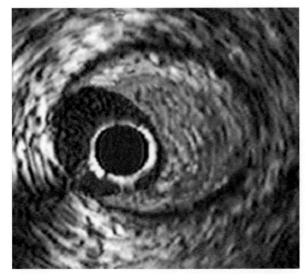

Figure Q27-14

(A) Directional atherectomy before stenting will result in greater acute lumen gain compared with direct stenting
(B) Adequate stent expansion cannot be achieved in this lesion without pretreatment with rotational atherectomy
(C) Because of the thrombotic nature of this lesion, aspiration thrombectomy is a reasonable alternate strategy
(D) In these lesions, ultrasound-guided debulking using directional or rotational atherectomy will reduce late lumen loss

27.15 All of the following statements regarding in-stent restenosis are correct, EXCEPT:
(A) Late lumen loss correlates strongly with tissue growth inside the stent
(B) Late lumen loss measured by IVUS correlates with angiographic late loss
(C) Negative remodeling is a major determinant of in-stent restenosis
(D) Late lumen loss is usually uniformly distributed along the stented segment
(E) Late lumen loss distal to the edge of the stent is most likely because of negative remodeling

27.16 IVUS imaging can be used to assess angiographically mild nonculprit lesions in patients undergoing coronary angiography for acute coronary syndromes. Figure Q27-16 represents four different nonculprit lesions. Assuming these lesions were not treated, which is more likely to result in an adverse cardiac event in the ensuing few years?

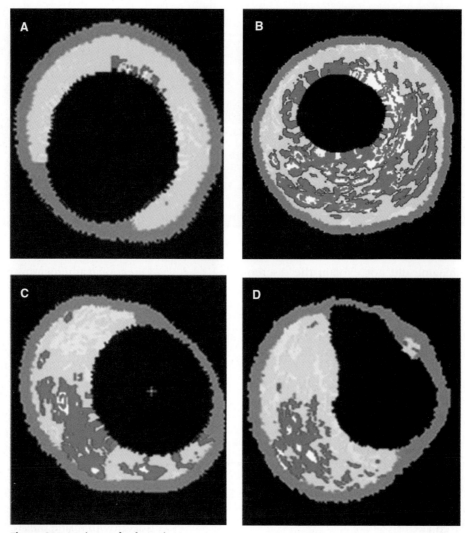

Figure Q27-16 (see color insert)

(A) Figure Q27-16A
(B) Figure Q27-16B
(C) Figure Q27-16C
(D) Figure Q27-16D

27.17 A 59-year-old patient presents with typical angina 8 months after undergoing primary angioplasty using a 33-mm-long sirolimus-eluting stent in the mid LAD in the setting of an acute anterolateral MI. The RCA and LCX are free of significant obstructions. The LAD angiogram is shown in Figure Q27-17A. IVUS imaging is performed; the image in Figure Q27-17B is obtained from the proximal

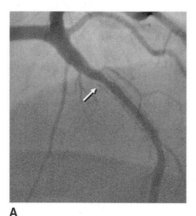

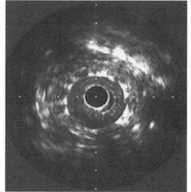

A   B

Figure Q27-17
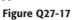

stent segment (see arrow). Which of the following statements is true regarding the IVUS findings?

(A) IVUS-defined diameter stenosis > 50% is commonly focal

(B) The diameter stenosis shown is primarily caused by intimal hyperplasia

(C) With drug-eluting stents of that length, IVUS-defined underexpansion is rare

(D) The mechanism of diameter stenosis is not related to the stent length

27.18 IVUS imaging is frequently used to assess the results of high-pressure stent deployment. Which of the following images of coronary stents is the LEAST likely to need the use of a larger balloon and/or higher inflation pressure (Fig. Q27-18A–D)?

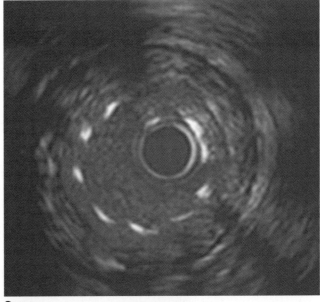

C

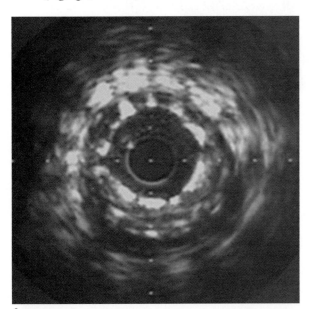

A

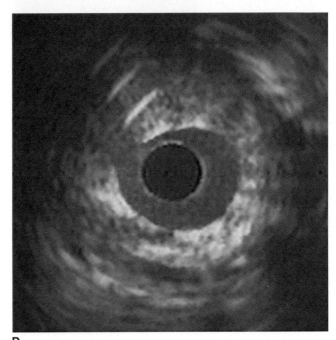

D

Figure Q27-18 (A-D)

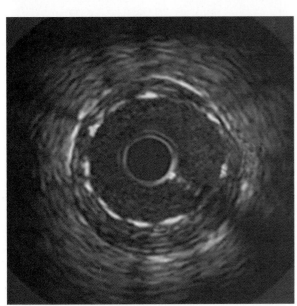

B

27.19 Which of the following IVUS findings is NOT associated with very late stent thrombosis after DES implantation?

(A) Longer stented segment

(B) Incomplete strut apposition

(C) Smaller reference segment vessel area

(D) Larger in-stent segment vessel area

27.20 A middle-aged hypertensive patient presents with atypical chest pain that is precipitated by effort and sometimes occurring at rest. Coronary angiography reveals slight luminal irregularities in the RCA and LCX arteries. A cranial projection shows an indeterminate lesion in the mid–distal LAD (Fig. Q27-20A). IVUS imaging is performed to evaluate the significance of the lesion and a representative image of the minimum lumen area is shown (Fig. Q27-20B). Which of the following statements is most accurate?

(A) IVUS findings suggest statin therapy is the most appropriate course of action

(B) The angiogram did not reveal the true severity of the lesion due to heavy calcification

(C) FFR across this lesion is most likely to be <0.75

(D) Percutaneous intervention on this lesion will reduce the risk of death or myocardial infarction

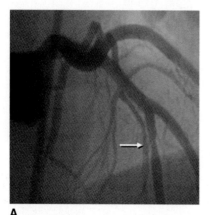
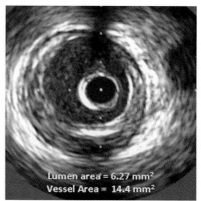

Lumen area = 6.27 mm²
Vessel Area = 14.4 mm²

A
B
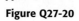

Figure Q27-20

27.1 **Answer B.** As a general rule, the measurements on ultrasound images are performed from the leading edge of an echo-dense layer to the leading edge of another echo-dense layer. The lumen area is defined as the area bound by the leading edge of the intima or the interface between the echo-dense intima and the echo-lucent blood elements in the lumen. The vessel area is the area bound by the external elastic membrane (EEM) that can be identified as the interface between the leading edge of the echo-dense adventitia and the echo-lucent medial layer (Line B on Figure Q27-1B). The difference between the lumen and EEM areas is the atheroma area. In fact, this area includes the atheroma and the thickness of the media. This has traditionally been accepted to avoid the inaccurate tracing around the trailing edge of the atheroma. In addition, the thickness of the medial layer is relatively unchanged by the presence or severity of disease. The minimum diameter between the lumen and the EEM tracings is measured to define the presence or the absence of disease (Line D on Figure Q27-1B). Several definitions have been used but, in general, a minimum diameter of 0.5 mm is considered abnormal. The minimum lumen diameter is the shortest line through the center point of the lumen (Line C on Figure Q27-1B) (*J Am Coll Cardiol* 2001;37:1478–1492; *Curr Probl Cardiol* 1999;24:541–566).

27.2 **Answer B.** In extensive coronary artery dissections, it is challenging to distinguish between the true and the false lumens. Usually this is the first most important step in bailout stenting, which is intended to restore flow in the true lumen and obliterate the false channel. Passage of the angioplasty wire in a side branch and injecting contrast through the distal tip of a balloon are some of the maneuvers used to confirm the position of the wire. However, this does not exclude the possibility of "fenestration" (i.e., that the wire passed from the false to the true lumens). An IVUS can assist in confirming the position of the wire before stenting. The two important features of the true lumen are the trilaminar appearance of the wall and the presence of side branches. Figure A27-2A shows a side branch (*arrow*) in continuity with the vessel lumen that is surrounding the

IVUS catheter, confirming the fact that the catheter is in a true lumen. Figure A27-2B reveals the characteristic trilaminar appearance (*arrows*) of the true lumen with an intra-arterial wall hematoma (*asterisk*) seen in the false lumen. These findings confirm the true lumen position of the wire, and proceeding with PTCA/stenting would be the appropriate next step.

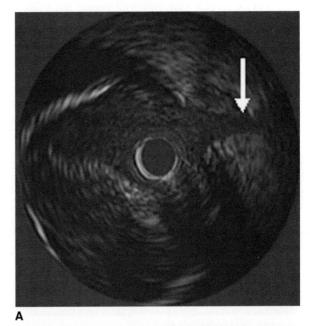

A

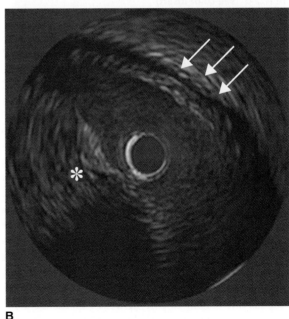

B

Figure A27-2

27.3   **Answer D.** IVUS-derived VH depends on advanced analysis of the radiofrequency backscatter of the ultrasound signal, using a larger number of parameters. Rather than just using the signal amplitude to define a shade of gray for each reflected line, this method utilizes a more complex mathematical autoregressive model to calculate the frequency spectrum from the region of interest (the coronary plaque) (*Circulation* 2002;106:2200–2206). The complex mathematical calculations do not lend themselves to quick interpretation by clinicians, hence the development of a simplified color-coded display (Fig. A27-3). Despite the improvement in differentiation between various tissue components of plaques, radiofrequency analysis remains unreliable in distinguishing between organizing thrombus and lipidic or soft plaques. The VH data provide incremental information from a more advanced analysis of the radiofrequency backscatter but do not directly influence the image resolution of the ultrasound image.

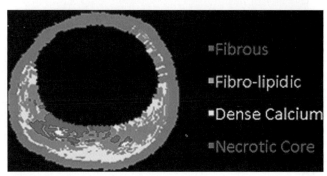

Figure A27-3 (see color insert)

27.4   **Answer C.** In the absence of a reference segment to compare with, defining stenosis severity can be difficult. This is true for all ostial lesions, particularly in cases of ostial left main disease. In addition to the angiographic appearance, the absence of backflow of contrast into the aortic cusp when the catheter is engaged is a worrisome sign that needs to be identified immediately. An additional clue is the pressure waveform, which is "ventricularized" or shows "dampening" if the catheter is obstructing flow into the ostial left main trunk. However, pressure dampening can occur in the absence of a severe obstruction if the catheter tip is directed toward and makes contact with the arterial wall. In most cases of suspicious left main lesions, an adjunctive modality is utilized to assess stenosis severity. This can be achieved by using a pressure wire and calculating the FFR or by an IVUS

imaging. Several studies have demonstrated the predictive value of the measurements obtained through either modality. An FFR ≥ 0.75 predicts a low risk of death or cardiac events in the ensuing 2 to 3 years on medical therapy alone. Similarly, when an IVUS left main lumen area ≥ 5.9 mm² is correlated with an FFR ≥ 0.75, both measures strongly predict an event-free survival over a 3-year period. Given the stable clinical presentation and the lumen area exceeding 7 mm², placing a balloon pump and sending the patient to surgery would not provide any clinical benefit compared with medical therapy alone. FFR measurement in equivocal left main stenosis is appropriate, and very useful in guiding therapy, but it would be redundant to perform both IVUS imaging and FFR measurement. With the availability of adjunctive modalities such as the pressure wire and IVUS imaging, the decision about hemodynamic significance of such lesions can be made in the catheterization laboratory (*Heart* 2001;86:547–552; *Circulation* 2004;110:2831–2836).

27.5   **Answer A.** There are several randomized trials that examined the role of IVUS guidance in bare-metal stenting in comparison to the standard angiography-guided approach. The majority of those studies demonstrated a trend favoring the IVUS-guided strategy in reducing the need for repeat revascularization, but most did not reach thresholds of statistical significance. However, a recent meta-analysis demonstrated that, in aggregate, an IVUS-guided strategy leads to larger acute lumen gain, less diameter reduction at follow-up, less angiographic restenosis, and less need for repeat revascularization (*Am J Cardiol* 2011;107:374–382). There was no conclusive evidence in any of the studies that the IVUS-guided strategy reduces the risk of myocardial infarction. In most studies, the IVUS-guided approach was associated with increased utilization of balloons and procedural time. Given the significantly lower risk of restenosis with drug-eluting stents, randomized studies addressing these questions will require much larger sample sizes and cost and thus are unlikely to ever be performed.

27.6   **Answer C.** On the basis of clinical and laboratory evidence, it is seen that this patient had sustained a myocardial infarction, probably a few days before presentation. The angiograms reveal an area of haziness in the mid LAD at the level of a diagonal bifurcation, although diameter reduction compared with the adjacent segments is not significant. Haziness could be the result of calcification of the arterial wall, but a more important differential diagnosis for haziness in this context would be plaque rupture and/or overlying intraluminal thrombosis (Fig. A27-6A,B). Another possibility is an eccentric lesion that is more severe than what the angiogram reveals in this projection. In these situations, an IVUS can be very helpful in making the diagnosis.

IVUS imaging of the mid-LAD segment revealed a large plaque burden (PB) with minimal calcification proximal to the diagonal bifurcation (Fig. A27-6A), but with a minimal lumen area of 3.4 mm², indicating a hemodynamically severe stenosis. At the level of the bifurcation (Fig. A27-6B), there is evidence of plaque rupture, with flow communication between the true LAD lumen (surrounding the IVUS catheter artifact) and the ulcerated plaque "underneath" the fibrocalcific cap (*arrow*). On the basis of these findings, percutaneous or surgical revascularization would be more appropriate than medical therapy. In acute myocardial infarction patients, the utility of FFR is not well studied, and with an area of 3.4 mm², one would expect the FFR to be <0.75. Given the severity of disease and the measured lumen area, it is likely that this patient will have postinfarction angina if the lesion is not treated (*Circulation* 1999;100:250–255; *Curr Probl Cardiol* 1999;24:541–566).

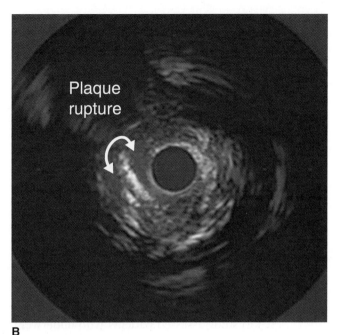

B

Figure A27-6B

27.7 **Answer C.** In the REVERSAL trial, patients were randomly assigned to receive a moderate lipid-lowering therapy of pravastatin 40 mg/d vs. a more intensive regimen of atorvastatin 80 mg/d. An IVUS assessment of a mildly diseased coronary segment was performed upon enrollment and after 18 months. The primary end point of the study was the percentage change in TAV, which was computed as

$$\frac{\text{TAV (follow - up)} \ \text{TAV (baseline)} \times 100}{\text{TAV (baseline)}}$$

The TAV was calculated as the sum of differences between EEM and lumen areas across all evaluable slices in the target segment. In the ASTEROID trial, a cohort of patients received 40 mg of rosuvastatin with IVUS imaging performed at baseline and after 24 months. The primary end point was change in PAV that was computed as

$$\left(\frac{\sum \left(\text{EEM}_{CSA} - \text{LUMEN}_{CSA} \right)}{\sum \text{EEM}_{CSA}} \right) \times 100$$

where EEM_{csa} is the EEM area and LUMEN_{csa} is the lumen area. For each patient, the change in PAV was computed as the difference between PAV at follow-up imaging and PAV at baseline imaging.

In the moderate lipid-lowering (pravastatin) group, there was a positive change in the TAV indicating net progression compared with

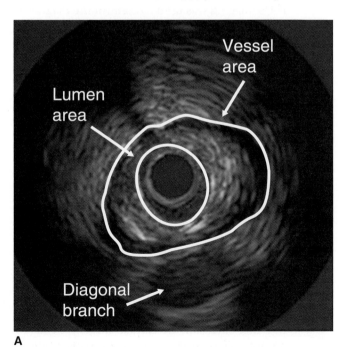

A

Figure A27-6A

baseline. In the intensive lipid-lowering (atorvastatin) arm, there was no evidence of progression in TAV compared with baseline. These findings suggested that intensive lipid lowering could result in arrest of disease progression. In the very intensive lipid-lowering (rosuvastatin) group, there was a significant reduction in PAV after 24 months of therapy, indicating regression of disease. Across all groups, there was a linear correlation between the change in measures of atheroma volume and the magnitude of reduction in LDL cholesterol. These studies were powered on the basis of the expected change in atheroma volume and did not enroll enough patients to detect differences in clinical outcomes (*JAMA* 2004;291:1071–1080; *JAMA* 2006;295:1556–1565).

27.8 Answer D. The serial ultrasound restenosis (SURE) study assessed patients who underwent coronary balloon angioplasty or atherectomy by serial angiographic and ultrasound examinations performed at preintervention, postintervention, 24-hour, 1-month, and 6-month follow-up. The serial examination of the treated lesion sites provided great insight into the remodeling responses and the mechanisms of late lumen loss or restenosis. Typically, lesions treated with PTCA or atherectomy undergo a biphasic remodeling response: A significant increase in vessel area between 24 hours and 1 month (adaptive remodeling) followed by a significant decrease (constrictive remodeling) between 1 and 6 months. At any point of time, the change in the vessel area (remodeling) was the most important determinant of the resultant lumen area. This correlation was much stronger than the correlation between changes in lumen area and those in plaque area. As for the mechanism of restenosis, the early adaptive remodeling response of the vessel was not different between lesions that did and did not develop restenosis, which meant that there was no apparent difference in vessel area at the 1-month time point. However, the constrictive remodeling response (between 1 and 6 months) was more significant in lesions that eventually developed restenosis compared with those that ended with a favorable outcome. In this study, IVUS imaging revealed a significant increase in lumen diameter between 24 hours and 1 month, which could not be identified by quantitative angiography (*Circulation* 1997;96:475–483).

27.9 Answer C. As initially described by Glagov et al. in a necropsy study, arterial remodeling is the

expansion of the EEM of the arterial wall at sites of atherosclerosis to accommodate atheroma volume and preserve lumen size. Stenoses develop when the ability of the artery to remodel is overcome by the progressive enlargement of the atheroma. This is known as *positive or adaptive remodeling*. Another form of arterial remodeling known as *negative (or constrictive) remodeling* is the local shrinkage of the vessel size at the site of disease, which has been implicated in the stenotic atherosclerotic lesions and restenosis after balloon angioplasty. The IVUS investigators examining the phenomenon of remodeling compare the lesion of interest with a proximal reference segment free of disease and express a "remodeling index," which is calculated as the ratio of the EEM area at the lesion site to the EEM area at the proximal reference site. A remodeling index of >1.05 is consistent with positive remodeling, <0.95 is consistent with negative remodeling, and 0.95 to 1.05 is consistent with absence of remodeling. A positively remodeled atheroma is usually larger in size and more likely to present with unstable coronary syndromes (*Circulation* 2000;101:598–603; *J Am Coll Cardiol* 2001;38:297–306).

27.10 Answer B. This is a case of left main trunk dissection on engagement with an extra backup guiding catheter. The clue to the diagnosis was the change in the angiographic appearance of the left main trunk after the difficult engagement, although the projection was identical. IVUS imaging was used to confirm the diagnosis. There are two false channels in Figure A27-10 (*arrows*), with the IVUS catheter artifact occupying the true lumen of the vessel. The false channels in cases of dissection and/or plaque rupture can be better visualized with saline or contrast injection while imaging, as this accentuates the difference in echo density between the lumen and the arterial wall structures. In addition, the injected fluid can be seen traveling from the true to the false lumen in real time. The left main coronary dissection requires urgent management. If the patient is hemodynamically stable or can be stabilized with the help of an intraaortic balloon pump, then urgent coronary bypass surgery is probably the treatment of choice. If the patient is considered too unstable (e.g., severe ongoing ischemia, hypotension, and/or life-threatening ventricular arrhythmia), emergent stenting of the left main may be an acceptable alternative. In either situation, the cardiac surgeon needs to be notified as soon as the diagnosis is made in the catheterization laboratory. Any elective PCI should be aborted and the situation should be managed immediately. A balloon pump would be helpful to support the patient's hemodynamics on the way to the surgery suite or if stenting of the left main trunk is considered, but not to support PCI of the circumflex artery.

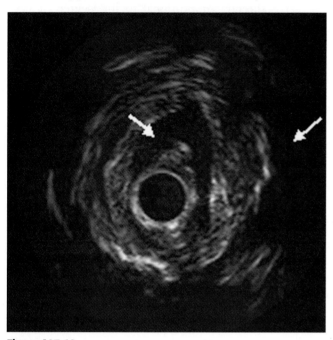

Figure A27-10

27.11   **Answer D.** IVUS imaging provides a detailed tomographic perspective of both the lumen and the wall of the artery. The IVUS findings frequently clarify and/or complement our understanding of the luminal silhouettes provided by contrast angiography. The American College of Cardiology/American Heart Association guidelines outline the clinical situations in which there is reasonable evidence for the benefit of IVUS imaging. These include assessment of the adequacy of stent deployment (measurement of the minimal in-stent lumen area and evaluating strut apposition), assessment of a suboptimal angiographic result after PTCA, determination of the mechanism of restenosis to enable appropriate management, evaluation of coronary anatomy at a location difficult to image angiographically, and the preinterventional assessment of the coronary calcium extent and distribution in which use of an atherectomy device is contemplated. IVUS imaging may also be considered in the assessment of coronary atherosclerosis in patients with both characteristic angina and positive functional study without a clear angiographic lesion. IVUS is also the gold standard for the accurate identification and quantification of cardiac allograft vasculopathy or transplant coronary disease. There is no role for IVUS when an angiographic diagnosis is clear and there is no planned intervention (*Circulation* 2006;113:156–175).

27.12   **Answer B.** Figure Q27-12A shows the struts of a slotted-tube stent, which are seen as bright ultrasound reflections around the circumference of the artery. The presence of a layer of echolucent tissue (distinct from the speckle of blood elements in lumen) is evidence of intimal hyperplasia within the boundaries of the stent, thereby indicating that this stent has been implanted in this artery in a prior procedure. In this section, the intimal hyperplasia appears nonobstructive. Figure Q27-12B is obtained from a tight stenosis in the middle of a 5-year-old vein graft. The atheroma is heterogeneous in density, but mostly echo lucent. Vein graft lesions are typically echo lucent in appearance and represent mixtures of lipid pools, collagen, and thrombotic material. In these lesions, heavy calcification is rare. The minimum lumen diameter is <2 mm. Figure Q27-12C is obtained from a native coronary artery at a bifurcation point. There is mild-to-moderate degree of atherosclerosis. The branch arising from the imaged vessel can be identified by following the continuity of the speckle of the blood elements around the IVUS catheter into the branch with an interruption of the layers of the wall (in the 5 o'clock direction). In this image, the wire artifact and its shadow are very apparent (in the 9 o'clock direction). Figure Q27-12D is obtained from a heavily calcified segment of a coronary artery. The arc of calcification occupies approximately three quadrants of the section and is seen as a bright echo with a shadow caused by the inability of the ultrasound beams to penetrate the tissue. Although this is not uncommon to see in native coronary arteries with advanced atherosclerosis, this degree of calcification does not develop in vein graft lesions (*Circulation* 1998;97:916–931).

27.13   **Answer C.** This is a case of a diffusely diseased LAD, in which the more severe segmental stenosis (shown in the Fig. Q27-13, left) is superimposed on a moderate and diffuse disease (shown in the Fig. Q27-13, middle and right). Coronary angiograms are traditionally interpreted in a segmental fashion, where the least stenosed segment is assumed to be the "normal" reference to which the other segments are compared. In the presence of diffuse disease, this segmental approach to interpretation results in underestimation of stenosis severity. Another problem with angiographic interpretation is the projection of usually complex lumen shapes within stenosed segments onto a two-dimensional screen. Angiographers compensate by obtaining orthogonal views, but the choice of those projections is still arbitrary. Therefore, it is conceivable that the projection that would be perfectly perpendicular to the minimum lumen diameter may not be obtained. In this case, IVUS imaging did demonstrate a severe stenosis in the midvessel with a minimum lumen diameter of <2 mm and an area of <4 mm². These measurements indicate a hemodynamically significant stenosis that is likely to cause ischemia on a stress test. This minimum lumen area by IVUS has a good correlation with an FFR of <0.75, which explains why the stress test was positive, despite the apparently "moderate" narrowing on angiography. The degree of narrowing in a bifurcation lesion can be difficult to angiographically assess, but that does not apply to a tomographic imaging modality such as IVUS. The branching point of the diagonal branch is not seen in any of the images shown here. In all the three images, the interruption of the circumference of the arterial wall is caused by the shadow of the wire artifact (*Circulation* 1999;100:250–255; *Curr Probl Cardiol* 1999;24:541–566).

27.14 **Answer A.** The IVUS image shows a heterogeneous plaque with areas of echo lucency suggesting a mixture of fibrous and fibrofatty tissues. These lesions, when located in proximal vessels, are ideal for directional atherectomy. Aggressive atherectomy guided by repeated ultrasound imaging will result in significant debulking and improved acute lumen gain; however, there has been no evidence of reduction in restenosis with this approach. Pretreatment with rotational atherectomy has not been shown to improve acute or late outcomes. It remains useful in heavily calcified lesions where stents cannot be delivered or adequately expanded. IVUS imaging is not a reliable tool for identification of intracoronary thrombus. The echogenic characteristics of thrombus are similar to heterogeneous plaque. In certain situations, a thrombus can be identified in the context of an acute myocardial infarction and when it is located within the lumen (*Am Heart J* 2004;148:663–669; *Am J Cardiol* 2004;93:953–958).

27.15 **Answer C.** In-stent restenosis is a result of neointimal tissue growth in the stent. Neointimal growth is uniformly distributed throughout the stent. In articulated stents (Palmaz-Schatz), immediate postprocedure tissue prolapse and subsequent neointimal hyperplasia tended to be worse at the central articulation point. Late lumen loss within the stented segments is directly proportional to the degree of neointimal hyperplasia. Slotted-tube stents abolish the negative remodeling response that is the primary driver of restenosis following balloon angioplasty. Therefore, the correlation between late loss and negative remodeling (shrinkage of the vessel area) is very weak in the stented segment. However, negative remodeling is more apparent in the few millimeters of the artery just distal to the edge of the stent and is the primary mechanism of late loss in this region of the artery. These changes are seen equally in native coronaries and saphenous vein grafts as well as in lesions treated with one or two stents. IVUS late lumen loss was found to correlate with, but was consistently smaller than, angiographic late lumen loss (*Circulation* 1996;94:1247–1254).

27.16 **Answer B.** In the PROSPECT trial, approximately 700 acute coronary syndrome patients underwent angiography and revascularization if needed. Three-vessel IVUS imaging and VH analysis were performed. Patients who developed events over the ensuing 3 years underwent repeat angiography and imaging. Adverse events were related to an originally nonculprit lesion in 11.6% of patients. Lesion characteristics that predicted development of future events included PB ≥ 70%, minimum lumen area (MLA) ≤4 mm², and thin-cap fibroatheroma (TCFA) on IVUS-derived VH. The presence of more than one feature increased the risk of future events (Fig. A27.16).

The VH images demonstrate a variety of plaque types. (A) is a fibrotic plaque consisting mainly of fibrotic plaque (dark green) with <10% necrotic core (red) and <10% dense calcification (white). (B) and (C) are thin-cap fibroatheromas (TCFA) characterized by the presence of >10% confluent necrotic core (red) and >30 degrees of the necrotic core abutting the lumen. (B) is more likely to cause future events because the PB is larger and the lumen is smaller. (D) is a thick-cap fibroatheroma (ThCFA), which contains >10% necrotic core (red), but that is separated from the lumen by a thicker fibrotic layer (green) (*N Engl J Med* 2011;364:226–235).

27.17 **Answer A.** This patient developed angina due to drug-eluting in-stent restenosis. IVUS imaging

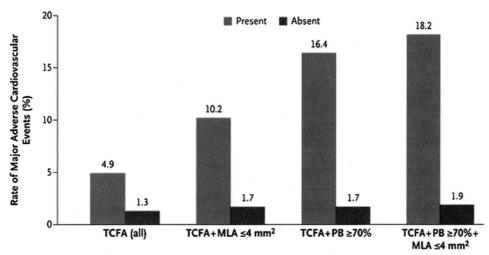

Figure A27-16

provided significant insight into mechanisms and patterns of DES restenosis. Although late loss is frequently diffusely distributed, significant intimal hyperplasia leading to >50% diameter reduction is focal in about half the cases. In the IVUS image shown, there are two mechanisms of restenosis: an underexpansion at the time of stent implantation and intimal hyperplasia that developed over time (Fig. A27-17A).

Underexpansion is defined as a stent area < 5mm², which is the area bound by the dashed black circle. Clearly, the stent could have been better expanded or a larger stent may have been used given the size of the concentric plaque between the stent border (dashed black circle) and the vessel border (solid white circle) (Fig. A27-17B). Intimal hyperplasia is significant when it occupies >50% of the stent area (area bound between the dashed black circle and the inner solid black circle demarcating the intimal

leading edge). In restenosis of longer stents, underexpansion is seen in more than a third of cases, and the mechanism of diameter reduction is frequently a combination of underexpansion and intimal hyperplasia, as shown here. In shorter stents (≤28 mm), restenosis is primarily driven by intimal hyperplasia alone. (*Circ Cardiovasc Interv* 2011;4:9–14)

27.18 **Answer B.** Following high-pressure stenting, a small postprocedure minimum in-stent lumen area is the most important predictor of target vessel revascularization. The various proposed IVUS criteria for optimal stent deployment emphasize achieving the largest possible in-stent lumen area. Increasing the in-stent lumen area usually requires larger balloons and/or higher inflation pressures; however, that would be limited by the reference vessel size. Panels A and B of the figure depict stents with relatively small lumen

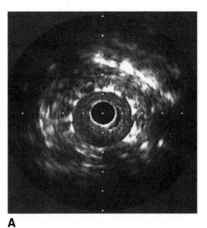

A

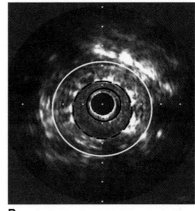

B

Figure A27-17

areas, which predispose a high risk of restenosis. Panels C and D depict a stent with gross malapposition of struts. Historically, such degrees of malapposition were commonly observed before routine use of high-pressure inflations and are considered a precipitating factor for stent thrombosis. In all three situations, operators typically resort to higher inflation pressures and/or balloon oversizing. The upper right figure depicts a well-expanded and well-opposed stent with a minimum area exceeding 7 mm². Even with bare-metal stents, such lumen areas are associated with target vessel revascularization rates in the single digits (*Eur Heart J* 1998;19:1214-1223; *J Am Coll Cardiol* 1994;24:996-1003; *Am Heart J* 2001;141:823-831).

27.19 **Answer C.** IVUS findings in DES patients presenting with very late stent thrombosis provide useful insights into the possible mechanisms of this serious clinical problem. IVUS findings in 13 DES patients with very late thrombosis were compared to 144 control DES patients who underwent imaging and had no documented stent thrombosis. Patients with very late stent thrombosis had longer stents, more overlapping stents, and more stents per lesion. The prevalence of incomplete strut apposition was 77% in the thrombosis group compared with 12% in the control group. There was no difference in reference segment vessel area, but the in-stent vessel area was significantly larger in the thrombosis group, indicating more positive remodeling (*Circulation* 2007;115:2426-2434). The high prevalence of incomplete strut apposition in stented segments presenting with late and very late thrombosis was confirmed in another small retrospective study that included 23 DES patients (*J Am Coll Cardiol* 2010;1936-1942).

27.20 **Answer A.** When an intermediate lesion is encountered, further assessment of the lesion can be accomplished either by functional assessment using pressure or flow measurements or by morphologic delineation using IVUS imaging. FFR cutoff values of 0.75 to 0.80 have been correlated with short- and long-term clinical data; lesions that do not meet this criterion are associated with favorable clinical outcomes with no need for revascularization. The cutoff values for IVUS measurements that identify hemodynamically significant lesions have mostly been determined by correlation with FFR. In a study of 51 lesions in 42 stable patients, the IVUS measurements that maximized the sensitivity and specificity of the correlation with IVUS were minimum lumen area <3.0 mm² and area stenosis >60%. The combination of both criteria (lumen area <3.0 mm² and area stenosis <0.60%) had 100% sensitivity and specificity (*Circulation* 1999;100:250-255). In another study of 53 lesions, a minimal luminal area of ≤4 mm² and an area stenosis >70% were the best indicators of hemodynamic significance, as determined by an FFR <0.75 (*Am J Cardiol* 2001;87:136-141). Retrospective analysis of 1-year clinical outcomes after deferring PCI (357 intermediate lesions in 300 patients), the only independent predictors of an event (death, MI, or target lesion revascularization) were IVUS minimum lumen area and area stenosis. In lesions with a minimum area ≥4.0 mm², the event rate was acceptably low to allow reasonably safe deferral of PCI (*Circulation* 1999;100:256-261). IVUS interrogation of this lesion reveals an eccentric heterogeneous plaque with minimal calcification. The lumen area and the area stenosis are consistent with a hemodynamically nonsignificant lesion that requires no revascularization but does warrant secondary prevention with statin therapy.

28

Approach to the Patient with Hemodynamic Compromise

Zoran S. Nedeljkovic and Alice K. Jacobs

QUESTIONS

28.1 A 50-year-old man presents to the hospital with worsening substernal chest discomfort that began 3 hours ago while shoveling snow. He has no significant past medical history and takes no medications. His risk factors for cardiovascular disease include current tobacco use and a family history of premature coronary artery disease. On arrival to the emergency room, his blood pressure is 100/70 mm Hg and heart rate is 84 beats/min. His lung fields are clear to auscultation and percussion, and cardiovascular examination is notable for normal heart sounds and no audible murmurs. His electrocardiogram shows 2 mm of ST-segment elevation in leads II, III, and aVF, with 1 mm of ST depression in V1–V3.

He is taken to the cardiac catheterization laboratory for emergency percutaneous revascularization. Angiography of the left coronary artery is normal. A single-frame cineangiogram of the right coronary artery before and after dilation of the stenosis with a 2.5-mm balloon is shown in Figure Q28-1A, B.

The patient subsequently complains of nausea and vomits. The hemodynamic tracing from the monitor is shown in Figure Q28-1C.

Which of the following would you do next?

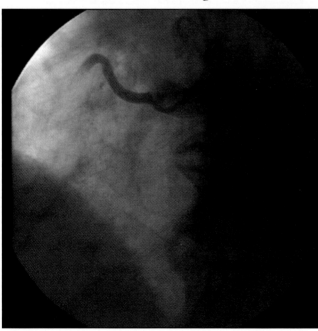

A

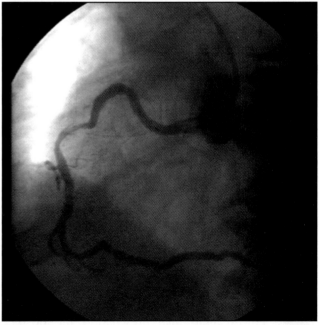

B

Figure Q28-1

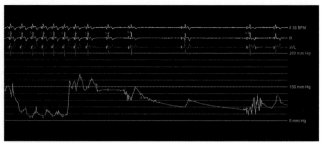

C
Figure Q28-1

   (A) Reinflation of the angioplasty balloon in the proximal segment of the coronary artery and preparation for emergency pericardiocentesis

   (B) Administration of atropine and intravenous fluids

   (C) Prompt insertion of a temporary transvenous pacemaker

   (D) Administration of dopamine

28.2 Which of the following hemodynamic profiles is most consistent with cardiogenic shock secondary to inferior wall myocardial infarction (MI) with right ventricular (RV) involvement?

Table Q28-2.

	RA	RV	PA	PCW	Ao	CO	SVR
A	3	20/3	20/8	7	88/56	3.2	1,590
B	15	35/14	36/15	15	85/60	3.0	1,800
C	2	22/3	24/8	8	82/40	7.2	600
D	15	50/18	52/28	30	90/62	2.9	1,550

(RA, RV, PA, PCW, and Ao denote right atrial, right ventricular, pulmonary arterial, pulmonary capillary wedge, and aortic pressure measured in mm Hg, respectively; CO denotes cardiac output expressed in L/min; SVR denotes systemic vascular resistance in dyne-s-cm^{-5})

28.3 Which of the following is associated with the greatest risk of coronary artery perforation during percutaneous coronary intervention (PCI)?

   (A) Rotational atherectomy of a stenosis in the midportion of a tortuous right coronary artery

   (B) Balloon angioplasty of a densely calcified proximal left anterior descending (LAD) artery stenosis using a high-pressure balloon

   (C) Stent placement in a stenosis in the proximal right coronary artery following failed fibrinolysis for an acute inferior wall MI

   (D) Stent placement in a stenosis in the midportion of a saphenous vein graft to the obtuse marginal branch

28.4 A 59-year-old man presents to the hospital with chest pain and is found to have anterior T-wave inversions and an elevated cardiac troponin. He is treated with aspirin, clopidogrel, and unfractionated heparin. He is taken to the cardiac catheterization laboratory, and following angiography of the left coronary artery he complains of severe chest pain with evidence of ST-segment elevation on the monitor. His blood pressure is 80/40 mm Hg with a heart rate of 90 beats/min. A single-frame cineangiogram of the left coronary artery in the right anterior oblique projection with caudal angulation is shown in Figure Q28-4. Which of the following should be done next?

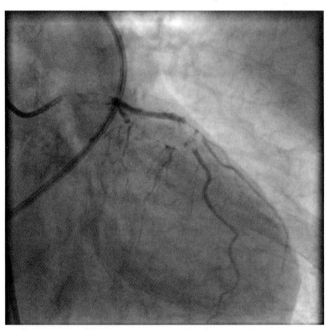

Figure Q28-4

   (A) Insertion of an intraaortic balloon pump (IABP)

   (B) Emergent coronary artery bypass surgery for dissection of the left main coronary artery

   (C) Administration of 100% oxygen

   (D) Administration of abciximab and preparation for emergency PCI of the left main and LAD arteries

28.5 A 68-year-old woman is undergoing rotational atherectomy of an angulated lesion in the mid right coronary artery with a 1.5-mm burr. Her blood pressure suddenly drops to 70/30 mm Hg, and angiography demonstrates contrast extravasation into the pericardial space. In preparation for emergency pericardiocentesis for cardiac tamponade, protamine sulfate should be given if which of the following antithrombotic agents had been used during PCI?

(A) Heparin
(B) Fondaparinux
(C) Bivalirudin
(D) Lepirudin

28.6 An 82-year-old woman with peripheral arterial disease is admitted to the catheterization laboratory for diagnostic catheterization following an acute coronary syndrome. She is given 1.0 mg of midazolam and 50 μg of fentanyl, both intravenously for conscious sedation. Following insertion of a sheath into the right femoral artery, a left diagnostic catheter is positioned over a wire into the ascending aorta. Prior to angiography of the left coronary artery, the patient is noted to be confused with incoherent speech. Her blood pressure is 108/80 mm Hg and heart rate is 78 beats/min. Which of the following would be the next most appropriate course of action?

(A) Emergent neurological evaluation
(B) Administration of flumazenil and naloxone
(C) Administration of an additional 0.5 mg of intravenous midazolam
(D) Administration of 0.5 mg of intravenous haloperidol

28.7 Which of the following agents should initially be used in the management of hypotension and cardiogenic shock secondary to stress-induced (Takotsubo) cardiomyopathy?

(A) Dobutamine
(B) Dopamine
(C) Phenylephrine
(D) Metoprolol

28.8 A 54-year-old man undergoes rescue angioplasty following unsuccessful reperfusion with fibrinolytic therapy for an acute anterior wall MI. Coronary angiography reveals thrombotic occlusion of the proximal LAD artery with no other significant epicardial coronary artery disease. Following initial balloon inflation across the stenosis in the proximal LAD artery, there is restoration of antegrade flow. The electrocardiogram and arterial pressure from the guiding catheter are shown in Figure Q28-8.

Which of the following should be done next?

(A) Administration of bolus and infusion of amiodarone
(B) Administration of bolus and infusion of lidocaine
(C) Observation
(D) DC cardioversion

28.9 An 80-year-old woman presents to a community hospital with unstable angina associated with transient inferolateral ST-segment depression. She is treated with aspirin, clopidogrel, enoxaparin, and eptifibatide. The serum cardiac troponin I is measured at 2.1 ng/mL. Her complete blood count, serum electrolytes, and renal function are normal. Diagnostic coronary and left ventricular (LV) angiography is performed in a catheterization laboratory in a community hospital that does not perform PCI. Findings revealed normal LV systolic function and single-vessel coronary artery disease with a 90% stenosis in the mid right coronary artery. The femoral arterial sheath is sutured in place, and she is transferred to a tertiary hospital where the lesion is dilated and treated with a drug-eluting stent with a successful angiographic result. The femoral arteriotomy site is closed using a collagen plug closure device. Eptifibatide is continued at the conclusion of the PCI.

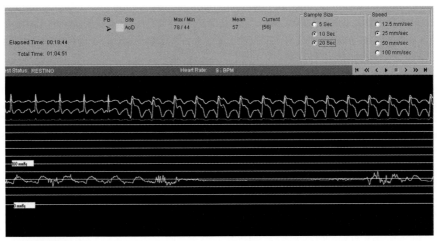

Figure Q28-8

Two hours later she complains of nausea, abdominal pain, and vague chest discomfort. Her blood pressure is 90/60 mm Hg and heart rate is 44 beats/min. She appears pale and diaphoretic. Her lungs are clear to auscultation and her cardiac exam is without murmurs, rubs, or gallops. Her abdomen is soft with no reproducible tenderness. Her right groin has a small hematoma with no evidence of bleeding. Her electrocardiogram shows nonspecific findings.

Following administration of 0.5 mg atropine intravenously and normal saline, her blood pressure and heart rate rise to 108/68 mm Hg and 70 beats/min, respectively. Which of the following should be done next?

(A) Computed tomography (CT) of the abdomen
(B) Continued observation
(C) Urgent coronary angiography to exclude acute stent thrombosis
(D) Discontinue eptifibatide and obtain stat CBC and type and crossmatch

28.10 Which of the following mechanisms is most likely responsible for hypotension resulting from RV MI?

(A) Increase in LV preload
(B) Increase in LV afterload
(C) RV diastolic dysfunction
(D) Pericardial constraint

28.11 A 74-year-old woman presents to the emergency room with 4 hours of substernal chest pain and shortness of breath. She has a history of long-standing hypertension and coronary artery disease, with a prior MI 6 years ago. At that time, a cardiac defibrillator (ICD) was implanted. On physical examination, her blood pressure is 100/40 mm Hg with a heart rate of 88 beats/min and a respiratory rate of 16 per minute. The lung fields are clear to auscultation, and the heart sounds are regular with a systolic flow murmur heard in the second right intercostal space.

The electrocardiogram shows an acute inferoposterior wall ST-segment elevation MI. The chest x-ray is shown in Figure Q28-11.

She is treated with aspirin, heparin, and a single intravenous dose of metoprolol and is taken to the cardiac catheterization laboratory for emergency PCI. Angiography of the left coronary artery reveals moderate disease in the mid LAD artery and diffuse mild disease in the left circumflex artery. The right coronary artery is occluded with thrombus in the midportion. The mid right coronary artery is successfully treated with a single drug-eluting stent with no residual

stenosis. However, following stent deployment there is grade 2 thrombolysis in myocardial infarction flow in the distal bed of the right coronary artery that does not improve despite multiple doses of intracoronary nitroprusside. The systemic blood pressure is 80/40 mm Hg. Right heart catheterization is performed and reveals a pulmonary arterial pressure of 44/16 mm Hg and a mean pulmonary capillary wedge pressure of 16 mm Hg. An IABP is placed, and there is appropriate diastolic augmentation and systolic unloading. Upon arrival to the coronary care unit, the patient rapidly develops severe shortness of breath with a blood pressure of 100/50 mm Hg and a heart rate of 110 beats/min. The electrocardiogram shows nonspecific changes. She is emergently intubated for pulmonary edema.

Which of the following is likely contributing the patient's sudden decompensation?

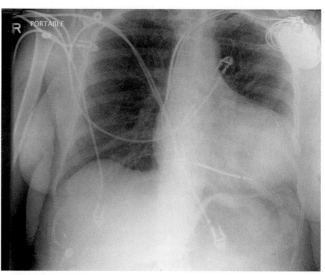

Figure Q28-11

(A) Acute stent thrombosis
(B) Acute severe mitral insufficiency
(C) Acute severe aortic insufficiency
(D) Acute ventricular septal rupture (VSR)

28.12 A 68-year-old woman with a past history of well-controlled hypertension presents to the hospital with several days of intermittent substernal chest pressure and shortness of breath. On arrival to the emergency room, her blood pressure is 90/70 mm Hg, her heart rate is 105 beats/min, and her respiratory rate is 26 breaths/min. She is diaphoretic and in visible respiratory distress. Cardiovascular examination is notable for a jugular venous pressure of 8 cm, rales at the bases of both lung fields, and a 3/6 harsh systolic

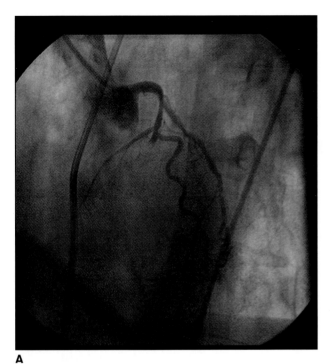

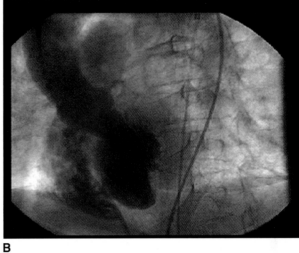

A

B

Figure Q28-12

murmur at the left sternal border. Her extremities are cool. Her electrocardiogram reveals sinus tachycardia with 2-mm ST-segment elevation in V1–V4 and 1-mm ST-segment depression in II, III, and aVF. Her baseline complete blood count, serum electrolytes, and renal function are normal.

She is given aspirin and heparin and undergoes endotracheal intubation for airway support. She is taken to the cardiac catheterization laboratory for emergency angiography. Single-frame cineangiogram in the LAO-cranial projection of her left coronary and LV angiogram are shown in Figure Q28-12A, B. The next most appropriate course of action would be:

(A) Administration of abciximab followed by primary PCI of the LAD artery
(B) Insertion of an IABP followed by primary PCI of the LAD artery
(C) Primary PCI of the LAD artery and referral for emergency cardiac surgery
(D) Insertion of IABP and referral for emergent cardiac surgery

28.13 A 36-year-old man undergoes diagnostic coronary and LV angiography for evaluation of chest pain. His cardiac examination is notable for the presence of a mid-peaking systolic ejection murmur, heard best at the left sternal border, without radiation. His lungs are clear to auscultation. His

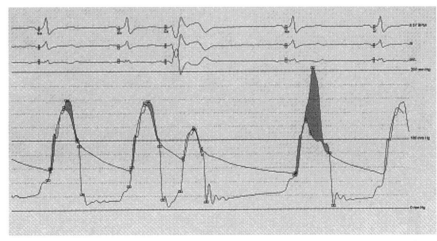

Figure Q28-13

electrocardiogram shows LV hypertrophy with secondary repolarization abnormalities. His coronary angiogram demonstrates normal left and right coronary arteries, and LV angiography reveals normal systolic function. A simultaneous LV and femoral arterial pressure tracing is shown in Figure Q28-13.

The procedure was uneventful, but later during recovery, the patient complains of chest pain and lightheadedness. On physical examination, his blood pressure is 70/50 mm Hg with a heart rate of 88 beats/min. He appears diaphoretic and the extremities are cool. In addition to administration of intravenous fluids, which of the following should be administered?

(A) Atropine
(B) Dopamine
(C) Dobutamine
(D) Phenylephrine

28.14 A 63-year-old man is admitted to the hospital for evaluation of exertional shortness of breath and chest pain. His risk factors for ischemic heart disease include hypertension, hyperlipidemia, and obesity. His initial treatment includes aspirin and unfractionated heparin. Cardiac enzymes are negative for MI, and the remainder of his laboratory values is normal. A pharmacologic nuclear study is performed and demonstrates a medium-sized, moderately severe perfusion defect in the inferolateral wall with near-complete reperfusion on the resting images. He presents to the cardiac catheterization laboratory for diagnostic right and left heart catheterization via the transfemoral approach. Using a balloon-tipped flotation catheter, right-sided pressures are recorded as below:

Table Q28-14.

Right atrial pressure (mean, mm Hg)	11
RV pressure (systolic, end diastolic, mm Hg)	52/10
Pulmonary arterial (systolic, diastolic, mean, mm Hg)	54/20, 31

The catheter is advanced into the left-sided pulmonary wedge position and the mean pressure is recorded at 18 mm Hg. Following deflation of the balloon, an appropriate rise in the mean pressure is seen, confirming that the catheter was in the wedge position. The patient suddenly develops hemoptysis with rapid oxygen desaturation. The most appropriate immediate management includes:

(A) Reinflation of the balloon-tipped catheter in the pulmonary artery for presumed rupture of the pulmonary artery

(B) Placement of the patient in the left lateral decubitus position and emergency thoracic surgical consultation for presumed rupture of the pulmonary artery

(C) Administration of protamine

(D) Surgical consultation for emergency chest tube insertion

28.15 A 66-year-old woman with a history of hypertension and hyperlipidemia undergoes diagnostic coronary angiography for an abnormal exercise stress test. The patient receives standard premedication for the procedure, including midazolam and fentanyl. The catheter is advanced smoothly around the aortic arch, and the left main coronary is engaged. The initial single-frame cineangiogram of her left coronary artery is shown in Figure Q28-15.

The patient suddenly complains of shortness of breath and chest pain. Physical examination is notable for a blood pressure of 82/50 mm Hg, a heart rate of 94 beats/min, a respiratory rate of 24 per minute, and an oxygen saturation of 92%. Cardiac examination reveals no murmurs or gallops, and her lungs demonstrate diffuse inspiratory and expiratory wheezing. Which of the following should be done next?

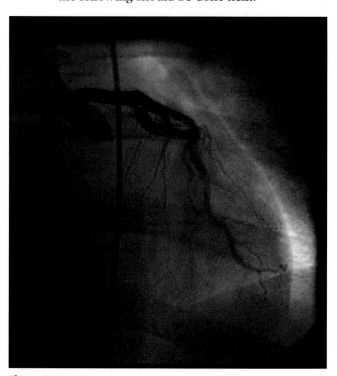

Figure Q28-15

(A) Switch to a lower-osmolar iodinated contrast agent

(B) Repeat left coronary angiography to exclude dissection of the left main coronary artery

(C) Administer diphenhydramine, antihistamines, and epinephrine

(D) Administer flumazenil to reverse the effects of the benzodiazepine

28.16 A 50-year-old female with a long history of cigarette smoking and hypertension undergoes coronary angiography for Class III stable angina and an exercise-echocardiogram notable only for anterolateral ischemia and normal LV function. Left coronary angiography reveals a 90% stenosis in the mid LAD artery and insignificant disease in the left circumflex artery. Following catheter placement in the right coronary ostium, the patient complains of severe angina. Blood pressure falls from 150/80 mm Hg to 80/40 mm Hg, and the heart rate increases to 90 beats/min. Angiography reveals a 95% stenosis of the proximal right coronary artery without signs of dissection. The patient continues to complain of severe chest pain, and the monitor reveals ST-segment elevation in leads II and III. Which of the following would you do next?

(A) Administer 100 μg of intracoronary nitroglycerin in the right coronary artery

(B) Administer atropine 0.6 mg IV and IV fluids

(C) Replace the diagnostic catheter with a guiding catheter and prepare for emergency PCI of the right coronary artery

(D) Insert an IABP in preparation for emergency PCI of the right coronary artery

28.17 An 82-year-old man with a history of hypertension, type 2 diabetes, and dyslipidemia is brought in by his family to the emergency room after being noted to be lethargic with difficulty breathing. On examination, he is diaphoretic with a blood pressure of 85/50 and a heart rate of 110 beats/min. His heart sounds are normal without any murmurs, and rales are present over the lower third of the lung bases. His electrocardiogram shows evidence of an evolving anteroseptal MI with Q waves in V1–V3 and 2- to 3-mm ST-segment elevation. What class of recommendation do the 2004 ACC/AHA Guidelines for the Management of Patients with ST-Elevation Myocardial Infarction assign to primary percutaneous intervention for this clinical situation?

(A) Class I

(B) Class IIa

(C) Class IIb

(D) Class III

28.18 In which of the following patients would a percutaneous circulatory assist device offer the greatest benefit?

(A) A 58-year-old woman with left ventricular ejection fraction (LVEF) 50% undergoing unprotected left main coronary angioplasty

(B) A 37-year-old man with fulminant myocarditis and cardiogenic shock despite high-dose inotropic support

(C) An 80-year-old man with LVEF 45% undergoing PCI on a 7-year-old saphenous vein graft to the posterior descending artery

(D) A 50-year-old man with recent anterior MI, LVEF 40%, undergoing PCI of a proximal LAD/diagonal artery bifurcation lesion

28.19 A 49-year-old woman undergoes diagnostic cardiac catheterization via the right femoral artery for evaluation of chest pain and an abnormal stress test. Coronary angiography reveals nonobstructive coronary artery disease. The 5-F arterial sheath is removed in the laboratory, and manual pressure is applied to achieve hemostasis. She is transferred to the recovery area and after 45 minutes develops nausea with an urge to void. Her blood pressure is 80/40 mm Hg and her heart rate is 60 beats/min. On examination, there is a small amount of blood saturating the dressing over the femoral arteriotomy but no hematoma. She is brought back into the laboratory, and angiography of the right femoral artery is performed via the contralateral approach (Fig. Q28-19). What should be the next step in the management of this patient?

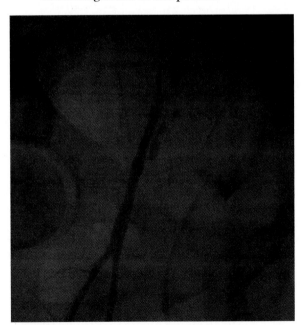

Figure Q28-19

(A) Surgical consultation for operative repair
(B) Prolonged manual pressure of the right femoral arteriotomy
(C) A trial of balloon occlusion with insertion of a covered stent if bleeding persists
(D) Transfusion of packed red blood cells and platelets

28.20 A 70-year-old man undergoes primary PCI of the proximal LAD artery in the setting of an acute MI complicated by cardiogenic shock. His blood pressure at the conclusion of the intervention is 80/50 mm Hg with a heart rate of 100 beats/min. Hemodynamics from right heart catheterization are as follows:

Table Q28-20.

Right atrial pressure (mean, mm Hg)	15
Pulmonary arterial (systolic, diastolic, mean, mm Hg)	54/28, 37
Pulmonary capillary wedge pressure (mean, mm Hg)	26
Cardiac output (L/min)	3.5

The patient has a history of aortobifemoral bypass surgery and is not a candidate for an IABP. Which of the following agents would be most appropriate initial agent for management of hypotension?

(A) Phenylephrine
(B) Norepinephrine
(C) Dobutamine
(D) Dopamine

28.21 A 40-year-old woman undergoes diagnostic LV angiography for evaluation of severe mitral insufficiency secondary to degenerative mitral valve disease. Following injection of radiographic contrast material at a rate of 15 mL/s for a total of 45 mL, she develops bradycardia associated with nausea and vomiting. What should be done next?

(A) Administer intravenous steroid and antihistamine
(B) Abort further angiography
(C) Switch to low-osmolar contrast agent
(D) Insert temporary transvenous pacemaker prior to further angiography

28.22 A 52-year-old man presents to the emergency department with 3 days of intermittent chest discomfort and progressively increasing fatigue and shortness of breath. Prior to being brought to the hospital, he had a near-syncopal episode. Four weeks prior, he underwent minimally invasive bioprosthetic aortic valve replacement for a bicuspid aortic valve and aortic stenosis. On examination, his blood pressure is 90/60 mm Hg, and auscultation reveals clear lung fields and no audible murmur. His electrocardiogram is shown in Figure Q28-22. Intravenous fluids are administered. What should be the next step in his management?

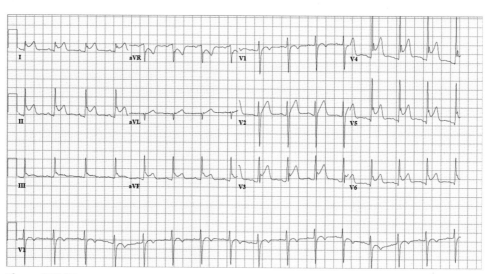

Figure Q28-22

(A) Administer aspirin and unfractionated heparin, and perform urgent coronary angiography
(B) Echocardiography
(C) Insertion of temporary transvenous pacemaker
(D) Prescribe nonsteroidal anti-inflammatory drug and discharge from emergency department

28.23 A 70-year-old man is transferred to a tertiary hospital with cardiogenic shock secondary to an anterior wall MI. He presented to the referring hospital with several days of intermittent chest discomfort that became persistent over the last 12 hours. His electrocardiogram showed anterior ST elevation in V1–V4 with Q waves in those leads. He is treated with aspirin, unfractionated heparin, and dopamine titrated to 5 μg/kg/min.

On arrival to the catheterization laboratory, his blood pressure is 90/60 mm Hg, and heart rate is 100 beats/min. A grade 3 systolic murmur is heard over the left sternal border, and crackles are heard over the lower lung fields.

What is the most appropriate sequence of events to be performed in the catheterization laboratory?

(A) Coronary angiography followed by PCI
(B) Coronary angiography followed by bypass surgery
(C) Right heart catheterization followed by coronary angiography
(D) No cardiac catheterization as presentation is beyond the window of myocardial salvage

28.24 A patient in the coronary care unit develops a retroperitoneal (RP) bleed following PCI of a diagonal branch of the LAD artery. In addition to aspirin and clopidogrel, unfractionated heparin and abciximab were administered for the procedure. The systolic blood pressure is palpated at 70 mm Hg. Intravenous fluid is administered through two peripheral lines, and two units of packed red blood cells are called for. The activated clotting time (ACT) is 170 seconds, and results of the complete blood count are shown below.

Table Q28-24.

White blood cell count	5,300/μL
Hemoglobin	7.0 g/dL
Platelet count	50,000/μL

Which of the following interventions would assist in helping restore hemostasis?

(A) Administer protamine 20 mg, intravenously
(B) Transfuse platelets
(C) Plasmapheresis
(D) Intravenous immunoglobulin G

28.25 In performing transjugular endomyocardial biopsy, which of the following patients is at highest risk of hemodynamic deterioration in the event of cardiac perforation?

(A) A 30-year-old man undergoing routine biopsy 12 months following cardiac transplantation with LVEF 60%
(B) A 22-year-old woman with HIV, idiopathic dilated cardiomyopathy, and normal RV size and systolic function
(C) A 58-year-old man with severe biventricular enlargement and dysfunction, and LVEF 20%
(D) A 60-year-old man with severely increased LV wall thickness and LVEF 55%

28.1 **Answer B.** Nausea and vomiting, often associated with hypotension and bradycardia, are common with MI, particularly with inferior wall infarction. Hypotension and bradycardia are attributed to direct activation of parasympathetic/vagal reflex pathways or LV stretch receptors (Bezold-Jarisch reflex) that lead to bradycardia and peripheral vasodilation, and are usually transient. The Bezold-Jarisch reflex commonly occurs, as in this case, following reperfusion of the infarct artery in a patient with an inferior MI.

28.2 **Answer B.** RA pressure is elevated with a mildly elevated PCW and SVR and with a low CO. In (A), filling pressures are all low and SVR is elevated, consistent with hypovolemic shock. In (C), filling pressures are also low, but CO is elevated and SVR is low, consistent with sepsis. In (D), PCW is elevated, CO is relatively low, and SVR is elevated, consistent with cardiogenic shock. This contrasts with shock secondary to predominant RV involvement, where the PCW is only mildly elevated.

28.3 **Answer A.** Coronary artery perforation is an infrequent occurrence following PCI. Perforations during PCI can occur as a result of guidewire manipulation ("wire exit") or improper sizing of the balloon. Elderly patients and women appear to be at increased risk. However, PCI following fibrinolytic therapy and PCI of a saphenous vein graft are not associated with increased risk of perforation. In a prospective study of the incidence of coronary artery perforation in the early 1990s, use of newer devices to treat coronary lesions by cutting or ablating tissue (atherectomy, laser) were associated with an increased incidence of perforation compared to balloon angioplasty alone (*Circulation* 1994;90:2725–2730). These investigators defined a scheme for classifying coronary artery perforations into one of three groups: Extraluminal crater without extravasation (Type 1), pericardial or myocardial blush without contrast extravasation (Type 2), or extravasation through frank (≥1-mm) perforation (Type 3). Type 1 and Type 2 perforations can usually be managed with prolonged balloon inflations and reversal of anticoagulation. Type 3

perforations are usually associated with a higher incidence of adverse events (death, MI, tamponade, or emergency cardiac surgery).

Prolonged balloon inflations may not be well tolerated, and perfusion balloons have been used in this setting to seal off the perforation and maintain adequate distal perfusion. Heparin anticoagulation is usually reversed with protamine and pericardial tamponade is treated with pericardiocentesis. If these measures fail, emergency surgery is needed. Polytetrafluoroethylene-covered stents have emerged as an attractive alternative in the nonsurgical management of coronary artery perforations, with promising results (*Circulation* 2000;102:3028–3031). If these measures fail, emergency surgery is needed.

28.4 **Answer C.** Coronary air embolus is a preventable complication of cardiac catheterization. When it does occur, treatment is usually supportive with administration of 100% inhaled oxygen. If the chest pain or ischemia persists despite oxygen, an IABP and pressor support may be necessary, although the ischemia is usually transient. Coronary artery bypass surgery is not indicated.

28.5 **Answer A.** Protamine sulfate is given intravenously to neutralize the anticoagulant effect of heparin. The usual dose is 1 mg of protamine sulfate for each 100 units of residual unfractionated heparin. Protamine partially neutralizes the effect of low-molecular-weight heparins (enoxaparin), but does not affect the pentasaccharide (fondaparinux). Neither direct thrombin inhibitors (bivalirudin or lepirudin) nor glycoprotein IIb/IIIa inhibitors are affected by protamine.

28.6 **Answer B.** Elderly patients are at increased risk for idiosyncratic reactions to benzodiazepines and narcotics. In the outlined scenario, one would be concerned about an acute cerebrovascular event (particularly since there has been manipulation of a guidewire and catheter in the ascending aorta and aortic arch); however, the initial management should include reversal of the benzodiazepine and narcotic. Additional sedatives or psychoactive medications should be avoided until the patient's neurological status is clarified.

28.7 **Answer D.** Stress-induced cardiomyopathy (also referred to as Takotsubo cardiomyopathy or transient apical ballooning syndrome) is characterized by transient LV dysfunction, usually involving the apical and midventricular segments. The condition mimics acute MI, but develops in the absence of acute coronary obstruction (*Circulation* 2008;118:2754–2762). Compensatory hypercontractility of the basal LV segments can lead to LV outflow tract obstruction and hypotension analogous to that seen with hypertrophic obstructive cardiomyopathy. Intravenous fluid should be administered initially to patients who do not have significant pulmonary congestion. Beta-blockers should be administered to reduce the contractility of the basal LV and relieve the LV outflow tract obstruction. Refractory hypotension that does not respond to fluids and/or beta-blocker can be managed with phenylephrine or with IABP counterpulsation.

28.8 **Answer C.** The initial portion of the electrocardiogram demonstrates sinus tachycardia with a rate of approximately 100 beats/min. The arterial pressure is 78/44 mm Hg. The wide-complex rhythm that develops is an accelerated idioventricular rhythm (AIVR) that is often seen following successful reperfusion in acute MI, either by pharmacologic or mechanical means, and is usually transient. Antiarrhythmic therapy is not indicated for AIVR. Likewise, electrical cardioversion is also not indicated.

28.9 **Answer D.** The patient likely has an acute RP bleed and should be treated with supportive care and discontinuation of the IIb/IIIa platelet receptor antagonist. Compression of the femoral arteriotomy site may be helpful, and blood transfusion should be performed for ongoing bleeding that is causing hemodynamic instability or that results in an unacceptably low hemoglobin. Urgent ileofemoral angiography can also be performed to identify the site of bleeding, and in some cases percutaneous treatment can be utilized (i.e., use of balloon or covered stent to seal the area of vessel injury and extravasation).

Femoral arterial puncture above the inguinal ligament (particularly with puncture of the back wall) may predispose to bleeding in the retroperitoneal space. This patient's diagnostic angiogram was performed in another hospital, and therefore, the information regarding the arterial access may not have been available. Continued administration of eptifibatide may have aggravated any ongoing bleeding. The diagnosis of retroperitoneal bleeding should be suspected in any patient following transfemoral catheterization who develops an unexplained vagal reaction or transient hypotension. The diagnosis can be confirmed with CT scanning, but the diagnosis is usually made on clinical grounds and the treatment is generally supportive with surgical exploration and repair seldom required.

28.10 **Answer B.** RV ischemia and infarction almost exclusively occur in the setting of infarction of the inferior wall of the left ventricle. This is most often seen with occlusion of the right coronary artery, proximal to the origin of the acute marginal branches. The characteristic triad of hypotension, clear lung fields, and elevation of the jugular venous pressure in the setting of an acute MI are classic features of RV infarction. Acute ischemia of the right ventricle leads to RV dilation, and in the presence of an intact pericardium, the interventricular septum shifts towards the left ventricle. This leads to RV systolic dysfunction and a decrease in LV preload, both of which can lead to hypotension. Initial management strategies should include optimization of RV preload with volume loading. Prompt revascularization is beneficial in relieving RV and LV ischemia. Other important features of the management of RV infarction include avoiding agents that may reduce preload, including nitroglycerin and diuretics. Inotropic agents (dobutamine) and IABP counterpulsation are sometimes needed to augment the cardiac output and improve hemodynamics (*N Engl J Med* 1994;330:1211–1217).

28.11 **Answer C.** Moderate or severe aortic insufficiency is a contraindication to an IABP. Inflation of the balloon during diastole raises the aortic pressure and increases coronary blood flow. Clues that this patient may have had chronic underlying aortic insufficiency are the presence of a wide pulse pressure, presence of a systolic murmur (due to overall increased blood flow across the aortic valve), and cardiomegaly on the chest x-ray. Placement of an IABP in this patient caused worsening acute, severe aortic insufficiency and pulmonary edema. An IABP would not be expected to cause clinical deterioration in the presence of an acute ventricular septal defect or acute severe mitral insufficiency. Acute stent thrombosis would not necessarily cause acute pulmonary edema, and is usually associated with chest pain and ST-segment elevation on the electrocardiogram.

28.12 **Answer D.** The patient is presenting with an acute anterior wall MI caused by thrombotic occlusion of the mid-LAD artery, complicated by rupture of the ventricular septum and cardiogenic shock. Percutaneous revascularization of the LAD artery should not be performed. This patient appears to be a surgical candidate and should have an IABP inserted, followed by emergency cardiac surgery and repair of the ventricular septum.

28.13 **Answer D.** The hemodynamic tracing demonstrates a typical finding in patients with hypertrophic obstructive cardiomyopathy and LV outflow obstruction. There is no LV outflow tract gradient at rest, but following a premature ventricular beat, there is augmentation of the LV contractility and outflow tract obstruction, which leads to a significant systolic pressure gradient and a narrowing of the pulse pressure (Brockenbrough-Braunwald sign). Following the procedure, he develops signs and symptoms of acute LV outflow obstruction that should initially be managed by bed rest and administration of intravenous fluids to augment preload. Refractory hypotension should be managed with intravenous phenylephrine (a pure α-agonist, vasoconstrictor). Dopamine should not be given as any inotropic agent may worsen the outflow tract obstruction and exacerbate hypotension. Atropine can be used for situations associated with increased vagal tone, but would not be appropriate in the acute management in this setting.

28.14 **Answer B.** Pulmonary artery rupture is a rare, but often lethal, complication of Swan-Ganz catheterization. Risk factors include older age, pulmonary hypertension, improper balloon inflation or positioning, manipulation of an inflated balloon-tipped catheter in the wedge position, and possibly anticoagulation (*Chest* 1995;108:1349–1352). Patients universally develop acute hemoptysis, which can be massive. Hemothorax can develop rapidly, and the patient should initially be turned to the side of the hemothorax to protect the unaffected lung. Immediate thoracotomy is likely the only life-saving therapy for patients who develop hemothorax. Reversal of anticoagulation is also reasonable once initial stabilizing measures have been performed. A chest tube can be inserted as a temporizing measure, but is not a substitute for prompt surgical correction.

28.15 **Answer C.** Reactions to iodinated contrast media occur in <1% of patients but may occur in 17% to 35% of patients with a prior contrast reaction (*Ann Intern Med* 2003;139:123–136). Common clinical manifestations can range from mild (pruritus and urticaria), to serious (bronchospasm and angioedema), to life threatening (shock). These manifestations are due to release of histamine from direct degranulation of tissue mast cells and circulating basophils and are anaphylactoid reactions in contrast to IgE-mediated true allergic reactions. Acute management of anaphylactoid contrast reactions in the catheterization laboratory includes administration of intravenous antihistamines (both anti-H_1 and anti-H_2) and corticosteroids (although the latter do not work immediately). Severe reactions that lead to respiratory and hemodynamic compromise should be treated with epinephrine (*Cathet Cardiovasc Diagn* 1995;34:99–104).

28.16 **Answer A.** Catheter-induced coronary spasm, most common in the proximal right coronary artery, should be considered in this patient based on the timing of the onset of symptoms. Although the chest pain could precipitate a vagal reaction and hypotension, the increase in heart rate makes this less likely. In addition, the absence of inferior ischemia on the stress test makes the diagnosis of coronary spasm more likely. Intravenous or intracoronary nitrates should be given prior to PCI whenever this diagnosis is suspected. Coronary spasm should be considered in the presence of a proximal stenosis in the right coronary artery that is smooth and concentric, particularly if the catheter deeply engages the artery.

28.17 **Answer B.** According to the ACC/AHA Guidelines for the Management of Patients with ST-Elevation Myocardial Infarction, emergency revascularization is given a Class I recommendation (conditions for which there is evidence and/or general agreement that a given procedure or treatment is beneficial, useful, and effective) for suitable patients <75 years of age who develop cardiogenic shock within 36 hours of MI, in whom revascularization can be performed within 18 hours of the onset of shock (*J Am Coll Cardiol* 2004;44:671–719). The SHOCK trial was a multicenter, randomized trial comparing emergency revascularization (either PCI or CABG) with initial medical stabilization (including an IABP) for patients with ST elevation or new left bundle branch block (LBBB) MI and cardiogenic shock. Although the 30-day mortality (primary end point) between the two groups was not statistically different, at 6 months and 1 year, mortality was better in the group assigned to emergency revascularization, compared to the group treated with initial medical stabilization (*N Engl J Med* 1999;341:625–634; *JAMA* 2001:285:190–192). A prespecified subgroup of patients <75 years of age similarly showed an overall benefit with emergency revascularization, with respect to 30-day mortality; however, of those >75 years (*n* = 56), there was no difference in mortality between the two treatment strategies. This might have been explained by the unexpectedly low mortality rate among elderly patients assigned to the initial medical stabilization arm, as their survival was similar to younger patients assigned to medical stabilization. Therefore, for patients >75 years of age, the ACC/AHA guidelines assign primary PCI a Class IIa (conditions for which there is conflicting evidence and/or divergence of opinion about the usefulness/efficacy of a procedure or treatment, but the weight of the evidence is in favor of such a procedure or treatment).

28.18 **Answer B.** Percutaneous circulatory assist devices are used in situations of severe cardiovascular hemodynamic compromise or collapse, such as fulminant myocarditis (as a bridge to cardiac transplantation). They are also commonly used in high-risk PCI in the setting of cardiogenic shock, severe LV dysfunction, or in intervention on the last remaining artery supplying viable myocardium.

28.19 **Answer C.** An RP bleed should be suspected in any patient who develops unheralded hypotension following transfemoral catheterization, even in the absence of visible bleeding in the groin. Femoral angiography prior to sheath removal is helpful in identifying whether the arterial puncture is above the inguinal ligament, in which case manual compression may be inadequate at achieving hemostasis. Angiography performed via the contralateral femoral artery can be performed to establish the site of bleeding and determine if suitable for percutaneous treatment. In this case, angiography confirmed suspected bleeding in the retroperitoneal space and identified contrast extravasation from the external iliac artery. Although vascular surgery can be performed to repair the site of bleeding, a trial of balloon occlusion, followed by insertion of a covered stent, would deliver more

immediate treatment and avoid higher morbidity associated with surgery. Manual pressure will likely be ineffective on its own with the location of bleeding above the femoral head. Transfusion of packed red blood cells may be needed but would depend on the initial hemoglobin and how quickly the bleeding is arrested.

28.20 **Answer D.** Vasopressors are commonly used to treat hypotension in various shock states. Phenylephrine is a potent α-adrenergic agonist, and raised mean arterial blood pressure through vasoconstriction and an elevation in systemic vascular resistance. Norepinephrine has potent α_1- and β_1-adrenergic activity ($\alpha > \beta$), and is commonly used to treat refractory hypotension in septic shock. Dopamine, at doses higher than 10 μg/kg/min, acts predominantly as an α-adrenergic agonist and potent vasoconstrictor. At doses <10 μg/kg/min but >3 μg/kg/min, it acts as a β-adrenergic agonist and positive inotrope. Dopamine is often used as a first-line agent for the treatment of persistent hypotension in cardiogenic shock. Dobutamine is a positive inotropic agent that also causes systemic vasodilation and is not a preferred agent for the treatment of persistent hypotension in cardiogenic shock.

28.21 **Answer C.** Side effects related to intravenous contrast agents may include bradycardia, hypotension, nausea, and vomiting. These are related to the tonicity of the agent used and occurred much more frequently when high-osmolar contrast agents were used in the past. These effects do not represent allergic reactions and should not be treated with steroids and/or antihistamines. The effect is usually transient, and the procedure can be continued.

28.22 **Answer B.** The electrocardiogram shows characteristic findings of acute pericarditis (diffuse, concave ST-segment elevation and PR-segment depression). Pericardial inflammation and effusion can develop several days to weeks following cardiac surgery, as part of the postpericardiotomy syndrome. Associated chest pain is pleuritic in nature, and a pericardial friction rub may be present on exam. The minimally invasive cardiac surgical technique may also be associated with more incomplete exposure and drainage of the pericardial space, as compared with the traditional full sternotomy incision. An echocardiogram should be obtained to assess for the presence of pericardial fluid and to further assess if tamponade is present. The history and the ECG are not consistent with an acute coronary syndrome, so anticoagulation and urgent angiography are not appropriate at this stage. While nonsteroidal anti-inflammatory agents are part of the management of uncomplicated pericarditis, this patient's recent cardiac surgery and current hypotension require further investigation.

28.23 **Answer C.** The case illustrates a late presentation following an acute anterior wall infarction complicated by cardiogenic shock. Symptoms had been present for several days, and the electrocardiogram as described shows evolving changes of a transmural, Q-wave infarction. The finding of a systolic murmur should alert the examiner to the possibility of a mechanical complication, in this case VSR. When VSR is suspected, right heart catheterization and sampling of blood for oximetry should be performed prior to angiography to assess for the presence of a left-to-right shunt. Echocardiography or LV angiography can also be performed to establish the diagnosis. If VSR is confirmed, coronary angiography can be performed prior to referral for cardiac surgery.

28.24 **Answer B.** Bleeding complications are common following PCI and can range from minor bleeding at the access site to life-threatening bleeding in the RP space. Reversal of anticoagulation may be warranted if bleeding occurs and leads to hemodynamic compromise. Protamine can be given to reverse the effects of heparin, but in this case would likely not be helpful when the ACT is already low. Abciximab is a monoclonal antibody that binds to the platelet glycoprotein IIb/IIIa receptor and inhibits platelet aggregation. Thrombocytopenia, leading to bleeding complications, can develop following exposure to abciximab and is more common than with eptifibatide and tirofiban (*Am Heart J* 2000;140(2):206–211). Abciximab should be discontinued, and platelets transfused, in patients who are actively bleeding. Plasma exchange is a treatment for thrombocytopenia resulting from thrombotic thrombocytopenic purpura, but is not used when thrombocytopenia is related to abciximab. Similarly, intravenous immunoglobulin is not used to treat this scenario.

28.25 **Answer C.** Serious complications associated with RV endomyocardial biopsy include chamber perforation and pericardial tamponade, supraventricular and ventricular arrhythmias, complete atrioventricular block (especially in the presence of left bundle branch block), and pulmonary embolism (*Circulation* 2007;116(19):2216–2233). The risk of such major complications are reported at <1% (*Circulation* 2008;118(17):1722–1728). Potential factors which may increase the risk of complications include RV chamber enlargement, elevated RV filling pressure, thrombocytopenia, or anticoagulation with heparin or warfarin. Prior cardiac surgery that involved excision of the pericardium may have a lower risk of tamponade in the event a perforation were to occur.

29

Peripheral Interventional Procedures

Arun Kalyanasundaram and Samir Kapadia

QUESTIONS

29.1 Which of the following patients is NOT an appropriate candidate for carotid artery stenting (CAS) according to the SAPPHIRE trial criteria?

(A) An 82-year-old woman with a recent history of transient ischemic attack (TIA), poorly controlled hypertension, and 60% stenosis of the internal carotid artery

(B) A 72-year-old man with a history of myocardial infarction (MI) 3 weeks ago and an 80% stenosis of the right internal carotid artery (ICA)

(C) A 60-year-old diabetic man with a history of cerebrovascular accident 6 weeks ago resulting in residual left upper extremity paresis with 90% left internal carotid stenosis

(D) An asymptomatic 85-year-old man with severe emphysematous lung disease, NYHA (New York Heart Association) class III congestive heart failure (CHF), and bilateral 80% stenosis of the internal carotid arteries

29.2 All of the following are complications of CAS, EXCEPT:

(A) Stroke
(B) Hypotension/Bradycardia
(C) MI
(D) Hyperperfusion Syndrome
(E) All of the above

29.3 The angiogram in Figure Q29-3 was performed on a 74-year-old diabetic patient with a recent hospitalization for transient left upper extremity paresis. On the basis of the data reported by large, randomized trials evaluating the efficacy of traditional carotid endarterectomy (CEA), which of the following statements is TRUE?

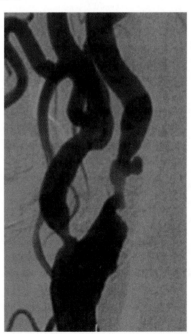

Figure Q29-3

(A) This patient is not an appropriate candidate for CEA because of his recent transient left upper extremity paresis and should be considered for CAS for an optimal outcome

(B) The patient would be appropriate for CEA and can expect a lower risk of any major or fatal ipsilateral stroke in the 2 years following the procedure at the expense of an initial increase in the 30-day risk of death and stroke as compared with medical therapy

(C) The patient is a candidate for CEA and can expect a lower risk of stroke or death immediately following the procedure but the benefit becomes insignificant at 2 years as compared with medical therapy

(D) The patient is a candidate for CEA and can expect a lower risk of any ipsilateral or contralateral stroke in the 2 years following the procedure

29.4 Periprocedural stroke during carotid stenting is most commonly attributable to distal embolization. During which portion of the procedure are distal embolic events most likely to occur?

(A) Wiring
(B) Predilatation
(C) Stenting
(D) Postdilatation
(E) Guide placement

29.5 Which of the following types of procedures has the least detectable amount of embolization by diffusion-weighted MRI?

(A) Carotid stenting with filter-on-wire emboli protection device
(B) Carotid stenting with distal-occlusion emboli protection device
(C) Carotid stenting with proximal occlusion emboli protection device
(D) carotid endarterectomy
(E) carotid stenting with initial predilation using a 2.0 Coronary balloon; followed by distal-occlusion emboli protection device

29.6 Which of the following statements regarding symptomatic peripheral arterial disease (PAD) is INCORRECT?

(A) Most patients participating in formal exercise rehabilitation programs have been shown to double their symptom-free walking period
(B) Because of their high rate of comorbid cardiovascular disease (CVD) and vascular events, all patients with PAD should be considered to have coronary artery disease (CAD) until proved otherwise, and initiated on drug therapy until their low-density lipoprotein C (LDL-C) levels are reduced to <100 mg/dL
(C) The presence of low ankle-brachial indices (ABIs) in hypertensive patients is a predictor of increased mortality
(D) The FDA has approved both pentoxiphylline and clopidogrel for the treatment of intermittent claudication (IC)

29.7 All of the following are acceptable indications for endovascular intervention to the superficial femoral arterial lesion shown in the following figure, EXCEPT:

(A) Incapacitating intermittent claudication
(B) Rest pain
(C) Development of nonhealing ulcerations or wounds of the lower extremity
(D) Presence of a 5-cm eccentric 80% lesion of the proximal superficial femoral artery (SFA) in a patient with mild intermittent claudication

29.8 The angiogram in Figure Q29-8 is that of a 65-year-old man who has a history of poorly controlled diabetes, hypertension as well as tobacco abuse, and complains of claudication symptoms after walking approximately 100 feet. His symptoms have been stable for more than 3 years, and he denies rest pain or chronic, nonhealing wound infections. Which of the following statements regarding this patient's future management is INCORRECT?

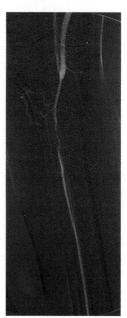

Figure Q29-8

(A) The patient should be counseled on risk factor modification, including smoking cessation, and should be referred to a formal exercise rehabilitation program
(B) Because of the high rate of complications during infrapopliteal interventions, including thrombosis and perforation, angioplasty of these lesions is contraindicated
(C) The indications for endovascular intervention of these lesions include critical limb ischemia, rest pain, nonhealing wounds, or limb salvage
(D) Long-term patency rates for infrapopliteal interventions are not as favorable as those for iliac or femoral procedures

29.9 A 75-year-old woman with an ongoing history of hypertension, hypercholesterolemia, tobacco abuse, and moderately severe claudication presents with a complaint of sudden onset, unbearable pain in the right lower extremity for the past 3 hours. An examination reveals a cool and mottled extremity with no popliteal arterial pulsation detected. Which of the following statements regarding this condition is INCORRECT?

(A) The most common etiologies of this condition are in situ thrombosis and embolism; however, the differential diagnosis must also include dissection, trauma, vasculitis, or abdominal aortic aneurysm (AAA) thrombosis or dissection

(B) Treatment options for this condition include primary surgical revascularization, intravenous thrombolysis, or percutaneous mechanical thrombectomy

(C) An initial approach of antithrombotics, such as heparin, should be considered

(D) Without rapid diagnosis and treatment, this patient is at high risk for amputation and/or mortality under any circumstance

29.10 All of the following are indications for renal arteriography, EXCEPT:

(A) Onset of hypertension in an individual younger than 30 or older than 55 years or rapidly accelerating hypertension in a previously well-controlled patient

(B) Azotemia after the initiation of an angiotensin-converting enzyme inhibitor (ACEI)

(C) Asymmetric kidney size as documented by noninvasive imaging in association with an unexplained elevation in creatinine (>1.5 mg/dL)

(D) The finding of an abdominal bruit on physical examination

(E) Following the completion of a diagnostic left-heart catheterization in a patient with severe coronary atherosclerosis with normal renal function

29.11 Which of the following is NOT an indication for percutaneous revascularization of the lesion seen in Figure Q29-11?

(A) Recurrent admission for decompensated heart failure or flash pulmonary edema in a medically compliant 72-year-old patient

(B) Hypertension refractory to >3, maximally dosed, antihypertensive medications

(C) Subacute renal failure (creatinine < 3.0 mg/dL) in normal-sized kidneys (>9 cm) on non-invasive imaging

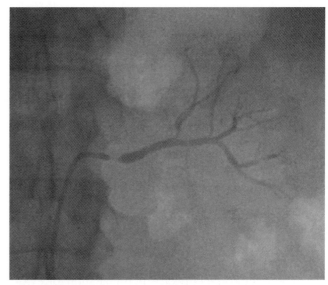

Figure Q29-11

(D) Chronic kidney disease in a 65-year-old non-diabetic requiring renal replacement therapy (i.e., dialysis) instead of an alternative etiology

(E) Severe coronary atherosclerotic disease to prevent worsening of renal function (current GFR > 60) in a male, diabetic patient

29.12 Which of the following statements regarding the treatment of renal artery stenosis (RAS) is TRUE?

(A) Trials evaluating percutaneous revascularization of significant RAS (>70% lesion) in patients with renovascular hypertension have demonstrated no reduction in blood pressure as compared with patients treated with medical therapy, although they help preserve renal function long-term

(B) Angioplasty with stent placement is superior to angioplasty alone in patients with fibromuscular dysplasia (FMD)

(C) Especially in patients with aorto-ostial or proximal RAS, angioplasty with stenting is superior to angioplasty alone

(D) ACEIs should not be used in patients with a significant unilateral RAS, secondary to a high risk of azotemia from the accentuated transglomerular pressure gradient

29.13 A 65-year-old diabetic man with a history of hypertension, hypercholesterolemia, and heavy tobacco use presents to his local emergency department complaining of increasing lower abdominal pain over the past 3 weeks. During his physical examination, a tender, pulsatile mass is detected in the lower abdomen with an associated systolic murmur. High-resolution computed tomography (CT) scan reveals an infrarenal AAA with a maximal diameter of 6 cm without evidence of rupture or leak. Which of the following statements regarding the management of this patient's condition is TRUE?

(A) Current data regarding the long-term efficacy of endovascular aneurysm repair (EVAR) indicates that this patient would likely have a significantly reduced all-cause mortality if he underwent EVAR as opposed to open surgical repair

(B) There is no long-term follow-up with EVAR and hence should not be considered in a person at this age, with open surgical repair being the preferred modality of treatment

(C) The CT was unwarranted. An abdominal angiogram should have been the diagnostic modality of choice, in preparation for EVAR

(D) Cardiac complications are the most common serious perioperative complication of EVAR and the most common cause of late death

(E) If records from the patient's primary care physician revealed that the AAA was actually discovered the previous year and was 5.5 cm in maximal diameter at that time (<0.5 cm/year), a reasonable management strategy would include aggressive medical management of the patient's hypertension, counseling for smoking cessation, and a repeat CT scan in 6 months to evaluate the AAA dimensions

29.14 Which of the following is NOT typically noted as a complication of AAA endovascular repair?

(A) Leaking of blood into the aneurysmal sac from either the proximal or distal sites of endograft attachment

(B) Accumulation of blood in the aneurysmal sac due to retrograde blood flow from patent lumbar or inferior mesenteric arteries

(C) Increased graft porosity resulting in slow permeation of blood across the endograft into the aneurysmal sac

(D) Renal, mesenteric, or iliac artery ischemia

(E) Spinal cord ischemia (SCI)

29.15 A 75-year-old man with a history of poorly controlled hypertension, PAD, chronic obstructive pulmonary disease (COPD), and a 60 pack per year history of tobacco abuse presents to his primary care physician's office noting development of dizziness, blurred vision, and gait instability after chopping wood. The patient's wife states that he had difficulty with his speech and appeared to be disoriented the previous week when he was

helping their son move. The patient's neurologic examination is unremarkable, with the exception of diminished radial pulse in the right upper extremity. Which of the following statements regarding this patient is TRUE?

(A) A noncontrast head CT would be the most informative diagnostic test and would likely reveal the etiology of the patient's symptoms

(B) The patient should be immediately transferred to the nearest emergency department for urgent neurologic evaluation and thrombolytic therapy

(C) After ordering a sedimentation rate and prescribing a course of oral steroid therapy, the patient should be referred to ophthalmology for an urgent slit lamp examination

(D) After obtaining a baseline electrocardiogram, complete blood count, basic metabolic panel, and coagulation studies (prothrombin time, activated partial thromboplastin time), the patient should be referred for an arch aortogram as soon as possible

(E) The patient should undergo a transthoracic echocardiogram with agitated saline to rule out patent foramen ovale

29.16 Which of the following does the angiogram in Figure Q29-16 show?

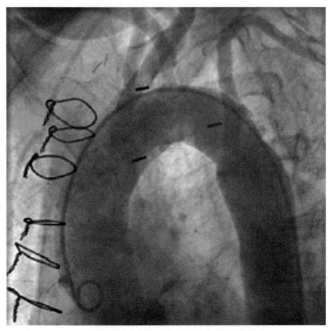

Figure Q29-16

(A) Right-sided aortic arch
(B) Retroesophageal right subclavian
(C) Anomalous origin of the left vertebral
(D) Normal aortic arch

29.17 A 26-year-old woman presents with low-grade fever over the past 6 to 8 weeks associated with weight loss, malaise, and nocturnal diaphoresis. The patient also notes that her right arm has become painful and "crampy" over the same time course. In addition, the patient states that since the previous week her vision seemed to have become blurred, and she is now concerned that she may be losing her sight altogether. Remarkable findings on examination include a temperature of 38°C, blood pressure 185/100, the presence of a left infraclavicular bruit, and a diminished right radial pulse. The angiogram in Figure 29-17 is of this patient. Which of the following statements regarding this patient's condition is TRUE?

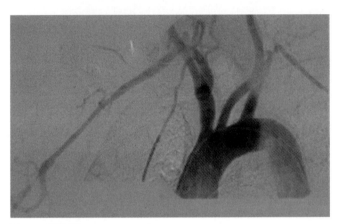

Figure Q29-17

(A) After obtaining a sedimentation rate, VDRL test, rheumatoid factor, antinuclear antibody, coagulation studies, and baseline blood chemistries, the patient should undergo urgent cerebral and aortic arch angiography for possible intervention

(B) Immediate, aggressive control of the patient's hypertension should be avoided in this situation

(C) Treatment for this condition should consist of high-dose glucocorticoids and cyclophosphamide

(D) Primary angioplasty offers a higher rate of cure for this condition

(E) Regardless of the mode of treatment, the patient faces a low relapse rate

29.18 Which of the following does the angiogram in Figure Q29-18 show?

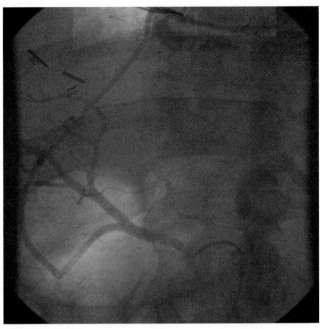

Figure Q29-18

(A) Superior mesenteric artery (SMA)

(B) Inferior mesenteric artery (IMA)

(C) Hepatic and in situ right gastroepiploic graft to posterior descending artery (PDA)

(D) Splenic artery

(E) Left gastric and in situ right gastroepiploic graft to PDA

29.19 A 73-year-old male patient who had treatment of his right SFA with balloon angioplasty 4 years ago and subsequent stenting 2 years ago has the following angiogram (Fig. Q29-19A–C).

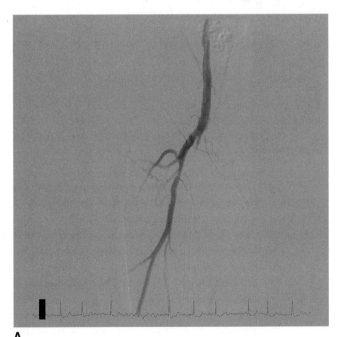

A

Figure Q29-19A

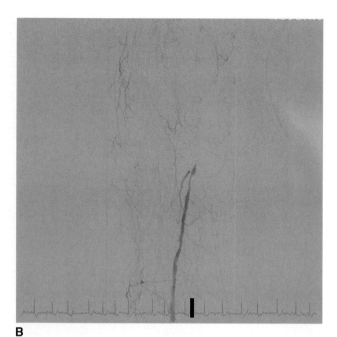

B

Figure Q29-19B

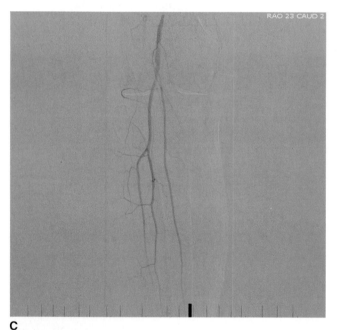

C

Figure Q29-19C

(A) This is a TASC B lesion and endovascular repair is a reasonable option for the patient if he has a high surgical risk

(B) This is a TASC C lesion and endovascular repair is a reasonable option if the patient has a high surgical risk

(C) This is a TASC D lesion and surgical option is clearly preferred

(D) This is a TASC B lesion. However, neither surgical nor endovascular options are viable given the poor distal run-off

29.20 Figure Q29-20 is classic for:

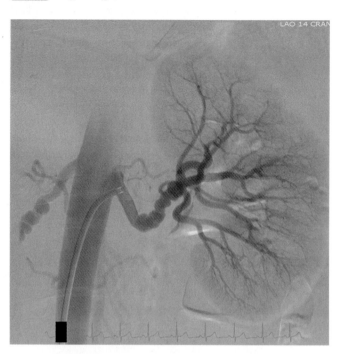

Figure Q29-20

(A) Fibromuscular dysplasia (FMD)

(B) Atherosclerotic renovascular disease

(C) Posttransplantation stenosis

(D) Neurofibromatosis

29.21 In lower extremity interventions, the device in Figure Q29-21 would be best suited for:

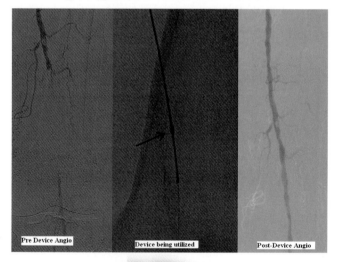

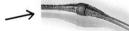

Figure Q29-21

(A) Focal noncalcified SFA lesions

(B) Ostial SFA lesion

(C) Heavily calcified lesions

(D) Bailout for treatment of perforations

29.22 All of the following can be concluded from the CREST trial among patients with symptomatic or asymptomatic carotid stenosis, EXCEPT:

(A) Risk of the primary outcome of stroke, MI, or death are not significantly different in the group undergoing carotid-artery stenting and the group undergoing CEA

(B) During the periprocedural period, there was a higher risk of minor stroke with stenting and a higher risk of MI with endarterectomy

(C) After the periprocedural period, the incidence of ipsilateral stroke was similar with carotid-artery stenting and with CEA

(D) The risk of ipsilateral stroke was higher with stenting during the periprocedural period and continues to increase after the periprocedural period

29.23 Which of the following statements is INCORRECT?

(A) PAD affects approximately 5 to 10 million adults in the United States, with an increased incidence in the elderly and in African Americans

(B) Despite the widespread prevalence and cardiovascular risk implications, only 25% of PAD patients are undergoing treatment

(C) In the general population, about a third with PAD have the classic symptoms of IC, and two-thirds have no leg symptoms

(D) The risk factors for PAD are similar to those for coronary heart disease (CHD), although diabetes and cigarette smoking are particularly strong risk factors for PAD

(E) PAD is a marker for systemic atherosclerotic disease. Persons with PAD, compared to those without, have four to five times the risk of dying of a cardiovascular disease event, resulting in two to three times higher total mortality risk

29.24 The angiogram in Figure Q29-24 was performed after an unsuccessful attempt to place a large 14F sheath in the left common femoral artery. The most important finding is:

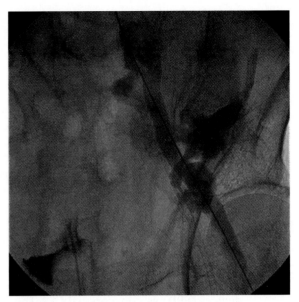

Figure Q29-24

(A) A severely diseased left external iliac artery

(B) Critical internal iliac artery stenosis that needs immediate intervention

(C) Small perforation that can be dealt with by placement of a larger sheath in the ipsilateral side

(D) Large perforation that needs immediate stenting from the ipsilateral side

(E) Large perforation that needs immediate balloon occlusion from contralateral side

29.25 A 65-year-old man presents with hypotension from pulmonary embolism after knee replacement surgery. Which one of the following is TRUE?

(A) Diagnosis is confirmed by angiography

(B) Aspiration thrombectomy is the first line of treatment

(C) Filter placement is optimal therapy considering recent knee surgery

(D) Hypercoagulable workup is necessary

(E) Three months of coumadin therapy is adequate if this is the first thromboembolic event

ANSWERS AND EXPLANATIONS

29.1 Answer C. Several large registries and one randomized clinical trial have demonstrated that the outcomes following CAS compare favorably with the traditional surgical endarterectomy (CEA) in select high-risk populations. The SAPPHIRE trial (*N Engl J Med* 2004;351:1493–1501) randomized 334 patients with symptomatic (>50% stenosis) or asymptomatic (>80% stenosis) carotid disease traditionally considered a high risk for surgical intervention to percutaneous carotid intervention with nitinol stents in conjunction with embolic protection devices (EPD) vs. conventional CEA. The results demonstrated the noninferiority of CAS as well as a 39% reduction in the primary end point of a composite of death, stroke, and MI within 30 days. Additionally, patients randomized to CAS enjoyed lower rates of target-vessel revascularization and a shorter hospital stay, as well as a significantly greater 1-year event-free survival (88% vs. 79%, *p* = 0.048). On the basis of the balance of evidence, the FDA has approved elective CAS only in the "high-risk" populations with symptoms, listed subsequently. Although trials evaluating lower-risk populations are currently ongoing, only patients meeting one or more of the following criteria are deemed candidates for CAS.

Clinical: Age > 80 years, CHF III–IV, known severe left ventricular dysfunction (ejection fraction < 30%), open heart surgery needed within 6 weeks, recent MI (>24 hours and <4 weeks), unstable angina (Canadian Cardiovascular Society class III/IV), severe pulmonary disease, contralateral laryngeal nerve palsy.

Anatomic: Previous CEA with recurrent stenosis, high cervical lesions or clear cell acanthoma lesions below the clavicle, contralateral carotid occlusion, radiation therapy to the neck, prior radical neck surgery, severe tandem lesions (*N Engl J Med* 2004;351:1493–1501).

Further, although age >80 years was a criterion for SAPPHIRE, a recent meta-analysis concluded that stenting for symptomatic carotid stenosis should be avoided in older patients (age ≥ 70 years) but might be as safe as endarterectomy in younger patients (*Lancet* 2010;376:1062–1073). The patient in choice C does not meet any high risk criteria.

29.2 Answer E. Data obtained from the high-risk carotid stenting registries indicate that the 30-day incidence of post-CAS stroke approaches 3%. The primary mechanism of procedure-related stroke is thought to be the distal embolization of atheromatous debris dislodged during the procedure. In addition, manipulation of wires, catheters, and guides in the aortic arch and common carotid artery are not protected by EPD and are frequently responsible for strokes outside the territory of the treated carotid artery.

Distention of the carotid sinus mechanoreceptors by angioplasty and stenting may activate the vasomotor center of the medulla through cranial nerve IX. Subsequent vagal activation results in peripheral vasodilatation with hypotension and bradycardia. This phenomenon is relatively common and occurs in up to 40% of the procedures involving internal carotid lesions. Interestingly, in the restenotic lesions after endarterectomy, this reflex is typically not encountered. Supportive therapy with IV fluids, atropine, pseudoephedrine (60 mg PO b.i.d.), and, infrequently, dopamine are needed to counter hypotension and bradycardia.

The incidence of MI within 30 days of carotid stenting in the high-risk cohort of patients in the SAPPHIRE trial was 1.9%, which was significantly lower than that seen after CEA in that trial (*N Engl J Med* 2004;351:1493–1501).

In a response to carotid occlusive disease and chronically decreasing cerebral perfusion pressures, the cerebral vessels may undergo a compensatory vasodilatation in an effort to maintain adequate blood flow to the brain. Following intervention to the carotid artery, there is a sudden concomitant increase in blood flow to the dilated vasculature and the net effect can be hyperperfusion to the brain with resultant edema. Presenting symptoms can include a throbbing, retro-orbital headache that lateralizes to the side of the intervention, nausea, vomiting, visual changes, focal motor deficits, and even seizures. Increased flow velocities by transcranial doppler in symptomatic patients even in the absence of any significant findings on CT imaging are suggestive of hyperperfusion. Aggressive control of blood pressure is necessary to prevent this complication (*J Am Coll Cardiol* 2004;43:1596–1601).

29.3 **Answer B.** The benefits of CEA in select patients with symptomatic carotid atherosclerosis (i.e., TIA, nondisabling stroke) have been well-documented by numerous randomized trials. The North American Symptomatic Carotid Endarterectomy Trial (*N Engl J Med* 1991;325:445–453) was a prospective, multicenter study that randomized 396 patients with a history of hemispheric or retinal TIA or a nondisabling stroke in the 4 months before entry with stenosis of 70% to 99% in the symptomatic carotid artery to either medical therapy or CEA. Although CEA was associated with a significantly higher risk of death or stroke at 30 days (5.8% vs. 3.3%), this was countered by a significantly lower risk of major or fatal ipsilateral stroke (13.1% vs. 2.5%, $p < 0.001$) as well as reduced risk of any ipsilateral stroke in the CEA group at 2-year follow-up. The overall benefit of CEA persisted even after perioperative stroke and death were included in the end point analysis. The European Carotid Artery Surgery Trial (*Lancet* 1998;351:1379–1387) randomized 2,518 patients with symptomatic, ipsilateral carotid stenosis, and also found that despite a 7% 30-day rate of stroke or death, patients with severe stenosis (70% to 99%) treated with CEA had a significantly lower risk of ipsilateral stroke (2.8% vs. 16.8%, $p < 0.0001$) by 3 years' follow-up. The benefit of CEA persisted even after including all perioperative strokes, death, or any other stroke in the analysis (12.3% vs. 21.9%). It is noteworthy that patients with mild stenosis (0% to 29%) did not realize significant benefit from CEA. Therefore, the patient *is* a good candidate for CEA given his recent TIA and >80% stenosis of the ipsilateral carotid (A). The preceding data would suggest that he could anticipate a slightly increased risk of perioperative stroke or death but would then likely be at a significantly reduced risk of ipsilateral or fatal stroke over the next 2 to 3 years (C). Currently, there is no evidence that CEA for symptomatic carotid stenosis reduces the risk of contralateral stroke.

29.4 **Answer D.** Although the rate of periprocedural stroke has been significantly reduced by the use of EPD, this is still a serious complication of CAS. Randomized trials comparing CAS with and without EPDs are not likely because of obvious ethical concerns; however, multiple retrospective studies have suggested efficacy of EPD in the prevention of stroke during CAS (*Stroke* 2003;34:813–819; *Eur Heart J* 2004;25:1550–1558).

Although there is a risk of distal embolization of dislodged debris during all the preceding noted portions of the intervention, postdilatation of the stent poses the greatest risk. Although postdilatation of heavily calcified lesions can result in the displacement of calcific plaque debris with subsequent embolization, lesions composed of softer plaque materials may respond to overaggressive postdilatation by extrusion of the plaque contents with resultant embolization.

29.5 **Answer D.** Filter-type devices are usually composed of a polyurethane netting with a fixed pore space (from 80 to 140 μm) fitted over a titanium–nickel (nitinol) frame and are currently the most widely used of the EPDs. In practice, the filter is delivered across the carotid lesion in a collapsed form on a 0.014-in. guidewire. Optimum positioning of the filter depends upon deployment in a portion of the vessel that is straight and free of significant disease. This is frequently found in the prepetrous portion of the cervical ICA, which is usually straight and free of disease. An advantage of the filter-type device is that it allows continuous antegrade blood flow during the intervention. It also allows adequate visualization of the artery during the procedure with dye injection.

Distal occlusion balloon devices are the next most common form of EPD. This device functions through a balloon that is inflated and deflated through a crush-resistant nitinol hypotube situated in a 0.014-in. guidewire. After crossing the stenotic lesion, a marker on the device is placed in the prepetrous portion of the cervical ICA. Subsequent to proper positioning, the balloon is inflated resulting in cessation of all antegrade blood flow. Following the intervention, the column of blood immediately proximal to the balloon is aspirated through a monorail export system thereby removing any debris dislodged during instrumentation.

Yet another system to prevent embolization during procedures includes a proximal occlusion device that creates retrograde flow in the ICA by establishing a continuous pressure gradient between the ICA and the femoral vein. This is accomplished by occluding both the proximal CCA and external carotid artery with balloon-mounted catheters resulting in cessation of antegrade flow. Blood is aspirated from the CCA through the catheter tip distal to the balloon and is returned to the femoral vein through a blood return system resulting in a continuous retrograde flow of blood in the ICA and removal of all plaque debris from cerebral circulation. However, patients in the stenting group using any of the EPDs have more ischemic lesions on diffusion-weighted imaging on posttreatment scans compared to CEA (*Lancet Neurol* 2010;9:353–362).

29.6 **Answer D.** Participation in a formal exercise rehabilitation program results in a significant improvement in the time to claudication pain and the time to maximal pain as demonstrated by Gardner and Poehlman in their meta-analysis of 33 trials evaluating walking distances in patients with PAD before and after rehabilitation. Program characteristics that were noted to correlate to increased pain-free distances were exercise duration >30 minutes per session, participation in at least three sessions per week, walking as a mode of exercise, and the use of near-maximal claudication pain as an end point, with participation in the program of >6 months. The only independent predictors of increased walking distances were the use of the claudication end point, program length, and mode of exercise ($p = 0.001$) (*JAMA* 1995;274:975–980).

On the basis of the results of numerous studies detailing the elevated crude rates of CHD in patients with PAD, the current National Cholesterol Education Program/Adult Treatment Panel III recommendations consider PAD as a CHD risk equivalent and advise that the goal LDL-C be lowered to <100 mg/dL with consideration of drug therapy in addition to lifestyle modifications to achieve this goal (*Circulation* 2004;110:227–239). The heart protection study prospectively randomized 20,536 patients with either CAD, diabetes mellitus, or PAD to either simvastatin 40 mg once daily vs. placebo and reported a reduction in all-cause mortality of 13% ($p = 0.0003$), major vascular events by 24%, coronary death by 18%, and nonfatal or fatal stroke by 25%. Most strikingly, the reduction in the event rates was also observed in the subgroups of patients without known coronary disease, including those with diabetes, cerebrovascular disease, and PAD (*Lancet* 2002;360:1623–1630).

Abnormal ABIs (<0.9), as a noninvasive diagnostic tool for PAD, have been shown to be associated with other traditional cardiovascular risk factors as well as more than a threefold increase in CHD and CVD mortality. In a prospective cohort study of 1,537 patients with systolic hypertension, 25.5% of participants recorded an ABI of <0.9. Abnormal ABI was statistically associated with the presence of other typical CAD risk factors. After 1- to 2-year follow-up, the presence of an abnormal ABI had an increased age–sex adjusted relative risk of mortality because of CHD of 3.8 (95% CI, 2.1 to 6.9), CVD of 3.7 (95% CI, 1.8 to 7.7), and total mortality of 4.1 (95% CI, 2 to 8.3) (*JAMA* 1993;270:487–489).

Currently, the only FDA-approved medications labeled for the purpose of relief of claudication because of PAD are pentoxifylline and cilostazol. Cilostazol, a type III phosphodiesterase inhibitor with direct action on the platelets and vascular smooth muscle, functions as a potent antiplatelet agent as well as vasodilator. A meta-analysis of eight randomized, placebo-controlled trials encompassing 2,702 patients with moderate to severe claudication demonstrated that cilostazol increased maximal and pain-free walking distances by 50% and 67%, respectively (*Am J Cardiol* 2002;90:1314–1319). Pentoxifylline, known to function by reducing the red blood cell viscosity, was shown to increase the pain-free walking distance by a mean of 29.4 m (95% CI, 13.0 to 45.9 m), and the absolute claudication distance by a mean of 48.4 m (95% CI, 18.3 to 78.6 m) in a total of 612 patients with moderate, IC symptoms at baseline (*CMAJ* 1996;155:1053–1059). Another study, however, indicated that cilostazol was more effective than pentoxifylline for increasing pain-free walking distances, but was associated with a greater incidence of side effects such as diarrhea and headache (*Am J Med* 2000;109:523–530).

29.7 **Answer D.** The current American Heart Association guidelines recommend that percutaneous endovascular interventions be reserved for patients who have developed severe, incapacitating claudication that significantly interferes with their lifestyle or work. Additional indications include the development of rest pain, presence of nonhealing ulcerations or wounds, or the development of lower extremity gangrene. Most patients with angiographic evidence of obstructive SFA disease do not have significant claudication symptoms and therefore do not warrant peripheral intervention on the basis of the presence of lesions alone (*J Am Coll Cardiol* 2006;47:1239–1312).

29.8 **Answer B.** Given that the long-term patency rates following infrapopliteal angioplasty are inferior to that of the larger vessels above the knee, percutaneous transluminal angioplasty (PTA) should be reserved for situations of acute limb ischemia (ALI), nonhealing wounds, or for limb salvage in patients who are not surgical candidates. Medical therapy with antiplatelet agents, such as aspirin, clopidogrel, or cilostazol, should be the first line of therapy. In addition to participation in a formal exercise rehabilitation program, risk factor modification including the aggressive management of diabetes and the cessation of tobacco use are also essential. Although the rate of progression to eventual limb loss or severe ischemia is 2% per year, diabetic patients with claudication symptoms have a greater likelihood of progressing to rest pain, developing gangrene, and eventual limb loss. Smokers also have increased rates of disease progression and have a 20% risk of limb loss if they continue to smoke (*J Am Coll Cardiol* 2006;47:1239–1312).

Although vessel perforation or thrombosis can occur during any interventional procedure involving a lower extremity vessel, the complication rate of PTA in the infrapopliteal vascular bed is not prohibitively high and, as noted in the preceding text, has clear indications. In a recent study evaluating the efficacy of below-the-knee stent-supported angioplasty to establish inline arterial flow in 82 patients with critical limb ischemia (68%) or lifestyle limiting claudication (32%), the technical success rate was 94% for de novo lesions, and there were no major adverse events such as death, MI, or limb loss reported. In addition, there was a significant increase ($p = 0.0001$) in the ABIs of both the groups following intervention, as well as a subjective improvement in wound healing and decreased rest pain (*J Am Coll Cardiol* 2004;44:2307–2314). Treating below-the-knee critical limb ischemia with DES may also be an effective and safe means of preventing major amputation and relieving symptoms (*J Am Coll Cardiol* 2010;55:1580–1589).

29.9 **Answer B.** This patient's presentation is consistent with that of ALI and should be treated as a medical emergency. Timely diagnosis and the institution of an appropriate therapy is crucial to prevent limb loss and even death, with the 30-day mortality rates approaching 15% and amputation rates between 15% and 30%. ALI is most frequently because of in situ thrombosis in the setting of preexistent atherosclerosis or embolism from a proximal source. All the treatment modalities listed in the preceding text are utilized for this condition; however, the delivery of thrombolytic therapy for the treatment of ALI should be catheter-based, not intravenous. This is because of the data showing increased rates of significant hemorrhage, and less successful target-vessel patency with the use of intravenous

thrombolytics as opposed to intra-arterial delivery. Percutaneous mechanical thrombectomy is largely reserved for patients with contraindications to thrombolysis but is also useful in debulking thrombus mass before thrombolytic therapy or for rescue therapy after failed lysis (*J Vasc Interv Radiol* 2005;16:585–595). Because of the large number of medical comorbidities that usually accompany patients with ALI, surgical treatment of ALI carries significant risk of mortality with figures approaching 30% in some series (*J Vasc Interv Radiol* 1996;7:57–6).

29.10 **Answer E.** The vast majority of RAS is because of either atherosclerotic disease or FMD, and is estimated to be present in up to 5% of hypertensive patients. In addition, RAS may be noted in up to 30% to 40% of patients with documented atherosclerosis of other vascular beds (*N Engl J Med* 2001;344:431–442). Atherosclerotic renal disease (>90% of RAS) typically involves the ostium or proximal third of the renal artery, progresses with age and is known to be associated with hypertension and renal insufficiency (*N Engl J Med* 2001;344:431–442). FMD (<10% of RAS) is most commonly found in women aged 15 to 50 years, and involves the distal two-thirds of the vessel with a characteristic "string of beads" appearance on angiography (*N Engl J Med* 2004;350:1862–1871). In addition to the preceding indications, other indications for renal arteriography include azotemia without clear etiology in a patient with evidence of atherosclerotic disease in other vascular beds, malignant hypertension refractory to the addition of three of more antihypertensive medications, or unexplained renal failure. Although it is generally a safe and well-tolerated procedure, renal arteriography should only be considered for patients in whom the operator has strong clinical suspicion of renovascular disease. Although uncommon, complications of renal arteriography include atheroembolism, renal artery ostial trauma, dissection, and contrast nephrotoxicity. Performing routine angiography of the renal vasculature in a patient without one of the preceding indications is not recommended.

29.11 **Answer E.** Given the paucity of randomized data comparing percutaneous intervention to medically based therapy for the treatment of RAS, there remains controversy over the exact indications for renal artery intervention. Because of the rather high perioperative mortality rate associated with surgical revascularization (2% to 13%

in varying reports), percutaneous revascularization is currently preferred over surgical intervention. In RAS secondary to atherosclerosis, stenting yields superior results to angioplasty alone and is definitely indicated for ostial lesions, restenosis, suboptimal results after angioplasty (>30% residual stenosis, gradient > 15 mm Hg), or in cases complicated by dissection (*Lancet* 1999;353:282–286). In RAS because of FMD, hypertension can typically be managed successfully with medical therapy including ACEI, and percutaneous intervention is not necessary. In situations where intervention is required, angioplasty alone provides a cure rate approaching 80%.

Therefore, in the presence of significant RAS (lesion >70% or >15 mm Hg pressure gradient), evidence of CHF, progressive or endstage renal disease, and malignant or medically refractory hypertension are the indications to proceed with percutaneous intervention. The mere presence of RAS that is not associated with any of the above is not an indication for intervention.

29.12 **Answer C.** Renal artery revascularization may be indicated in patients with hemodynamically significant lesions who have resistant hypertension, malignant hypertension, an inability to tolerate antihypertensive medications, recurrent episodes of flash pulmonary edema, and perhaps unstable angina (*Circulation* 2006;113:e463).

Given the suboptimal outcomes often seen with angioplasty of aorto-ostial and proximal renal arterial lesions, the use of angioplasty with stenting has become a common practice in many institutions. In a prospective study of 85 patients with ostial atherosclerotic RAS randomized to either angioplasty plus stenting or angioplasty alone, the primary success rate of angioplasty was 57% as compared with 88% in the stenting group (31%; 95% CI, 12 to 50) with no significant differences in the complication rate (*Lancet* 1999;353: 282–286). This difference was maintained through the 6-month follow-up with primary patency rate of angioplasty reported at 29% as compared with 75% in the stent group (46%; 95% CI, 24 to 68). Similar to the clinical experience, restenosis was reported in 48% of the angioplasty group as opposed to only 14% in the stenting group (34%; 95% CI, 11 to 58); however, after rescue stenting, long-term follow-up of vessel patency was similar in both groups.

It has been shown that among patients with unilateral RAS and renovascular hypertension, the use of ACEIs are particularly effective for blood pressure control, especially in patients with unilateral RAS (*Am J Kidney Dis*

1999;33:675–681). Although the vasodilatory effect on the glomerular efferent arteriole may result in a transglomerular pressure drop, this is usually compensated for by the contralateral kidney and results in a stable serum creatinine. It should be noted, however, that acute renal failure can result from the use of ACEI in the setting of RAS, and the patients treated in this fashion require a close and serial follow-up.

29.13 **Answer D.** Preprocedural planning is the most critical component of a technically successful endovascular AAA repair. CT provides the backbone for evaluating patient candidacy. In addition to the indications of either an asymptomatic aneurysm of appropriate maximal diameter or a small aneurysm with features putting it at increased risk of rupture, patients being considered for EVAR must fulfill several anatomic criteria. These include: (1) iliofemoral access vessels that will allow safe insertion and deployment of the device, adequate seal, and sufficient length to provide axial support for the graft; and (2) an infrarenal aortic neck of adequate length, limited angulation, and appropriate diameter. These anatomic features, as well as the presence or absence of thrombus and calcium at each level, can be evaluated using CT. The short-term results from the EVAR in patients with AAA (EVAR-1) trial that randomized 1,082 patients aged 60 years and older with aneurysms >5.5 cm in diameter to either surgical or endovascular repair showed a significant reduction in 30-day mortality in the endovascular repair group (1.6% vs. 4.7%, 0.33 0.15 to 0.74, $p = 0.007$) (*Lancet* 2004;364:843–848). However, long-term follow-up data from EVAR-1 revealed that 4 years after randomization, all-cause mortality between the groups was similar with that of the endovascular repair group experiencing higher overall rates of complication (17.6/100 person years vs. 3.3/100 person years, 95% CI, [3.5 to 6.8], $p < 0.0001$) and needed reintervention (6.9/100 person years vs. 2.4/100 person years, 95% CI, 2.7 1.8 to 4.1, $p < 0.0001$) (*Lancet* 2005;365:2187–2192). Similar results were reported in the smaller Dutch Endovascular Aneurysm Management (DREAM) trial that randomized 351 patients with an aneurysm >5 cm to endovascular or open surgical repair. As in EVAR-1, there was a significant reduction in 30-day mortality in the endovascular group (1.2% vs. 4.6%; 95% CI, 0.1 to 4.2), but this difference was no longer significant by 6 months' follow-up (*N Engl J Med* 2004;351:1607–1618). Although the recently published long-term follow-up results of the DREAM trial revealed a significant reduction in aneurysm-related mortality benefiting the endovascular group (2.1 vs. 5.7; 95% CI, –0.5 to 7.9), there was no significant difference in the cumulative survival between endovascular and open repair groups (89.7% vs. 89.6%). In contrast to the EVAR-1 trial, however, the rates of severe complication, aneurysm rupture, and reintervention were similar in both groups (*N Engl J Med* 2005;352:2398–2405).

With longer follow-up now being achieved after EVAR, >97% 5-year and >94% 9-year rupture-free survival have been observed (*Ann Surg* 2006;244:426–438).

Although there is no randomized data to support the optimum time for aneurysmal repair, general expert opinion suggests that the larger the aneurysm, the greater the risk of rupture. Other independent risk factors for AAA rupture include COPD, hypertension, female gender, smoking, and symptoms including abdominal tenderness or back pain. Additionally, aneurysms that expand >0.6 cm in 1 year are at a high risk of rupture. Therefore, this patient would likely not do well with medical management and should be strongly considered for repair, either surgical or endovascular. Finally, cardiac complications are the most common serious perioperative complication of EVAR (*N Engl J Med* 2004;351:1607–1618) and the most common cause of late death (*Lancet* 2005;365:2179–2186.).

29.14 **Answer E.** A dreaded complication, spinal cord ischemia (SCI) is an infrequent complication of open surgical repair of thoracic aortic aneurysm repair, although it can be seen following endovascular repair as well. SCI is typically not a complication of AAA repair. Artery of Adamkiewicz is the largest anterior segmental medullary artery. When damaged or obstructed, it can result in anterior spinal artery syndrome, with loss of urinary and fecal continence (*Eur J Cardio-Thorac Surg* 19:203–213) and impaired motor function of the legs; sensory function is often preserved to a degree. Option A describes a type I endoleak, which can be because of undersizing of the stent, poor proximal or distal fixation, neck dilation, stent fracture or separation, or aneurysms with short, angulated necks. With rare exceptions, the presence of a type I endoleak requires immediate treatment that could include stenting at the location of the leak, further angioplasty of the graft, or open surgical repair. Option B describes a type II endoleak, which is considered a more benign complication with treatment typically reserved for cases where the aneurysmal

sac continues to enlarge. Option C describes a type IV endoleak that is most commonly seen in conjunction with thin-walled Dacron grafts, and is also not thought to be at high risk for causing significant clinical complications. Not mentioned in the preceding text is type III endoleak that results from limb separation or fabric wear and may require the deployment of an additional cuff to adequately treat. As one might expect, embolization of thrombus or plaque debris during EVAR is a feared, but an unfortunately real complication that can result in ischemia of any distal vascular bed. Perforation and/or dissections of the iliac artery are fortunately decreasing in recent years partly because of increased flexibility and easier insertion of the delivery device (*Br J Surg* 2005;92:937–946).

29.15 **Answer D.** The group of symptoms described in the preceding text is referred to as the subclavian steal syndrome, and can often be confused for TIA, stroke, migraine headache, intracranial mass, or temporal arteritis. The etiology of the symptom complex is vertebrobasilar insufficiency due to the presence of a proximal subclavian stenosis that results in retrograde blood flow in the ipsilateral vertebral artery. In addition to the symptoms mentioned in the preceding text, common presenting symptoms are that of upper extremity claudication, paresthesia, numbness, ataxia, confusion, diplopia, nystagmus, and visual symptoms. A rare, but well-documented phenomenon, is that of coronary steal due to retrograde blood flow in the ipsilateral internal mammary artery thereby causing ischemia in the targeted coronary vascular bed. Indications for revascularization of the subclavian artery include symptomatic steal syndromes, disabling upper extremity weakness, vertebrobasilar insufficiency, preservation of flow to the in situ internal mammary grafts, or evidence of embolic phenomenon in the upper extremities thought secondary to the subclavian disease. The presence of subclavian disease in the absence of symptoms is not an indication for intervention and should be avoided. Although ultrasound and magnetic resonance angiography can help diagnose this problem, angiography would be the most efficient and precise strategy to diagnose and treat the subclavian steal syndrome.

29.16 **Answer A.** There are many different variations of the right-sided aortic arch. The most commonly seen right-sided aortic arch has the left carotid as the first branch. The left subclavian is the last branch. The easiest way to understand

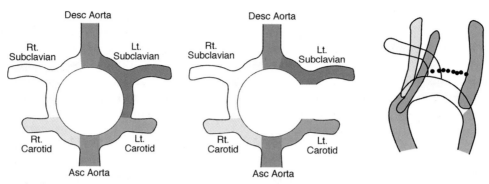

Figure A29-16 (see color insert)

the right-sided aortic arch is to be familiar with embryology. As shown in Figure A29-16, normally, the segment between the right subclavian and the descending aorta disappears, but in right-sided arch that is most commonly encountered within adults, the segment between the left carotid and subclavian disappears.

29.17   Answer C. The clinical presentation described in the preceding text is consistent with Takayasu's arteritis—a chronic, idiopathic disease that is characterized by inflammation of the aorta and its main branches. The disease affects almost exclusively female patients, is more common in Asian persons, and the mean age at presentation is 25 years. The symptoms at clinical presentation are because of the limb or organ ischemia due to the progressive stenosis of involved arteries. In a prospective cohort study of 60 patients with confirmed Takayasu's arteritis after a mean follow-up of 5.3 years (*Ann Intern Med* 1994;120:919–929), it was reported that the most common presenting symptoms included arm claudication (63%), light-headedness (33%), visual changes (often bilateral), constitutional complaints such as weight loss and fever, and less commonly chest pain and myalgias. Physical findings included carotid bruit (80%), diminished or absent radial pulse (53%), carotodynia (32%), visual aberration, and less commonly aortic insufficiency (due to aortic root inflammation and distention). Hypertension was noted in 33% of the patients at some point of their disease course and was highly associated with either unilateral or bilateral RAS. Angiography demonstrated aortic lesions in 65% of these patients, 32% of these lesions involved the aortic arch and its branches, and 68% involved the aortic vasculature above and below the diaphragm. Interestingly, no patient was noted to have sole involvement of the abdominal aorta. Medical therapy usually consisted of oral steroids dosed at 1 mg/kg for up to 3 months with the addition

of a cytotoxic agent such as cyclophosphamide or azathioprine, if the steroid dose is unable to be weaned. Surgical treatment was indicated in patients with refractory hypertension due to RAS, extremity ischemia, cerebrovascular ischemia, or critical (>70%) stenosis of at least three cerebral vessels, moderate or severe aortic regurgitation, or cardiac ischemia due to angiographically proven coronary artery stenosis. Angioplasty was less commonly performed and was most often employed in the revascularization of the subclavian and renal vessels. Approximately half of the interventions were successful on the first attempt and only one-third on the second with restenosis being a common problem.

29.18   Answer C. Originating from the anterior portion of the aorta inferior to the aortic hiatus of the diaphragm, the celiac artery is a short arterial trunk that courses anteriorly and divides into three larger branches—the left gastric, the hepatic, and the splenic arteries (Fig. A29-18).

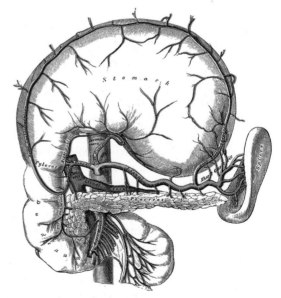

Figure A29-18 (see color insert)

The smallest of the three vessels, the left gastric artery, courses superiorly and branches into numerous subdivisions to provide blood flow to portions of the esophagus and the cardiac portion of the stomach before passing along the lesser curvature of the stomach to the pylorus, where it commonly anastomoses with the right gastric artery.

The hepatic artery courses to the porta hepatis and branches into the right and left hepatic arteries, thereby supplying blood flow to both lobes of the liver.

Running along the greater curvature of the stomach, the right gastroepiploic artery anastomoses with the left gastroepiploic branch of the splenic artery and provides blood flow to both surfaces of the stomach. Given its large caliber and close proximity to the inferior aspect of the heart, the right gastroepiploic artery is amenable for grafting to the distal right coronary artery (RCA) and PDA as is seen in the preceding angiogram.

The SMA and IMA are large branches that arise from the aorta inferior to the celiac trunk and are not visualized in this angiogram.

29.19 **Answer B.** This patient has had two prior interventions (and the lesion is likely at least 15 cm in length). This makes it at least a TASC C lesion. However, there is no involvement of the popliteal artery. Hence, it is not a TASC D lesion. The distal run-off is good (all three vessels, i.e., anterior tibial, peroneal, and posterior tibial are patent). For aortoilliac and femoral popliteal disease, endovascular repair is the recommended treatment of choice for type A lesions and is preferred for type B lesions, whereas open surgical repair is best suited for type D lesions. Type C lesions remain in a gray zone, with endovascular repair reserved for patients with a high surgical risk (*Eur J Vasc Endovasc Surg* 2007;33(Suppl 1):S1–S75).

29.20 **Answer A.** FMD lesions typically show a beading pattern. With the most common subtype of FMD, medial fibroplasias, the dilated arterial segments are often larger in diameter than the original vessel. This is not the case with perimedial fibroplasias, in which the beads are up to, but not greater than, the caliber of the original vessel. In posttransplant RAS, there could be a variety of reasons—faulty surgical technique, arterial injury during donor nephrectomy or perfusion preservation, chronic rejection, and atherosclerotic disease (*N Engl J Med* 2004; 350:1862–1871).

29.21 **Answer B.** For focal noncalcified lesions, angioplasty alone often provides an excellent angiographic result. For ostial SFA lesions, or disease that extends into the popliteal artery, where stenting should certainly be avoided, atherectomy (using Silverhawk LS and LX catheters in the SFA, and Silverhawk MS catheter in the popliteal artery) with adjunctive low pressure angioplasty (2–4 atm) may be the preferred strategy. For heavily calcified lesions, a low threshold for primary stenting (following initial angioplasty) is reasonable, because of the poor results typically achieved with angioplasty alone, and the difficulty of current generation atherectomy catheters to effectively treat heavily calcified plaque (CATH SAP 3: Ivan Casserly, John Messenger. **Chapter 12: Peripheral Vascular Disease.** *Lower Extremity Angiography and Interventions*)

29.22 **Answer D.** In the CREST trial, there were no significant difference in the estimated 4-year rates of the primary end point between carotid-artery stenting and CEA (7.2% and 6.8%, respectively; hazard ratio for stenting, 1.11; 95% CI, 0.81 to 1.51; $p = 0.51$). During the periprocedural period, the incidence of the primary end point was similar with carotid-artery stenting and CEA (5.2 and 4.5%, respectively; hazard ratio for stenting, 1.18; 95% CI, 0.82 to 1.68; $p = 0.38$), although the rates of the individual end points differed between the stenting group and the endarterectomy group (death, 0.7% vs. 0.3%; $p = 0.18$; stroke, 4.1% vs. 2.3%; $p = 0.01$; MI, 1.1% vs. 2.3%; $p = 0.03$). After the periprocedural period, the incidence of ipsilateral stroke was similarly low with carotid-artery stenting and with CEA (2.0% and 2.4%, respectively; $p = 0.85$). Note that the increased incidence was not in major strokes but in minor strokes. (CREST Investigators. Stenting vs. Endarterectomy for Treatment of Carotid-Artery Stenosis. *N Engl J Med* 2010;363:11–23.)

29.23 **Answer C.** A study from the NHANES 1999 to 2000 data found that PAD affects approximately 5 million adults. Prevalence increases dramatically with age and disproportionately affects blacks (*Circulation* 2004;110:738–743). Experts in the field generally agree that PAD affects approximately 8 million Americans (*JAMA* 2001;286:1317–1324; *NEJM* 1992;326:381–386). PAD affects 12% to 20% of Americans age 65 and older. Despite its prevalence and cardiovascular risk implications, only 25% of PAD patients are undergoing treatment (*J Vasc Interv Radiol* 2002;13:7–11). In the general population, *only about* 10% of persons with PAD have the classic symptoms of IC. About 40% do not complain of leg pain, while the remaining 50% have a variety of leg symptoms different from classic claudication (*JAMA* 2001;286:1317–1324; *Circulation* 1985;71:516–522). However, in an older, disabled population of women, as many as two-thirds of individuals with PAD had no exertional leg symptoms (*Circulation* 2001;104:504.). The risk factors for PAD are similar to those for CHD, although diabetes and cigarette smoking are particularly strong risk factors for PAD (*Am J Epidemiol* 1989;129:1110–1119.). Persons with PAD have impaired function and quality of life. This is true even for persons who do not report leg symptoms (*Ann Intern Med* 2002;136:873–883; *JAMA* 2004;292:453–461). PAD is a marker for systemic atherosclerotic disease. Persons with PAD, compared to those without, have four to five times the risk of dying of a cardiovascular disease event, resulting in two to three times higher total mortality risk (*NEJM* 1992;326:381–386; *JAMA* 1993;270:487–489).

29.24 **Answer E.** This was a significant perforation during attempted placement of a large arterial sheath. It is of critical importance to reverse anticoagulation and achieve contralateral access, followed by balloon occlusion from the contralateral side. This could be followed by treatment of a covered stent should there be inadequate results from the balloon treatment alone.

29.25 **Answer E.** If proven, this would be considered a first provoked thromboembolic event. Patients with a first episode of PE or DVT who have a reversible or temporary risk factor that has resolved should receive warfarin therapy for at least 3 months. Typically, hypercoagulable workup is best reserved for patients with thrombosis that is unprovoked, a positive family history, or recurrent venous thrombosis. An IVC filter is not the default treatment in the postoperative setting and should be considered only if there is a clear contraindication to anticoagulation.

30 Cerebrovascular Interventions

Debabrata Mukherjee

QUESTIONS

30.1 A 67-year-old Caucasian male presents to your office for evaluation. He states that he has had three episodes of transient ischemic attacks (TIAs) in the last year. His medical history is significant for hypertension and dyslipidemia. His laboratory evaluation shows evidence of left ventricular hypertrophy on his ECG, a creatinine of 1.3, and LDL of 98. He is currently taking amlodipine for hypertension and simvastatin for dyslipidemia.

He denies any history of coronary or peripheral vascular disease. Antiplatelet regimen for stroke prevention may include all of the following, EXCEPT:

(A) Aspirin monotherapy
(B) Aspirin and extended-release dipyridamole
(C) Clopidogrel monotherapy
(D) Aspirin and clopidogrel

30.2 In assessing carotid artery atherosclerosis, all the following statements are true, EXCEPT:

(A) When performed by a trained sonographer, the sensitivity and specificity of Doppler ultrasonography and B-mode imaging approaches 90%
(B) Peak end-diastolic velocity above 135 cm/s and peak end-systolic velocity above 240 cm/s are suggestive of stenosis >80%
(C) Carotid duplex scans can provide similar assessment of near-complete occlusive lesions as CE-MRA
(D) Contrast-enhanced MRA is superior to carotid duplex in assessing long internal carotid lesions (more than 3 cm)

(E) Angiography should be used when the results of the noninvasive tests are inconclusive or yield conflicting results and/or if percutaneous intervention is planned

30.3 A 73-year-old man presents with history of frequent TIAs. His medical history is significant for prior myocardial infarction, hypertension, and dyslipidemia. Baseline labs are unremarkable. A CT angiogram was ordered by his primary care physician to assess for carotid stenosis. All the following may render carotid endarterectomy (CEA) difficult or not feasible, EXCEPT:

(A) Prior radiation to the neck or previous radical neck surgery
(B) Severe tandem lesion
(C) Aorto-ostial or proximal common carotid artery lesion
(D) Lesion location is distal cervical (C2 level and above)

30.4 A 59-year-old woman with history of coronary artery disease, and prior left CEA, presented with a history of two episodes of slurred speech and right-sided weakness. These episodes lasted for < 1 hour, and the patient recovered completely. The patient's medications include aspirin, lisinopril, and atorvastatin. A carotid angiogram is shown in Figure Q30-4. The most appropriate option for the management of this patient is:

351

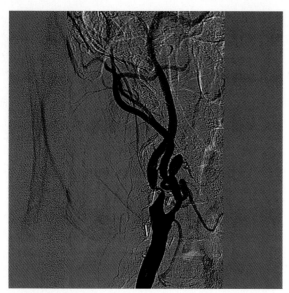

Figure Q30-4

    (A) Repeating CEA
    (B) Carotid artery stenting (CAS)
    (C) Adding clopidogrel to the current regimen
    (D) Initiating warfarin

30.5 A 77-year-old woman presents with history of an ischemic stroke 4 weeks ago. She has now completely recovered from the stroke and does not have any residual neurological deficit. Her neurologist has ordered an MRA, which showed a Type 3 aortic arch (Fig. Q30-5) and a severe 90% stenosis of the ostium of the internal carotid artery. MRA also revealed a moderate-size pedunculated thrombus in the left internal carotid artery. All of the following are considered high-risk factors during CAS in her, but stenting is still considered feasible, EXCEPT in:

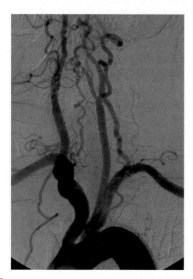

Figure Q30-5

    (A) Age > 75
    (B) Type 3 aortic arch

    (C) Pedunculated thrombus
    (D) Stenosis involving the ostium of the internal carotid artery

30.6 A 67-year-old man presents with episodes of dizziness and diplopia for the last 3 weeks. His past medical history is significant for diabetes and hypertension. Carotid and vertebral artery ultrasound are performed and reveal <30% stenosis of bilateral carotid arteries, a small diminutive left vertebral artery, and severe stenosis of the origin of a large dominant right vertebral artery. Subsequent angiography confirms a 90% ostial narrowing of a large right vertebral artery (Fig. Q30-6). In discussing with the patient his therapeutic options regarding his severe vertebral artery stenosis, all of the following are true, EXCEPT:

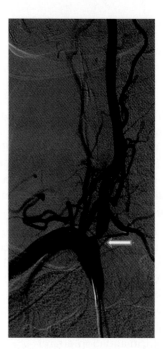

Figure Q30-6

    (A) The data are primarily limited to case series on the role of percutaneous intervention for vertebral artery stenosis
    (B) Embolic events involving the brain stem can be life threatening
    (C) About 25% of patients with vertebrobasilar insufficiency have an associated significant carotid artery disease, the management of which may relieve the symptoms
    (D) The risk of recurrent stroke in the acute phase of a vertebrobasilar TIA is low; however, the risk is high for recurrent CVA on longer-term follow-up

30.7 A 71-year-old gentleman undergoes carotid stenting for severe symptomatic right internal carotid artery stenosis. His blood pressure remains in the 80 to 90 systolic range even after 18 hours of the procedure. All of the following factors may have been possible predictors of persistent hypotension following his carotid stenting, EXCEPT:

(A) History of myocardial infarction
(B) Distance from the carotid bifurcation <10 mm
(C) History of ipsilateral CEA
(D) Intraprocedural hypotension

30.8 A 67-year-old man with history of hypertension, prior radiation to the neck in the context of thyroid cancer, and hyperlipidemia presented with recurrent short-lived episodes of visual loss in his left eye. His ECG shows normal sinus rhythm with left ventricular hypertrophy. A bilateral carotid duplex study was done, which was suggestive of total occlusion of the right internal carotid artery and severe stenosis of the left internal carotid artery. A carotid angiogram was done (Fig. Q30-8). What is the best route of action in the management of this patient?

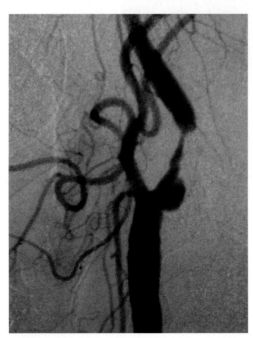

Figure Q30-8

(A) Proceed with CAS
(B) Arrange a vascular surgery consultation for possible CEA
(C) Initiate anticoagulation with heparin followed by warfarin for 4 to 6 weeks with reevaluation with angiography at that time
(D) Initiate anticoagulation and plan reevaluation with angiography in 48 hours

30.9 A 61-year-old man was referred to the interventional cardiology service for a second opinion regarding the management of a newly diagnosed carotid disease. The patient underwent, prior to his referral, a carotid duplex study to assess a bruit over the left carotid artery. This study was soon followed by an angiography by the local cardiology group (Fig. Q30-9). The patient has been experiencing occasional headache over the past 2 months. His BP is 140/88 in your office. His total cholesterol is 220, and his LDL is 150. The patient was advised to consider undergoing CEA. What would be your recommendation to this patient at this point?

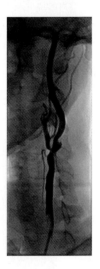

Figure Q30-9

(A) The patient should undergo endarterectomy as he is at a low risk (<4%) for such procedure
(B) Proceed with carotid stenting with the use of a filter wire to protect the distal circulation
(C) Initiate aspirin 162 mg PO QD, atorvastatin 80 mg PO QHS, and ramipril 2.5 mg PO QD
(D) Initiate aspirin 162 mg PO QD, clopidogrel 75 mg PO QD, atorvastatin 80 mg PO QHS, and ramapril 2.5 mg PO QD

30.10 Following a postdilatation of a carotid stent, the patient became acutely hemiparetic and aphasic. Figure Q30-10A–D shows the sequence of angiography, stenting, and postdilatation of the stent. What would be the best route of action in this situation?

(A) Remove the filter wire and reassess
(B) Inject intracarotid urokinase
(C) Use a larger balloon to further dilate the stent
(D) Use an export catheter to aspirate

30.11 A 69-year-old gentleman presents with unstable angina, and coronary angiography reveals severe three-vessel obstructive coronary artery disease. A carotid ultrasound is ordered by the surgical

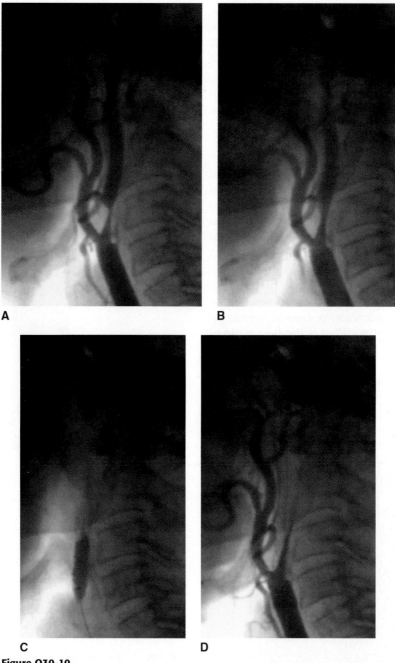

Figure Q30-10

team, which shows <50% stenosis in the right coronary artery and 80% stenosis in the left internal carotid arteries. There is mild nonobstructive disease of bilateral vertebral arteries. In patients such as this individual with concomitant coronary artery disease and carotid disease, all of the following are true, EXCEPT:

(A) The risk of perioperative neurological event following coronary artery bypass grafting (CABG) is about 9% for individuals with internal carotid artery disease with >50% stenosis

(B) Randomized clinical trials have confirmed that carotid stenting followed by CABG (staged) carries the lowest risk for perioperative neurological events when compared with simultaneous CEA and CABG (combined)

(C) Retrospective reports showed little difference between the staged and the combined approaches for revascularization

(D) Asymptomatic >75% internal carotid artery stenosis carries a 14% risk of perioperative stroke in patients undergoing CABG

30.12 In assessing carotid artery severity according to the North American Symptomatic Carotid Endarterectomy Trial (NASCET), all the following statements are true EXCEPT:

(A) Percent Stenosis = (Presumed Normal Segment diameter – Diseased segment diameter)/ Presumed Normal Segment diameter × 100

(B) The normal segment is defined as the diameter of the segment just distal to the carotid bulb and not the carotid bulb itself or the poststenotic area distal to the lesion

(C) The normal segment is defined as the estimated diameter of the carotid bulb as it was prior to the atherosclerotic narrowing

(D) Percent of stenosis by the European Carotid Surgery Trial (ECST) is always more severe than the percent stenosis given by NASCET method

30.13 A 76-year-old diabetic with documented three-vessel disease underwent a carotid duplex study that was suggestive of total occlusion of the right internal carotid artery and high-grade left carotid artery disease. The surgeons are reluctant to proceed with CABG until the patient's left carotid artery is further assessed and treated. Carotid angiogram confirmed the total occlusion of the right internal carotid artery and the noted anatomy on the left carotid artery (Fig. Q30-13). What would be the best route of action in this patient among the following?

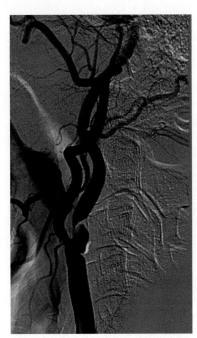

Figure Q30-13

(A) Anticoagulation for 1 month and then reassessment of the left internal carotid artery at that point

(B) Proceed with stenting with the placement of 7 French Cook Shuttle catheter in the common carotid artery, then cross the lesion with a 0.014 in. coronary guidewire, with subsequent predilatation and then stenting with a self-expanding stent

(C) CEA is the only option for such a lesion as it is unfavorable for carotid stenting

(D) Proceed with stenting with the placement of 7 French Cook shuttle catheter in the common carotid artery, then cross the lesion with a filter-based embolic protection device, followed by predilatation and then stenting with a self-expanding stent

30.14 A 73-year-old woman with long-standing hypertension presents with recurrent TIAs despite being on antiplatelet therapy. A carotid angiogram is performed at the request of her neurologist, which reveals 80% ostial stenosis of the left common carotid artery (Fig. Q30-14). In performing carotid stenting in this individual, all the following technical principles are recommended, EXCEPT:

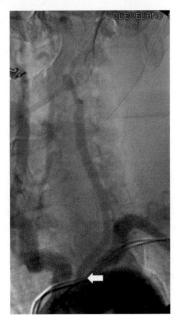

Figure Q30-14

(A) The larger catheter should be advanced into the carotid in a stepwise and coaxial fashion over the smaller catheter and always over a guidewire

(B) Predilatation is recommended to confirm the ability to adequately dilate the stenosis

(C) Self-expanding stents are preferred for the carotid bifurcation

(D) Self-expanding stents are preferred for ostial common carotid artery

30.15 A 68-year-old woman underwent carotid angiography for evaluation of recurrent TIAs. Angiography revealed an ulcerated stenosis with heavy plaque burden (Fig. Q30-15). A closed-cell design stent (NexStent, Xact) may offer the following advantages in this patient, EXCEPT:

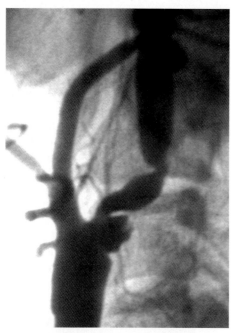

Figure Q30-15

(A) Greater plaque coverage than open-cell stents
(B) Reduced risk of delayed embolism due to plaque protrusion
(C) Flexibility
(D) Higher radial strength

30.16 The Carotid Revascularization Endarterectomy vs. Stenting Trial (CREST) randomly assigned patients with symptomatic or asymptomatic carotid stenosis to undergo carotid artery stenting or CEA. The primary composite end point was stroke, myocardial infarction, or death from any cause during the periprocedural period or any ipsilateral stroke within 4 years after randomization. The study demonstrated that:

(A) The risk of the composite primary outcome of stroke, myocardial infarction, or death did not differ significantly in the group undergoing carotid artery stenting and the group undergoing CEA
(B) The risk of the composite primary outcome of stroke, myocardial infarction, or death was significantly higher in the group undergoing carotid artery stenting compared to the group undergoing CEA

(C) The risk of the composite primary outcome of stroke, myocardial infarction, or death was significantly lower in the group undergoing carotid artery stenting and the group undergoing CEA
(D) The trial was stopped prematurely due to lack of funding

30.17 A major difference between coronary and cerebral arteries that interventionalists need to be aware of is that:

(A) Cerebral arteries have a thicker tunica media
(B) Cerebral arteries have no external elastic lamina
(C) Cerebral arteries have thick supportive adventitia
(D) Cerebral arteries have less tortuosity

30.18 A 58-year-old woman presented to the emergency room with a left hemiparesis. Upon evaluation, the patient had a blood pressure of 132/78, an altered level of alertness, mild left hemineglect, a left homonomous hemianopsia, subtle impairment of upgaze, and a mild left hemiparesis and left hemianesthesia. The diagnosis of probable posterior cerebral artery (PCA) occlusion was made on clinical grounds. The patient was immediately taken to the catheterization laboratory, and cerebral angiography was performed (Fig. Q30-18). The angiogram shows:

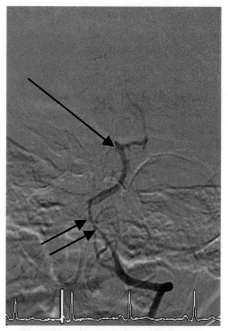

Figure Q30-18

(A) Occluded right posterior cerebral artery
(B) Occluded right middle cerebral artery
(C) Occluded right anterior cerebral artery
(D) Occluded right inferior cerebellar artery

30.19 A 53-year-old man with diabetes mellitus, hypertension, coronary artery disease, and cigarette smoking developed recurrent, crescendo left middle cerebral artery (MCA) TIAs despite treatment with clopidogrel. Carotid angiography (Fig. Q30-19) reveals:

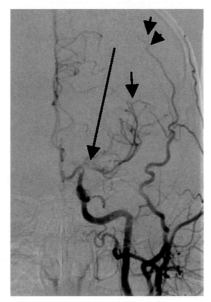

Figure Q30-19

(A) 90% left common carotid stenosis
(B) 90% left ostial internal carotid artery stenosis
(C) 90% left ICA terminus stenosis extending into the MCA
(D) 90% left external carotid artery stenosis

30.20 A 71-year-old man presents with symptoms of dizziness and lightheadedness for 3 weeks. The patient also gives history of a drop attack 4 days ago. An ultrasound study was suggestive of a severe stenosis in one of the blood vessels to the brain. An angiogram performed (Fig. Q30-20) shows:

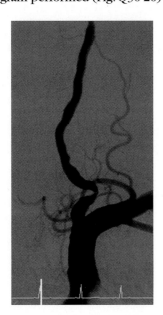

Figure Q30-20

(A) Severe stenosis of the proximal left vertebral artery
(B) Severe stenosis of the left carotid artery
(C) Severe stenosis of the right carotid artery
(D) Severe stenosis of the proximal right vertebral artery

30.21 At the present time, Medicare covers PTA of the carotid artery concurrent with the placement of an FDA-approved carotid stent with embolic protection for the following, EXCEPT:

(A) Patients who are at high risk for CEA and who also have symptomatic carotid artery stenosis ≥70%
(B) Patients who are at high risk for CEA and have symptomatic carotid artery stenosis between 50% and 70%, in accordance with the Category B IDE clinical trials regulation
(C) Patients who are at high risk for CEA and have asymptomatic carotid artery stenosis ≥80%, in accordance with the Category B IDE clinical trials regulation
(D) Coverage is limited to procedures performed using FDA-approved carotid artery stents and with or without FDA-approved or cleared embolic protection devices

30.22 Regarding training for carotid stenting, the SCAI/SVMB/SVS guideline specifies that:

(A) Operators perform a minimum of 30 supervised diagnostic cervicocerebral angiograms (at least 15 as a primary operator) and a minimum of 25 supervised carotid interventions (at least 13 as a primary operator) prior to performing CAS independently
(B) Operators perform a minimum of 50 supervised diagnostic cervicocerebral angiograms (at least 25 as a primary operator) and a minimum of 45 supervised carotid interventions (at least 23 as a primary operator) prior to performing CAS independently
(C) Operators perform a minimum of 100 supervised diagnostic cervicocerebral angiograms (at least 50 as a primary operator) and a minimum of 50 supervised carotid interventions (at least 26 as a primary operator) prior to performing CAS independently
(D) Operators perform a minimum of 30 supervised diagnostic cervicocerebral angiograms (at least 5 as a primary operator) and a minimum of 25 supervised carotid interventions (at least 10 as primary operator) prior to performing CAS independently

30.23 A 59-year-old man presents with vertigo and diplopia. As part of his evaluation, his neurologist orders ultrasound of both vertebrals, which reveals small occluded left vertebral. Doppler of the right vertebral (Fig. Q30-23) is suggestive of:

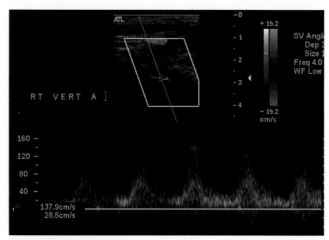

Figure Q30-23

(A) Normal flow in the right vertebral artery
(B) Severe stenosis of the right vertebral artery
(C) Moderate nonobstructive stenosis of the right vertebral artery
(D) Mild stenosis of the right vertebral artery

30.24 A 63-year-old man presents to your inpatient cardiology ward with unstable angina. Risk factors include hypertension and smoking history. On physical examination, he has a left carotid bruit, an S4 gallop, and diminished dorsalis and posterior tibial pulses in the left leg and absent dorsalis pedis in the right leg. Coronary angiography reveals 70% left main stenosis, severe (80%) mid left anterior descending artery stenosis, and 70% stenosis in the midportion of the right coronary artery. Left ventriculography reveals mild systolic dysfunction with an estimated ejection fraction of 50% and LVEDP of 17 mm Hg. A carotid ultrasound is indicated prior to CABG based on all of the following, EXCEPT:

(A) Peripheral arterial disease
(B) Carotid bruit
(C) Age > 60 years
(D) Smoking history
(E) Left main stenosis

30.25 Current guidelines for CEA in symptomatic and asymptomatic patients state that:

(A) CEA is indicated in symptomatic patients with stenosis 60% to 99%, if the risk of perioperative stroke or death is <5%. For asymptomatic patients, guidelines recommend CEA for stenosis 60% to 99%, if the risk of perioperative stroke or death is <2%
(B) CEA is indicated in symptomatic patients with stenosis 70% to 99%, if the risk of perioperative stroke or death is <6%. For asymptomatic patients, guidelines recommend CEA for stenosis 80% to 99%, if the risk of perioperative stroke or death is <3%
(C) CEA is indicated in symptomatic patients with stenosis 50% to 99%, if the risk of perioperative stroke or death is <6%. For asymptomatic patients, guidelines recommend CEA for stenosis 60% to 99%, if the risk of perioperative stroke or death is <3%
(D) CEA is indicated in symptomatic patients with stenosis 70% to 99%, if the risk of perioperative stroke or death is <5%. For asymptomatic patients, guidelines recommend CEA for stenosis 80% to 99%, if the risk of perioperative stroke or death is <3%

30.1 **Answer D.** The 2008 Update to the AHA/ASA Recommendations for the Prevention of Stroke in Patients With Stroke and Transient Ischemic Attack recommends that aspirin (50 to 325 mg/d) monotherapy, the combination of aspirin and extended-release dipyridamole, and clopidogrel monotherapy are all acceptable options for initial therapy (Class I, Level of Evidence A) (*Stroke* 2008;39:1647–1652). Based on ESPRIT trial, the combination of aspirin and extended-release dipyridamole is recommended over aspirin alone (Class I, Level of Evidence B). The efficacy of dual antiplatelet therapy with aspirin and clopidogrel was tested in the Management of Atherothrombosis With Clopidogrel in High-Risk Patients With Recent TIA or Ischemic Stroke (MATCH) trail. The MATCH trial did not show additional clinical value of adding aspirin to clopidogrel in high-risk patients with transient ischemic attack or ischemic stroke, and the risk of life-threatening or major bleeding is increased with the combination of aspirin and clopidogrel (*Lancet* 2004;364:331–337).

30.2 **Answer C.** Carotid duplex is inferior to CE-MRA in assessing near-complete occlusive disease, calcified lesions, high carotid bifurcation, and long (>3 cm) lesions. (*J Vasc Surg* 2005;41:962–972; *Neuroimaging Clin N Am* 2005;15:351–365). All other statements are true.

30.3 **Answer B.** CEA is generally technically challenging or not feasible in patients with prior radiations to the neck, prior neck surgery or ipsilateral CEA (the so-called hostile neck), aortoostial or proximal common carotid disease. CEA is associated with higher risk in patients with restenosis following CEA, contralateral ICA occlusion, severe comorbidities, and contralateral laryngeal nerve palsy. Severe tandem lesions can be effectively treated with endarterectomy.

30.4 **Answer B.** The risk of a stroke is quite high in this patient with recurrent hemispheric TIA and a high-grade ICA disease (10% in the first year and about 30% in 5 years). Among the high-risk features for recurrent stroke are hemispheric TIA, recent TIA, increasing frequency of TIA, and high-grade carotid stenosis. The patient's anatomy is suitable for CAS, which may be the best route of action in this scenario. Prior CEA in this patient increases the risk of complications with a second CEA but may also be considered, depending on local expertise. The use of clopidogrel or warfarin in addition to aspirin will offer the patients an inferior therapeutic intervention when compared to carotid artery revascularization. While patients with restenosis following CEA were not included in the NASCET and Asymptomatic Carotid Atherosclerosis Study (ACAS) trials, such history was a qualifying criterion for inclusion in the SAPPHIRE trial (*N Engl J Med* 2004;351:1493–1501), which focused on high-risk patients with severe carotid disease and showed that CAS was noninferior to CEA.

30.5 **Answer C.** Presence of pedunculated thrombus is an absolute contraindication for both carotid stenting and endarterectomy, and neither should be attempted till thrombus is resolved. Older age, Type 3 arch may make the procedure technically challenging but still feasible in experienced hands.

30.6 **Answer D.** The risk of recurrent stroke is extremely high in the acute phase (up to 7 days after the presenting symptoms); however, the risk of death and stroke is relatively low thereafter (*Cochrane Database Syst Rev* 2005;(2)).

30.7 **Answer C.** Predictors of hypotension during and/or after carotid stenting include history of MI, proximity to the carotid sinus, and intraprocedural hypotension (*Stroke* 1999;30:2086–2093; *Am J Surg* 2005;190:691–695).

30.8 **Answer C.** Presence of pedunculated thrombus is an absolute contraindication for both CAS and CEA (*Curr Cardiol Rep* 11:384–390). Anticoagulation should be initiated and a reassessment with angiography should be postponed for at least 4 to 6 weeks.

30.9 **Answer A.** While the efficacy of CAS in the management of low-risk severe asymptomatic carotid atherosclerosis is under evaluation, CEA remains the standard of care in the management of patients with severe asymptomatic carotid artery disease who are at an acceptable surgical risk (<4%). The risk of stroke in this patient (with >60% stenosis) is 3.2% per year. In the ACAS, 1,659 patients with asymptomatic carotid stenosis of at least 60% were randomized to CEA vs. medical therapy (*JAMA* 1995;273:1421–1428; *Lancet* 2004;363:1491–1502). The perioperative stroke or death reported in this study was 2.3%.

30.10 **Answer D.** No-reflow is a serious complication of carotid stenting. It is attributed to a large thrombus burden that overwhelms the filter wire leading to stagnant forward circulation and essentially no flow distal to target lesion. Aspirating this thrombus column, while the filter wire is in place, is the recommended strategy in this situation. Retrieving the filter wire will release the thrombotic debris and result in distal embolization. The use of urokinase can further complicate this precarious situation with intracerebral bleeding. Larger balloon inflation will not resolve this complication and is likely to result in dislodgement of more thrombotic debris distally (*J Am Coll Cardiol* 2005;46:1466–1472; *Cardiovasc Surg (Torino)* 2005;46:261–265).

30.11 **Answer B.** The evidence for the most appropriate strategy is derived from retrospective analysis. The risk of stroke is reported to be 3% to 4% in the staged approach as opposed to 2.8% to 3.3% in the simultaneous approach. The reversed staged approach (to proceed with CABG followed by CEA) is associated with 14% risk of stroke (*Semin Thorac Cardiovasc Surg* 2001;13:192–198; *Am J Cardiol* 2005;96:519–523).

30.12 **Answer C.** All the statements are accurate statements with the exception of C. In the ECST, normal segment was defined as the estimated diameter of the carotid bulb as it was prior to the atherosclerotic narrowing (Fig. A30-12). (*J Neurosurg* 1995;83:778–782; *J Mal Vasc* 1993;18:198–201).

NASCET | ECST

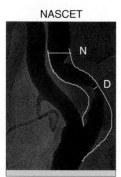 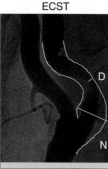

Percent stenosis = [(N-D/N) X 100]

NASCET = 67 % stenosis   ECST = 84 % stenosis

Figure A30-12

30.13 **Answer D.** The angiogram shows severe ulcerated stenosis of the left internal carotid artery without any evidence of thrombus. Several mechanical approaches have been developed in an attempt to prevent distal embolization during carotid stenting. The use of distal balloon occlusive device (PercuSurge GuardWire, Medtronic, Santa Rosa, CA) has been studied in a large series of CAS reporting a 30-day stroke and death risk of 2.7%. The use of Accunet (Guidant, Indianapolis, IN) was assessed in the ARCHER registry of 437 patients with symptomatic stenosis of at least 50% or asymptomatic stenosis of >80% but with high-risk features of surgery. The composite risk of stroke, death, or myocardial infarction at 30 days was reached in 7.8% in the overall cohort but was 1.4% in the 141 patients with restenosis following CEA.

The use of embolic protection devices has not entirely eliminated periprocedural strokes. Such devices are not operational during the diagnostic phase of the procedure nor are they operational during the final phase of the procedure. Nevertheless, the use of such device is widely adopted and recommended during CAS (*AJNR* 2005;26:854–861; *Catheter Cardiovasc Interv* 2008;72:309–317).

30.14 **Answer D.** Balloon expandable stents are for aorto-ostial disease (*Cardiovasc Intervent Radiol* 2002;25:109–114). Self-expanding stents should be used for the carotid bifurcation and other compressible lesions.

30.15 **Answer C.** Closed-cell stents are characterized by fully connecting struts and may offer greater plaque coverage than open-cell stents—with both connecting and nonconnecting struts—potentially reducing the risk of delayed embolism due to plaque protrusion. Therefore, this type of stents may be preferred for soft or ulcerated plaques with high embolic potential. Finally, closed-cell stents have higher radial strength, an important feature in severely calcified lesions. Open-cell stents are more flexible, conform better to the artery, and result in better wall apposition. Therefore, this stent type may be preferred in tortuous arteries and in lesions extending into the common carotid artery.

30.16 **Answer A.** The CREST trial demonstrated that among patients with symptomatic or asymptomatic carotid stenosis, the risk of the composite primary outcome of stroke, myocardial infarction, or death did not differ significantly in the group undergoing carotid artery stenting and the group undergoing CEA. During the periprocedural period, there was a higher risk of stroke with stenting and a higher risk of myocardial infarction with endarterectomy, but overall risk was similar (*N Engl J Med* 2010;363:11–23).

30.17 Answer B. There are major differences between the cerebral vessels and the coronary arteries or other muscular arteries. The cerebral vessels are histologically different: they have no external elastic lamina, and they have a thinner tunica media and trivial adventitia; this makes these vessels quite fragile. They also differ from the coronary arteries in being partly (i.e., the petrous and cavernous carotids) surrounded by bone or rigid and fibrous tissue (i.e., the dura mater). Combined with significant tortuosity in their proximal segments, this makes the navigation of endovascular devices to the intracranial vessels extremely difficult, if not impossible at times, which greatly increases the risk of vessel injury and perforation during endovascular therapy.

30.18 Answer A. A left vertebral angiogram was then performed, confirming that the right PCA was in fact occluded (*arrow*). Note, however, that the left vertebral artery is hypoplastic intracranially (*double arrow*) and the BA curves towards it, suggesting that the dominant vessel is the right vertebral artery. A microcatheter was placed just proximal to the PCA and fibrinolysis was initiated. In this case, the patient's age, low blood pressure, short duration of ischemia, and relatively small clot burden were all factors in favor of fibrinolysis. Over a period of 30 minutes, 4 units of Retavase were infused 1 unit at a time. Final angiography revealed complete recanalization of the right PCA. The patient made a significant recovery before the arteriotomy was closed, and by the next morning she was entirely normal.

30.19 Answer C. An AP view left common carotid angiogram shows a severe terminal ICA restenosis extending into the MCA (*long arrow*). The stenosis was severely flow-limiting comparing the extent of MCA filling (*short arrow*) with that of the occipital artery (*double arrow*). A 014″ microwire was advanced into the inferior division of the left MCA. A 2.0- × 9-mm balloon was advanced into the lesion and angioplasty was performed. An angiogram revealed significant lesion recoil with slow flow into the ACA. A 3.0- × 15-mm Wingspan stent was delivered. The patient's symptoms resolved, and at follow-up, he was asymptomatic.

30.20 Answer A. The angiogram shows severe stenosis of the left vertebral artery. This was treated with angioplasty and stenting and subsequent resolution of his symptoms.

30.21 Answer D. Effective March 17, 2005, Medicare covers PTA of the carotid artery concurrent with the placement of an FDA-approved carotid stent with embolic protection for the following:

- Patients who are at high risk for CEA and who also have symptomatic carotid artery stenosis ≥70%. Coverage is limited to procedures performed using FDA-approved CAS systems and FDA-approved or FDA-cleared (effective December 9, 2009) embolic protection devices. If deployment of the embolic protection device is not technically possible and not performed, then the procedure is not covered by Medicare (effective December 9, 2009);
- Patients who are at high risk for CEA and have symptomatic carotid artery stenosis between 50% and 70%, in accordance with the Category B IDE clinical trials regulation (42 CFR 405.201), as a routine cost under the clinical trials policy (Medicare NCD Manual 310.1), or in accordance with the NCD on CAS postapproval studies (Medicare NCD Manual 20.7);
- Patients who are at high risk for CEA and have asymptomatic carotid artery stenosis ≥80%, in accordance with the Category B IDE clinical trials regulation (42 CFR 405.201), as a routine cost under the clinical trials policy (Medicare NCD Manual 310.1), or in accordance with the NCD on CAS postapproval studies (Medicare NCD Manual 20.7).

Coverage is limited to procedures performed using FDA-approved carotid artery stents and FDA-approved or FDA-cleared embolic protection devices. The use of an FDA-approved or FDA-cleared embolic protection device is required. If deployment of the embolic protection device is not technically possible, and not performed, then the procedure is not covered by Medicare.

30.22 Answer A. The SCAI/SVMB/SVS document (*J Am Coll Cardiol* 2005;45:165–174) specifies that new operators perform a minimum of 30 supervised diagnostic cervicocerebral angiograms (at least 15 as a primary operator) and a minimum of 25 supervised carotid interventions (at least 13 as a primary operator) prior to performing CAS independently. Fewer studies required by the cardiology and vascular surgery organizations reflect their belief that previous experience with coronary (minimum of 300 diagnostic coronary angiograms and 250 coronary interventions) and peripheral interventional procedures (minimum of 100 diagnostic peripheral angiograms and 50 peripheral interventions) are transferable to neurovascular interventions.

"Primary operator" means that the trainee is handling the catheter, guidewire, EPD, balloon, and stent, under the direct supervision of the mentoring physician. Furthermore, only one trainee can be considered the primary operator on any one carotid stenting procedure (*J Am Coll Cardiol* 2007;49:126–170).

30.23 **Answer B.** Normal peak systolic velocity (PSV) for the vertebral artery is approximately 20 to 60 cm/s. A focal PSV of >100 cm/s (as in this case) is indicative of a significant stenosis (Zwiebel WJ. Ultrasound vertebral examination. In: *Introduction to vascular ultrasonography*. 4th ed. Philadelphia, PA: WB Saunders Company, 2000:167–176). Note that, due to asymmetry in vertebral artery diameter (present in >70% of normal individuals), there can be considerable difference in PSV between an individual's (normal) VA. A normal VA diameter on ultrasound is regarded as approximately 4 mm, with a tendency for the left VA to be usually larger than the right. The right vertebral duplex ultrasonography figure demonstrates PSVs of 137 cm/s with broadening of the spectral waveform suggestive of severe stenosis.

30.24 **Answer C.** In asymptomatic patients, there are no guidelines to support routine screening for carotid artery stenosis, except for some patients scheduled for CABG. Prior to CABG, carotid duplex screening is recommended in asymptomatic patients with age >65 years, left main coronary stenosis, peripheral arterial disease, history of smoking, history of TIA or stroke, or carotid bruit (*J Am Coll Cardiol* 2007;49:126–170).

30.25 **Answer C.** Current AHA guidelines recommend CEA in symptomatic patients with stenosis 50% to 99%, if the risk of perioperative stroke or death is <6% (*Circulation* 1998;97:501–509). For asymptomatic patients, AHA guidelines recommend CEA for stenosis 60% to 99%, if the risk of perioperative stroke or death is <3%. The 2005 guidelines from the American Academy of Neurology recommend that eligible patients should be 40 to 75 years old and have a life expectancy of at least 5 years (*Neurology* 2005;65:794–801).

Percutaneous Valve Repair and Replacement

Thomas Gehrig and Thomas M. Bashore

QUESTIONS

31.1 A 79-year-old female presents to her local physician with 3 months of progressive shortness of breath and 1 week of substernal chest pressure while walking up two flights of stairs. Her past medical history is significant for severe emphysema (on home oxygen for 5 years) as well as the prior resection of a right upper lobe for stage 1 squamous cell carcinoma. Her pulmonary function tests are quite poor, with both obstructive and restrictive lung disease. Echo/Doppler reveals significant aortic valve calcification with a peak instantaneous gradient of 4.2 m/s, no significant aortic regurgitation, and normal left ventricular (LV) function. Cardiac catheterization shows insignificant coronary disease.

As she is considered high risk for aortic valve replacement (AVR) due to her lung disease, you are asked to consider balloon aortic valvuloplasty.

Based on current data regarding this procedure, a successful balloon aortic valvuloplasty procedure would be expected to result in which of the following outcomes?

(A) A greater improvement in symptoms if the baseline ejection fraction (EF) is diminished
(B) A long-term sustained benefit superior to AVR and without the surgical risk
(C) An improvement in NYHA functional class only if there is improvement in LV diastolic function
(D) Improvement in her clinical status to allow her to now safely undergo AVR later

31.2 Mitral stenosis (MS) results in a gradient between the left ventricular end diastolic pressure (LVEDP) and the pulmonary capillary wedge (PCW) pressure. Each of the following disorders can also cause an elevated gradient between the PCW pressure and the LVEDP, EXCEPT:

(A) Shone syndrome
(B) Primary pulmonary hypertension
(C) Pulmonary venoocclusive disease
(D) Cor triatriatum sinister
(E) Pulmonary vein stenosis

31.3 A 60-year-old woman with prior mitral commissurotomy for rheumatic MS is undergoing percutaneous mitral valvuloplasty. Following an Inuoe 28 mm balloon dilation of the mitral valve, the LA mean pressure changes as shown in Figure Q31-3. The next most appropriate course of action is to:

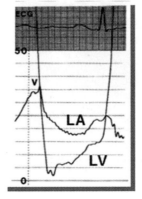 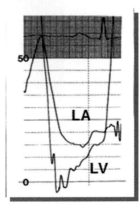

Figure Q31-3. The preproceural left atrial (LA) and left ventricular (LV) tracings are compared to the postprocedural tracings.

(A) Remove the balloon and deem the procedure a success

(B) Upsize to a larger balloon for further dilation

(C) If the patient is hemodynamically unstable, place an intraaortic balloon pump and obtain urgent surgery consultation

(D) Hemodynamically support with phenylephrine

(E) Re-zero the pressure transducer to ensure its accuracy

31.4 Which of the following characteristics of the rheumatic mitral valve is not considered in the MGH echocardiographic scoring system?

(A) Severity of mitral valve regurgitation

(B) Leaflet mobility

(C) Valvular thickening

(D) Valvular calcification

(E) Subvalvular thickening and fibrosis

31.5 The echocardiogram in Figure Q31-5 is obtained on a 40-year-old woman with a prior history of rheumatic fever as a child. The echocardiographer noted mild to moderate calcium in the leaflets and commented on reduced leaflet mobility. The patient is experiencing progressive dyspnea with exertion. She is referred for possible percutaneous balloon mitral valvuloplasty. She has had atrial fibrillation for at least 2 years. Based on the echocardiographic findings, you would suggest:

(A) Proceed with percutaneous mitral valvuloplasty

(B) Increase her diuretics and see her back in 4 to 5 weeks

(C) Add amiodarone and attempt direct current cardioversion (after transesophageal echocardiogram [TEE] is performed)

(D) Refer her for surgical mitral valve replacement

(E) Refer her for surgical mitral commissurotomy

31.6 In a patient with severe MS, which one of the following is not an indication for percutaneous balloon mitral valvuloplasty based on the current ACC/AHA valvular heart disease guidelines?

(A) Progressive dyspnea on exertion

(B) New onset atrial fibrillation

(C) Severe pulmonary hypertension

(D) Tricuspid valve regurgitation

(E) Left ventricular dysfunction

31.7 A 55-year-old male presents to your office in severe right heart failure. Thirteen years ago, he had two-vessel coronary artery bypass, a mitral valve replacement with a bileaflet mechanical mitral valve, and a tricuspid valve replacement with a porcine bioprosthesis. He has no angina but some dyspnea, and he has noted a progressive enlargement of his abdomen with peripheral edema above his ankles. You obtain an echocardiogram that includes the following (Fig. Q 31-7). Based on the echo/Doppler above, you would suggest:

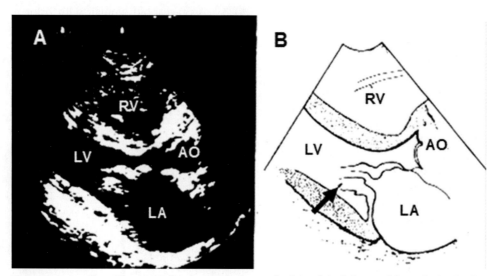

Figure Q31-5. The still echocardiogram of the long axis view of the left ventricle and mitral valve is shown with an anatomic diagram of the same view accompanying for clarification.

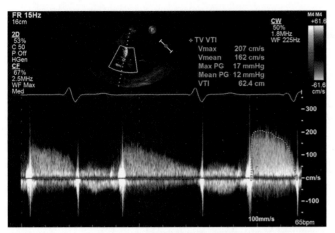

Figure Q31-7. A representative echo Doppler tracing through a prosthetic tricuspid valve replacement with mean gradient of 12 mm Hg. (see color insert)

(A) A cardiac MRI to better assess his right ventricular (RV) function, as echocardiography may be misleading in this situation

(B) A cardiac catheterization to assess his anatomy and hemodynamics and then likely the performance of percutaneous tricuspid valvuloplasty

(C) A cardiac catheterization to assess his anatomy and hemodynamics and be referred for surgical tricuspid valve replacement

(D) An increase in his diuretics, and an exercise sestamibi performed to determine if he has ongoing coronary ischemia

31.8 Figure Q31-8 represents a TEE. There is spontaneous echo contrast noted within the left atrial chamber. You are asked if the patient is a candidate for percutaneous mitral valvuloplasty with this finding. Which of the following is TRUE regarding the presence of spontaneous left atrial contrast?

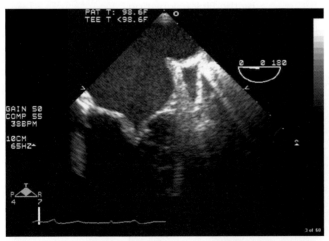

Figure Q31-8. Still frame image of a transesophageal echo study evaluating severe rheumatic mitral stenosis.

(A) It is most often associated with severe MR

(B) It is an indication of the need for immediate valvuloplasty or valve replacement

(C) It is often associated with a left atrial appendage thrombus

(D) The presence of "smoke" in the left atrium (LA) contraindicates mitral valvuloplasty due to the high risk of embolic stroke

(E) It should be treated with long-term antiplatelet therapy

31.9 Which of the following is a valid statement regarding the results of a successful percutaneous balloon mitral valvuloplasty procedure?

(A) It allows for the cessation of antibiotic endocarditis prophylaxis

(B) A successful procedure can be defined as a postprocedural valve area >1.5 cm^2 with no more than 2+ MR

(C) A successful procedure prevents any recurrence of commissural fusion

(D) A successful procedure prevents early occurrence of atrial fibrillation in the future

(E) Even if there is a low echo score for the mitral valve anatomy (<8), restenosis at 10 years can be expected in over 50%

31.10 An 80-year-old is referred to you for possible aortic valvuloplasty. He has chronic obstructive lung disease and has had a prior biventricular pacer with implantable defibrillator placed due to congestive heart failure and an LV EF of 28%. The biventricular pacemaker has not improved his symptoms. His PFTs reveal moderate obstructive lung disease. His resting pO$_2$ is 91%. His estimated GFR is 60 mL/min. He has been a heavy alcohol user in the past and knew about an aortic murmur for many years. Over the past few months, he has developed progressive symptoms of dyspnea and chest pressure. A cardiac catheterization in his local community revealed a 25 mm Hg mean aortic gradient with no aortic insufficiency and an aortic valve area (AVA) of 0.7 cm^2. He has no coronary artery disease. His brain natriuretic peptide (BNP) is elevated at 620 pg/mL.

He undergoes a second cardiac catheterization, during which time he is given intravenous dobutamine while simultaneously determining his cardiac output and valve gradient. The relevant hemodynamics of the aortic and LV pressures with graded doses of dobutamine are shown (Fig. Q31-10). Based on the above hemodynamics result, he should be considered for which of the following?

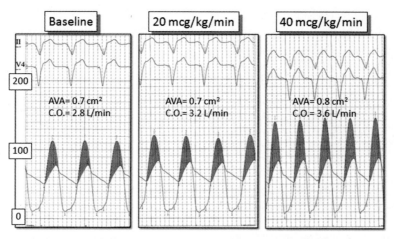

Figure Q31-10. Series of hemodynamic tracings comparing left ventricular and aortic pressures at baseline and with increasing doses of intravenous dobutamine in a patient with low output low gradient AS. Valve areas calculated as indicated.

(A) Aortic valve replacement
(B) Medical therapy only
(C) Percutaneous aortic valvuloplasty
(D) He should be referred to a center that has access to a percutaneous aortic valve stent

31.11 A 22-year-old college student is referred because of a murmur. On exam and by echocardiography, she has a classic doming pulmonary valve with a peak pulmonary valve gradient by echocardiography of 80 mm Hg. She is minimally symptomatic, but the decision is made to proceed with pulmonary valvuloplasty based on the hemodynamics. The procedure goes smoothly, but she becomes hypotensive immediately after the balloons are removed. The preprocedural and postprocedural right ventriculograms are shown (Figure Q31-11). What is the most likely cause for hypotension in this setting?

(A) The pulmonary valve has ruptured and there is severe pulmonary regurgitation
(B) A ventricular septal defect has been caused by the procedure
(C) Relief of the pulmonary valve stenosis has resulted in severe subpulmonic dynamic stenosis with low output
(D) There is obvious tamponade due to rupture of the pulmonary artery

31.12 Pulmonary hypertension associated with mitral valve stenosis:

(A) Completely resolves following surgical valve correction, but not with percutaneous treatment
(B) Is associated with a soft P2 on physical exam
(C) Is an absolute contraindication to percutaneous valvuloplasty
(D) May lead to a falsely elevated cardiac output by the Fick calculation
(E) Can lead to significant concomitant tricuspid regurgitation

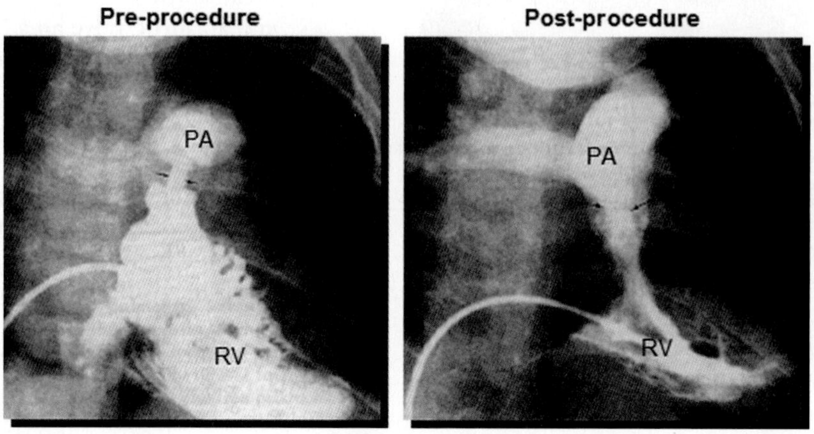

Pre-procedure

PA

RV

Post-procedure

PA

RV

Figure Q31-11. The right ventricular (RV) angiogram before pulmonary valvuloplasty is shown on the left and the immediate postprocedural RV angiogram on the right.

31.13 You have just performed a second balloon inflation across a congenitally stenotic pulmonary valve using a single balloon technique. The preprocedural and postprocedural pressure curves are obtained and are shown in Figure Q31-13. Based on the hemodynamics, next most appropriate action would be to:

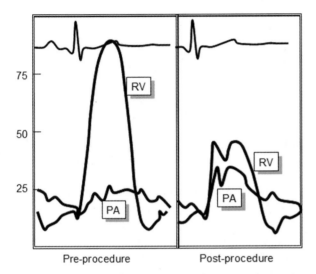

Pre-procedure   Post-procedure

Figure Q31-13. The preprocedural RV and PA pressures are shown on the left and compared with the postprocedural pressures.

(A) Conclude the procedure is a success

(B) Upsize to a larger balloon to improve the valvular area

(C) Place an intraaortic balloon pump and call for emergent pulmonary valve replacement

(D) Perform an emergent TEE to assess whether there is severe pulmonary regurgitation

(E) Add low-dose dobutamine for support given the drop in the RV pressures

31.14 A 14-year-old Caucasian male sees you for consultation regarding a murmur. He had been followed for this by his local pediatric cardiologist prior. He has been feeling fine, except he notes some increased fatigue lately after an hour or so of pickup basketball. He denies any chest pressure or presyncope. On exam, he has the murmur of aortic stenosis (AS) with mid-to-late peaking. You obtain an echocardiogram: his LV function is normal and the Doppler across his aortic valve reveals the following (Fig. Q31-14). What should be your next course of action?

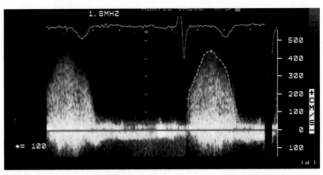

Figure Q31-14. Continuous wave Doppler signal through aortic valve showing peak velocity of 450 cm/s.

(A) He is asymptomatic clinically, and he needs no further studies

(B) He should be considered for percutaneous aortic valvuloplasty

(C) He should undergo a cardiac catheterization to confirm the AS and evaluate his coronary arteries

(D) He should be started on beta-blockers and followed with an echocardiogram every 6 months

(E) He should be referred for surgical valve replacement

31.15 You are asked to see a 23-year-old woman who is 27 weeks pregnant. She has had little prenatal care. She has no known heart condition but is getting progressively short of breath as the pregnancy continues. She finally saw an internist that obtained an echocardiogram (Fig. Q31-15). On exam, she has a loud opening snap with an easy to discern diastolic rumble. No MR is audible. She has early congestive heart failure but remains in normal sinus rhythm. The mitral valve appears to move well, but there is evidence for thickening of the mitral valve and some calcium. The submitral apparatus looks reasonably good. You decide she has an echo score of 8 to 9. Based on these data, your best therapeutic option in this situation is to use which of the following strategies?

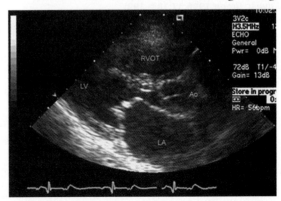

Figure Q31-15. Parasternal transthoracic echo image of a patient with moderate mitral stenosis.

(A) Heart failure therapy using diuretics, ACE inhibitors, beta-blockers, and digoxin
(B) Put her to complete bed rest until she delivers the baby
(C) Consult cardiac surgery for mitral valve commissurotomy or replacement
(D) Consider percutaneous balloon valvuloplasty
(E) Consider abortion of the pregnancy

31.16 During percutaneous mitral valvuloplasty, the Inoue balloon initially inflates distally and then the balloon is pulled into the mitral annulus and inflation to a maximal balloon diameter is subsequently achieved. Figure Q31-16 reflects a common problem encountered during this procedure. What problem is being encountered during this procedure?

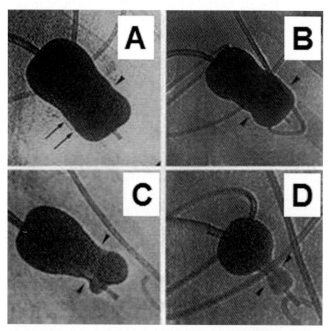

Figure Q31-16. The Inoue balloon is shown inflated in the mitral apparatus. Panels A to D represent the shape of the balloon during these inflations. (Modified from Hung JS, Lau KW. Pitfalls and tips in inoue balloon mitral commissurotomy. *Cathet Cardiovasc Diagn* **1996;37:188–199).**

(A) There is submitral scarring that is preventing the balloon from fully inflating
(B) There is a defect in the distal Inoue balloon that is preventing full inflation
(C) There is an obstruction in the Inoue catheter that is preventing full inflation
(D) The operator is using an improper mixture of radiographic contrast to inflate the balloon

31.17 Which of the following procedures can be successfully approached by percutaneous balloon techniques?

(A) Calcific mitral valve stenosis (nonrheumatic)
(B) Parachute mitral valve with stenosis

(C) Subaortic membranous stenosis
(D) Cor triatriatum membrane
(E) Bicuspid aortic valve in young patients

31.18 A 90-year-old female presents to the catheterization laboratory for elective percutaneous aortic valvuloplasty. She has severe AS with preserved LV function and symptoms of dyspnea. You explain to her the most common complication from the procedure is:

(A) Aortic regurgitation
(B) Left ventricular perforation
(C) Heart block
(D) Access site bleeding requiring transfusion
(E) Death

31.19 Transcatheter aortic valve replacement (TAVI) is currently being evaluated in the United States. In the nonsurgical arm of the PARTNER's trial, evaluating the Sapien balloon expandable AVR, patients were randomly assigned to TAVI vs. medical treatment. Compared to medical therapy in this high-risk group, which statement is true regarding TAVI therapy?

(A) There is a 1-year mortality improvement
(B) There is a 30-day mortality improvement
(C) Aortic valve regurgitation worsens over the course of the first year
(D) Hemolysis across the implanted valve worsens over the course of the first year

31.20 A variety of approaches have been evaluated for implantation of a percutaneous stented aortic valve. Among these approaches to the aortic valve are all of the following, EXCEPT:

(A) Antegrade following transseptal catheterization
(B) Retrograde from the subclavian artery
(C) Retrograde from the radial artery
(D) Antegrade via the LV apex
(E) Retrograde from the femoral artery

31.21 In the Endovascular Valve Edge-to-Edge Study (EVEREST) II of percutaneous mitral valve repair, patients were randomized in a 2:1 fashion to MitraClip percutaneous repair vs. open surgical procedure. Results at 1 year suggested:

(A) Equivalent efficacy in reduction of MR at 1 year
(B) Similar rates of bleeding with either procedure
(C) Higher risk of endocarditis with a surgical approach
(D) Similar NYHA and quality-of-life indices at 1 year

31.22 In patients with high surgical risk due to comorbidities, transcatheter AVR with the Sapien valve vs. standard medical therapy in the PARTNER trial showed:

(A) A mortality advantage of percutaneous valve replacement over standard medical care at 1 year

(B) A high rate of valve deterioration at the 1-year echocardiographic follow-up

(C) A 4% periprocedural mortality of percutaneous valvular placement

(D) No improvement in the NYHA Functional Class at 1 year between the two groups

31.23 The pulmonary angiogram in Figure Q31-23 reveals the results from percutaneous pulmonary valve replacement in a prior surgical RV-to-PA conduit. Which of the following is not considered a potential complication from this procedure?

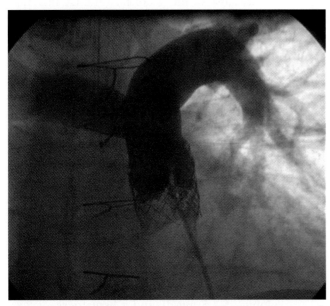

Figure Q31-23. Pulmonary angiogram with percutaneous pulmonary valve in place.

(A) Injury to the right coronary artery

(B) Rupture of the pulmonary artery

(C) Complete heart block

(D) Tricuspid regurgitation

(E) Pulmonary regurgitation

31.24 The percutaneous aortic valve, CoreValve, is shown in Figure Q31-24. Its deployment may be accomplished via all of the following approaches, EXCEPT:

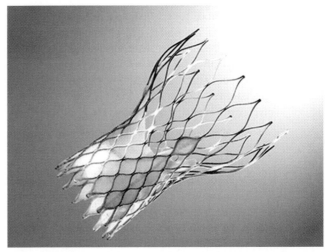

Figure Q31-24. Medtronic percutaneous aortic CoreValve. (see color insert)

(A) Percutaneous via the right common femoral artery

(B) Performed via surgical cutdown to the right external iliac artery

(C) Transapically through a small thoracotomy

(D) Through a surgical cutdown at the right subclavian artery

31.25 A 49-year-old has had long-standing MS without MR and moderate aortic regurgitation with trivial AS. She has had a progressive increase in dyspnea and palpitations and is brought to the cardiac catheterization lab for hemodynamic confirmation of her diagnosis and possible mitral valvuloplasty. In the cardiac catheterization laboratory, the following data were obtained:

Heart rate of 62
RA mean pressure: 5 mm Hg
PA pressure of 55/25 with a mean of 35 mm Hg
PCW pressure of 26 mm Hg
LV: 150/10 mm Hg
Aorta: 130/80 (95)
Mitral gradient: mean 16 mm Hg
Aortic gradient: mean 10 mm Hg
Cardiac output: 3 L/min using the Fick method
LV angiogram: no MR and normal LV function
Aortic angiogram: 2+ aortic regurgitation
The cardiology fellow in the laboratory determines the MVA is 0.8 cm².
Which of the following is a correct statement regarding the hemodynamic findings?

(A) She has both mild AS and mild MS

(B) She has mild AS and moderate MS

(C) The MVA cannot be calculated from these data due to the associated aortic regurgitation

(D) She has mild AS and severe MS

31.26 Novel methods for less invasive mitral valve repair continue to be under active investigation. The EVEREST trial utilizes a mitral valve clip to create a double orifice mitral valve similar to one surgical option (the Alfieri approach). All of the following approaches are undergoing various stages of investigation at this time, EXCEPT which one?

(A) An approach that reduces the annular size by placing clips along the inner surface of the mitral annulus (from a catheter in the LV guided by one in the coronary sinus) and then pulling the mitral annulus toward a central clip to reduce the annular size

(B) An approach using a catheter in the coronary sinus to reduce the annular size by a cinching method

(C) An approach to reduce the mitral annular size by placing external epicardial buttons from the anterior LV wall through the LV and onto the posterior LV wall to reduce the A-P mitral annular diameter

(D) An approach with a left atrial basket with hooks to snag the mitral annulus and reduce its overall size

31.27 A 72-year-old woman consults you regarding progressive symptoms of dyspnea. She had a porcine mitral valve replacement 14 years ago for mitral valve endocarditis. Her post-op course was complicated due to mediastinitis. She does not want to undergo another surgical procedure.

She has a 16 mm Hg mean mitral gradient across the prosthetic mitral valve, but only trivial MR. In the course of your evaluation, you obtain the following TEE (Fig. Q31-27).

Based on the results of the TEE results and your knowledge of the effectiveness of percutaneous balloon mitral valvuloplasty, which of the following recommendations is most appropriate?

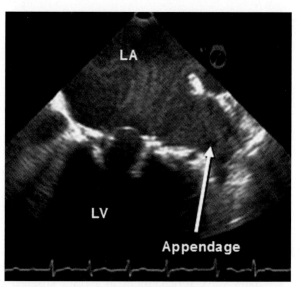

Figure Q31-27. Transesophageal echo image of a left atrium with spontaneous echo contrast and prosthetic mitral valve.

(A) She needs surgical mitral valve replacement. Because of the "smoke" in the LA, this must be done through a median sternotomy

(B) She needs surgical mitral valve replacement. This can be done through a minithoracotomy in this situation

(C) She can undergo percutaneous mitral valvuloplasty but needs to be on warfarin at least several weeks before the procedure due to the "smoke" in the LA

(D) She can undergo percutaneous mitral valvuloplasty now, since the LA appendage appears to be without thrombus

31.28 A 64-year-old woman with severe MR is seeing you 6 months following mitral valve replacement with a St. Jude bileaflet mitral valve. She initially did well after surgery, but now she has new anemia. She was seen by her family practice physician who found she had a hemoglobin of 7.5 mg/dL and a hematocrit of 24%. A haptoglobin was undetectable and the LDH was four times the upper limit of normal. On your exam, she has a loud holosystolic murmur and the echocardiogram confirms severe paravalvular MR. After being given iron, folate, and weekly erythropoietin, she continues to be anemic.

All of the following are options to consider, EXCEPT:

(A) Continue anemia therapy until redo mechanical mitral valve replacement

(B) Continue anemia therapy until replacement of the mechanical mitral valve with a bioprosthetic mitral valve

(C) Immediate surgical repair of the perivalvular regurgitation

(D) Continue anemia therapy and withhold warfarin for 8 weeks to see if the perivalvular regurgitation will thrombose prior to repeat surgery

(E) Attempt closure of the perivalvular leak with an occluder device now

31.29 A 40-year-old woman with severe mitral stenosis and an echocardiographic valve score of 7 is taken to the catheterization laboratory for percutaneous balloon mitral valvuloplasty. The procedure is going well, but just as the Inoue balloon catheter is placed in the LA, the patient becomes hypotensive.

The following 12-lead ECG is obtained (Fig. Q31-29). Based on these data, the next appropriate action should be:

(A) Pericardiocentesis

(B) Protamine to reverse the effect of heparin

(C) Coronary angiography

(D) Immediate balloon mitral valvuloplasty

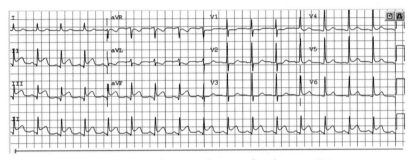

Figure Q31-29.   Twelve-lead electrocardiogram showing acute MI.

ANSWERS AND EXPLANATIONS

31.1 **Answer C.** In a 3-year follow-up review of patients with aortic valvuloplasty, Davidson CM, et al. (*Am J Cardiol* 1991;68:75–80) found the baseline EF an important echocardiographic predictor of postprocedural 1-year survival and improvement in symptoms. Functional improvement was found to be related to diastolic improvement despite early aortic valve restenosis even at 6 months (*J Am Coll Cardiol* 1990;16:795–803). Answer A is therefore inaccurate (low EF) and in no series has there been superiority of percutaneous balloon aortic valvuloplasty vs. surgery in an elderly population. After aortic valvuloplasty, postprocedural 30-day mortality was noted to be 14% with 11% cardiac in nature, suggesting most patients succumb to cardiac death. Overall survival in the NHLBI Balloon Valvuloplasty Registry of 674 patients was poor at 55% at 1 year, 35% at 2 years, and 23% at 3 years of follow-up, though functional improvement was noted in the majority of those who did survive with 78% of patients NYHA class 1 or 2 at 1 year of follow-up and was related to improvement in diastolic function (*Circulation* 1994;89:642–650).

31.2 **Answer B.** There are several explanations for an elevated PCW to left ventricle (LV) diastolic gradient. While rheumatic MS is the leading cause, other rarer causes may occur. A mitral web may exist just above the mitral valve and be part of a syndrome with multiple and variable levels of obstruction (*Am J Cardiol* 1963;11:714–725). This syndrome includes a parachute mitral valve (that can result in MS) and/or the supramitral valve ring. In *cor triatriatum sinister*, a membrane divides the LA into an accessory venous chamber and an LA chamber contiguous with the mitral valve. *Pulmonary venoocclusive disease* (*J Am Coll Cardiol* 2004;43:5S–12S) is obliterative disease of the pulmonary venous bed or pulmonary veins themselves. In most cases, the cause is unknown but may be related to viral infection or connective tissue diseases such as lupus or Calcinosis Raynaud's syndrome Esophageal dysmotility Sclerodactyly Telangiectasia (CREST) syndrome. It may also be a complication of certain hematologic cancers such as leukemia or lymphoma, or due to chemotherapy. It presents clinically as pulmonary hypertension but will show elevated and usually differential gradients throughout the pulmonary vasculature due to the patchy distribution of this illness. *Pulmonary vein stenosis* may be primary or secondary to fibrosing mediastinitis, iatrogenic related to atrial fibrillation ablations, surgical instrumentation (lung transplant) and chest radiation. The presentation may also exhibit differential wedges across the lung bed, as blood flow may only go to the least affected areas. If suspected, it is important to obtain a PCW pressure in all four quadrants of the lung. Wedge angiograms done by initially injecting contrast in the distal pulmonary artery occluded by a balloon-tipped catheter and then allowing the contrast to clear in order to visualize each pulmonary vein separately may be helpful in evaluating these disorders. Primary pulmonary hypertension patients have intrinsic disease of the pulmonary bed and have precapillary smooth muscle hypertrophy. These patients have a normal PCW, an elevated pulmonary vascular resistance, and no significant PCW/LV gradient.

31.3 **Answer C.** This tracing clearly shows a large V wave within the atrial tracing consistent with severe mitral regurgitation (MR) as a complication of the balloon valvuloplasty procedure. Large V waves may only reflect impaired LA compliance, however, and thus the importance of comparing this to the preprocedural tracing. Mitral regurgitation during mitral valvuloplasty is a known complication, occurring in about 3% of patients. This is usually due to rupture of a chord in the heavily scarred subvalvular apparatus or to a tear in the leaflet itself. A progressive increase in the V wave during the procedure has a sensitivity of 79% and specificity of 89% for worsening MR (*Am J Cardiol* 1998;82:1388–1393). More than 2+ MR means that the procedure has been unsuccessful. One would not upsize the balloon diameter in the face of severe MR. Phenylephrine increases afterload on the LV and would increase the V wave in the LA tracing. While re-zeroing of the transducer may be useful, it would not negate the presence of a V wave of this magnitude. Depending on the severity and baseline clinical status, the appropriate course would be to place an intraaortic balloon pump and proceed to urgent surgery if the patient is hemodynamically compromised. Otherwise elective surgery is indicated.

31.4 **Answer A.** Four characteristics are taken into account in the scoring system, with each given a 0- to 4-point value based on severity (*Br Heart J* 1988;60:299–308).

(A) Leaflet Mobility
1. Highly mobile valve with only leaflet tip restriction
2. Midportion and base of leaflets with reduced mobility
3. Valve leaflets move forward in diastole mainly at the base
4. No or minimal forward movement of the leaflets in diastole

(B) Valvular Thickening
1. Leaflets minimally thickened (4–5 mm)
2. Mid-leaflet thickening, pronounced thickening of the margins
3. Thickening extends through the entire leaflets (5–6 mm)
4. Pronounced thickening of all leaflet tissue (>8 mm)

(C) Subvalvular Thickening
1. Minimal thickening of chordal structures just below the valve
2. Thickening of the chordae extending up to 1/3 of the chordal length
3. Thickening extending to the distal third of the chordae
4. Extensive thickening and shortening of all chordae extending down to the papillary muscles

(D) Valvular Calcification
1. A single area of increased echo brightness
2. Scattered areas of brightness confined to the leaflet margins
3. Brightness extending to the midportion of the leaflets
4. Extensive brightness throughout most of the leaflet tissue

A "0" score implies normal valve morphology. A total valve score of ≤8 implies a mobile valve readily amenable to percutaneous valvuloplasty. Progressively higher total valve scores result in less favorable results after valvuloplasty, both acutely and in the long term. (*J Am Coll Cardiol* 2002;39: 328–334). Neither MR severity nor mitral valve area (MVA) is a component of the valve score. In general, however, only those patients with <2+ MR are acceptable candidates for the procedure.

31.5 **Answer D.** Based on the echocardiographic scoring system, even the still echocardiographic image reveals significant submitral scarring (see arrow) and a thickened mitral valve. This alone would give her an echo score of 7 to 8. While calcium and mobility cannot be defined from this still frame, the comments of the echocardiographer add further points to the valve scoring system, making it further *unlikely* this is a valve that would respond to percutaneous valvuloplasty methods. Increasing the diuretics may help in the short term, as might the return to normal sinus rhythm if feasible after this long a period and with what is an enlarged LA. She is now symptomatic, and a surgical intervention is appropriate. The valve morphology for a surgical commissurotomy is precisely the same as for percutaneous valvuloplasty, so that is not an option. The appropriate option is surgical valve replacement at this time.

31.6 **Answer D.** The indications for percutaneous balloon valvuloplasty for MS include the presence of moderate to severe MS defined as an MVA of ≤1.5 cm² and the absence of an LA appendage thrombus and <2+ mitral insufficiency (*J Am Coll Cardiol* 2008;52:e1–e142).

Class I indication: Symptomatic (FC III or IV) MS with favorable valvular anatomy (Ia)
Class II indication: Asymptomatic MS with favorable valve morphology and a pulmonary systolic pressure of >50 mm Hg at rest or >60 mm Hg with exercise (IIa)
Class II indication: Patients with significant symptoms and less favorable valve anatomy who are at high risk for surgery (IIa)
Class II indication: Patients with new atrial fibrillation (IIb)
Tricuspid valve regurgitation may be primary, due to rheumatic involvement, or, more often, secondary, due to RV enlargement from pulmonary hypertension. Neither the presence of TR nor some LV dysfunction excludes patients from the procedure; by the same token, they are not part of the primary indication to proceed

31.7 **Answer C.** While a cardiac MRI does provide better information regarding RV mass and function, and RV dysfunction may be playing a role in his symptoms, a preserved RV by echocardiography is adequate to exclude this and the important finding in the image shown is the presence of porcine tricuspid valve stenosis (TS). The normal tricuspid valve area is about 10 cm² and any gradient over 2 mm Hg is considered abnormal, with severe TS diagnosed when the mean gradient is >5 mm Hg. He clearly has severe TS (mean gradient 12 mm Hg) with right heart failure due to degeneration of his bioprosthesis valve. In the tricuspid position, these valves can be expected to remain functional from 10 to 12 years. Degeneration usually results in both tricuspid regurgitation and stenosis. There is very little experience with percutaneous balloon valvuloplasty for a stenotic tricuspid bioprosthetic valve, but what information is available suggests that there is an extremely high risk of valvular tearing and that severe tricuspid regurgitation can be expected (*J Heart Valve Dis* 2010;19:159–160). Given his clinical situation, redo tricuspid valve replacement is the best clinical option to resolve his situation. While constrictive pericarditis may also be potentially playing an associated role in this situation, the high tricuspid valve gradient points primarily to the tricuspid valve as the main culprit here.

31.8 **Answer C.** The meaning of spontaneous echo contrast remains obscure. It typically represents slow atrial flow (*J Am Soc Echocardiogr* 1991;4:648–650) and while the phenomenon is clearly not circulating thrombi, it is often associated with a left atrial appendage or mural thrombus and a higher risk for embolization (*J Am Coll Cardiol* 2005;45:1807–1812). At this time, there is no specific recommendation for anticoagulation based on this finding unless concomitant thrombus is visualized in the LA or LA appendage or the patient has intermittent or sustained atrial fibrillation. In that situation, warfarin therapy and not antiplatelet therapy is recommended. Patients referred for percutaneous mitral valvuloplasty frequently have spontaneous left atrial contrast and, if there is no evident atrial appendage thrombus, the patient can safely undergo the procedure.

31.9 **Answer B.** The patient risk for endocarditis has not been shown to be reduced following mitral valvuloplasty. Based on the latest guidelines, the patient would not be candidate for endocarditis prophylaxis anyway.

Successful mitral valvuloplasty should be attained in a high percentage (up to 95%) of cases with the excellent valve morphology that results in a valve score of <8 (*Am Heart J* 1995;129:1197–1203). While several definitions of success are possible, a common one defines success as a valve area >1.5 with no more than 2+ MR. Others have used a >50% increase in the baseline valve area or a >50% decrease in the valve gradient.

There are no data that mitral valve procedures reduce the risk of atrial fibrillation though left atrial size does help predict who can maintain sinus rhythm (*Am J Cardiol* 2006;97:1045–1050) and amiodarone (*J Heart Valve Dis* 2002;11:802–809) has had some success in this population. In addition, it is known that chronic atrial fibrillation portends a poorer long-term result from the procedure compared to those in sinus rhythm (*J Heart Valve Dis* 2005;14:727–734). Rheumatic carditis has often been postulated as to why the onset of atrial fibrillation does not always correlate with the severity of the MS.

Unfortunately, the majority of patients will ultimately have the recurrence of stenosis. In a serial echocardiographic study (*J Am Coll Cardiol* 2002;39:328–334) as expected, echocardiographic restenosis was more frequent than clinical symptoms of restenosis. By serial echocardiography at 5 years, 20% had restenosis if the baseline echocardiographic score was <8, but 60% had restenosis if the baseline echocardiographic score was ≥8. Clinical restenosis occurs at a later time, but the anatomic features also predict clinical outcome. In a recent study with a 10-year follow-up, clinical restenosis was present in 23% of those with an echo cardiographic score of ≤8, 55% of those with an echocardiographic score of 9 to 11, and 50% of those with an echocardiographic score of ≥12.

31.10 **Answer A.** Low-gradient, low-output AS is defined as a mean gradient <30 mm Hg and an AVA < 1.0 cm². In this case, the fundamental decision is whether his poor LV function is due to his aortic valve (true stenosis) or due to his underlying cardiomyopathy (pseudostenosis). The Gorlin equation is unreliable at low outputs, and the valve area may appear severe in both instances. Using nitroprusside or dobutamine to increase the cardiac output provides a means to sort true stenosis from pseudostenosis. Using dobutamine in this situation increased his aortic valve gradient but changed his AVA trivially. His stroke volume increased by >20%, the definition of preserved cardiac reserve. These data suggest that despite the low gradient, the primary limitation is the stenotic aortic valve and not the underlying cardiomyopathy (*Circulation* 2002;106:809–813). He would therefore benefit from AVR if he is an acceptable candidate otherwise.

His low LVEF suggests percutaneous aortic valvuloplasty is a poor option. There are data that the elderly who best benefit from aortic valvuloplasty are those with a preserved EF (*Am J Cardiol* 1990;65:72–77). Patients with a preserved LVEF also do well with surgery, though. Since aortic valvuloplasty has been shown to provide very limited short- or intermediate-term survival benefit or symptomatic relief in the elderly (*J Am Coll Cardiol* 1995;26:1522–1528), its use is therefore very limited and would not be the best choice in this situation.

His BNP is mildly elevated though, and this may suggest his benefit from AVR will be less than one might expect. In the multicenter TOPAS (Truly or Pseudo-Severe Aortic Stenosis) trial, those patients with high BNP levels (>550 pg/mL) did not appear to have the same benefit from surgical AVR when compared to those with BNP levels <550 pg/mL (*Circulation* 2008;118:S234–S242). For this patient, this might not bode well.

The indications for percutaneous AVR are evolving. If his comorbidities are prohibitive for surgical AVR, that is likely to be a potential option where available. In this case, surgical AVR is preferred as his risk appears acceptable.

31.11 **Answer C.** A classic domed pulmonary valve responds excellently to percutaneous balloon valvuloplasty techniques. On an average, the peak gradient can be expected to fall from about 90 to 29 mm Hg. The procedure has low risk, generally in the range of 1% to 2% and complications include pulmonary edema (presumably from increasing flow to previously underperfused lungs), perforation of a cardiac chamber or vessel, high-grade AV block, pulmonary valve regurgitation, or the "suicide RV" shown in the figure. Sudden relief of the pulmonary valve obstruction can produce transient dynamic RV outflow obstruction as shown in the postprocedural image. This is usually readily treated with intravenous beta-blockers, calcium blockers, and fluids. It is important not to give inotropic agents as these will worsen the dynamic obstruction.

31.12 **Answer E.** Pulmonary hypertension in patients with mitral valve stenosis often is higher than one would expect from the passive rise in the pulmonary venous pressure alone (*N Engl J Med* 1956;254:829–830). Both reactive vasoconstriction and more fixed morphologic changes may occur. Early in the course of the disease, the changes are reversible with the lowering of the pulmonary venous pressure following mitral valvuloplasty or valve replacement. Later on, the changes become more fixed and

are characterized by fibrinoid necrosis, loss of smooth muscle cell nuclei, fibrin deposition, and eventually the plexiform lesion similar to that seen in primary pulmonary hypertension or in Eisenmenger's physiology. The time course of the reduction of pulmonary hypertension is often initially acute with a gradual continued reduction over the ensuing months following the procedure (*J Am Coll Cardiol* 2002;39:328–334).

The elevated pulmonary pressure is associated with a loud or sharp P_2 on physical exam and occasionally pulmonary insufficiency (the Graham-Steele murmur). There is often an associated RV lift and tricuspid regurgitation. In this setting, the tricuspid valve may develop regurgitation either due to annular dilation and chordal displacement as the RV enlarges or due to rheumatic valvular involvement or a combination. Pulmonary hypertension does not affect the Fick output measures, though associated TR and pulmonary insufficiency can alter cardiac output determined by indicator-dilution methods, such as right heart thermodilution techniques. While not a contraindication to percutaneous treatment, special care in balloon size and dilation should be made in MS patients with pulmonary hypertension, since they may be less tolerant to any increase in MR that may occur during the procedure.

31.13 **Answer A.** This tracing clearly shows a decrease in the gradient, which marks a successful procedure. A successful procedure is generally considered one in which the gradient has been reduced to <20 mm Hg. Pulmonary valvuloplasty has a success rate of over 90% and complications are rare (*Cathet Cardiovasc Diagn* 1997;40:427–430). It is performed by using one or two balloons side-by-side to dilate to annular size of 1.2 to 1.4 times the measured annulus, as there is much elastic recoil in the pulmonary artery. Recently the Inoue mitral valvuloplasty balloon has been used with excellent results. The figure represents a successful result and no further action is needed.

31.14 **Answer B.** The echo/Doppler reveals a peak aortic velocity gradient of 4.5 m/s. This corresponds to a peak instantaneous aortic valve gradient of 81 mm Hg. The calculated valve area is 0.6 cm² by the continuity equation. Based on his activity level and early symptoms, he needs an intervention. While percutaneous balloon aortic valvuloplasty has not proven to be an effective procedure in elderly patients, there are better data that it is useful in the adolescent age group. The success rate of valvuloplasty in this subset is high (90%) with a procedural mortality of <2% and an average reduction in the aortic gradient of about 60 (*J Pediatr* 2010;157:445–449). Progressive regurgitation or restenosis occurs in about half the patients by 8 to 9 years, though, and careful follow-up is warranted. Successful valvuloplasty in this age group allows deferral of surgical intervention to a later date and is particularly important in young women who wish to have children.

He does not need catheterization to confirm the diagnosis or for an evaluation of his coronary artery disease. If a percutaneous approach cannot be performed technically, he should consider surgical intervention. Surgery is usually done with a bioprosthetic valve (often an aortic homograft or his own pulmonary autograft as part of the Ross procedure), though young patients have earlier restenosis with bioprosthetic valves than older patients (*J Am Coll Cardiol* 2008;52:e1–e142).

31.15   **Answer D.** During pregnancy, many hemodynamic events occur, including a 25% increase in the red blood cell mass and a 30% to 50% increase in the blood volume. As a result, there is relative anemia. There is a reduction in systemic vascular resistance as well as pulmonary vascular resistance. The cardiac output increases until about the 32nd week of pregnancy where it levels out at from 30% to 50% higher than prepregnancy. During the latter stages of pregnancy, the stroke volume declines and the cardiac output is maintained by an increase in the heart rate. In MS, the increase in blood volume and stroke volume required markedly increases the mitral gradient. In the final trimester, the increasingly rapid heart rate also reduces diastolic time and further increases the mitral gradient. This can lead to progressive symptoms of heart failure. The use of ACE inhibitors is relatively contraindicated in pregnancy, though the risk is less in the last trimester. Complete bed rest has been used in the past, but patients become progressively deconditioned and its use is much less now. Surgical commissurotomy or replacement can be done, but there is substantial fetal loss if the patient is placed on the heart–lung machine for any length of time. Abortion at this stage would not be appropriate due to the advanced age of the fetus.

Percutaneous balloon valvuloplasty has been done quite safely (*Am J Cardiol* 2006;98:812–816)

during pregnancy and would be the procedure of choice here despite the borderline echocardiographic score of 8 to 9. She already has had heart failure, and it would be to the fetus' advantage to mature further before delivery.

31.16   **Answer A.** In each frame, the Inoue balloon in unable to fully inflate due to rigid submitral apparatus scar and fibrosis. The procedure should be terminated when this is seen to prevent rupture of any of the submitral apparatus and severe MR. Careful observation of the inflated balloon can thus provide important information that may prevent valve rupture (*Circulation* 2009;119:e211–e219; *Catheter Cardiovasc Interv* 1999;47:213–217).

31.17   **Answer E.** Calcific MS is the consequence of mitral annular calcium with invasion onto the mitral leaflets. This produces rigidity and creates an obstruction to LV inflow. As the commissures are not fused, the valve is not susceptible to balloon valvuloplasty techniques. A parachute mitral valve includes a single papillary muscle with all the thickened and shortened chordae tendineae inserting onto it. While attempts have been made to balloon these, they have generally been unsuccessful. A subaortic membrane may be present below the aortic valve with attachments to both the ventricular septum and the anterior leaflet of the mitral valve. It often recurs even after surgical correction, and though attempts have been reportedly successful, it is generally not amenable to percutaneous balloon methods. In cor triatriatum, a membrane separates the pulmonary venous chamber from the LA. Again occasional reports of successful tearing of the opening into the LA have been reported, but this is generally considered a surgical problem.

A bicuspid aortic valve in the adolescent can respond to percutaneous balloon procedures (*Circulation* 2008;117:1201–1206). Once it has significantly calcified, the results are not different from the poor results with calcific tricuspid aortic valve stenosis.

31.18   **Answer D.** In the NHLBI experience (*Circulation* 1994;89:642–650), acute complications of aortic valvuloplasty occurred in 57% of patients, with severe complications in 25% and procedural mortality of 3%. Perforation of the ventricle occurred in 10 patients (1.3%), heart block in 30 patients (4%), and bleeding requiring transfusion in 136 patients (20%).

31.19 **Answer A.** Patients in the palliative portion of the PARTNER trial (*N Engl J Med* 2010;363:1597–1607) were not felt to be surgical candidates as their Society of Transthoracic Surgeons risk scores were >10%. Patients randomized to TAVI showed a 1-year mortality of 30.7% compared with that of medically treated patients at 49.7%. However, due to periprocedural issues, there was slightly higher 30-day mortality with TAVI (5% vs. 2.8% for medically treated patients). Aortic regurgitation with moderate-to-severe paravalvular leak was noted in 11.8% of patients at 30 days and 10.5% at 1 year. Hemolysis from the valve was not a detectable issue.

31.20 **Answer C.** Of the two percutaneous devices that have undergone clinical trials to date, one (the Edwards SAPIEN valve) is placed within the architecture of the stenotic aortic valve and fixed in position via an expandable balloon inflation. This device can be placed either retrograde across the aortic valve or antegrade from the LV side via either entry into the LV from the LA (transseptal approach) or via an LV puncture (LV apical approach using a minithoracotomy) or a transaxillary approach (*Eur J Cardiothorac Surg* 2011;40:49–55). The CoreValve device is a nitinol self-expanding stented valve that requires the proximal portion of the stent to approximate the ascending aortic root. This requires the valve be placed only in a retrograde manner across the aortic valve. While the sheath size requirement for both valves continues to fall, the smallest sheath is still an 18-F sheath—much too large to consider placement from the radial artery at this time.

31.21 **Answer D.** The Everest II trial (*J Am Coll Cardiol* 2009;54:686–94; American College of Cardiology Scientific Session, *Conference Proceeding* 2010.) randomized 279 patients with 3+ to 4+ MR to percutaneous close with the MitraClip device vs. open surgical repair. The procedural safety end point, a composite that included death, major stroke, reoperation, urgent/emergency surgery, myocardial infarction, renal failure, and blood transfusion, favored MitraClip with a 10% event rate vs. 57% for surgery at 30 days. The majority of events were needed for transfusion in 8.8% of those with the MitraClip vs. 53.2% in surgical group. While surgical repair clearly demonstrated better results in reduction of MR at 1 year (over half patients with MitraClip had 2+ to 4+ MR vs. 16% of surgical patients), quality of life scores were similar in the two groups. There was no evidence of increased valvular infection with either procedure.

31.22 **Answer A.** The nonsurgical arm of the PARTNER trial (*N Engl J Med* 2010;363:1597–1607) evaluated a group of patients with a predicted surgical mortality of >50% at 30 days as judged by at least two cardiac surgeons. In this population, 358 patients were randomized to SAPIEN valve replacement versus optimal medical care. The trial showed a periprocedural mortality of 6.4% at 30 days vs. 2.8% in the standard therapy arm. However, at 1 year, the mortality in the TAVI group was 30.7% vs. 50.7% in the standard medical arm, showing a clear mortality advantage to treatment. Echocardiographic follow-up showed moderate-to-severe aortic paravalvular insufficiency in 11.8% of patients at 30 days, dropping to 10.5% at 1 year. The TAVI group showed clear improvement in functional class at symptoms at 1 year with 74.8% vs. 42% in NYHA class I/II at the 1-year anniversary.

31.23 **Answer D.** The placement of a percutaneous pulmonary valve has been associated with all of the complications listed, except for tricuspid regurgitation (*Semin Thorac Cardiovasc Surg Pediatr Card Surg Annu* 2009;112–117). The procedure can also be done in those with percutaneous valve failure (valve-in-valve procedure) (*Eur Heart J* 2008;29:810–815). Right coronary artery compression can be avoided by performing careful MRI/CT angiography before the procedure to assess the distance between the conduit (and site of stent valve implantation) and the coronary artery ostia.

31.24 **Answer C.** The Medtronic CoreValve is a tissue valve suspended in a self-expanding nitinol cage. The valve comes in an 18-F system, smaller than Edwards' SAPIEN balloon expandable valve. This may make the valve easier to insert in elderly patients or women with smaller vessels. It virtually "hangs" from the ascending aorta and spans the coronary arteries. However, unlike the Edwards' valve, which can be mounted for an antegrade approach, the CoreValve can only be placed in a retrograde fashion at the aortic position and therefore cannot be placed via an LV apical approach. The apical approach is shown in Figure A31-24.

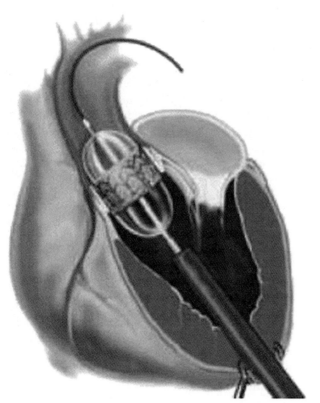

Figure A31-24. Cartoon depicting transapical placement of a percutaneous SAPIEN aortic valve. (see color insert)

31.25 **Answer D.** She has minimal aortic gradient and the AS is quite mild. The determination of an estimated valve area depends on knowledge of the amount of forward flow (cardiac output) across the valve in question and the mean gradient across the valve. From the Gorlin equation (*Am Heart J* 1951;41:1–29)

Mitral valve area =

$$\frac{\text{cardiac output}/(\text{diastolic filling period} \times \text{heart rate})}{44.3 \times 0.85 \times \left(\sqrt{\text{mean mitral gradient}}\right)}$$

Since all of these data were not obvious from the information provided, one can estimate the valve area quickly to confirm the fellow's finding by using the Hakki method (*Circulation* 1981;63:1050–1055):

The Hakki method can be applied to other valves and is a simplified calculation. Using this method

$$\text{Hakki Mitral valve area} = \frac{\text{Cardiac output}}{\left(\sqrt{\text{mean gradient}}\right)}$$

In this case, the cardiac output (3 L/min) by the square root of the mean gradient (4 mm Hg) results in a valve area of 0.75 cm² and is simpler to remember than the classic Gorlin formula.

Both depend on knowing the true flow across the mitral valve and on determining the

mean gradient. The Gorlin formula examines the amount of time in a minute that forward flow is occurring (diastolic filling time × heart rate), uses 44.3 as the gravitational constant, and adds a constant (in this case 0.85 for the mitral valve) that was found to be needed to increase the accuracy of the measurement when the results were compared to autopsy findings.

In this instance, determination of the flow across the mitral valve is not directly impacted by the presence of aortic regurgitation, as the flow across the mitral valve is the same as the Fick-determined cardiac output flow. If there was MR, then the amount of the regurgitant flow would need to be added to the Fick forward flow to determine the total flow across the mitral valve during diastole. If there is both AR and MR, then one should only report the gradients across the valves, since one cannot determine the amount of flow across each valve with any accuracy.
Mitral valve area
Normal: 4 to 6 cm²
Mild MS: 1.5 to 2.5 cm²
Moderate MS: 1.0 to 1.5 cm²
Severe MS: <1.0 cm²

31.26 **Answer D.** Percutaneous approaches to MR continue, though there remain little clinical data with only a few patients being reported. One of the more complete trials, the phase I EVEREST I trial, enrolled 47 patients (*J Am Coll Cardiol* 2009;54:686–694). Phase II has now been completed (American College of Cardiology Scientific Session, *Conference Proceeding* 2010). Besides the percutaneous clip approach, efforts are continuing to develop coronary sinus cinching devices (*Circ Cardiovasc Interv* 2009;2:277–284) to reduce the mitral annular size or to attempt annuloplasty using stitches inserted into the mitral annulus from the ventricular side (*Herz* 2009;34:444–450). All of these devices are in very early trials, and the data are too premature as to the advantage, or even the safety and efficacy, of any particular approach. In the transventricular method (*Herz* 2009;34:444–450), a magnetic-tipped catheter is placed into the coronary sinus and used to locate the tip of a second catheter placed through the aortic valve into the LV and shaped to abut against the mitral annulus. Stitches are implanted into the mitral annulus at various locations identified by the two catheters. Each stitch site is then pulled toward each other to reduce the mitral annular size. Another approach has been to reduce the anteroposterior LV diameter using a transventricular chord attached to anterior and posterior epicardial pads (Coapsys method) (Fig. A31-26).

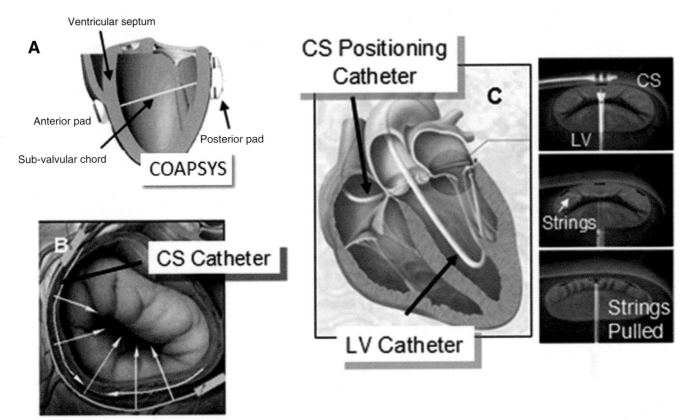

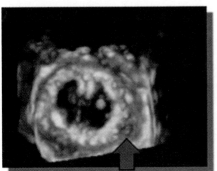

Figure A31-26. Cartoon depicting percutaneous therapies for MR including reducing ventricular diameter (A), coronary sinus circumference reduction (B), and intraventricular annular reduction (C).

31.27 **Answer B.** The patient has severe MS due to prosthetic valve stenosis. There are only anecdotal cases (*Catheter Cardiovasc Interv* 2004;63:503–506) suggesting this lesion is amenable to percutaneous mitral valvuloplasty, as the degenerative porcine valve has little commissural fusion. Percutaneous mitral valvuloplasty has no real role to play in this lesion (*J Am Coll Cardiol*

2008;52:e1–e142). The presence of "smoke" with no appendage thrombus suggests low flow in the atrium but does not affect the surgical approach.

31.28 **Answer D.** The perivalvular regurgitation likely represents dehiscence of a portion of the surgical ring from the mitral annulus. The anemia is due to destruction of the RBCs from the turbulence

St. Jude MVR with Leak   **Catheter in Perivalvular Hole**   **Final Result**

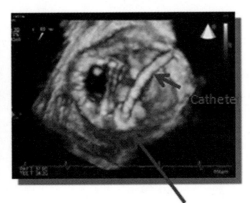

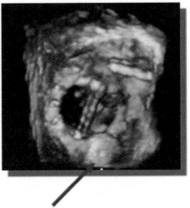

Amplatzer Occluder in Perivalvular Hole

Figure A31-28. Three-dimensional echo imaging of a St. Jude prosthetic valve with a perivalvular leak and subsequent occlusion with an Amplatzer percutaneous occlusion plug.

created through the perivalvular leak. While initial therapy with folate, iron, and erythropoietin may resolve the issue in patients with only mild hemolysis, this did not occur in our patient. Definitive repair usually requires surgical intervention, though there are now increasing reports of success using percutaneous occluder devices. One example is shown in Figure A31-28 (*JACC Cardiovasc Imaging* 2009;2:771–773). Withholding warfarin in this situation puts the patient at great risk for thrombosis on the mechanical prosthetic valve, and that strategy would not be appropriate.

31.29 **Answer C.** Complications following transseptal and the insertion of a catheter in the LA are uncommon (<5%) in experienced centers. The immediate differential should include a vagal reaction, perforation of a cardiac structure with tamponade, bleeding from the groin insertion site, or a coronary embolus (from either thrombus material or air). If a vagal reaction had occurred, one would expect the heart rate to be lower. If a retroperitoneal or access site bleed had occurred, then one would expect a high heart rate. Proceeding with the procedure would not make sense until the cause of the hypotension has been discovered. In this instance, the ECG suggests acute inferoposterior myocardial injury, and coronary angiography would be appropriate to determine if there is a coronary embolus.

QUESTIONS

32.1 Which of the following statements is CORRECT regarding the atrial septal defect (ASD) demonstrated in the angiogram (Fig. Q32-1)?

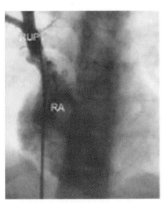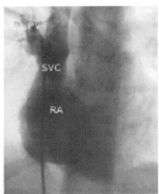

Figure Q32-1

(A) This defect is commonly associated with anomalous connection of the left pulmonary veins (PVs)

(B) This type of defect accounts for approximately 25% of ASDs

(C) Approximately half of these patients have a P-wave axis < 30 degrees

(D) Percutaneous closure of this defect is favored over the Warden procedure

(E) This defect is located posterior to the fossa ovalis

32.2 The following statements regarding Ebstein anomaly are true, EXCEPT:

(A) ASD or patent foramen ovale is usually present

(B) There is characteristic displacement of the septal and anterior leaflets into the right ventricle (RV)

(C) ECG may reveal right atrial (RA) enlargement

(D) RV preload reserve is diminished

(E) 25% to 30% of these patients will have paroxysmal atrioventricular reentrant tachycardia

32.3 A 47-year-old male presents to your clinic with progressive shortness of breath. He notes that he "just doesn't have the stamina" that he used to and finds himself easily tired with his routine exercise. His vitals are BP 135/75, P 70, RR 15, and SpO_2 95%. His height, weight, and body surface area are 177 cm, 77 kg, and 1.94 m². There is a 2/6 systolic murmur heard best in the left infraclavicular space. He displayed no peripheral edema, and his distal pulses are 2/2 throughout. Lab work demonstrates hemoglobin of 14.5 g/dL and hematocrit of 42%. Transthoracic echocardiography demonstrates a normal RV, a mildly dilated left ventricle with normal function, an estimated RV systolic pressure of 75 mm Hg, and a 5-mm patent ductus arteriosus (PDA) with predominately left to right shunt flow. The patient is brought to the catheterization laboratory for complete hemodynamic assessment:

RA mean: 11 mm Hg
RV: 76/5 mm Hg
PA: 90/20 mm Hg, PA mean: 45 mm Hg
PCWP mean: 10 mm Hg
Ascending aorta: 130/85 mm Hg
IVC saturation: 70%
SVC saturation: 68%

RA saturation: 66%
RV saturation: 65%
MPA saturation: 78%
Aortic saturation: 96%

Calculate this patient's shunt flow and $Q_p{:}Q_s$ assuming oxygen consumption of 125 mL/kg while breathing room air.

(A) 1.2 L/min; 1.5:1
(B) 2.2 L/min; 1.5:1
(C) 2.6 L/min; 1.7:1
(D) 2.8 L/min; 1.7:1
(E) 3.2 L/min; 1.9:1

32.4 This patient's pulmonary vascular resistance is:

(A) 3.7 Wood units
(B) 5.1 Wood units
(C) 7.6 Wood units
(D) 8.9 Wood units
(E) 11.1 Wood units

32.5 The next best step in management for the patient in Question 32.3 is:

(A) Clinical follow-up
(B) Clinical follow-up with endocarditis prophylaxis
(C) Percutaneous device closure
(D) Percutaneous device closure with endocarditis prophylaxis
(E) Surgical evaluation

32.6 A 26-year-old female presents to your clinic with palpitations. Over the last few years, she has noticed frequent pulmonary infections but otherwise "feels fine" and takes no medications. She has a strong family history of coronary heart disease. Her vitals are BP 125/85, P 70, RR 15, and SpO$_2$ 98%. Her height, weight, and body surface area are 158 cm, 70 kg, and 1.72 m². On exam, she has a wide, fixed, split S2 and a 2/6 systolic flow murmur heard best in the second left intercostal space. ECG demonstrates RA enlargement and right axis deviation, but a 24-hour Holter monitor was nondiagnostic. Transthoracic echocardiography shows a dilated right atrium and right ventricular dilation with paradoxical motion of the ventricular septum. There is a 20-mm centrally located ASD with a 10-mm rim of residual tissue around the defect. The PVs appear to drain normally. Right ventricular pressure is estimated to be 15 mm Hg. The patient is brought to the catheterization laboratory for complete hemodynamic assessment. Precatheterization lab work demonstrates hemoglobin of 13.2 g/dL and hematocrit of 40%:

RA mean: 8 mm Hg
RV: 40/5 mm Hg
PA: 40/10 mm Hg, PA mean: 20 mm Hg
PCWP mean: 5 mm Hg
Ascending aorta: 120/80 mm Hg
IVC saturation: 78%
SVC saturation: 70%
RA saturation: 92%
RV saturation: 90%
MPA saturation: 89%
Aortic saturation: 99%

This patient's mixed venous saturation is:

(A) 70%
(B) 72%
(C) 74%
(D) 76%
(E) 78%

32.7 Calculate this patient's shunt flow and $Q_p{:}Q_s$ assuming oxygen consumption of 125 mL/kg while breathing room air.

(A) 5.0 L/min; 1.7:1
(B) 6.9 L/min; 1.7:1
(C) 6.9 L/min; 2.7:1
(D) 7.2 L/min; 2.7:1
(E) 7.2 L/min; 3.0:1

32.8 Percutaneous ASD closure in adults should be considered in all of the following circumstances, EXCEPT:

(A) Asymptomatic and otherwise unexplained RA enlargement
(B) Platypnea–orthodeoxia
(C) QP:QS < 1.5:1
(D) Chronic atrial tachyarrhythmia
(E) Left to right shunting and pulmonary arterial pressure 40% of systemic arterial pressure

32.9 A 40-year-old woman is referred to your office for increased shortness of breath and cyanosis. She has a history of complex congenital heart disease including D-transposition of the great arteries, a large VSD with overriding tricuspid valve, and a mildly hypoplastic RV. She has had regular cardiology follow-up until she lost her medical insurance at age 35. She has not been seen by a cardiologist since. She notes that she has had chest pain "all her life," but recently experienced severe chest pain that sent her to the emergency department. An echocardiogram at that time revealed an LVEF of 30% and a peripheral oxygen saturation of 80%. She has noticed that her fingers and toes are often blue or grey and she now becomes "winded" while doing household chores. She takes no medications and smokes about 1 pack/day. Her vitals are BP 80/50 (left arm), P 87, RR 20, and SpO$_2$ 88% on 4 L O$_2$. Her height, weight, and body surface area are 165 cm, 37 kg, and 1.35 m^2. On room air, her saturation dropped to 68% upon walking 50 ft. She has digital clubbing and moderate cyanosis. She has a prominent S2 with a 3/6 systolic murmur heard at the right upper sternal boarder. Imaging confirmed her congenital diagnosis and found her systemic ventricular EF to be 40%. Labs reveal hemoglobin of 19.8 g/dL and hematocrit of 60.0%. She is taken to the catheterization laboratory for complete hemodynamic assessment.

RA mean: 7 mm Hg
RV: 109/4 mm Hg
PA: 102/32 mm Hg, PA mean: 59 mm Hg
PCWP mean: 18 mm Hg
IVC saturation: 70%
SVC saturation: 67%
RA saturation: 68%
RV (systemic ventricle) saturation: 81%
Aortic saturation: 80%
PV saturation: 96%
LV (pulmonary ventricle) saturation: 81%
MPA saturation: 79%

Calculate this patient's shunt flow, Q_p:Q_s, and pulmonary vascular resistance assuming oxygen consumption of 125 mL/kg while breathing room air.

(A) 1.3 L/min; 0.75:1; 10.5 Wood units
(B) 1.3 L/min; 0.67:1; 11.0 Wood units
(C) 1.8 L/min; 0.75:1; 11.5 Wood units
(D) 1.8 L/min; 0.67:1; 12.0 Wood units
(E) 2.0 L/min; 0.5:1; 12.5 Wood units

32.10 The patient above is administered 40 ppm nitric oxide for 5 minutes. Her catheterization data now reveals:

PA: 89/26 mm Hg, PA mean: 49 mm Hg
PCWP mean: 18 mm Hg
Aortic saturation: 92%
PA saturation: 93%

What is the next best step in management?
(A) Heart–lung transplantation
(B) Arterial switch with VSD closure
(C) Pulmonary artery banding
(D) Pulmonary vasodilator therapy
(E) Home oxygen therapy

32.11 A 36-year-old male with tetralogy of Fallot (TOF) is referred to your office for progressive fatigue and palpitations. A palliative Blalock-Taussig shunt was placed at age 6 months, and

he underwent total correction at age 2 years with shunt takedown. When he was 21 years old, an RV to PA valved conduit was placed. His vitals are BP 130/80 (left arm), P 80, RR 15, and SpO$_2$ 98% on room air. His height and weight are 170 cm and 64 kg. ECG is notable for paroxysmal atrial fibrillation. Echocardiography reveals mild LV dysfunction, moderate AI, and a moderately stenotic conduit. He is brought to the catheterization laboratory for further assessment, and his descending angiogram is shown (Fig. Q32-11).

What is the most likely cause of his symptoms?

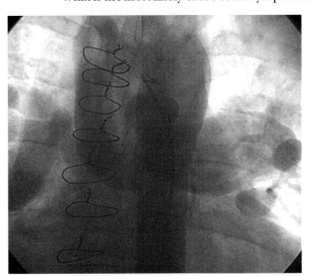

A

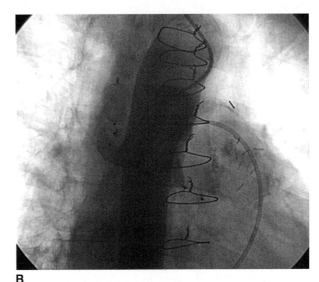

B

Figure Q32-11

(A) Free pulmonary insufficiency and right heart failure
(B) Pulmonary arteriovenous fistula
(C) Residual Blalock-Taussig shunt flow
(D) Cameral fistula
(E) Aortopulmonary collaterals

32.12 Angiography is performed on a 21-year-old patient who presents with shortness of breath (Fig. Q32-12). What is the diagnosis?

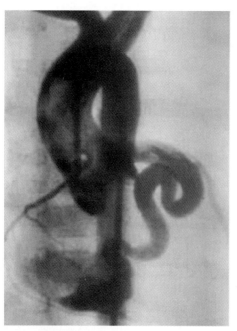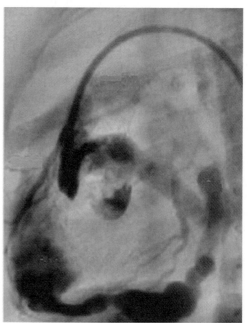

Figure Q32-12

(A) Pulmonary fistula draining into the RV
(B) Pulmonary fistula draining into the LV
(C) Venovenous collateral
(D) Coronary artery fistula draining into the RV
(E) Coronary artery fistula draining into the coronary sinus

32.13 A 32-year-old female is referred to your clinic with a 6-month history of progressive dyspnea on exertion and fatigue. Her history is notable for multiple hospital admissions for pneumonia, and 3 months ago she became increasingly short of breath after delivery of a healthy baby boy. Her echocardiogram showed a grossly dilated RV with mildly reduced function and RVSP of 85 mm Hg. A cardiac MRI is performed as part of her workup and a portion is shown in Figure Q32-13. In addition to what is shown, the scan is notable for a hypoplastic right PV and a large aortopulmonary collateral to the right pulmonary artery. This constellation of findings is likely related to which syndrome?

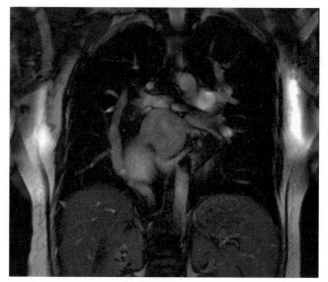

Figure Q32-13

(A) Noonan's syndrome

(B) Scimitar syndrome

(C) Holt-Oram syndrome

(D) Kartagener's syndrome

(E) Down's syndrome

32.14 A 67-year-old female is referred to your clinic after suffering a left MCA stroke resulting in motor deficits and memory problems. Since the stroke, she has had a number of transient ischemic attacks while on aspirin therapy. She has no other medical problems, and her age is her only atherosclerotic risk factor. Her neurologist found no embolic source after an extensive workup. Her transthoracic and intracardiac echocardiograms are shown in Figure Q32-14A,B and report no structural abnormalities. What is the most likely source of this patient's neurologic problems?

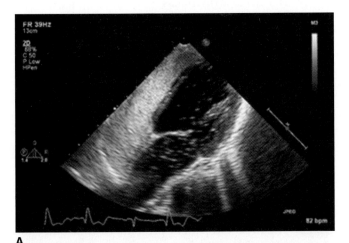

A

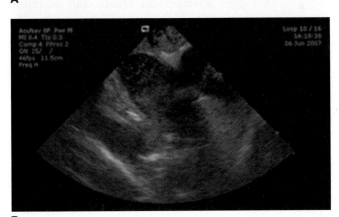

B

Figure Q32-14

(A) Unroofed coronary sinus

(B) Sinus venous ASD with partial anomalous venous return

(C) Pulmonary arteriovenous malformation

(D) PDA

(E) Aortic atheroma

32.15 A 53-year-old male is referred to your office for new onset chest pain and exercise intolerance. He has a history of coarctation of the aorta that was surgically repaired at 3 years of age. He remembers having a cardiac catheterization procedure when he was a teenager but does not remember the results. He follows up regularly with his primary care physician who treats his hypertension and dyslipidemia. His family history is notable for coronary artery disease. His vitals are BP 140/78 (right arm) 135/75 (left arm) 120/60 (left leg), P 58, RR 12, and SpO2 99%. His height and weight are 175 cm and 86 kg. On exam, he has a 2/6 systolic ejection murmur heard at the left upper sternal border and a 2/6 systolic ejection murmur heard over the left posterior thorax. Transthoracic echocardiography demonstrates normal ventricular function with trivial aortic insufficiency. Discrete narrowing of the descending aorta is noted. The patient is brought to the catheterization laboratory for complete hemodynamic assessment.

In which of the following situations is balloon angioplasty and/or stent placement not indicated?

(A) Significant aortopulmonary collateral flow

(B) Peak gradient of 25 mm Hg

(C) Long-segment coarctation

(D) Presence of bicuspid aortic valve

(E) Prior primary surgical repair with resection and end-to-end anastomosis

32.16 In addition to recoarctation and the need for transcatheter intervention, the following are possible late findings associated with aortic coarctation, EXCEPT:

(A) Cerebral aneurysm

(B) Elevated renin levels

(C) Premature coronary disease

(D) Aortic dissection

(E) Ventricular arrhythmia

32.17 The most common coronary artery anomaly is which of the following?

(A) Single coronary artery

(B) Origin of the left circumflex coronary artery from the right coronary artery

(C) Origin of the left anterior descending coronary artery from the right coronary sinus

(D) Origin of the left main coronary artery from the right coronary sinus

(E) Origin of the left main coronary artery from the pulmonary artery

32.18 A patient is found to have doming pulmonary valve stenosis on echocardiography with 1+ pulmonary regurgitation. After proper consenting, she is taken to the catheterization lab for formal hemodynamic assessment.

RA mean: 13 mm Hg
RV: 85/7 mm Hg
PA: 34/22 mm Hg, PA mean: 28 mm Hg
PCWP mean: 14 mm Hg
Ascending aorta: 130/80 mm Hg
CO: 4.5 L/min

The next best step in management is:

(A) Immediate pulmonary balloon valvuloplasty
(B) Refer the patient for surgical valvotomy
(C) Follow-up echocardiogram in 3 to 6 months
(D) Follow-up catheterization in 1 year
(E) No further treatment is recommended

32.19 A patient with long-standing, severe pulmonary stenosis underwent successful balloon valvuloplasty. Right ventricular pressure suddenly rises to near-systemic levels following the procedure. The most likely cause is:

(A) Valve leaflet avulsion
(B) Severe pulmonary insufficiency
(C) Puncture of the main pulmonary artery
(D) Restenosis
(E) Infundibular spasm

32.20 A 43-year-old female with a history of TOF presents to your clinic with moderate chest discomfort, exercise intolerance, and fatigue. She had a palliative Blalock-Taussig shunt placed at 4 months of age and underwent a complete repair at age 2 years including a VSD patch and a subpulmonary resection. She has been followed intermittently for the past two decades but does not report any other health conditions. ECG reveals a PR interval of 180 ms, QRS of 183 ms, and a QTc of 415 ms. Echocardiography reveals right ventricular dilation, moderately decreased right ventricular function, severe pulmonary insufficiency, moderate tricuspid valve regurgitation with an RVSP of 45 mm Hg, and a small residual VSD. She is sent for a cardiac MRI to better assess her anatomy.

Pulmonary valve peak velocity: 1.5 m/s
Pulmonary valve forward volume: 99 mL/beat
Pulmonary valve reverse volume: 38 mL/beat
Pulmonary valve regurgitant fraction: 39%
Right ventricular end diastolic volume: 197 mL (113 mL/m2)
Right ventricular end systolic volume: 91 mL (52 mL/m2)

Right ventricular stroke volume: 105 mL (60 mL/m2)
Cardiac index 6.5 L/min/m²

All of the following are indications for pulmonary valve replacement in this patient, EXCEPT:

(A) Symptoms
(B) ECG findings
(C) Ventricular function on echocardiography
(D) Presence of residual VSD
(E) Right ventricular dimensions on CMR

32.21 The Fontan procedure or total cavopulmonary anastomosis is used as a palliative procedure in patients with single ventricle physiology. All of the following would be clinical evidence of Fontan failure, EXCEPT:

(A) Ascites
(B) Peripheral edema
(C) Atrial arrhythmias
(D) High cardiac output heart failure
(E) Protein-losing enteropathy (PLE)

32.22 A patient referred to your clinic has a screening echocardiogram that reveals dilation of the coronary sinus. The person is otherwise doing well. The most likely associated finding will be:

(A) Tricuspid stenosis
(B) TOF
(C) Primum ASD
(D) Persistent left-sided SVC
(E) Maternal alcohol ingestion failure

32.23 A 24-year-old patient presents to your office for chest pain, shortness of breath, and dizziness on exertion. An echocardiogram reveals subaortic stenosis. Your discussion with the patient includes the following statements, EXCEPT:

(A) This lesion is amenable to a percutaneous intervention
(B) This lesion is typically discrete
(C) This lesion can reform following surgical intervention
(D) Surgery is the most effective option for this patient
(E) This lesion can lead to aortic regurgitation that can progress over time

32.24 Spontaneous bacterial endocarditis prophylaxis should only be observed in which of the following situations?

(A) Cleft mitral valve
(B) TOF repair with a pericardial VSD patch and infundibular resection >10 years ago
(C) Percutaneous PFO closure 3 months ago
(D) Bicuspid aortic valve
(E) PDA occluder placed 1 year ago

32.25 Congenital rubella is associated with all of the following cardiovascular abnormalities, EXCEPT:

(A) Ebstein anomaly
(B) PDA
(C) VSD
(D) Transposition of the great arteries
(E) Tricuspid atresia

32.1 **Answer E.** The angiogram depicts an anomalous right upper pulmonary vein associated with a sinus venosus ASD. Injection of this vein fills the right atrium and RV with contrast. Due to the superior nature of the defect, it can be difficult to cross with a catheter and the predominant left to right shunt limits opacification of the left atrium. The three main forms of ASDs are ostium secundum, ostium primum, and sinus venosus defects. Ostium secundum defects are the most prevalent, accounting for approximately 75% of all ASDs, and are located near the fossa ovalis. Ostium primum defects account for approximately 15% of all ASDs and are located just above the atrioventricular canal. Sinus venosus defects account for approximately 5% to 10% of ASDs. These defects are located posterior to the fossa ovalis and often only have adjacent septal rim tissue anteriorly and inferiorly. Two very rare forms of ASD include coronary sinus defects and inferior vena caval forms of sinus venosus defects (*Circulation* 2006;114:1645–1653).

Sinus venosus defects are almost always associated with anomalous drainage of the right-sided PVs, which often drain to the right atrium or to the superior vena cava (as shown in the angiogram). Sinus node involvement is common in these patients resulting in left axis deviation (and inversion) of the P wave (*Am Heart J* 1973;85:177–185). Unlike ostium secundum ASDs, sinus venosus defects are not amenable to catheter-based closure and therefore require surgical intervention. The Warden procedure transects the superior vena cava above the anomalous PV connections, followed by anastomosis to the RA appendage. The ASD and superior vena caval orifice is then baffled to the left atrium with a patch (*Ann Thorac Surg* 2007;84:1651–1655).

32.2 **Answer B.** Ebstein anomaly represents the most common congenital anomaly of the tricuspid valve. In Ebstein anomaly, the anterior leaflet arises from the normal position on the tricuspid valve annulus. However, the septal and posterior leaflets are displaced into the RV to varying degrees. This results in a portion of the RV becoming "atrialized." The anterior leaflet may be redundant, resulting in a "sail-like" appearance. Usually an atrial level communication is present (either PFO or ASD) permitting right to left shunting. Ebstein morphology promotes atrial level shunting by at

least two mechanisms. Tricuspid valve leaflets are often elongated leading to atrial level shunting (*Circulation* 2008;117:1340–1350). Patients with right to left shunting do not easily develop systemic venous congestion from right-sided heart failure compared to those with an intact septum, but the price paid is often exertional hypoxemia.

Management of Ebstein anomaly is driven by symptoms; asymptomatic patients require no specific therapy. Accessory conduction pathways are present in up to 30% of these patients and may dictate medical management or catheter ablation (*Circulation* 1996;94:376–383). Patients who present with exertional cyanosis secondary to atrial level shunting may benefit from percutaneous device closure. Temporary balloon occlusion of the defect may lead to elevation of RA pressure and a drop in cardiac output. In patients with favorable hemodynamics, these changes will be minimal and closure may be performed. If significant changes in RA pressure or cardiac output occur, the communication should be left patent (*Heart* 2006;92:827–831). Patients with severe symptoms requiring surgical management almost always present during childhood. Surgical management includes tricuspid valve repair (if possible) or replacement, shunt closure, ventricular plication, atrial reduction, and antiarrhythmic surgery. The bidirectional Glenn procedure has also been employed in these patients to unload the right heart (*Curr Opin Pediatr* 2009;21:565–572).

Figure A32-2 shows a right ventricular inflow view of echocardiogram of patient with Ebstein anomaly. The arrow on the left points to an apically displaced posterior leaflet. The arrow on the right points to an elongated anterior leaflet that attaches to the valve annulus.

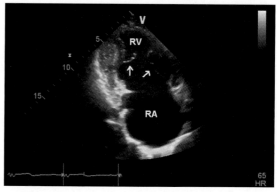

Figure A32-2

32.3 **Answer D.** This patient has a PDA with left to right flow. Signs and symptoms supporting this diagnosis include dyspnea on exertion, widened pulse pressure, and a left subclavicular murmur (classically a continuous "machinery" murmur). Over time, chronic pulmonary volume overload will lead to remodeling of the pulmonary vasculature and increased pulmonary vascular resistance. This patient has elevated pulmonary artery pressures (mean = 45 mm Hg). Pulmonary arterial pressures will eventually reach or exceed systemic pressures and flow through the shunt will become predominantly right to left, a condition known as Eisenmenger's syndrome (ES). Body surface area was calculated using the DuBois method (*J Clin Anesth* 1992;4:4–10)

$$BSA(m^2) = 0.007184 \times weight^{0.425}(kg) \times height^{0.725}(cm)$$

$$BSA(m^2) = 0.007184 \times 77^{0.425}(kg) \times 177^{0.725}(cm)$$

$$= 1.94\,m^2$$

The first step in solving this problem is to localize the oxygen saturation step-up. Blood flow from the IVC, SVC, and coronary sinus mix in the right atrium. Each stream has different oxygen saturations, so measurements will vary depending on the sampling location in the atrium and the degree of mixing that occurs. A "positive" step-up in oxygen saturation between the systemic veins and the RA must be ≥7% (absolute difference in mean saturation values). As blood has more time to mix, saturation becomes more homogeneous, and a "positive" step-up in oxygen saturation between the RA and RV or RV and PA need only be ≥5% (*Am J Cardiol* 1980;46:265–271). This patient has a 14% step-up in oxygen saturation between the RV and PA consistent with a significant left to right shunt. The Fick method is used to calculate the pulmonary blood flow assuming oxygen consumption of the lungs to be 125 mL/m².

$$Q_P = \frac{O_2\ Consumption}{(PV - PA)O_2\ Content}$$

$$\approx \frac{(125\,mL/m^2)(1.94\,m^2)}{(0.96 - 0.78)\left(\dfrac{14.5\,g\,Hgb}{100\,mL\,blood}\right)\left(\dfrac{1.36\,mL\,O_2}{g\,Hgb}\right)}$$

$$= 6.8\,L/min$$

If aortic saturation is ≥95%, it may safely be substituted for pulmonary venous saturation. If aortic saturation is <95%, right to left shunt must be ruled out with a hyperoxygen challenge. If right to left shunting is present, pulmonary venous oxygen saturation may be assumed to be 98% if there is no underlying pulmonary disease. The Fick method is also used to calculate systemic blood flow.

$$Q_S = \frac{O_2\ Consumption}{(SA - MV)O_2\ Content}$$

$$\approx \frac{(125\,mL/m^2)(1.94\,m^2)}{(0.96 - 0.65)\left(\dfrac{14.5\,g\,Hgb}{100\,mL\,Blood}\right)\left(\dfrac{1.36\,mL\,O_2}{g\,Hgb}\right)}$$

$$= 4.0\,L/min$$

To determine systemic blood flow, the Fick method is used again, though with one important caveat. The mixed venous value must be obtained proximal to the shunt location (pulmonary artery saturation is *not* mixed venous saturation in this instance). The shunt is located in the pulmonary artery, so the RV saturation is used. If significant pulmonic regurgitation is present, it would be reasonable to use RA saturation instead.

Once QP and QS are known, shunt flow and QP:QS are easily calculated.

$$Q_{Shunt} = Q_P - Q_S = 6.8 - 4.0 = 2.8/min$$

$$Q_P : Q_S = 6.8/4.0 = 1.7/1$$

Alternatively QP:QS may be quickly calculated as follows:

$$\frac{Q_P}{Q_S} \approx \frac{\dfrac{O_2\ Consumption}{(PV - PA)O_2\ Content}}{\dfrac{O_2\ Consumption}{(SA - MV)O_2\ Content}}$$

$$= \frac{(SA - MV)O_2\ Content}{(PV - PA)O_2\ Content} = \frac{0.96 - 0.65}{0.96 - 0.78}$$

$$= \frac{0.31}{0.18} = 1.7/1$$

32.4 **Answer B.** Pulmonary vascular resistance is calculated as follows:

$$PVR = \frac{P_{\overline{PA}} - P_{\overline{PV}}}{Q_P} = \frac{45\,mm\,Hg - 10\,mm\,Hg}{6.8\,L/min}$$

$$= 5.1\,Wood\ units$$

32.5 **Answer D.** For patients with a small PDA and no evidence of left heart volume overload, clinical follow-up every 3 to 5 years is appropriate. Endocarditis prophylaxis is not recommended for patients with unrepaired PDA who are not cyanotic. Closure of a PDA is indicated if there is evidence of left atrial or left ventricular (LV) enlargement, net left to right shunting, or history of endarteritis. This patient has multiple indications for closure of his PDA. He is symptomatic, has evidence of right ventricular enlargement, and is beginning to develop pulmonary arterial disease. Patients with indications for closure should be referred to an adult congenital heart disease specialist and evaluated for device closure. PDAs in adults tend to be highly calcified and present additional risk during surgical closure. Even if a patient is to undergo additional cardiac surgery, percutaneous PDA closure prior to surgery presents the lowest procedural risk to the patient. Endocarditis prophylaxis is indicated in this patient under two circumstances. Patients should receive prophylaxis for the first 6 months after repair if prosthetic materials are used (surgical or interventional repair). Second, patients should receive prophylaxis if residual shunt is present adjacent to any prosthetic material. Asymptomatic patients should also be considered for device closure to prevent unavoidable pulmonary vascular disease and left heart enlargement. PDA closure is contraindicated for patients with clear pulmonary arterial hypertension and evidence of right to left shunting (ES) (*Circulation* 2008;118:e714–e833).

Figure A32-5 shows a lateral angiogram after delivery of an Amplatzer ductal occluder (St. Jude Medical; St. Paul, MN) as designated by the arrow.

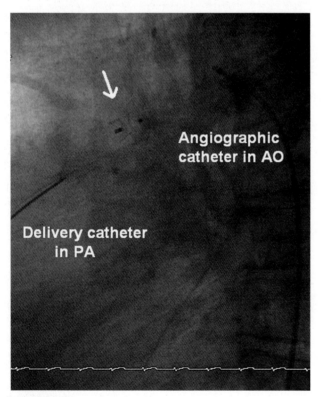

Figure A32-5

32.6 **Answer B.** This patient has a secundum ASD with left to RA shunting.

ASDs typically present with shortness of breath or palpitations in the adult population or are discovered incidentally on chest x-ray or echocardiography or during workup for stroke (from paradoxical embolization).

As discussed in Question 32.3, the first step in answering the question is to localize the shunt. This patient has an oxygen step-up at the level of the right atrium. A "positive" step-up in oxygen saturation at the atrial level must be $\geq 7\%$ (absolute difference in mean saturation values). A "positive" step-up in oxygen saturation at the ventricular or arterial levels must be $\geq 5\%$ (*Am J Cardiol* 1980;46:265–271). The Fick method is used to calculate the pulmonary blood flow assuming oxygen consumption of the lungs to be 125 mL/m². But which systemic venous saturation do we use? The saturation in the IVC is typically higher than the saturation in the SVC (the kidney receives 25% of the cardiac output and consumes less oxygen than other organs) which is higher still than the saturation in the coronary sinus. The Flamm formula is used to estimate mixed venous saturation in this situation.

$$\text{MV\%} \approx \frac{(3 \times \text{SVC\%}) + \text{IVC\%}}{4} = \frac{(3 \times 70) + 78}{4} = 72\%$$

32.7 **Answer C.** Once the mixed venous saturation is estimated, the Fick method may be used to determine Q_P, Q_S and Q_{shunt}.

$$Q_P = \frac{\text{O}_2 \text{ Consumption}}{(\text{PV} - \text{PA})\text{O}_2 \text{ Content}}$$

$$\approx \frac{(125\,\text{mL/m}^2)(1.72\,\text{m}^2)}{(0.99 - 0.89)\left(\dfrac{14.5\,\text{g Hgb}}{100\,\text{mL blood}}\right)\left(\dfrac{1.36\,\text{mL O}_2}{\text{g Hgb}}\right)}$$

$$= 10.9\,\text{L/min}$$

$$Q_S = \frac{\text{O}_2 \text{ Consumption}}{(\text{SA} - \text{MV})\text{O}_2 \text{ Content}}$$

$$\approx \frac{(125\,\text{mL/m}^2)(1.72\,\text{m}^2)}{(0.99 - 0.72)\left(\dfrac{14.5\,\text{g Hgb}}{100\,\text{mL blood}}\right)\left(\dfrac{1.36\,\text{mL O}_2}{\text{g Hgb}}\right)}$$

$$= 4.0\,\text{L}$$

$$Q_{Shunt} = Q_P - Q_S = 10.9 - 4.0 = 6.9\,\text{L/min}$$

$$Q_p : Q_s = \frac{10.9}{4.0} = \frac{2.7}{1}$$

Or,

$$\frac{Q_P}{Q_S} \approx \frac{\dfrac{O_2 \text{ Consumption}}{(PV - PA)O_2 \text{ Content}}}{\dfrac{O_2 \text{ Consumption}}{(SA - MV)O_2 \text{ Content}}}$$

$$= \frac{(SA - MV)O_2 \text{ Content}}{(PV - PA)O_2 \text{ Content}} = \frac{0.99 - 0.72}{0.99 - 0.89} = \frac{0.27}{0.10} = \frac{2.7}{1}$$

32.8 Answer D. ASDs are one of the most common adult congenital heart diseases encountered. In asymptomatic children, ASDs that are <3 mm in diameter are likely to close spontaneously within a few years. Closure is only pursued if symptoms develop or spontaneous closure does not occur during the follow-up period (*Pediatric Cardiol* 1999;20:195–199). In adults, defects <5 mm with no evidence of right ventricular volume overload or paradoxical embolism are thought to present no additional risk and do not warrant closure. Small defects (<10 mm) may become symptomatic but generally not until the fourth or fifth decade of life.

Hemodynamic studies have shown that the magnitude and direction of flow through an ASD depends on the relative compliance of the ventricles. Large ASDs are said to be unrestrictive if left and RA pressures are equal. Initially right ventricular compliance is far greater than LV compliance, and the shunt flow tends to be left to right. If the RV dilates due to chronic volume overload, compliance will decrease and the magnitude of the shunt may decrease. However, insignificant shunts that did not lead to ventricular remodeling early may become problematic late in life if LV compliance decreases due to comorbidities such as hypertension, coronary disease, or left-sided valve disease.

According to the most recent guidelines, ASD closure is indicated when there is evidence of RA or right ventricular enlargement, paradoxical embolism or platypnea–orthodeoxia. Closure may be considered for net left to right shunting with pulmonary artery pressure < 2/3 systemic pressure, pulmonary vascular resistance < 2/3 systemic vascular resistance, or when responsive to pulmonary vasodilator therapy or following a successful balloon occlusion test (*Circulation* 2008;118:e714–e833). Furthermore, appropriate anatomy must be present for percutaneous closure. This includes one (or at most a few) defects that are <4 cm in diameter located centrally in the atrial septum with at least a 4-mm rim of tissue surrounding the defect(s) to ensure proper sealing of the occlusion device. Sinus venosus

defects and primum septal defects are not amenable to percutaneous closure. Traditionally, a $Q_P:Q_S$ ratio of 1.5:1 has been used to define a shunt that should be closed. While this definition may be useful in children and young adults, it may not be the best definition for adults with long-standing right ventricular volume overload and pulmonary overcirculation. The latter may increase right-sided pressures and decrease the shunt magnitude as discussed above, likely as a harbinger of ES (*Clev Clin J Med* 2007;74:137–147).

Medical management should be pursued for a patient with atrial tachyarrhythmia to restore sinus rhythm. If atrial fibrillation is present, anticoagulation should also be considered.

Figure A32-8 depicts an Amplatzer atrial septal occluder (St. Jude Medical; St. Paul, MN) on PA angiography. The arrow in the picture points out the AcuNav ultrasound catheter (Johnson & Johnson-Biosense Webster; Diamond Bar, CA) used to assist in device delivery. The delivery sheath filled with contrast sits in close proximity to the probe.

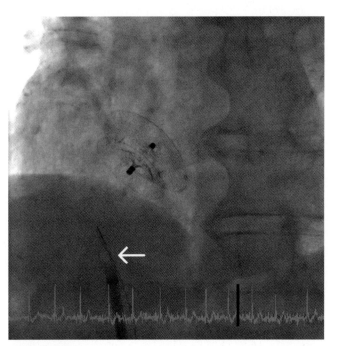

Figure A32-8

32.9 Answer A. Understanding the anatomy of this patient is the first step to understanding the solution. In d-TGA, there is atrioventricular concordance with ventriculoarterial discordance. In isolated d-TGA, the pulmonary and systemic circulations are completely separate. The presence of a communication (in this case a large VSD) between the two circulations is necessary for survival. This patient likely remained asymptomatic for much of her life as the shunt flow was predominately left to right. Now this patient has signs and symptoms of ES with right to left shunting. Once again, the Fick method is used to calculate pulmonary blood flow, systemic blood flow, and shunt flow.

$$Q_p = \frac{O_2 \text{ Consumption}}{(PV - PA)O_2 \text{ Content}}$$

$$\approx \frac{(125\,\text{mL}/\text{m}^2)(1.35\,\text{m}^2)}{(0.96 - 0.80)\left(\frac{19.8\,\text{g Hgb}}{100\,\text{mL Blood}}\right)\left(\frac{1.36\,\text{mL O}_2}{\text{g Hgb}}\right)}$$

$$= 3.9\,\text{L}/\text{min}$$

$$Q_s = \frac{O_2 \text{ Consumption}}{(SA - MV)O_2 \text{ Content}}$$

$$\approx \frac{(125\,\text{mL}/\text{m}^2)(1.35\,\text{m}^2)}{(0.80 - 0.68)\left(\frac{19.8\,\text{g Hgb}}{100\,\text{mL blood}}\right)\left(\frac{1.36\,\text{mL O}_2}{\text{g Hgb}}\right)}$$

$$= 5.2\,\text{L}/\text{min}$$

$$Q_{shunt} = Q_s - Q_p = 5.2 - 3.9 = 1.3\,\text{L}/\text{min}$$

$$Q_p : Q_s = \frac{3.9}{5.2} = \frac{0.75}{1}$$

Alternatively $Q_p:Q_s$ may be quickly calculated as follows:

$$\frac{Q_p}{Q_s} \approx \frac{\dfrac{O_2 \text{ Consumption}}{(PV - PA)O_2 \text{ Content}}}{\dfrac{O_2 \text{ Consumption}}{(SA - MV)O_2 \text{ Content}}}$$

$$= \frac{(SA - MV)O_2 \text{ Content}}{(PV - PA)O_2 \text{ Content}} = \frac{0.80 - 0.68}{0.96 - 0.80}$$

$$= \frac{0.12}{0.16} = \frac{0.75}{1}$$

Pulmonary vascular resistance is calculated as follows:

$$PVR = \frac{P_{\overline{PA}} - P_{\overline{PV}}}{Q_P}$$

$$= \frac{59\,\text{mm Hg} - 18\,\text{mm Hg}}{3.9\,\text{L}/\text{min}} = 10.5\,\text{Wood units}$$

32.10 **Answer D.** Pulmonary overcirculation from left to right shunting causes pulmonary *vascular* remodeling that leads to increased pulmonary vascular resistance and pulmonary arterial hypertension. Subpulmonary ventricular failure and increased right-sided pressures lead to reversal of the shunt and consequent cyanosis. Surgical or percutaneous correction of defects resulting in significant pulmonary overcirculation should take place as early as possible to

prevent irreversible pulmonary vascular disease. Ideally, significant shunts from VSDs would be repaired prior to 2 years of life while atrioventricular canal defects and conotruncal abnormalities (as in this case) would receive corrective surgery before 6 months of life (*Am J Cardiol* 1974;34:75–82). ES is classified with other forms of pulmonary arterial hypertension according to the World Health Organization based on similarities in clinical presentation, morphology, and response to treatments (Dana Point Classification). Although patients with ES have a longer life expectancy than those with idiopathic pulmonary arterial hypertension (77% survival vs. 35% survival at 3 years, untreated), the prognosis is still quite grim (*J Heart Lung Transplant* 1996;15:100–105).

This patient demonstrated some reversibility of her pulmonary vascular disease and might benefit from selective pulmonary vasodilator therapy such as endothelin antagonists, prostacyclin analogs or phosphodiesterase 5 inhibitors (*Semin Respir Crit Care Med* 2009 Aug;30:421–428). Heart–lung transplant is performed in end-stage ES treatment. Late surgical correction with an arterial switch procedure and VSD closure after the development of pulmonary vascular disease would carry significant mortality risk now that pulmonary vascular disease has developed. Restricting flow to the pulmonary vascular bed with pulmonary artery banding has not been shown to alter the disease course. Administration of 100% oxygen to a patient with right to left shunting will not significantly improve systemic oxygen saturation. Furthermore, long-term oxygen therapy in ES has not been shown to improve symptoms, functional capacity, or survival (*Am J Respir Crit Care Med* 2001;164:1682–1687).

32.11 **Answer E.** TOF is characterized by pulmonic stenosis, ventricular septal defect (VSD), right ventricular hypertrophy, and an overriding aortic valve, all of which are caused by anterior displacement of the conal septum. In the past, many centers employed palliative Blalock-Taussig shunts to augment pulmonary blood flow and then waited for some years to perform a "complete" repair. The complete repair consisted of pulmonary outflow tract resection usually with a transannular patch, VSD closure, and takedown of any surgically placed shunts. As operative techniques and patient management have improved, the complete repair is now performed as the initial procedure early in life. Relief of right ventricular outflow tract obstruction generally results in some degree of pulmonary insufficiency. Many late complications of surgically repaired TOF are a result of long-standing pulmonic insufficiency. The right heart dilates and eventually fails. Pulmonary valve repair or placement with a valved conduit is common, but necessitates frequent reoperations for valve replacements throughout life when a tissue valve is used. Now that determinants of late outcomes after TOF repair have become more apparent, there has been a trend towards "valve-sparing" procedures during initial repair to prevent PI altogether. Percutaneous pulmonic valve implantation is also on the horizon and will undoubtedly have a positive impact in these patients.

Another frequent complication encountered in adults with TOF, particularly those with pulmonary atresia, is the formation of aortopulmonary collaterals. Initially, they develop in response to decreased pulmonary blood flow, but over time this adaptation causes LV volume overload and pulmonary overcirculation. Collaterals can be singular or multiple and often follow a tortuous branched course. This patient has developed significant aortopulmonary collaterals as shown on the angiogram in the question, and these are likely the cause of his symptoms.

Percutaneous closure of collaterals is often undertaken to treat symptoms of pulmonary overcirculation and left heart volume overload. Collateral closure is also performed in preparation for open heart surgery, because collateral flow may compromise a bloodless field. The angiogram shows markedly decreased collateral flow after placement of vascular plugs in the collateral vessels.

32.12 **Answer D.** This angiogram depicts a coronary artery fistula draining into the RV. These are also known as *coronary–cameral fistulas* as they drain into a cardiac chamber. Coronary fistulae most often originate from the left coronary artery, but may also originate from the right coronary artery or both. The majority of coronary fistulae terminate on the right side of the heart (approximately 90%), most often in the RV (approximately 40%). Other termination locations include the right atrium, pulmonary arteries, or left-sided structures. Cameral fistulae are typically small and do not affect myocardial oxygen supply. However, coronary steal may cause myocardial ischemia distal to the fistula and cause compensatory dilation proximal to the fistula. This may manifest as shortness of breath, angina, myocardial infarction, arrhythmia, or thrombosis. Lesions

tend to enlarge with age, and clinical symptoms have been reported in 63% of patients over the age of 20 (*Circulation* 1979;59:849). Excellent long-term outcomes have been demonstrated with surgical repair, but percutaneous closure has also been demonstrated to be safe and effective in addition to being less invasive.

32.13 **Answer B.** Scimitar syndrome is a rare disorder characterized by hypoplasia of the right lung, anomalous right pulmonary venous drainage to the inferior vena cava, and aortopulmonary collateral flow to the right lung. The cardiac MRI image shows an anomalous PV (on the left side of the image) draining to the base of the right atrium—the so-called scimitar vein for its appearance that mimics the look of a sword. Noonan's syndrome is an autosomal dominant disease notable for short stature, minor dysmorphic facial features, pulmonic stenosis, and hypertrophic cardiomyopathy. Kartagener's syndrome is a form of primary ciliary dyskinesia with coexistent situs inversus, sinusitis, and bronchiectasis. Holt-Oram syndrome is an autosomal dominant disorder notable for upper body limb deformities and ASDs. Down's syndrome is associated with many cardiovascular anomalies, but anomalous pulmonary venous drainage is not one.

32.14 **Answer C.** Patent foramen ovale is thought to be the link between venous thrombus and arterial embolization. Serpiginous thrombi have even been captured in transit through the PFO tunnel. In this case, PFO was excluded in the stem of the question. However, the contrast echocardiograms both demonstrate right to left shunting. The next most likely cause of right to left shunting is the presence of pulmonary AVMs. Pulmonary AVMs are often congenital and associated with hereditary hemorrhagic telangiectasia (Rendu-Weber-Osler syndrome), but a small percentage of these are idiopathic (*J Vasc Interv Radiol* 2006;17:35–44). The majority of pulmonary AVMs are "simple" where one or a few arteries from the same pulmonary segment feed the malformation. "Complex" lesions have multiple feeder vessels and may be diffuse.

An unroofed coronary sinus defect is a rare lesion that could permit right to left shunting and paradoxical embolization but would likely have been diagnosed on echocardiogram. An ASD could also permit transient right to left shunt and cause paradoxical embolization but would be evident on echocardiography. A PDA could also cause paradoxical embolization in the setting of ES. ES would be highly unlikely as this patient does not display any signs or symptoms of the disease. Aortic atheroma is a common source for embolization, especially during cardiac surgery, but this patient does not have risk factors for atheroma, making this choice less likely.

Figure A32-14 depicts a selective pulmonary angiogram demonstrating a pulmonary arteriovenous malformation, which then empties into the left atrium (arrows designate the path of blood through the AVM).

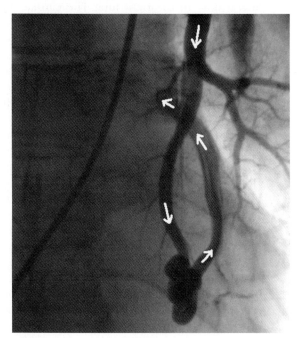

Figure A32-14

32.15 **Answer C.** Coarctation of the aorta accounts for approximately 4% of all congenital heart disease, and more than 80% have additional cardiac anomalies such as bicuspid aortic valve, aortic stenosis, ventricular defects, or complex cyanotic defects. Medical texts and review books frequently report the site of coarctation as either "preductal" or "postductal," but in reality, the vast majority are located opposite from the duct, or "juxtaductal." Most patients with coarctation are diagnosed in infancy because of coexistent cardiac defects, but some remain asymptomatic into adulthood because of significant collateral flow. In adults, coarctation is usually diagnosed during the workup for secondary hypertension.

Management of coarctation combines both surgery and interventional strategies. The mode of primary repair is controversial, but at most centers, primary repair is surgical. Recoarctation is common following primary repair, and most

reinterventions are performed percutaneously. Indications for balloon angioplasty and/or stent placement include a gradient of 20 mm Hg or more (*Circulation* 2008;118:e714–e833). Stent placement in long-segment coarctation may be considered, but long-term studies of safety and efficacy are lacking. Bicuspid aortic valve is present in approximately 50% of coarctation patients. Bicuspid aortic valve alone does not preclude balloon angioplasty or stent placement. The type of surgical repair does not appear to influence outcomes for balloon dilation or stent placement in patients with residual coarctation or recoarctation (*Am Heart J* 2000;139:1054–1060). The most often used surgical technique for isolated coarctation is resection with end-to-end anastomosis.

Figure A32-15 shows a BIB catheter (NuMed; Hopkinton, NY) inflation of a Genesis XD stent (Johnson & Johnson-Cordis Corp.; Warren, NJ) in the descending aorta at the site of recoarctation.

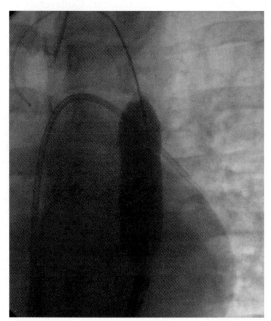

Figure A32-15

32.16 **Answer E.** The pathophysiology of hypertension in patients with coarctation of the aorta is multifactorial. One mechanism involves activation of the renin–angiotensin–aldosterone system as a result of decreased renal blood flow. This system does not always return to baseline after primary repair. Due to elevated systemic blood pressures, patients with aortic coarctation are predisposed to coronary artery disease and aortic dissection. Cerebral aneurysms have been reported in approximately 10% of adults with aortic coarctation, the rupture of which may be the presenting symptom for long-term asymptomatic patients (*Mayo Clinic Proceedings* 2003;78:1491). Development of ventricular arrhythmia is not associated with aortic coarctation.

32.17 **Answer B.** Origin of the left circumflex from the right coronary artery is the most common congenital coronary anomaly. Single coronary arteries occur in approximately 5% to 15% of coronary anomalies and are seen in conditions such as truncus arteriosus, transposition of the great arteries, and TOF. Origin of the left main coronary artery from the right sinus of Valsalva carries important clinical significance as the course can lead between the ascending aorta and the MPA. This can result in compression of the artery with resultant sudden cardiac death. Origin of the left main coronary artery from the PA is also known as Bland-Garland-White syndrome (*Congenit Heart Dis* 2009;4:239–251).

Figure A32-17 shows a right anterior oblique angiographic image of an anomalous left main coronary artery (vessel on superior portion of the image), which originates from the right coronary cusp (the right coronary artery is in the lower half of the image traveling downward) in this case and travels between the great vessels. This lesion has been associated with an increased risk of sudden death in children and young adults.

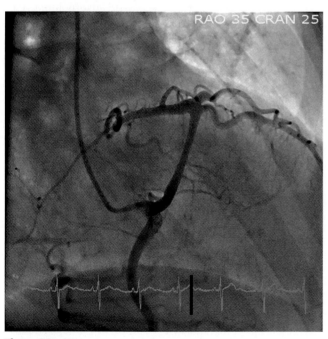

Figure A32-17

32.18 **Answer A.** This patient has a peak-to-peak pressure gradient of 54 mm Hg. Current guidelines recommend valvuloplasty in asymptomatic patients with a peak-to-peak gradient >40 mm Hg and in symptomatic patients with a peak-to-peak gradient >30 mm Hg with less than moderate pulmonary regurgitation. Asymptomatic patients with a peak-to-peak gradient <30 mm Hg may be safely observed. Patients with valvular pulmonic stenosis, right ventricular systolic pressure >80 mm Hg, and dysplastic valve morphology should be referred for surgical valvotomy (*Circulation* 2008;118;e523–e661;*Circulation* 2008;118;e714–e833).

32.19 **Answer E.** The so-called suicide right ventricle occurs when stenosis at the level of the valve is relived and hypertrophied musculature along the infundibulum dynamically obstructs the right ventricular outflow tract. This only tends to occur when right ventricular pressures exceed 100 mm Hg (*Am Heart J* 1989;118:99–103). Pulmonary balloon valvuloplasty is a remarkably safe procedure with a very low complication rate. The death rate has been estimated at 0.24% and major complication rate at 0.35% (*Am J Cardiol* 1990;65:775–783). Transient systemic hypotension occurs during periods of balloon inflation along with bradycardia and premature ventricular contractions.

Figure A32-19 shows a lateral projection of an Inoue balloon (Toray Industries; Houston, TX) inflated in the right ventricular outflow tract and splitting the commissures of the valve (at central waist).

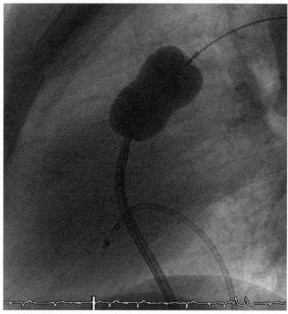

Figure A32-19

32.20   Answer E. There are a variety of anatomical and functional abnormalities associated with the heart after repair of TOF. Repair of the right ventricular outflow tract often compromises the integrity of the pulmonary valve apparatus leading to pulmonary valve insufficiency. Chronic volume overload leads to right ventricular dilation, increased pulmonary insufficiency, and ventricular dysfunction. Right ventricular dysfunction promotes arrhythmia, fibrosis, RVOT aneurysm formation, LV dysfunction, and declining functional status. Ideally, valve replacement would take place prior to the onset of symptoms and before RV function begins to decline. This must be balanced with the expectation that a bioprosthetic valve has a median life span of 10 years and repeat surgeries will likely be necessary throughout the patient's life. Indications for valve replacement include symptoms of exercise intolerance or heart failure, QRS duration >180 ms, QRS prolongation > 3.5 ms/year, sustained arrhythmia, right ventricular end systolic volume >85 mL/m², right ventricular end diastolic volume >170 mL/m², residual shunt defects, or residual right ventricular outflow tract obstruction (RVSP ≥ 2/3 systemic pressure) (*Congenit Heart Dis* 2007;2:386–403). Her RV volume indices (right ventricular end diastolic volume: 113 mL/m² and right ventricular end systolic volume: 52 mL/m²) do not quite meet the criterion for surgery.

32.21   Answer D. Single ventricle physiology is marked by the obligation of one functional ventricle (either right or left) to generate sufficient cardiac output to traverse blood through both the systemic and pulmonary vasculature. As there is no generation of force as the blood passes from the systemic venous return into the pulmonary arterial bed through the Fontan circuit or the total cavopulmonary anastomosis, flow into the lungs is passive. Elevation of pressures in the pulmonary vasculature from ventricular failure, AV valve regurgitation, increased pulmonary blood flow or resistance, or arrhythmias can result in congestion in the Fontan circuit and a "failing Fontan." Evidence of Fontan failure can be seen with right-sided failure signs, such as peripheral edema, ascites, and PLE. PLE is postulated to be secondary to bowel edema and resultant protein loss in the stool. As venous pooling occurs, this can result in low cardiac output states (Fig. A32-21). Previous surgeries and scar formation can result in atrial arrhythmias.

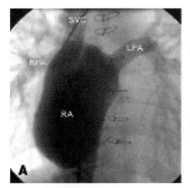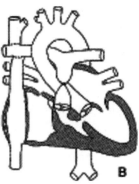

Figure A32-21

32.22   Answer D. Dilation of the coronary sinus should prompt the physician to consider the possibility of a persistent left-sided vena cava (LSVC). The physiology of this finding is completely normal, and there are no clinical manifestations. Persistent LSVC may also be associated with TOF and other cyanotic cardiac defects, but this was not the case in this clinical scenario. Persistent LSVC becomes a consideration if patients are to undergo cardiac surgery or if they were to have a catheterization with a venous approach from the left upper extremity.

32.23   Answer A. Subaortic stenosis is more common in men and can be difficult to differentiate from valvar aortic stenosis. Echocardiography, particularly transesophageal, is the best technique to evaluate this lesion. Surgical intervention is the standard approach as percutaneous techniques have been ineffective. Aortic insufficiency can develop secondary to thickening or impaired mobility of the valve leaflets and can worsen over time. Current guidelines recommend surgical intervention in subaortic stenosis for a peak instantaneous gradient of 50 mm Hg, a mean gradient of 30 mm Hg on echocardiography, or less if the LV end systolic diameter is >50 mm or LV ejection fraction is <55% or aortic regurgitation becomes progressive. Even with surgical resection, this lesion can recur (*Circulation* 2008;118:e714–e833).

32.24   Answer C. The most recent guidelines set forth by the ACC/AHA recommend SBE prophylaxis for patients with implanted prosthetic materials, patients with a history of infective endocarditis, unrepaired cyanotic congenital heart disease including patients with palliative shunts and conduits, repaired congenital heart disease with residual defects adjacent to prosthetic material, or completely repaired congenital heart disease with prosthetic material by surgery or cardiac catheterization for 6 months following the procedure. (*J Am Coll Cardiol* 2008;52:676–685).

32.25 **Answer A.** Congenital rubella is not typically associated with Ebstein anomaly. It is, however, associated with peripheral pulmonary arterial stenosis, PDA, ASD, VSD, TOF, transposition of the great arteries, tricuspid atresia, and coarctation of the aorta. In addition to cardiovascular abnormalities, congenital rubella is associated with microcephaly, cataracts, and deafness. Rubella has also been documented as a viral cause of myocarditis.

33 Patent Foramen Ovale and Atrial Septal Defect

Howard C. Herrmann

QUESTIONS

33.1 Figure Q33-1 shows a pictorial diagram of the heart with a patent foramen ovale (PFO) shown by an arrow. Which of the following statements correctly identifies other anatomic structures?

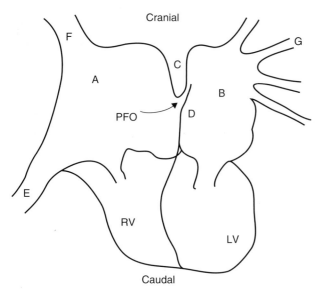

Figure Q33-1

(A) A=left atrium, C=septum secundum, G=inferior vena cava

(B) B = right atrium, A = left atrium, F = superior vena cava

(C) G = right upper pulmonary vein, D = septum secundum

(D) A = right atrium, B = left atrium, E = inferior vena cava

(E) A = right atrium, B = left atrium, G = left subclavian vein

33.2 Current indications for closure of a PFO may include all of the following, EXCEPT:

(A) Recurrent paradoxical embolism

(B) Hypoxemia due to right-to-left shunting

(C) Pulmonary hypertension

(D) Decompression illness

(E) Orthodeoxy–platypnea syndrome

33.3 A 50-year-old man suffers an occipital stroke. His neurologic workup reveals no obvious cause for his stroke (cryptogenic). A transesophageal echocardiogram is done to look for a cardiac source of embolism and reveals only a PFO with right-to-left shunting after injection of agitated saline. He is referred to you for percutaneous device closure of his PFO. In your discussion with the patient, which of the following statements is accurate?

(A) The CardioSEAL closure device is US Food and Drug Administration (FDA)-approved for PFO closure

(B) Off-label PFO closure can be performed with any approved atrial septal defect (ASD) device as long as the physician recommends it and the patient consents

(C) Several devices have humanitarian device exemption approval for patients with recurrent paradoxical embolism on warfarin anticoagulation.

(D) The Institutional Review Board (IRB) approval is needed for any PFO procedure

33.4 Percutaneous PFO closure is being considered for each of the patients below. For which one of the following patients is percutaneous closure most reasonable?

(A) A 46-year-old man with lung cancer who suffers a stroke and has deep vein thrombosis in his right leg

(B) A 75-year-old man with recurrent transient ischemic attacks (TIAs) despite aspirin therapy. His transthoracic echocardiogram (TTE) shows mitral stenosis and a PFO

(C) A 42-year-old woman who suffers a stroke and has a PFO. Her workup reveals lupus and a positive anticardiolipin antibody

(D) A 45-year-old man who has had a presumed embolic stroke with no obvious risk factors for stroke. His magnetic resonance imaging (MRI) shows a recent as well as a remote infarct in two distinct areas. His TEE shows a PFO and an atrial septal aneurysm

33.5 A 33-year-old woman with a PFO, migraine headaches, and a cryptogenic stroke comes to you for a second opinion about closure after being told by another physician not to have it done. You review her history and echocardiographic studies and are concerned about several high risk features that, in your opinion, may warrant devise-based closure. Which of the following factors is NOT considered to increase the likelihood of recurrent stroke in patients with a presumed paradoxical embolism through a PFO?

(A) Large shunt

(B) Residual shunt after percutaneous closure

(C) Lipomatous septum secundum

(D) Prominent Eustachian valve and right atrium strands

(E) Event occurring on warfarin anticoagulation.

33.6 A patient is referred to you for percutaneous device closure of a PFO. During the procedure, the cine image reproduced in Figure Q33-6 is obtained. The figure illustrates which of the following findings and treatment strategies?

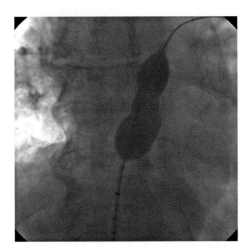

Figure Q33-6

(A) A sizing balloon is used to stretch and/or measure a long "tunnel"

(B) A sizing balloon is used to document the absence of a significant left-to-right shunting

(C) A percutaneous occluding device is being deployed by balloon inflation

(D) Pulmonary vein isolation is used to prevent atrial fibrillation before PFO closure

33.7 You are closing a PFO in a patient with a presumed paradoxical embolism. At the beginning of the procedure, you obtain the following echocardiographic image during injection of agitated saline (bubble study) in the right femoral vein (Fig. Q33-7). Which of the following is TRUE about this image?

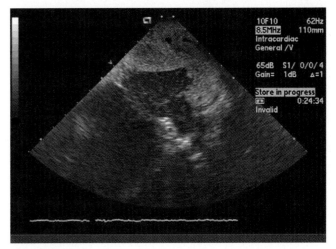

Figure Q33-7

(A) It is an intracardiac echo (ICE) image with the right atrium on top, left atrium below, head to the right, and feet to the left. It demonstrates right-to-left shunting through a PFO

(B) It is an ICE image with the left atrium on top and right atrium below. It demonstrates right-to-left shunting

(C) It is an ICE image with right atrium on top, left atrium below, head to left, and feet to right. There is opacification of the right atrium, but no obvious shunting

(D) It is a transesophageal echocardiogram image with left atrium on top and right atrium below. Left-to-right shunting is visible

33.8 Which of the following are possible explanations for the low rates of recurrent stroke and TIA after percutaneous device closure?

(A) The devices prevent thrombi from crossing the PFO

(B) Most trials of device closure have enrolled younger patients than in trials of medical therapy for stroke (selection bias)

(C) Concomitant medical therapy

(D) All of the above

33.9 Figure Q33-9A–C features three images of closure devices. Which of the following statements correctly identifies an image?

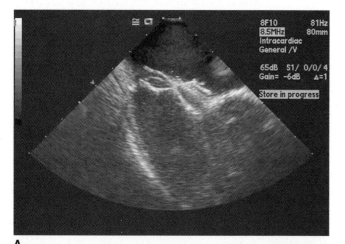

A

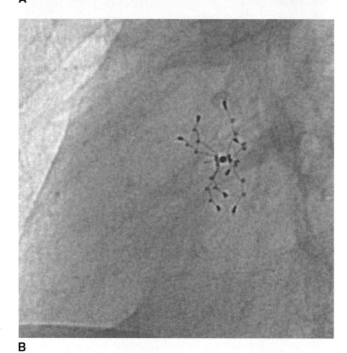

B

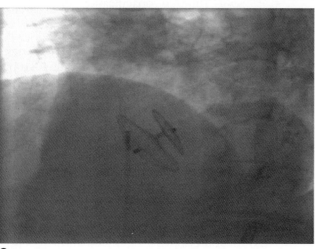

C

Figure Q33-9

(A) A = fluoroscopic image of a Gore HELEX device in a PFO
(B) B = fluoroscopic image of a CardioSeal device deployed in a PFO
(C) C = fluoroscopic image of an Amplatzer atrial septal occluder device
(D) A = ICE image of an Amplatzer atrial septal occluder device

33.10 A 40-year-old woman suffers a cryptogenic stroke and is referred to you after a TTE with contrast injection demonstrates right-to-left shunting. You see the patient in the office and review her study noting that the bubbles enter the left atrium more than five heart beats after their appearance in the right atrium. The most appropriate explanation for this finding is:

(A) Coexistent mitral stenosis
(B) Failure of the patient to provide a good Valsalva maneuver
(C) A pulmonary arterial-venous malformation (AVM)
(D) A persistent left superior vena cava

33.11 A 19-year-old male college student suffers a TIA and is referred to you for workup by his neurologist who hears a heart murmur. You examine the patient and hear a soft systolic ejection murmur at the left upper sternal border with a fixed split S2. You suspect that he has an ASD and discuss with him and his parents the need for further imaging evaluation with a transesophageal echocardiogram to confirm the diagnosis and determine the type of ASD. Which of the following statements about ASDs and percutaneous closure is FALSE?

(A) Secundum ASDs are the most common type and are usually located in the septum secundum
(B) Sinus venosus ASDs are often associated with one or more anomalous pulmonary veins
(C) Septum primum ASDs may be associated with ventricular septal defects (VSDs)
(D) Most ASDs can now be closed percutaneously

33.12 The transesophageal echo (TEE) on the patient in Question 33.11 confirms your suspicion that he has a septum secundum ASD. The anatomy appears favorable for percutaneous device closure with adequate rims on all sides. However, you explain to the patient that not all ASDs need to be closed. Current indications for ASD closure may include which of the following?

(A) Dyspnea

(B) Pulmonary hypertension

(C) Right-sided chamber enlargement

(D) Paradoxical embolism

(E) Qp:Qs > 1.5:1, even if asymptomatic

(F) All of the above

33.13 In order to obtain more information about the need for ASD closure on the patient in the above two questions, you decide to perform a right heart catheterization. On the basis of the oximetry measurements, you decide NOT to proceed with immediate closure of his defect. Which of the following measurements (see Table Q33-13) explains your hesitation?

Table Q33-13.

	SVC Saturation (%)	IVC Saturation (%)	Pa Saturation (%)	Aortic Saturation (%)
A	75	79	85	97
B	72	80	85	100
C	75	76	81	92
D	70	71	91	99

IVC, inferior vena cava; SVC, superior vena cava.

33.14 The ICE image (Fig. Q33-14) demonstrates which of the following?

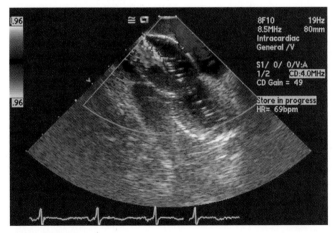

Figure Q33-14

(A) Balloon deployment of an Amplatzer atrial septal occlusion device

(B) Balloon sizing of an ASD

(C) Percutaneous balloon valvuloplasty for mitral stenosis

(D) Atrial septostomy to increase the ASD size before closure

33.15 A patient with a secundum ASD diagnosed on echo and right sided chamber enlargement is referred for device closure. After placement of the ICE catheter to guide deployment you obtain the image in Figure Q33-15. Which of the following statements best describes what you see?

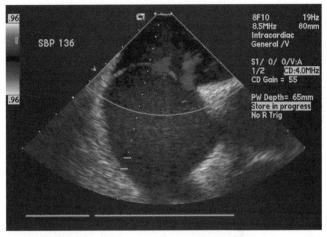

Figure Q33-15

(A) A septum primum defect with both an ASD and a VSD

(B) A fenestrated ASD that will require a surgically placed patch

(C) Echocardiographic reverberations from a bidirectional ASD

(D) Two discrete secundum defects potentially closable percutaneously

33.16 You are consenting a patient for device closure of an ASD. Which of the following complications (<30 days) and their incidence is INCORRECT for ASD device closure procedures?

(A) Perforation/Tamponade, <1%

(B) Stroke, <1%

(C) Device embolization, <1%

(D) Cardiac arrhythmia, approximately 5%

(E) Allergic reactions to nickel, approximately 5%

(F) Unsuccessful procedure, 2% to 3%

33.17 A 16-year-old teen has an incidentally discovered ASD and undergoes percutaneous device closure at your local children's hospital. He is subsequently lost to follow-up and is referred at age 29 to your hospital's adult congenital heart disease clinic. The cardiologist who sees the patient discusses the natural history of a successfully closed ASD. Which one of the following statements is TRUE in short-term and medium-term follow-up after percutaneous ASD closure?

(A) Most patients will not experience further enlargement or deterioration in right ventricular (RV) function

(B) Most patients will eventually require surgery to permanently close their defects

(C) Endocarditis prophylaxis and anticoagulation are required life-long

(D) Pulmonary hypertension will return to normal over 1 to 3 months

33.18 A 32-year-old woman has a large secundum ASD with dyspnea, right atrial and RV enlargement, and a 2.2:1 left-to-right shunt. Left ventricular function is normal. You bring her to the catheterization laboratory for percutaneous device closure under ICE and fluoroscopic guidance. Balloon sizing until color flow ceases demonstrates a diameter of 30 mm. You place, with some difficulty, a 30-mm-diameter amplatzer atrial septal occluder device. However, during the "push–pull" it easily pulls through the defect into the right atrium, and you decide to size up to a 32-mm-diameter device. During the removal and reinsertion of the new device, you notice ST elevation in the inferior leads with PVCs that resolve over about 5 minutes. You attribute this to an air embolism and proceed with insertion of the 32-mm-diameter device, which is successful. A follow-up echo 2 hours later demonstrates no LV wall motion abnormalities and telemetry shows no PVCs. However, 4 hours later you are called to see her after the patient has repeated runs of nonsustained ventricular tachycardia (NSVT). Her BP is normal. Which of the following should you do?

(A) Call for a stat echo and make immediate arrangements for transfer to the catheterization laboratory for PCI

(B) Call for a stat echo, surgical consultation, and make immediate arrangements for transfer to the catheterization laboratory for device retrieval

(C) Call for a stat echo and perform a bedside emergent pericardiocentesis

(D) You are not concerned, as this likely represents continued effects of the air embolism

33.19 Which of the following tests can be used to detect a right-to-left shunt?

(A) Transthoracic echo with peripheral intravenous contrast (e.g., agitated saline microbubbles) injection

(B) Transesophageal echo with contrast injection

(C) Transcranial doppler (power mode) ultrasonography with contrast injection

(D) Green dye indicator dilution curves

(E) Intracardiac echocardiography (ICE) with femoral venous contrast injection

(F) All of the above

33.20 Which of the following structural heart defects cannot be successfully closed with a percutaneous device?

(A) Secundum ASD

(B) Muscular VSD

(C) Postinfarction VSD

(D) Patent ductus arteriosus

(E) Sinus venosus ASD

33.1 **Answer D.** The foramen ovale is an interarterial communication defect present in up to 20% of normal adults. It is a small channel between the septum secundum (C) and septum primum (D) that may allow passage of blood or thrombotic emboli from the right atrium (A) to the left atrium (B) of the heart (paradoxical embolism).

33.2 **Answer C.** Most patients who undergo percutaneous (or surgical) PFO closure do so to prevent recurrent paradoxical embolism of a venous thrombus. However, a less common indication is hypoxemia due to positional right-to-left shunting (orthodeoxy-platypnea) (*J Interv Cardiol* 2005;18:227–232). Right-to-left shunting of dissolved gas after deep scuba diving can result in decompression illness and may be an indication for closure in some technical divers. Pulmonary hypertension alone is not an indication to close a PFO unless it results in hypoxemia due to right-to-left shunting. It may result secondarily because of left-to-right shunting through an ASD, but left-to-right shunting through a PFO is never severe enough to cause pulmonary hypertension.

33.3 **Answer B.** No device is FDA-approved for PFO closure. The HDE exemption had previously allowed closure with devices for patients with recurrent paradoxical embolism following failure of warfarin anticoagulation under IRB supervision, but has now been revoked. ASD occluders can be utilized by a physician in an off-label fashion to close a PFO, and IRB approval in addition to standard procedural consent is not required for this situation.

33.4 **Answer D.** This patient has evidence for recurrent paradoxical embolism with a high-risk anatomy. However, it must be recognized and discussed with the patient that the only randomized trial that has been completed failed to demonstrate that percutaneous closure is superior to medical therapy with either antiplatelet or anticoagulant therapy. The other patients have other potential causes for stroke or accepted indications for chronic anticoagulation with warfarin.

33.5 **Answer C.** Lipomatous septum secundum has not been shown to be a factor for recurrent paradoxical embolism. All of the other characteristics have been associated with recurrent paradoxical embolism.

33.6 **Answer A.** The segment of overlap between septum primum and secundum may be discrete, or have substantial overlap. In the latter case, the overlap segment or "tunnel" may be quite stiff thereby preventing optimal deployment of certain devices. In this case, stretching or tearing of the tunnel with a balloon can facilitate device placement.

33.7 **Answer A.** This is a standard ICE image projection with the transducer in the right atrium (top of image) looking across the septum to the left atrium. It is oriented with the feet to the left and the head of the patient to the right. The entire right atrium is opacified with contrast, which is flowing briskly through the PFO into the upper portions of the left atrium.

33.8 **Answer D.** All of the factors, that is, prevention of thrombus crossing the PFO, concomitant medical therapy, and younger age of patients are potential explanations although efficacy of PFO in stroke prevention has not been established in randomized trials.

33.9 **Answer B.** The figure in A is an ICE image of a deployed CardioSEAL device. The figure in B is the fluoroscopic image of the same device. The figure in C is a fluoroscopic image of an amplatzer PFO occluder (note the thin connecting waist that differentiates this image from an ASD device).

33.10 **Answer C.** Although a Valsalva maneuver (or sniffing) can increase the detection of a PFO by increasing right atrium (relative to left atrium) pressure, most shunts will be visible because of normal respiratory variation within five cardiac cycles. Patients with a pulmonary AVM may have an extracardiac shunt that is only visible once the contrast has traversed the pulmonary circulation. These can also be a cause of paradoxical embolism and can be diagnosed by chest computed tomography and MRI.

33.11 **Answer A.** Secundum ASDs are the most common form of ASD (70%) and most can now be closed percutaneously (hence, D is true). Secundum ASDs are (paradoxically) located in the primum portion of the atrial septum (Fig. A33-11). The ostium primum defects are associated with abnormalities of the endocardial cushion, and may involve the upper portion of the ventricular septum.

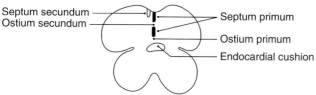

Figure A33-11

33.12 **Answer F.** All of these are reasonable indications for ASD closure in the presence of a significant left-to-right shunt. Traditionally, a Qp:Qs ratio >2 has been considered a cutoff for surgical closure in asymptomatic patients. However, it has been shown that percutaneous closure can increase peak oxygen consumption during exercise even in some apparently asymptomatic patients with Qp:Qs <2 (*J Am Coll Cardiol* 2004;43:1886–1891).

33.13 **Answer C.** Patients A, B, and D all have significant left-to-right shunts ranging from 1.7 to 3.6 calculated using a mixed venous saturation = ([3 × SVC + IVC])/4 and the shunt formula of Qp:Qs = (Aortic saturation – mixed venous saturation)/(Aortic saturation – Pulmonary artery saturation). Patient C has systemic desaturation that can reflect associated lung disease or right-to-left shunting. In the latter case, the bidirectional shunt formula must be utilized. Eisenmenger syndrome (right heart failure leading to reversal of flow across the ASD) must be assessed to ensure that closure does not result in acute or progressive right heart failure.

33.14 **Answer B.** This ICE image shows a balloon inflated in a secundum ASD, which is an important part of percutaneous ASD closure. The balloon forces the defect into a circular configuration, and is expanded until the color flow doppler evidence of left-to-right shunting ceases. An atrial septal occluder is then chosen such that either its central diameter is 1 to 2 mm greater than the waist measurement on the balloon or a disc diameter is >2 times the waist diameter.

33.15 **Answer D.** Secundum ASDs may have multiple defects or fenestrations. In some cases, these defects can be closed percutaneously by

placing an ASD device in the largest fenestration (cribriform device) or by using multiple septal occluder devices. In the illustrated case, these two discrete defects were closed using two ASD devices placed in an overlapping or "sandwich" approach (Fig. A33-15).

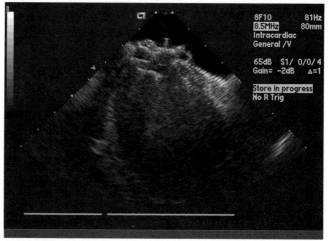

Figure A33-15

33.16 **Answer E.** Procedural success in the pivotal study was >97%, but does depend on how patients are selected preprocedure (should have at least 5 mm of tissue rim on all sides and diameter <38 mm). Major complications are rare, but atrial arrhythmias occur in up to 5% of patients within the first month. Allergic reactions are usually related to concomitant medications (especially clopidogrel), and true allergies to the nickel contained in the device that is made of a nickel–titanium alloy (nitinol) are extremely rare (<1/1,000). (AGA physician manual available at *http://www.Fda.gov/ ohrms/dockets/ac/01/briefing/3790b1_02_ sponsor.doc*)

33.17 **Answer A.** In general, percutaneous closure of an ASD is a definitive therapy that eliminates the left-to-right shunt causing RV enlargement, pulmonary hypertension, and the stimulus to further RV hypertrophy. However, some patients with pulmonary hypertension will have developed permanent changes that prevent the pressure from returning to normal (fixed pulmonary hypertension). Antiplatelet medications are usually administered for 6 months following device closure after which endothelialization reduces the risk of thrombus formation and infection. Anticoagulation is rarely necessary unless there is a separate indication such as chronic AF.

33.18 **Answer B.** Although air embolism can be a devastating complication, a small air embolism is usually well-tolerated, resolves rapidly, and has no lasting effects. The most likely explanation for the NSVT is that the device was not sufficiently oversized and embolized to the RV causing ectopy. This can be confirmed on echo and plans for device retrieval with a snare and cardiac surgical back-up is the most appropriate therapy. Perforation with tamponade can be ruled out by echo but would be unlikely without some hemodynamic compromise.

33.19 **Answer F.** A, B, and C are the usual preprocedure methods utilized. ICE is often used during the procedure to confirm the shunt before closure. Indocyanine green dye dilution curves can also be used to assess cardiac output and to detect shunts. If dye is injected into the femoral vein, early appearance in a femoral artery sample due to bypass of the pulmonary circulation is evidence of a right-to-left shunt (Fig. A33-19) (*Diagnostic and Therapeutic Catheterization* 1994; 388–390).

Because these calculations are somewhat cumbersome, this method has been replaced by imaging modalities with contrast injections. Currently, power mode transcranial doppler and transesophageal echocardiogram are considered more sensitive than TTE, although the patient position, injection site, and the use of maneuvers (e.g., Valsalva and Mueller) affect the sensitivity and specificity of shunt detection (*J Neuroimaging* 2004;14:342–349; *J Neuroimaging* 2003; 13:356–358).

33.20 **Answer E.** Sinus venous defects are in the upper portion of the septum and are often associated with anomalous pulmonary vein drainage into the right atrium. The lack of a rim of tissue superiorly and the frequent need to baffle the anomalous pulmonary venous flow to the left atrium make these defects not suitable for currently available closure devices.

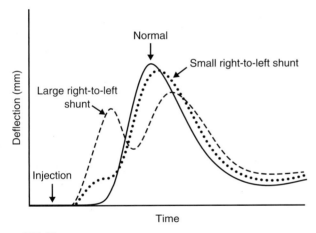

Figure A33-19

34

Percutaneous Balloon Pericardiotomy for Patients with Pericardial Effusion and Tamponade

Andrew O. Maree, Hani Jneid, and Igor F. Palacios

QUESTIONS

34.1 A 61-year-old woman with recent tricuspid valve repair presents with increasing dyspnea, orthopnea, and presyncope. The patient was hypotensive, with distended jugular veins and distant heart sounds on physical examination. On the basis of the hemodynamic tracing from the right ventricle (RV) shown in the Figure Q34-1, which of the following statements is INCORRECT?

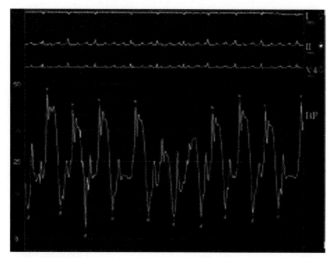

Figure Q34-1

(A) Pulsus paradoxus is likely to be present
(B) Presence of right ventricular collapse lasting more than one third of diastole is a more sensitive echo finding in this condition than right atrial collapse

(C) Blunt or absent Y descent on the right atrial pressure tracing is typically described in this condition
(D) Ventricular interdependence may be accentuated

34.2 Cardiac tamponade in the absence of pulsus paradoxus is described with all of the following, EXCEPT:

(A) Aortic incompetence
(B) Severe rheumatoid spondylitis
(C) Constrictive pericarditis
(D) Large atrial septal defect

34.3 Regarding the intervention depicted in Figure Q34-3, which of the following statements is INCORRECT?

(A) Left pleural effusion occurs in 1% to 2% of cases
(B) A pericardiocutaneous fistula is a potential complication
(C) It is recommended that the balloon be inflated until the waist disappears
(D) Biplane fluoroscopy is recommended

34.4 All of the following are relative contraindications to percutaneous balloon pericardiotomy, EXCEPT:

(A) Marginal respiratory reserve
(B) Presence of a large pleural effusion
(C) Thrombocytopenia
(D) Malignant pericardial effusion

34.5 Which of the following catheterization finding most reliably supports a diagnosis of pericardial constriction over restrictive cardiomyopathy?

(A) Pulmonary artery systolic pressure < 50 mm Hg

(B) A prominent Y descent

(C) Equalization of right and left heart late diastolic pressures

(D) Ventricular interdependence

34.6 Regarding pericardiocentesis, which of the following statements is MOST accurate?

(A) It is advisable to drain <500 mL at a time to avoid acute right ventricular dilatation

(B) Recurrence rate with drainage of large idiopathic pericardial effusions is no better than with conservative management

(C) Major complications occur during 1.3% to 1.6% of pericardiocenteses

(D) Effusions measured by echo tend to be larger than those measured by computed tomography (CT) or magnetic resonance imaging (MRI)

34.7 In the setting of aortic dissection, which of the following statements is INCORRECT?

(A) Pericardial effusion coincides with 17% to 45% of cases

(B) Pericardial tamponade occurs most frequently with a DeBakey type I dissection

(C) Pericardiocentesis may cause extension of the dissection

(D) Surgery should be performed as soon as possible

34.8 In patients with large malignancy-related pericardial effusion treated with percutaneous balloon pericardiotomy, which of the following is INCORRECT?

(A) Fever occurs in approximately one third of patients postprocedure

(B) Recurrence rate at 4 months is approximately 50%

(C) Results with immediate and deferred procedures are similar

(D) Lung and breast cancer–associated effusions are most common

34.9 A 64-year-old man with a history of alcohol dependency presented to the emergency room with increasing dyspnea, chronic cough, hemoptysis, and persistent fever. Echocardiography confirms

the presence of a large pericardial effusion. Simultaneous right atrial pressure and pericardial opening pressure are shown in Figure Q34-9. Regarding this hemodynamic tracing, which of the following statements is INCORRECT?

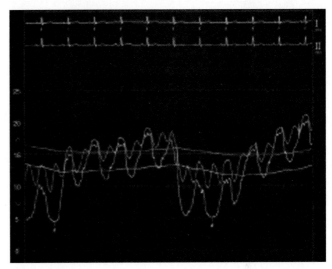

Figure Q34-9

(A) The X descent during ventricular systole is the dominant waveform

(B) The right atrial and pericardial pressures fall during inspiration

(C) With increased pericardial fluid accumulation, the X descent will become less prominent and the Y decent more pronounced

(D) RV mid-diastolic pressure may be elevated and equal to the right atrial and pericardial pressure

34.10 The patient discussed in Question 34.9 had a cardiac CT (short axis shown in Figure Q34-10) on admission. He had a reasonable symptomatic response to pericardiocentesis and his pericardial pressure returned to zero post-tap; however, his right atrial pressure remained elevated. On the basis of his findings on cardiac CT scan and his hemodynamic parameters, a presumptive diagnosis of effusive-constrictive pericarditis was made. Which of the following findings does NOT support this diagnosis?

(A) Equalization of the right and left ventricular end diastolic pressures

(B) A prominent dip and plateau waveform in the right ventricular tracing

(C) Concordance between the left and the right ventricular systolic pressures

(D) Right ventricular end systolic pressure <50 mm Hg

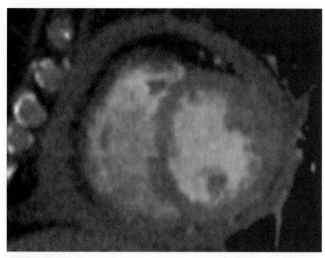

Figure Q34-10

34.11 *Mycobacterium tuberculosis* was found in the same patient's (discussed in Questions 34.9 and 34.10) pericardial fluid. Which of the following statements regarding tuberculous pericarditis is INCORRECT?

(A) Pericardial constriction occurs in 10% to 15% of cases

(B) The mortality rate approaches 85% in untreated cases

(C) A rapid diagnosis can be made from a small volume fluid sample by polymerase chain reaction (PCR)

(D) The tuberculin skin test is falsely negative in 25% to 30% of cases

34.12 A patient with a history of tuberculous pericarditis presents with progressively increasing dyspnea and undergoes the noninvasive study depicted in Figure Q34-12. Regarding this investigative study, which of the following statements is CORRECT?

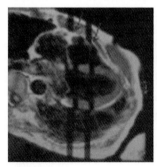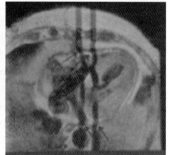

Figure Q34-12

(A) The image on the left represents evidence of pericardial constriction and tethered movement of the heart

(B) The images represent CT scan tagging, which can be used to diagnose pericardial constriction

(C) Pericardial thickening is absent in approximately 18% of cases of constrictive pericarditis

(D) Pericardiectomy for constrictive pericarditis has a mortality rate of 1% to 2%

34.13 Which of the following statements regarding endomyocardial biopsy or temporary pacemaker lead placement is FALSE?

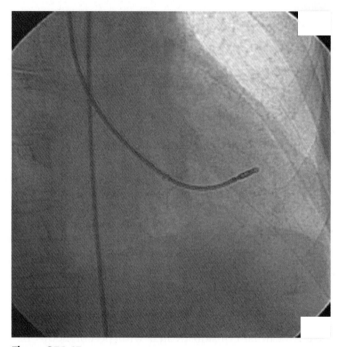

Figure Q34-13

(A) The rate of perforation during right ventricular biopsy is 0.3% to 5%

(B) Tamponade and circulatory collapse follow right ventricular perforation 75% of the time

(C) Pericardial hemorrhage complicates 0.1% to 3.3% of left ventricular biopsies

(D) Presence of right rather than left bundle-branch block configuration suggests pacemaker lead penetration of the RV

34.14 During insertion of an implantable cardioverter defibrillator, the patient becomes acutely hypotensive and an echo confirms the presence of an effusion. Which finding in the hemodynamic tracing in Figure Q34-14 does NOT support a diagnosis of pericardial tamponade?

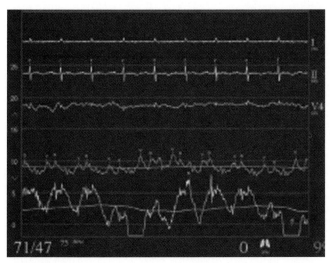

Figure Q34-14

(A) Presence of an elevated right atrial pressure
(B) Blunting of the Y descent in expiration
(C) Absence of respiratory variation in the right atrial tracing
(D) Pericardial pressure approaching right atrial diastolic pressure in expiration

34.15 Which of the following statements regarding the pericardium is INCORRECT?

(A) The pericardial space contains 15 to 35 mL serous fluid
(B) Pericardial inflammation may produce vagal-mediated responses
(C) The parietal pericardium is attached to both the diaphragm and the sternum
(D) Aspirin is more effective at reducing symptoms and recurrence of acute pericarditis than colchicine

34.16 With regard to an association between the procedure depicted in Figure Q34-16 and pericardial tamponade, which of the following is TRUE?

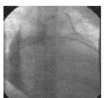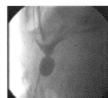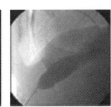

Figure Q34-16

(A) Performing the procedure in a biplane catheterization laboratory does not reduce the association with tamponade
(B) Presence of a small left atrium is associated with a greater incidence of tamponade

(C) Onset of symptoms of tamponade rarely occurs more than an hour after the procedure
(D) Tamponade occurs without associated chest pain in most cases

34.17 Which of the following parameters significantly determines pericardial pressure in the setting of a pericardial effusion?

(A) Volume of the effusion
(B) Rate of accumulation of the effusion
(C) Pericardial elasticity
(D) All of the above

34.18 Among patients with an active malignancy or a history of cancer and a significant pericardial effusion, which of the following statements is CORRECT?

(A) Pericardial disease is the most common indication for cardiology consultation among patients with cancer who are hospitalized
(B) Presence of abnormal fluid cytology is not associated with a significant reduction in survival
(C) Patients with malignancy-related pericardial effusions are twice as likely to require repeat pericardial intervention as those with non–malignancy-related effusions
(D) Pericardial fluid cytology is abnormal in approximately 75% of cases

34.19 Regarding percutaneous approach to pericardiocentesis, which of the following statements is FALSE?

(A) A right xiphocostal approach is associated with right atrium and inferior vena cava injury
(B) Puncture of the left pleura and lingual is more frequent with an apical approach
(C) Puncture of the left anterior descending coronary artery and left internal mammary artery is more common with the parasternal approach
(D) Left chest wall approach should not be used when performed with echo-guided procedures

34.20 Regarding percutaneous balloon pericardiotomy, which of the following is INCORRECT?

(A) Thoracocentesis is required following balloon pericardiotomy in 30% to 40% of cases

(B) Drainage of >100 mL fluid per 24 hours, 3 days after standard catheter drainage indicates the need for more definitive intervention

(C) Surgical window may be preferred if a loculated fibrinous effusion is present

(D) Reaccumulation of pericardial fluid with recurrent tamponade is considered a strong indication for performing percutaneous balloon pericardiotomy

34.21 Which of the following statements regarding pericardial effusion following cardiac surgery is FALSE?

(A) Postoperative pericardial effusion occurs in 50% to 85% of cases

(B) Cardiac tamponade occurs in 1% to 2% of patients who undergo cardiac surgery

(C) Cardiac tamponade occurs most frequently within 48 hours of surgery

(D) Nonsteroidal anti-inflammatory drugs do not reduce the risk of pericardial tamponade

34.22 Which of the following statements with regards to perforation by an implanted lead of a cardiac perforation electronic device is TRUE?

(A) The incidence is approximately <1%

(B) Late perforation is defined as perforation of the lead through the myocardium more than one week after implantation

(C) A fall in lead impedance is typical of lead perforation

(D) All of the above

34.23 Which of the following statements with regards to transseptal puncture and pericardial effusion is TRUE?

(A) Transseptal left heart catheterization is increasingly performed

(B) The incidence of cardiac tamponade is approximately 3.2%

(C) Newer technologies aimed at reducing complications include echocardiographic and CT guidance and radiofrequency and laser-facilitated puncture

(D) All of the above

34.24 Which of the following statement with regards to pericardial effusion in patients with systemic autoimmune disease is false?

(A) The pericardium may be involved in different systemic autoimmune diseases (i.e., systemic lupus erythematosus, rheumatoid arthritis, progressive systemic sclerosis, mixed connective tissue disease, Sjogren's syndrome, polyarteritis, giant cell arteritis, other systemic vasculitides)

(B) The pericardial involvement may occur either in a symptomatic form (usually during the active phase of the disease) or as asymptomatic pericardial effusion

(C) Pericardial effusion is a common manifestation of rheumatoid arthritis

(D) Pericarditis is frequent in patients with rheumatoid arthritis. It is usually asymptomatic, but cases of constrictive pericarditis or, more rarely, tamponade have been reported. In such cases, the study of pericardial fluid is of special interest for the etiological diagnosis

(E) Elevated rheumatoid factor is present in rheumatoid pericardial effusion

(F) A low glucose concentration is typically present in patients with rheumatoid pericardial effusion

34.1 **Answer B.** The hemodynamic trace depicts an elevated RV pressure with exaggerated respiratory variation consistent with pericardial tamponade. Echocardiographic evidence of right ventricular collapse lasting more than one third of diastole is a more specific but less sensitive sign of cardiac tamponade than right atrial collapse (*Circulation* 1984;70:966–971). Pulsus paradoxus, which is an exaggeration of the normal respiratory variation in blood pressure and is defined as a >10 mm Hg drop in the systolic arterial pressure during inspiration, is likely to be present. Blunting or loss of the right atrial pressure Y descent with a well-preserved X descent and enhanced ventricular interdependence are well-described findings in pericardial tamponade.

34.2 **Answer C.** Constrictive pericarditis is a well-described cause of pulsus paradoxus. Pericardial tamponade in the presence of the other three conditions may occur in the absence of pulsus paradoxus. In the presence of aortic incompetence, which may accompany aortic dissection, the left ventricle fills from the aorta during inspiration. The increase in systemic venous return during inspiration is balanced by a decrease in left-to-right shunting by a large atrial septal defect, which results in minimal change in the right ventricular volume and thereby a minimal displacement of the interventricular septum. Severe thoracic skeletal disease prevents wide changes in intrathoracic pressure (*J Postgrad Med* 2002;48:46–49).

34.3 **Answer A.** Left pleural effusion occurring within 24 to 48 hours of percutaneous balloon pericardiotomy is a common occurrence, which occurs in up to 50% of patients. Thoracentesis or chest tube placement is required in up to 16% of cases (*J Am Coll Cardiol* 1993;21:1–5). When carrying out the procedure, care must be taken to advance the balloon so that it straddles the parietal pericardium (Fig. A34.3); however, its proximal end needs to be clear of the skin and subcutaneous tissue to avoid pericardiocutaneous fistula formation. Biplane fluoroscopy is recommended to confirm the position of the balloon in two planes before inflation. Two to three balloon inflations are generally performed ideally resulting in complete obliteration of the waist caused by the parietal pericardium (*Textbook of interventional cardiology*. 1999:869–877).

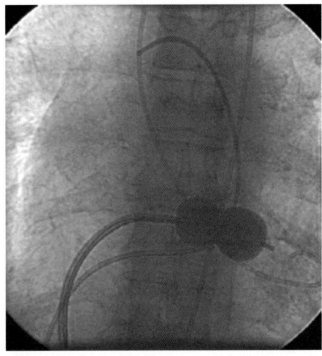

Figure A34-3

34.4 **Answer D.** If a large pleural effusion precedes percutaneous balloon pericardiotomy, then the chances of requiring thoracocentesis are high and procedure benefit must outweigh this risk. It is ill-advised to perform the procedure in patients with marginal pulmonary reserve such as in those postpneumonectomy owing to the risk of further compromise by a pleural effusion. Platelet or coagulation abnormalities are relative contraindications for the procedure because excessive bleeding from trauma to pericardial vessels may require surgical intervention (*J Am Coll Cardiol* 1993;21:1–5). The procedure is of particular benefit in patients with recurrent malignant pericardial effusions (*Cathet Cardiovasc Diagn* 1991;22:244–249). In the presence of a pyopericardium due to bacterial or fungal infection, percutaneous balloon pericardiotomy should not be performed.

34.5 **Answer D.** Dynamic respiratory variation consistent with ventricular interdependence is the best hemodynamic parameter for distinguishing pericardial constriction from a restrictive cardiomyopathy. During inspiration, the right ventricular systolic pressure increases and the left ventricular systolic pressure decreases and the inverse occurs during

411

expiration. This finding is >90% sensitive and specific in distinguishing the two conditions (*Circulation* 1996;93:2007–2013). A prominent Y descent in the right atrial pressure tracing is described with constriction along with equalization of right and left heart diastolic pressures; however, these are less reliable distinguishing parameters. In the presence of a restrictive cardiomyopathy, the left ventricular end diastolic pressure generally exceeds that of the RV. Pulmonary hypertension with a pulmonary artery systolic pressure <50 mm Hg is more typical of a restrictive process (*Circulation* 2006;113:1622–1632).

34.6 **Answer C.** Major complications are reported in 1.3% to 1.6% of cases of pericardiocentesis (*Eur Heart J* 2004;25:587–610). Drainage of more than 1 L of pericardial fluid at a time may be associated with right ventricular dilatation (*Am Heart J* 1984;107:1266–1270). Pericardial catheter drainage on large idiopathic effusions is associated with lower recurrence rate than with conservative treatment (*Am J Cardiol* 2002;89:704–710). Effusions measured by CT or MRI tend to be larger than when studied by echocardiography.

34.7 **Answer B.** Tamponade is more common with DeBakey type II (18% to 45%) than type I (17% to 33%) or type III (6%) aortic dissections (*N Engl J Med* 1992;327:500–501). Pericardial effusions are confirmed in 17% to 45% of patients presenting with aortic dissection and in 48% at autopsy (*Heart* 2001;86:227–234). Pericardiocentesis is contraindicated in these patients due to the risk of further hemorrhage and extension of the dissection (*Eur Heart J* 2001;22:1642–1681).

34.8 **Answer B.** Percutaneous balloon pericardiotomy in patients with large malignancy-related pericardial effusions is highly successful with approximately 88% freedom from recurrence at 4 months. Malignancy-related effusions are most commonly associated with lung and breast cancer. Results with immediate or deferred intervention are comparable and the procedure is associated with fever in approximately one third of patients (*Chest* 2002;122:893–899).

34.9 **Answer C.** The patient has elevated right atrial and pericardial pressures. The pericardial pressure approaches right atrial pressure in expiration and thereby represents early pericardial tamponade. The X descent, which occurs after the A wave and before and after the C wave, represents systolic decline in atrial pressure. It is well preserved during cardiac tamponade unlike the Y descent. The Y descent follows the V wave (venous filling of atrium in late systole) and represents diastolic decline in atrial pressure. The Y descent is initially blunted and then obliterated as pericardial pressure rises with increasing pericardial fluid accumulation. Both pericardial and right atrial pressures fall during inspiration and increase during expiration. Right ventricular mid-diastolic pressures are elevated and may equal the right atrial and pericardial pressures. Ultimately, diastolic equalization of pressures occurs and interventricular dependence becomes more apparent.

34.10 **Answer C.** Effusive-constrictive pericarditis exists when constrictive pericardial hemodynamic findings result after a pericardial effusion is treated. Pericardial constriction results in increased ventricular interdependence and discordance between the right and the left ventricular pressures. This is the best hemodynamic parameter for distinguishing constriction from a restrictive cardiomyopathy. The right and left ventricular end diastolic pressures usually differ by <5 mm Hg and a classic dip and plateau pattern is seen in diastole. Right ventricular end systolic pressure is usually <50 mm Hg unlike in restrictive cardiomyopathy where it can often be higher (*Curr Treat Options Cardiovasc Med* 1999;1:63–71).

34.11 **Answer A.** Pericardial constriction occurs in 30% to 50% of patients with tuberculous pericarditis. Mortality rate can be as high as 85% if untreated and the disease follows a relapsing and remitting course. Use of PCR to identify *M. tuberculosis* deoxyribonucleic acid is rapid and highly sensitive and can be performed on very limited samples. The tuberculin skin test is falsely negative in 25% to 33% of patients (*J Am Coll Cardiol* 1988;11:724–728).

34.12 **Answer C.** Pericardial thickening (>2 mm) was found to be absent in 18% of operatively proven cases of constrictive pericarditis (*Circulation* 2003;108:1852–1857). The mortality rate for pericardiectomy to treat constrictive pericarditis is approximately 6% to 12% (*Circulation* 1999;100:1380–1386). The images represent MRI tagging and show a normal heart on the left and an example of pericardial constriction on the right. The arrows accompanying the image on the left indicate normal pericardial sliding and those on the right indicated tethered pericardium in the presence of constriction. The ventricles on the right are classically tubular in appearance supporting the diagnosis.

34.13   Answer B. Tamponade and circulatory collapse follow right ventricular perforation in <50% of cases. Endomyocardial biopsy is complicated by right ventricular perforation in 0.3% to 5% of cases and left ventricular perforation in 0.1% to 3.3% of cases. Perforation of the RV by a pacemaker lead results in a right rather than left bundle-branch block pattern (*Eur Heart J* 2004;25:587–610).

34.14   Answer C. Exaggerated respiratory variation in the right heart pressure trace is expected in the setting of pericardial tamponade. Elevated right atrial pressure, blunted Y descent, and gradual narrowing in the difference between the pericardial and the right atrial pressures are all consistent with early evidence of pericardial tamponade.

34.15   Answer D. Pericardial pain is typically referred to the scapular ridge through the phrenic nerve and is relieved by sitting forward. Use of colchicine is supported by the results of the recent Colchicine for Acute Pericarditis Trial, in which colchicine gave greater symptom relief and was associated with less recurrence than aspirin (*Circulation* 2005;112:2012–2016).

34.16   Answer B. The image depicts mitral valvuloplasty, which requires puncture of the interatrial septum. Presence of a small left atrium and performance of the procedure without biplane imaging are associated with increased incidence of pericardial tamponade. Puncture of the left atrial free wall is associated with immediate chest pain; however, symptoms of tamponade may be delayed for 4 to 6 hours.

34.17   Answer D. Pericardial pressure increases in proportion to the effusion volume. Rapidly accumulating effusions can cause tamponade at a relatively low volume, whereas a slowly accumulating large volume chronic effusion is often well tolerated (*N Engl J Med* 2004;351:2195–2202). The parietal pericardium is fibroelastic; however, it can become fibrotic and less distensible with chronic inflammatory processes. Pericardial pressure increases more acutely if the pericardium is inelastic.

34.18   Answer A. Pericardial disease, either related or unrelated to malignancy or radiotherapy, is the most common indication for cardiology consultation among patients with cancer who are hospitalized. Pericardial fluid cytology is abnormal in approximately 50% of cases and presence of abnormal cytology is a significant predictor of decreased survival. These patients are five times more likely to require repeat intervention when compared with those with non–malignancy-related effusions (*J Clin Oncol* 2005;23:5211–5216).

34.19   Answer D. Multiple approaches to pericardiocentesis can be taken and include subxiphisternal, right xiphocostal, apical, and parasternal approaches. The left chest wall approach is often favored with echo-guided pericardiocentesis. Trauma to the right atrium and inferior vena cava is more with right xiphocostal approach, trauma to the left pleura and lingual with the apical approach, and puncture of the left anterior descending coronary artery and left internal mammary artery with the parasternal approach.

34.20   Answer A. Thoracocentesis is required following approximately 10% to 15% of cases of percutaneous balloon pericardiotomy. Continuous drainage of >100 mL in 24 hours, 3 days postprocedure and reaccumulation of an effusion with tamponade both indicate the need for a more definitive percutaneous or surgical procedure. A primary surgical approach may be preferred if a loculated fibrinous effusion is present (*Cathet Cardiovasc Diagn* 1991;22:244–249).

34.21   Answer C. Pericardial effusion occurs commonly after coronary artery bypass surgery and has an incidence of 50% to 85% (*Circulation* 1984;69:506–511). Cardiac tamponade occurs in approximately 1% to 2% of cases. It is typically insidious in onset and occurs most frequently more than a week postoperatively (*Chest* 1999;116:322–331). Evidence would indicate that nonsteroidal anti-inflammatory drug use neither reduces the size of the effusion nor reduces the risk of tamponade (*Ann Intern Med* 2010;152:137–143).

34.22   Answer A. The incidence of cardiac perforation by an implanted lead of a cardiac implantable electronic device is <1%. Late perforation is defined as perforation of the lead through the myocardium more than 1 month after implantation. Although early perforation is more common, late perforation is increasingly recognized (*Pacing Clin Electrophysiol* 2005;28:251–253). Typically, lead impedance will increase and there may be a failure to pace and sense or an increase in the pacing threshold. Lead perforation is commonly associated with a pericardial effusion and is a recognized cause of pericardial tamponade.

34.23 **Answer D.** A survey in Italy reported a 60-fold increase in transseptal left heart catheterization by electrophysiologists between 1992 and 2003 (*J Am Coll Cardiol* 2006;47:1037–1042). The incidence of incipient or clinically significant tamponade as a result of transseptal puncture is approximately 3.2% (*Clin Cardiol* 1986;9:21–26). A variety of newer techniques have evolved to improve safety and these include echo- and CT-guided approaches and the use of radiofrequency and laser to facilitate puncture.

34.24 **Answer C.** Pericardial effusion is a rare manifestation of patients afflicted with rheumatoid arthritis. Typically, the pericardial fluid of patients with rheumatoid effusion has a low glucose concentration and elevated rheumatoid factor titer. The pericardial involvement may occur either in a symptomatic form (usually during the active phase of the disease) or as asymptomatic pericardial effusion. Pericardial involvement in rheumatoid arthritis can present as pericardial effusion with tamponade, constrictive–effusive or constrictive disease.

35 Percutaneous Alcohol Septal Ablation for Hypertrophic Cardiomyopathy

Evan Lau, Amy Elsass, and E. Murat Tuzcu

QUESTIONS

35.1 A 43-year-old man with hypertrophic cardio-myopathy (HCM) and a resting left ventricular outflow tract (LVOT) gradient of 60 mm Hg is referred to you for alcohol septal ablation. He has dyspnea when walking rapidly up a flight of stairs or more than two blocks on level ground. His blood pressure is 140/80 mm Hg and his heart rate is 85 bpm. His exam is consistent with dynamic LVOT obstruction; however, there are no signs of heart failure. He is taking 12.5 mg of Toprol XL daily. You should:

(A) Arrange for left heart catheterization to be followed by alcohol ablation if severe coronary artery disease is not present

(B) Increase his Toprol XL to 25 mg daily and have him follow-up with his cardiologist for uptitration of β-blockers as tolerated and then reevaluate the symptoms

(C) Refer him for surgical consultation because he is too young for alcohol ablation

(D) Tell him that he should not be considered for alcohol ablation unless he develops New York Heart Association (NYHA) Class IV symptoms

35.2 A 57-year-old patient with HCM presents to your office because she is short of breath upon minimal exertion. Echocardiography demonstrates mild systolic anterior motion (SAM) of the mitral valve leaflet tips, mild mitral regurgitation, and a resting LVOT gradient of 10 mm Hg. What should you do next?

(A) Perform alcohol septal ablation

(B) Refer her for myectomy

(C) Arrange for a stress echocardiogram to determine if the LVOT gradient increases with exercise

(D) Tell her that her symptoms are unlikely related to LVOT obstruction

35.3 A 70-year-old HCM patient with resting and provokable LVOT gradients of 30 and 160 mm Hg, respectively, comes to you for alcohol septal ablation. She has NYHA functional Class IV symptoms in spite of maximal medical therapy. Her echocardiogram demonstrates normal left ventricular function, severe asymmetric left ventricular hypertrophy with an upper septal diameter of 2.0 cm, and SAM of the anterior mitral valve leaflet. The anterior mitral valve leaflet is excessively long and there is posterior mitral valve leaflet override as a result. There is moderate to severe MR at rest. Left heart catheterization shows mild, nonobstructive coronary artery disease. What would you recommend?

(A) Refer her for myectomy and repair of the mitral valve

(B) Proceed with alcohol septal ablation because you feel that her septal and valvular anatomy is ideal for this form of therapy

(C) Proceed with alcohol septal ablation because she does not have significant obstructive coronary artery disease that requires coronary artery bypass (CABG) surgery

35.4 Mortality following myectomy is much higher than that following alcohol septal ablation.

(A) True

(B) False

35.5 A 75-year-old man with HCM and severe LVOT obstruction comes to you because he wants alcohol septal ablation. He heard that it was a non-invasive procedure that will provide him with complete and immediate relief of his symptoms. He is NYHA functional Class III on maximum tolerated doses of verapamil and disopyramide, has SAM of the anterior mitral valve leaflet that is responsible for his LVOT obstruction, and has no unfavorable anatomical features to suggest that he would be better served by myectomy. How would you proceed?

(A) Schedule him for alcohol septal ablation because you feel confident that it will result in an immediate reduction in his LVOT gradient and therefore immediate resolution of his current symptoms

(B) Explain to him that while alcohol septal ablation is less invasive than myectomy, the reduction in LVOT gradient is not as complete immediately after alcohol ablation as that following myectomy. As a result, he initially may not experience a dramatic decrease in his symptoms

(C) Tell him that LVOT gradients are reduced significantly following alcohol septal ablation; however, the gradients gradually increase to preprocedure levels within a year's time

35.6 The most common conduction abnormality following PTSMA is:

(A) Complete heart block
(B) Left bundle branch block
(C) Right bundle branch block
(D) Alternating right and left bundle branch block

35.7 Which patients should have a temporary transvenous pacemaker placed prior to performing alcohol septal ablation?

(A) Patients without preexisting conduction abnormalities on ECG
(B) Patients in whom you feel you may need to ablate more than one septal perforator
(C) Patients with a preexisting left bundle branch block on ECG
(D) All of the above

35.8 What imaging modality has become standard practice to help with identification of the most appropriate septal branch targets for alcohol septal ablation?

(A) Intracardiac echocardiography
(B) Cardiac CT
(C) Myocardial contrast echocardiography (MCE)
(D) Cardiac MRI

35.9 What step is necessary prior to instillation of alcohol into the targeted septal branch?

(A) No steps are necessary once the targeted branch is identified
(B) Iodinated contrast must be injected into the central lumen of the balloon to make sure that alcohol will only go to the intended target
(C) A second flexible guidewire must be placed into the distal LAD, and a balloon inflated over that wire, just distal to the origin of the targeted septal artery. This will prevent extravasation of alcohol into the mid and distal portions of the LAD beyond the targeted branch
(D) None of the above

35.10 Approximately 10 mL of ethanol is necessary for successful ablation of a single septal perforator.

(A) True
(B) False

35.11 Once the procedure is complete, the operator must do all of the following, EXCEPT:

(A) Place the patient in the intensive care unit for at least 24 to 48 hours
(B) Remove the temporary pacemaker wire if complete heart block did not occur during the course of the procedure
(C) Cycle cardiac biomarkers until they have peaked
(D) Obtain a transthoracic echocardiogram prior to discharge for postprocedure gradient measurements

35.12 What features of this hemodynamic tracing distinguish it as HCM with LVOT obstruction rather than aortic stenosis (Fig. Q35-12)?

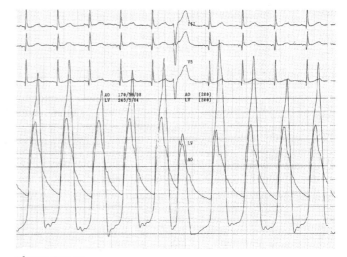

Figure Q35-12

(A) There is a decrease in aortic pulse pressure following a premature ventricular contraction

(B) There is an increase in the gradient between the left ventricle and aorta following a premature ventricular contraction

(C) There is a significant reduction in the gradient between the aorta and left ventricle in the beat of the PVC

(D) A and B

35.13 A 30-year-old female with HCM and a resting LVOT gradient of 70 mm Hg comes to you for alcohol septal ablation. She is otherwise healthy and has NYHA Class III symptoms in spite of maximal medical therapy. There are no anatomic reasons to suggest that she would be better served by a myectomy. You should:

(A) Schedule her for alcohol septal ablation and explain that her risk of developing a lethal ventricular arrhythmia is equivalent to that following myectomy

(B) Schedule her for a myectomy because there is a much higher risk of developing lethal ventricular arrhythmias following alcohol septal ablation

(C) Discuss with her that we do not yet know the true risk of lethal ventricular arrhythmias following alcohol septal ablation. Long-term data about the myectomy is more robust. She is young and at a surgical center that has extensive experience and excellent outcomes following myectomy; therefore, you would recommend at this point in time that she has a myectomy

(D) Schedule her for alcohol septal ablation because the risk of lethal ventricular arrhythmias following myectomy is much higher in young patients

35.14 Which of the following guidewires would be the least acceptable for use during alcohol septal ablation?

(A) HI-Torque Balance Middle Weight Wire (Guidant)

(B) HI-Torque Whisper Wire (Guidant)

(C) HI-Torque Cross-IT 200XT Wire (Guidant)

(D) HI-Torque Balance Heavy Weight (Guidant)

35.15 The following angiograms (Fig. Q35-15) were taken to document the key steps used during alcohol septal ablation in a 60-year-old patient with HCM and severe LVOT obstruction. A 0.014-in.

flexible guidewire followed by an over-the-wire balloon (2 × 10 mm) was introduced into the first major septal perforator prior to documenting the angiograms below. Before alcohol injection, the operator used MCE to confirm septal perfusion at the appropriate locations. The patient developed severe chest pain and an anterior ST elevation in multiple anterior leads following alcohol injection. Based on the information above and the angiograms below, what was the most likely cause?

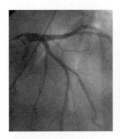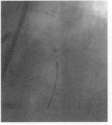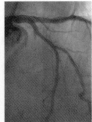

Figure Q35-15

(A) Plaque in the proximal LAD was disrupted by the guidewire during initial wiring of the septal perforator

(B) The guidewire caused dissection of the proximal LAD

(C) There was spillover of alcohol into the LAD beyond the septal perforator

(D) The septal perforator supplied portions of the anterior wall of the left ventricle

35.16 In looking at the following angiograms, which patient will likely have the best result in terms of LVOT gradient reduction following alcohol septal ablation?

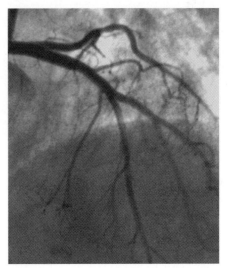

A

Figure Q35-16A

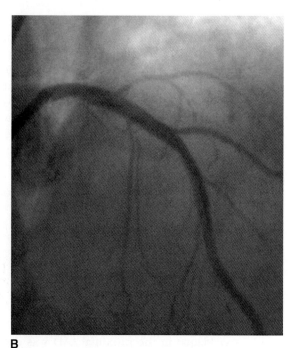

B

Figure Q35-16B

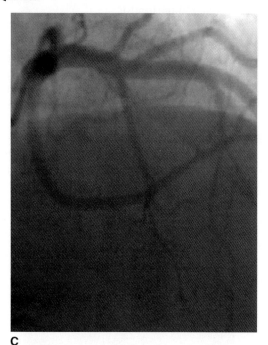

C

Figure Q35-16C

(A) Figure Q35-16A
(B) Figure Q35-16B
(C) Figure Q35-16C
(D) Unable to determine

35.17 Alcohol septal ablation has surpassed myectomy as the gold standard mechanical intervention for treatment of HCM with LVOT gradient obstruction.

(A) True
(B) False

35.18 Specific hemodynamic criteria exist to determine when the procedure is complete.

(A) True
(B) False

35.19 If a patient experiences chest pain and transient ST elevation in V1 and V2 during alcohol infusion, what should you do?

(A) Immediately stop the infusion of alcohol
(B) Immediately deflate the balloon
(C) Administer an intravenous analgesic agent like fentanyl
(D) Administer sublingual nitroglycerin

35.20 How should alcohol be administered into the central lumen of the balloon?

(A) As a rapid bolus injection
(B) At a rate of 1 mL/60–120 s
(C) At a rate of 1 mL/30 s
(D) At a rate of 1 mL/10 s

35.21 You are referred a 61-year-old patient with HCM and an LVOT gradient of 65 mm Hg. He has NYHA Class III symptoms despite optimal β-blocker therapy. You determine that he has anatomy suitable for both alcohol septal ablation and surgical septal myectomy. After discussing the patient's options, he chooses to go forward with alcohol septal ablation. Compared to septal myectomy, this patient undergoing alcohol septal ablation is more likely to have which of the following:

(A) Improved short-term mortality
(B) Improved long-term mortality
(C) Increased risk for ventricular tachyarrhythmia
(D) Increased risk for pacemaker implantation

35.22 The rationale for left atrial appendage occlusion is based on the theory that most left atrial thrombi originate from the left atrial appendage. What percentage of thrombi occur in the left atrial appendage?

(A) 60%
(B) 70%
(C) 80%
(D) >90%

35.23 Which of the following is a known complication of surgical left atrial appendage closure?

(A) Left atrial appendage tear
(B) Residual communication between the appendage and the left atrium
(C) Residual stump of the appendage
(D) All of the above

35.24 A 73-year-old man has just undergone placement of a Watchman (Atritech, Plymouth, MN) left atrial appendage occlusion device. What is the appropriate antithrombotic strategy after device placement?

(A) Aspirin 325 mg daily and plavix 75 mg daily for 6 months, followed by aspirin indefinitely

(B) Coumadin, with a goal INR of 2.0 to 3.0, for 45 days, followed by aspirin and clopidogrel up to 6 months, followed by aspirin indefinitely

(C) Coumadin, with a goal INR 2.0 to 3.0, for 6 months, followed by aspirin indefinitely

(D) Coumadin, with a goal INR of 1.5 to 2.0, for 6 months, followed by aspirin indefinitely

35.25 Which of the following was the most common adverse event in the device intervention arm of the PROTECT AF trial?

(A) Vascular complication

(B) Bleeding, requiring transfusion of >2 units.

(C) Pericardial effusion

(D) Stroke

35.26 How does the operator choose the appropriate size of the PLAATO (ev3, Plymouth, MN) left atrial appendage occluder?

(A) LA appendage ostial diameter by TEE

(B) LA appendage ostial diameter by angiography

(C) LA appendage volume by TEE

(D) LA appendage length by angiography

(E) A and B

35.1 **Answer B.** Percutaneous Transluminal Septal Myocardial Ablation (PTSMA) for the relief of LVOT obstruction in HCM should not be considered until a patient develops drug refractory severe symptoms. This patient is currently NYHA functional Class II without optimal medical therapy, which makes him an inappropriate candidate for mechanical intervention. Uptitration of Toprol XL would be the next step. This is important because drug refractory symptoms, a criteria for mechanical intervention, implies that the patient is on maximum tolerated doses of negative inotropic agents used to reduce the degree of LVOT obstruction (*Circulation* 2004;109:452–456; *JAMA* 2002;287:1308–1320; *J Am Coll Cardiol* 2003;42:1687–1713). These medications include β-blockers, non-dihydropyridine calcium channel blockers, and the antiarrhythmic disopyramide.

35.2 **Answer C.** For many years it was felt that LVOT obstruction occurred in 25% of the HCM population. However, recent literature and expert opinion suggests that it is much more common and occurs in up to 70% of HCM patients when both resting and provokable gradients are considered (*J Am Coll Cardiol* 2005;45:161). It is always important to assess for provokable LVOT gradient obstruction. This can be done with provocative maneuvers designed to decrease preload, decrease afterload, or increase cardiac contractility. Amyl nitrate, which decreases afterload, is routinely used with echocardiography to assess for a provokable LVOT gradient in HCM patients. Stress echocardiography is also helpful because changes in the degree of LVOT obstruction and mitral regurgitation at peak stress can be correlated with a patient's symptoms. Alcohol septal ablation should only be considered when there is a resting or provokable LVOT gradient of 50 mm Hg or more (*JAMA* 2002;287:1308–1320).

35.3 **Answer A.** In spite of maximal medical therapy, 15% of HCM patients with LVOT obstruction will develop debilitating heart failure and should be considered for mechanical intervention designed to relieve outflow tract obstruction (*Am J Cardiol* 1992;70:657–660). Several factors must be considered in order to determine the most appropriate form of mechanical intervention. For PTSMA to be effective, the mechanism of LVOT obstruction must be SAM of the anterior mitral valve leaflet with leaflet to ventricular septal contact (*J Am Coll Cardiol* 2003;42:1687–1713). In addition, there should be no structural abnormalities of the mitral valve and/or its apparatus, severe coronary artery disease amenable to CABG, or atypical patterns or excessive degrees of septal hypertrophy (*J Am Coll Cardiol* 2003;41:145; *Circulation* 2004;109:452–456; *J Am Coll Cardiol* 2003;42:1687–713). While this patient does have LVOT obstruction secondary to SAM of the anterior mitral valve leaflet, the leaflet is excessively long and allows for posterior mitral valve leaflet override. This is contributing to the degree of mitral regurgitation and cannot be corrected by alcohol septal ablation. Thus, this patient would be better served with myectomy and valvular repair or replacement.

35.4 **Answer B.** While mortality associated with both myectomy and alcohol septal ablation is center dependent, both are similar. The mortality associated with myectomy is 0% to 3%, while that associated with alcohol septal ablation is 1% to 4% with incidences of 0% to 2% at more experienced centers (*Circulation* 1999;100:1380–1386; *J Am Coll Cardiol* 2003;42:1687–1713; *J Am Coll Cardiol* 2005;46:470–476; *Circulation* 1994; 90:1781–1785; *Circulation* 2005;111:2033–2041; *J Am Coll Cardiol* 2010;55:823–834).

35.5 **Answer B.** Since the start of alcohol septal ablation in 1995, several observational studies have shown that both resting and provokable gradients following the procedure are reduced by more than 50%, with a majority being reduced by 90% or more (*Heart* 2000;83:326–331; *Circulation* 1999;98:2415–2421; *Eur Heart J* 1999;20:1342–1354; *Circulation* 1997;95:2075–2081; *J Am Coll Cardiol* 2000;36:852–855; *Circulation* 1998;98:1750–1755; *Circulation* 2001; 103:1492–1496; *J Thorac Cardiovasc Surg* 1999;47:94–100; *Lancet* 1995;346:211–214). However, the decrease in LVOT gradient following myectomy is more complete and immediate than that following alcohol septal ablation (*J Am Coll Cardiol* 2001;38:1994–2000). Three meta-analyses have compared outcomes in patients following alcohol septal ablation and surgical myectomy (*Eur Heart J* 2009;30:1080–1087; *J Am Coll Cardiol* 2010;55:823–834; *Circ Cardiovasc Interv* 2010;3:97–104). Although short- and long-term mortality has been consistently shown to be equivalent in patients undergoing alcohol septal ablation and surgical myectomy, it does appear that in patients undergoing surgical myectomy, the reduction in LVOT gradient is more robust. The clinician must also consider the time course of LVOT obstruction as well. For patients undergoing alcohol septal ablation, infarction and remodeling of the septum requires some time to mature; thus, the permanent result of the procedure is not determined until approximately 3 months following (*Am J Cardiol* 2006;97:1511–1514). Alternatively, in surgical myectomy, the LVOT obstruction is relieved immediately following the procedure.

35.6 **Answer C.** The most common conduction abnormality following alcohol septal ablation is right bundle branch block. Its high incidence of approximately 60% can be explained by the location of the right bundle branch in relation to the myocardial infarction created by alcohol septal ablation (*Am J Cardiol* 2004;93:171–175; *J Am Coll Cardiol* 2004;44:2329–2332). Unlike the left bundle, when the right bundle enters the muscular portion of the interventricular septum, it remains as a discrete cord-like structure located deep within its mid portion and does not begin to branch until it reaches the level of the papillary muscles. This is unlike the left bundle branch, which enters the muscular portion of the interventricular septum as multiple branches in a sheet-like array that are located much closer to the septum's endocardial surface throughout its anterior, mid and inferior portions (*J Am Coll Cardiol* 2004;44:2329–2332). During alcohol septal ablation, a transmural infarction is created in the mid portion of the septum, which often contains the right bundle branch and spares the more subendocardially located left bundle branch. It is important to keep in mind, however, that individual septal perfusion patterns do vary and a variety of conduction abnormalities can occur.

35.7 **Answer D.** A temporary pacemaker wire must be placed in the right ventricle prior to alcohol septal ablation in all patients, regardless of whether there is preexisting conduction disease and/or the operator feels that it may be necessary to ablate additional septal perforators. This is because complete heart block can occur transiently in up to 50% of patients undergoing the procedure (*J Am Coll Cardiol* 2003;42:296–300). Stable and reliable pacing thresholds are of utmost importance and some operators will utilize screw-in leads for this purpose. While all patients can develop this complication, there are risk factors for its development. Preexisting conduction disease, particularly, preexisting left bundle branch block, appears to place patients at greatest risk (*J Am Coll Cardiol* 2003;42:296–300; *Am J Cardiol* 2004;93:171–175). In addition, female gender, rapid injection of ethanol, and ablation of more than one septal perforator have been associated with higher incidences of complete heart block (*J Am Coll Cardiol* 2003;42:296–300).

35.8 **Answer C.** Prior to the use of MCE, operators determined the most appropriate septal branches by assessing the impact that temporary balloon occlusion had on the LVOT gradient. If balloon occlusion caused an acute and significant reduction in the LVOT gradient, typically ≥50%, the branch was selected if unwanted areas of myocardium were not at risk (*Eur Heart J* 1999;20:1342–1354). In addition to this technique, MCE has become standard to aid in selecting the most appropriate target branches. After the septal branch has been wired and a balloon placed over the wire in its most proximal portion, the guidewire is removed and the balloon inflated. One to two mL of an echocardiographic contrast agent is then injected into the balloon's central lumen and transthoracic echo images are obtained (*Circulation* 1999;98:2415–2421; *J Am Coll Cardiol* 1998;32:225–229; *Textbook of Interventional Cardiology* 2003:987–995). The contrast defines the myocardial territory supplied by the branch and delineates the area of planned infarction. The branch is chosen if the area of SAM-septal contact is opacified at the area of maximal flow acceleration and remote regions of the left and right ventricle are not involved (*Circulation* 1999;98:2415–2421; *Textbook of Interventional Cardiology* 2003:987–995). When compared to routine probatory balloon occlusion, ablations utilizing MCE result in smaller infarcts, greater LVOT gradient reductions, faster atrioventricular nodal recovery times, more significant reductions in NYHA functional class, and reduced incidences of recurrent LVOT obstruction (*Textbook of Interventional Cardiology* 2003:987–995).

35.9 **Answer B.** If spillover of alcohol occurs during infusion, a myocardial infarction secondary to abrupt closure of the LAD distal to the targeted branch can occur (*Circulation* 1997;95:2075–2081; *J Am Coll Cardiol* 2001;38:1707–1710). This highlights the need to confirm precise balloon positioning in the proximal portion of the branch and exclude reflux of dye into the LAD through contrast injection while the balloon is inflated, prior to alcohol infusion.

35.10 **Answer B.** Ten mL of ethanol is excessive for alcohol ablation. There is a higher incidence of complete heart block and permanent pacemaker implantation when large volumes are used, and typically, 1 to 2 mL is adequate as long as the appropriate target septal perforator branch is chosen (*J Am Coll Cardiol* 2003;42:296–300; *J Am Coll Cardiol* 2003;42:1687–1713; *Textbook of Interventional Cardiology* 2003;987–995).

35.11 **Answer B.** Following completion of the procedure, the temporary pacemaker wire must remain in place due to the high incidence of complete heart block that can occur transiently, during or following the procedure. If complete heart block is going to occur, it typically occurs intraprocedurally. Heart block occurring for the first time 24 to 48 hours after the procedure is rare (*J Am Coll Cardiol* 2003;42:296–300; *Circulation* 1999;98:2415–2421; *J Am Coll Cardiol* 2000;36:852–855; *Circulation* 1998;98:1750–1755). If the patient remains free of any concerning AV conduction abnormalities for up to 48 hours, the temporary wire can be removed. Monitoring should occur in an intensive care unit for the first 48 hours, and telemetry continued for the duration of the patient's stay. Cardiac biomarkers should be cycled and follow a pattern similar to that seen following an acute myocardial infarction. It is important to obtain a transthoracic echocardiogram to assess baseline postprocedure gradients prior the patient's discharge.

35.12 **Answer D.** This hemodynamic tracing demonstrates many of the features characteristic of the dynamic LVOT obstruction that occurs with HCM. What distinguishes it from aortic stenosis, which is a fixed obstruction to left ventricular outflow, is the decrease in the aortic pulse pressure and increase in LVOT gradient in the beat following a PVC. The former is referred to as the Brockenbrough-Braunwald-Morrow sign. When a PVC occurs, there is an increase in cardiac contractility and typically, although not present in this tracing, a compensatory pause that allows for an increase in left ventricular end diastolic volume. In a patient without a dynamic LVOT obstruction or in a patient with a fixed obstruction at the level of the aortic valve, the increase in contractility and increased end-diastolic volume will lead to an increase in the aortic pulse pressure. In HCM with LVOT obstruction, the increase in cardiac contractility following a PVC increases the degree of LVOT obstruction and the aortic pulse pressure decreases. This will occur even in situations where a compensatory pause allows for increased LV filling. The other feature in this tracing that will distinguish it from a patient with a fixed outflow obstruction as in aortic stenosis, is the tremendous increase in the left ventricular to aortic gradient following a PVC. This, too, is a result of a worsening of the outflow tract obstruction with an increase in cardiac contractility.

35.13 **Answer C.** The risk of sudden death following alcohol septal ablation continues to be controversial. There is concern that scar tissue as a result of the infarction may serve as substrate for the development of lethal ventricular arrhythmias, which would be an undesirable complication in a group of patients already prone to their occurrence (*Circulation* 2004;109:452–456; *JAMA* 2002;287:1308–1320; *J Am Coll Cardiol* 2003;42:1687–1713). The results of programmed electrical stimulation in a group of patients before and after alcohol septal ablation are mixed, and there have been two case reports of patients developing monomorphic ventricular tachycardia 1 to 2 weeks following alcohol septal ablation (*N Engl J Med* 2004;351:1914–1915; *Eur Heart J* 1999;20:1342–1354; *Am J Med Sci* 2004;328:185–188). The most recent studies examining the risk of sudden death and ventricular tachyarrhythmia following alcohol septal ablation have suggested that there is no increase in the attributable risk of sudden death (*J Am Coll Cardiol* 2010;55:823–834; *J Am Coll Cardiol* 2008;52:1718–1723). However, some would argue that these studies did not have adequate comparison groups to show that the rates of sudden death, arrhythmia, and/or ICD discharges should not be attributed to the alcohol septal ablation procedure. Furthermore, the follow-up period for these patients remains short, when considering the years of risk exposure for young patients undergoing this procedure. Conversely, after many years of experience with surgical myectomy, there has not been a significant concern over the risk of sudden death following this procedure. In fact, observational data for septal myectomy demonstrates that there may actually be a decreased risk of sudden death in patients who undergo surgical myectomy (*J Am Coll Cardiol* 2005;46:470–476; *Eur Heart J* 2007;28:2583–2588). These studies have not been randomized comparisons and should not be taken as definitive evidence of the sudden death risk following either procedure. However, the weight of experience appears to favor surgical myectomy, with regards to the risk of sudden cardiac death, particularly when considering options for a young patient. Therefore, because she is young, otherwise healthy, and has access to an experienced surgical myectomy center, it would be prudent to refer her for myectomy.

35.14 Answer C. Appropriate guidewire selection for alcohol septal ablation is of great importance for procedural success. Engaging and navigating through the septal branches can be challenging because they often take off at a 90 degree or greater angle from the LAD. In addition, the vessels can be small and tortuous. Ideally, one would like to use the safest guide wire with gradual tapering of its core that will provide flexibility and allow for the balloon to be inserted into and easily manipulated within the target vessel (*Textbook of Interventional Cardiology* 2003;987–995). The HI-Torque Cross-IT 200XT Wire is a poor choice for alcohol septal ablation because it has the least degree of flexibility of any of the wires listed. Not only will this increase the risk of vessel dissection and perforation, but engaging the vessel will also be quite challenging.

35.15 Answer C. While not frequently reported, myocardial infarction, most commonly involving the LAD territory, can occur at sites beyond the intended septal region (*J Am Coll Cardiol* 2001;38:1707–1710). The operator in this scenario failed to ensure proper balloon positioning within the proximal portion of the septal artery and did not ensure that there was no spillover of contrast into the LAD prior to injecting alcohol. A short balloon was used and this is important because these are easier to position solely within septal branches, which will decrease the risk of LAD dissection upon balloon inflation. Positioning of the balloon can then be confirmed by inflating the balloon within the septal branch and injecting contrast into the LMT. It is also important to confirm that the diameter of

the balloon is adequate to completely occlude the proximal portion of the septal branch during alcohol injection. This is done by injecting contrast into the central lumen of the balloon while it is inflated. This step, which was not performed during this procedure, will exclude the reflux of contrast into the LAD.

35.16 Answer D. Not only is it impossible to determine the degree of LVOT gradient reduction one will achieve with alcohol septal ablation by looking at an angiogram alone, it is impossible to determine which vessel(s) are appropriate for ablation. Individual septal perfusion patterns vary widely, as do the anatomical features related to LVOT obstruction. This is why it is important to assess the physiologic impact that temporary balloon occlusion has on the LVOT gradient, in addition to employing MCE, which will confirm that the septal artery(ies) supply the region where the mitral valve leaflets contact the septum and maximal flow acceleration occurs.

35.17 Answer B. The current gold standard mechanical intervention remains surgical myectomy. It involves excision of approximately 5 g of muscle from the basal anterior portion of the interventricular septum to just beyond the distal margins of the mitral valve leaflets (*Circulation* 2004;109:452–456; *JAMA* 2002;287:1308–1320; *J Am Coll Cardiol* 2003;42:1687–1713). Removal of the hypertrophied tissue decreases the degree of outflow tract obstruction and frequently improves the severity of MR secondary to SAM. Surgical treatment also allows for concomitant correction of intrinsic mitral valve and papillary muscle abnormalities. Mortality is 0% to 3% and patients experience long lasting symptomatic improvement that often includes an enhanced exercise capacity (*Am J Cardiol* 1992;70:657–660; *JAMA* 2002;287:1308–1320; *J Am Coll Cardiol* 2003;42:1687–1713; *J Am Coll Cardiol* 2005;46:470–476; *Circulation* 1994;90:1781–1785; *Circulation* 2005;111:2033–2041). Alcohol septal ablation was developed as a less invasive alternative to this procedure because elderly patients and those with multiple comorbidities are not always optimal candidates for surgery. In addition, the excellent results following myectomy come from a small number of North American and European medical centers, which highlights the fact that there is limited accessibility to this modality of treatment. Thus, while alcohol septal ablation appears to be a safe and effective technique, until long-term follow-up is available, it is most useful in selected patients, such as those with high surgical risk or those without access to a high volume surgical center with a track record for excellent outcomes, including a surgical mortality of ≤2%.

35.18 Answer B. No specific criteria are used to determine when to end the procedure, and practice patterns differ. Some interventionalists continue to ablate additional branches until the LVOT gradient is at a particular value, typically <50% of its baseline or <20 mm Hg (*Circulation* 2004;109:452–456; *J Am Coll Cardiol* 2000;36:852–855). Others stop the procedure after some reduction in the gradient as long as they are satisfied that the anatomic location of the alcohol bathed territory, as demonstrated by MCE, involves the area of SAM-septal contact and maximal flow acceleration.

35.19 Answer C. It is not uncommon for patients to experience chest pain during and several hours following alcohol infusion. This typically responds to intravenous analgesic agents, not sublingual nitroglycerin. Alcohol infusion should only be stopped if there is evidence of acute infarction in territories other than the septum. The balloon should not be deflated in response to chest pain because alcohol in the septal perforator can spill into the LAD and can cause abrupt occlusion of this vessel.

35.20 Answer B. Alcohol is not given as a rapid bolus injection as this leads to higher incidences of complete heart block (*J Am Coll Cardiol* 2003;42:296–300). Rather, alcohol is infused into the central lumen of the balloon at a rate of 1 mL per 60–120 seconds and the balloon should remain inflated for 5 to 10 minutes (*Textbook of Interventional Cardiology* 2003:987–995).

35.21 Answer D. To date, there are no randomized controlled trials comparing alcohol septal ablation and septal myectomy. A recently published meta-analysis (*J Am Coll Cardiol* 2010;55:823–834) examines outcomes from nonrandomized studies. In this pooled analysis, there was no statistically significant difference in short-term or long-term mortality. There has been a theoretic concern for increased ventricular tachyarrhythmia risk following alcohol septal ablation because of the scar created by infarction. To date, the studies examining this have not corroborated this hypothesis (*J Am Coll Cardiol* 2010;55:823–834; *J Am Coll Cardiol* 2008;52:1718–1723; *Am*

J Cardiol 2009;104:128–132). There has been an established difference in risk for postprocedural need for permanent pacemaker implantation, with those undergoing alcohol septal ablation demonstrating higher rates for this complication.

35.22 Answer D. In one series of 229 patients with atrial fibrillation undergoing TEE, surgery was used as the gold standard for identification of left atrial appendage thrombus (*Ann Int Med* 1995;123:817–822). In this cohort, 14 patients with left atrial appendage thrombus were identified, 13 of the 14 patients had thrombus that involved the left atrial appendage (92%). In most patients (12 of 14), the thrombus was confined completely in the appendage. A second transesophageal echocardiography series of 272 patients with atrial fibrillation identified 19 patients with left atrial thrombus; all of these patients had thrombus that was confined to the left atrial appendage or involved the orifice of the appendage (*J Am Coll Cardiol* 1994;24:755–762).

35.23 Answer D. The LAAOS trial was the first randomized trial of surgical closure of the left atrial appendage in patients at risk for atrial fibrillation (*Am Heart J* 2005;150:288–293). This was a small trial of 77 patients, looking at early, postoperative outcomes. During the procedure, 17% of patients suffered an atrial tear; most of these were related to a stapling device and were repaired intraoperatively. Eight weeks following surgical closure, patients underwent follow-up transesophageal echocardiography. This demonstrated that 44% of patients had inadequate closure, defined as residual blood flow into the appendage or a >1 cm residual stump of the appendage. Failure due to ongoing communication was more common with suture-based closure, while failure associated with the stapling device was related to distal deployment of the staples and a large residual stump at the base of the appendage. An observational study performed at the Cleveland Clinic showed that up to 60% of surgical appendage closures were a failure (*J Am Coll Cardiol* 2008;52:924–929). New surgical techniques and devices are being developed, including the Atriclip (Atricure, Inc, Westchester, OH), which was approved for use by the FDA in June 2010.

35.24 Answer B. PROTECT-AF (*Lancet* 2009;374:534–542) is the first randomized trial examining the use of the Watchman left atrial appendage occluder versus conventional warfarin therapy in patients with CHADS2 scores of 1 or more. Following placement of the device, patients were placed on warfarin for 45 days, at which point they were examined with transesophageal echocardiograms. If TEE demonstrated complete appendage closure or only a small peridevice leak, the patient was taken off of warfarin and started on aspirin (81 to 325 mg) and plavix 75 mg up to the 6 month follow-up. Following that, the patient was placed on aspirin indefinitely. The safety of placing the Watchman device without postprocedural use of warfarin is unknown.

35.25 **Answer C.** The incidence of serious pericardial effusion, defined as the need for drainage, was 4.8% in the intervention arm of the PROTECT AF trial (*Lancet* 2009; 374:534–542), making it the most common serious adverse event. This is thought to be related in part to operator experience. In the subsequent PROTECT CAP registry (*Circulation.* 2011;123:417–424), the rates of serious pericardial effusion decreased to 2.2%. Major bleeding (3.5%) and ischemic stroke (1.1%) are also listed as important adverse events. The rate of ischemic stroke is thought to be related to air embolism through the transseptal sheath. This is also thought to be related to operator experience, as subsequent registry data shows a 0% incidence in 460 patients.

35.26 **Answer E.** The appropriate size of the PLAATO device is determined by choosing a device whose size is 20% to 50% larger than the left atrial appendage ostial diameter, as determined by TEE and angiography (*J Am Coll Cardiol* 2005;46:9–14). Prior to final deployment, adequate occlusion of the appendage is determined by contrast injection through the central lumen of the device, contrast injection into the left atrium, and color Doppler flow of blood by TEE. The investigators created grading scales for residual leaks as seen angiographically and by TEE; mild residual leak was deemed acceptable for final device deployment.

QUESTIONS

36.1 A 40-year-old female airline pilot presents with a 2-month history of intermittent chest pain. Her symptoms arise in her left inframammary region. They can be reproduced with physical exertion, but can also occur spontaneously and in the postprandial state. The symptoms do not reliably dissipate with rest. She inquires about whether she should have a coronary angiogram. Select the BEST management:

(A) Calcium-channel antagonists
(B) Invasive coronary angiography
(C) Reassurance that her symptoms are not typical for angina pectoris
(D) Treadmill stress echocardiogram

36.2 A 74-year-old man with type II diabetes and a 3-month history of stable angina undergoes coronary angiography (Fig. Q36-2). Select the correct statement in regard to this patient's case:

(A) Coronary artery bypass grafting (CABG) is preferred over multivessel angioplasty
(B) An initial strategy of balloon angioplasty results in similar survival in comparison to CABG
(C) Drug-eluting stenting results in similar survival in comparison to bypass grafting
(D) An insulin-sensitization program is preferred over insulin provision

36.3 A 55-year-old woman is referred to your office with mild dyspnea. Six weeks ago, she suffered a myocardial infarction and did not undergo reperfusion therapy. Her referring physician had obtained a viability study with positron emission tomography, and those images are shown in Figure Q36-3. The study is interpreted as showing a large area of nonviable myocardium involving the anterior, apical, septal, and inferior regions.

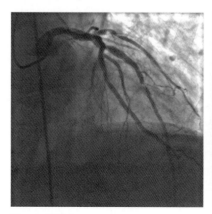
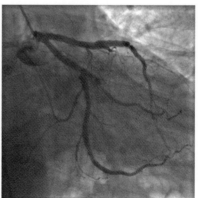

Figure Q36-2

There was also severe left ventricular and moderate right ventricular enlargement. No myocardial ischemia is found. Her ejection fraction is calculated to be 22%. Select the BEST management:

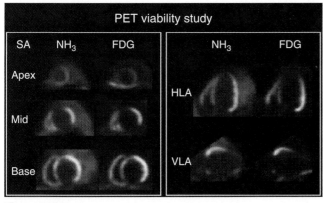

Figure Q36-3

(A) Coronary angiography and percutaneous revascularization
(B) Coronary angiography and CABG
(C) Medical therapy only
(D) Dobutamine stress echocardiogram

36.4 A 69-year-old man is referred for evaluation of chest pain. He exercises frequently, and his symptoms of angina occur near the completion of his regular 3-mile run. On a treadmill study with the Bruce protocol, he exercises for 7 minutes with no electrocardiographic evidence of ischemia or precipitation of angina. The patient takes no medications. He undergoes coronary angiography (Fig. Q36-4). Select the BEST management for this patient:

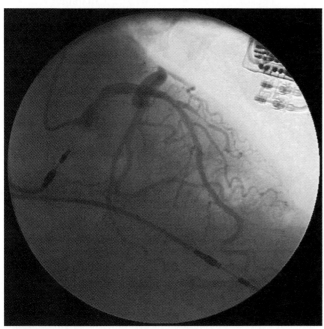

Figure Q36-4

(A) Initiation of a statin drug
(B) Referral to a cardiac surgeon
(C) Percutaneous coronary intervention (PCI)
(D) Stress echocardiography

36.5 A 60-year-old man is referred for angina. His symptoms began 3 months ago and progressed to where they have interfered with his job as a construction worker for the past 3 weeks. Apart from nicotine dependence, he has no other health problems. A recent echocardiogram showed his ejection fraction to be 50%. His coronary angiogram is shown in Figure Q36-5. Select the true statement in regard to this patient:

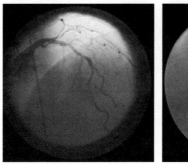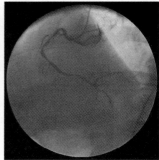

Figure Q36-5

(A) Randomized trials have shown equivalent long-term survival for CABG as compared to the initial strategy of PCI with stenting for similar patients
(B) Randomized trials of PCI vs. CABG frequently enrolled much older and severely symptomatic patients with abnormal ventricular function
(C) Balloon angioplasty alone results in more repeat procedures, whose cumulative costs exceed those of an initial strategy of bypass grafting

36.6 A 78-year-old man is referred for evaluation of 3 months of progressive angina. During an exercise treadmill study, the patient developed angina with an ischemic electrocardiogram with 2-mm horizontal ST-segment depression during stage 2 of the Bruce protocol. His comorbidities include hypertension, hyperlipidemia, and chronic obstructive pulmonary disease, which has been stable with steroid inhalers. His coronary angiogram is shown in Figure Q36-6. Select the CORRECT statement:

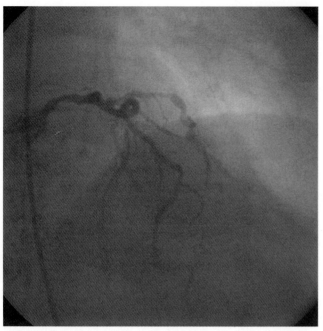

Figure Q36-6

(A) CABG is the preferred mode of revascularization in patients with significant left main disease

(B) The absence of distal left main disease indicates that the outcomes after revascularization with PCI or CABG would be comparable

(C) PCI is contraindicated

(D) Intravascular ultrasound or fractional flow reserve should be performed to determine the need for revascularization

36.7 Among randomized trials of PCI vs. CABG for patients with multivessel disease, what is the frequency of repeat revascularization in those undergoing surgery during long-term follow-up?

(A) 1% to 2%

(B) 5% to 6%

(C) 10%

(D) 15%

36.8 Which of the following is a true statement with regard to periprocedural rise in cardiac biomarkers among patients undergoing elective PCI?

(A) Positive linear relation exists between the risk of cardiac mortality and peak creatinine kinase (or CK-MB) for intermediate (1.5 to 3.0 times normal) and higher (>3 times normal) levels of rise

(B) A positive linear relation exists between the risk of cardiac mortality and elevation of troponin isoforms (I or T) at intermediate levels of elevation (<5 times normal)

(C) Elevation of troponin isoforms is common and not of prognostic value

(D) In comparisons of CABG to PCI, studies have utilized the same levels of cardiac biomarker rise in defining the rates of periprocedural myocardial infarction for both procedures

36.9 Which of the following is a true observation in randomized trials of stenting vs. bypass surgery for multivessel disease?

(A) Comparable 1- to 3-year survival has been observed, including among patients with severe ischemia and high-risk features for adverse outcomes with surgery

(B) Bypass surgery results in superior freedom from death or myocardial infarction

(C) In comparison to previous balloon angioplasty trials, there has been approximately a 90% reduction in need for repeat revascularization with stenting

(D) Because of the need for repeat procedures, patients undergoing PCI have demonstrated a small, but statistically significant, lower survival rate

36.10 A 57-year-old man is referred for angina. His symptoms began 2 months ago when he was shoveling heavy snow. He is able to clear his driveway without stopping, but he is worried that he could "drop dead." On a treadmill exercise study with the Bruce protocol, he exercised for 12 minutes and developed 1-mm horizontal ST-segment depression without chest pain. His only medication is atenolol, which he takes for hypertension. His angiogram is shown in Figure Q36-10. Select the BEST management:

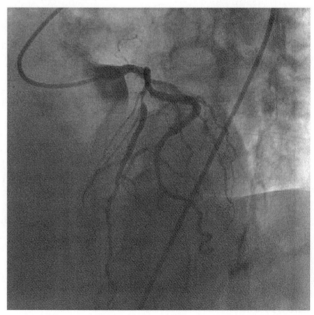

Figure Q36-10

(A) Intensification of medical therapy and lifestyle modification

(B) Bypass surgery with placement of an internal mammary graft to his LAD artery

(C) Percutaneous coronary revascularization

(D) External extracorporeal counterpulsation

36.11 A 64-year-old woman undergoes angiography for recent onset of mild angina. A tubular 70% stenosis in her mid LAD is found, and she undergoes successful percutaneous treatment with a 4.0/12 mm bare-metal stent. What is the probability of need for repeat target lesion revascularization in the next 4 years?

(A) ≤5%

(B) 8% to 20%

(C) >20%

(D) None of the above

36.12 A 45-year-old male executive undergoes a treadmill study with nuclear perfusion imaging as part of an annual exam. He recently began exercising for health maintenance and has no cardiovascular symptoms. He exercises for 4 minutes and develops 1.5-mm horizontal ST-segment depression that returns to normal after 5 minutes of recovery. He has no chest pain during the study. His nuclear imaging demonstrates impaired coronary flow reserve in the anterior and anterolateral walls of his left ventricle with mild dilatation on the poststress images. Select the BEST management:

(A) Medical therapy with more primary prevention measures

(B) Stress echocardiography

(C) Coronary angiography and revascularization

(D) Cardiac MRI with gadolinium for delayed hyperenhancement

36.13 A 64-year-old diabetic woman returns for follow-up after elective PCI for stable angina. She has been free of angina following the successful intervention. Currently indicated pharmacotherapy to prevent death or myocardial infarction in this patient include all of the following, EXCEPT:

(A) Aspirin

(B) β-Receptor antagonists

(C) Angiotensin-converting enzyme inhibitor (ACEI)

(D) Calcium-channel blockers

(E) Lipid-lowering therapy

36.14 A 56-year-old woman returns 6 months after having elective PCI of a proximal left circumflex lesion. She had entered a cardiovascular health program near her home after the

procedure and reports no symptoms with good functional capacity. Before the intervention, she had inquired about the possibility of restenosis during follow-up. She now wants to have a stress test to evaluate the status of the intervention. Select the BEST next step:

(A) Exercise electrocardiogram

(B) Stress echocardiography

(C) Invasive coronary angiography

(D) Cardiac CT angiogram

(E) Reassurance

36.15 Which of the following is a TRUE statement?

(A) Approximately 30% of saphenous vein grafts become occluded within 1 year after surgery

(B) Perioperative and long-term treatment with platelet inhibitors does not significantly improve the patency rate of saphenous vein grafts

(C) Use of the internal thoracic artery in place of a saphenous vein significantly improves long-term graft patency

(D) Aggressive lipid-lowering therapy does not significantly decrease vein graft atherosclerosis

36.16 A 66-year-old man recently underwent successful balloon angioplasty of a mid-LAD lesion after having a 2-month history of severe angina. His past medical history consisted of hyperlipidemia, but there was no history of diabetes or heart failure. Currently he is asymptomatic with an excellent functional capacity. The physical examination is normal. He undergoes electrocardiography (Fig. Q36-16). Select the most appropriate method for evaluating left ventricular function:

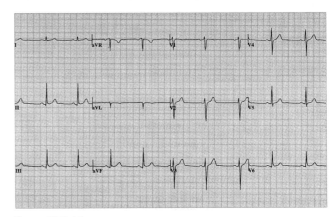

Figure Q36-16

(A) Transthoracic echocardiography

(B) Radionuclide angiography

(C) Cardiac MRI with gadolinium hyperenhancement

(D) Left ventriculography

(E) No further evaluation

36.17 A 72-year-old asymptomatic man presents for a second opinion regarding his CAD. As part of a general medical evaluation, he performed a treadmill study with the Bruce protocol where he exercised for 11 minutes. His electrocardiogram became positive for ischemia at 10 minutes of exercise with 1-mm, horizontal ST-segment depression. There was no accompanying chest pain. The patient subsequently underwent coronary angiography (Fig. Q36-17). He was advised to undergo PCI of this lesion, but was reluctant because he felt that the interventionalist was being "pushy." Select the CORRECT statement:

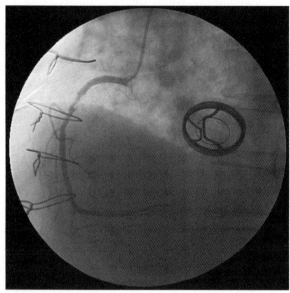

Figure Q36-17

(A) Revascularization of this lesion will reduce the risk of nonfatal infarction
(B) Surgery is preferred due to the complexity of the lesion
(C) Intensive medical therapy will result in similar long-term outcome compared to PCI

36.18 Which of the following findings on noninvasive testing is consistent with a high rate of annual cardiovascular events (>3% per year)?

(A) Left ventricular ejection fraction (LVEF) < 35%
(B) Single moderate-sized, lateral wall defect on stress thallium imaging
(C) New apical and inferior hypokinesis occurring at a heart rate of 130 bpm during dobutamine echocardiography
(D) A Duke treadmill score of −8

36.19 A 78-year-old man with a history of stable angina suffers an out-of-hospital cardiac arrest due to ventricular fibrillation. He was resuscitated immediately and has suffered no neurological sequelae. His medical history consists of hypertension, hyperlipidemia, and nicotine dependence. The patient undergoes coronary angiography (Fig. Q36-19). Select the correct statement(s):

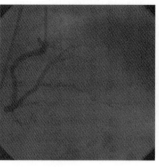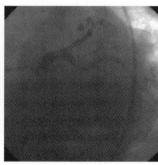

Figure Q36-19

(A) PCI is preferred over surgery
(B) Surgical revascularization is preferred over PCI
(C) Surgical revascularization and PCI are preferred equally
(D) Revascularization is not indicated

36.20 A 43-year-old man is referred for coronary angiography. He recently underwent an exercise echocardiogram. During exercise, he had developed mild pain in his right lower chest after 8 minutes of exercise on the Bruce protocol. Both the exercise ECG and stress echocardiographic images showed no evidence of ischemia. The exercise test is interpreted as equivocal, and he undergoes angiography. This demonstrates a 40% left main lesion. Using intravascular ultrasound, the minimal lumen area is determined to be 8.9 mm². Select the BEST management:

(A) CABG
(B) Balloon angioplasty only
(C) PCI with drug-eluting stenting
(D) Reassurance and no revascularization

36.21 Which of the following are false statements concerning the randomized trials of CABG vs. medical therapy?

(A) The majority of patients had severe symptoms and left ventricular dysfunction
(B) The survival advantage of the patients initially treated with surgery persisted to 10 postoperative years
(C) There was a 40% crossover rate to surgery by the medical therapy patients during follow-up
(D) Patients with single-vessel proximal LAD disease had better survival with surgery than with medical therapy

36.22 A 58-year-old healthy man is referred for treatment of his coronary disease. The patient states that he exercises regularly and reports no cardiovascular symptoms. He has a remote history of smoking but no other comorbidities. As part of a general medical evaluation, he underwent a CT scan of his chest, which suggested significant coronary atherosclerosis. Subsequently, an angiogram demonstrates a 50% lesion in the distal left main with good distal targets. Intravascular ultrasound of the left main lesion demonstrates the minimal lumen area to be 5.0 mm². Select the BEST management:

(A) CABG
(B) PCI with drug-eluting stenting
(C) Stress echocardiography
(D) Medical therapy only

36.23 A 62-year-old woman is referred for a 3-month history of worsening angina. Two years ago, she underwent PCI of a diagonal lesion with placement of a 3.0- × 13-mm sirolimus-eluting stent. Presently, walking a distance of 15 ft from her front door to the mailbox reliably precipitates her symptoms, but there are no unstable features. She has been faithfully taking her previously prescribed medications, including metoprolol (75 mg twice daily), isosorbide dinitrate (40 mg twice daily), aspirin (81 mg daily), atorvastatin (20 mg daily), and clopidogrel (75 mg daily). Which one of the following would be the appropriate next step?

(A) Treadmill study
(B) Stress radionuclide imaging
(C) Stress echocardiography
(D) Coronary angiography
(E) B, C, and D

36.24 A 77-year-old man with a 4-year history of stable angina is admitted to your hospital with dyspnea. On examination, crackles are auscultated in the lower halves of both lung fields. The first heart sound is slightly diminished, and a third heart sound is heard. His chest x-ray shows a cardiothoracic ratio of 0.6 with mild bilateral pulmonary infiltrates. Select the most appropriate next step:

(A) Intravenous diuresis
(B) Intravenous diuresis and ACEI therapy
(C) Intravenous diuresis, ACEI therapy, and coronary angiography

36.25 Which of the following therapies have Class I indications for revascularization in patients with stable angina?

(A) Left main disease for CABG
(B) Three-vessel disease for CABG
(C) Two-vessel disease with proximal LAD involvement and LV dysfunction for CABG
(D) Two- or three-vessel disease with suitable anatomy and no diabetes or LV dysfunction for PCI
(E) One- or two-vessel disease with a large area of viable myocardium and high-risk criteria on stress testing for PCI
(F) Restenosis after PCI with a large area of area of viable myocardium or high-risk criteria on stress testing for CABG or repeat PCI
(G) All of the above

36.26 A 72-year-old diabetic woman is referred for evaluation of exertional angina, which has been present for 2 months. Her cardiopulmonary examination is consistent with mild mitral regurgitation. On echocardiography, the LVEF is 55%. During exercise, the midanterior, apical, and inferoapical walls become hypokinetic after 6 minutes on the Bruce protocol. She undergoes coronary angiography, which is shown in Figure Q36-26. Select the BEST next step:

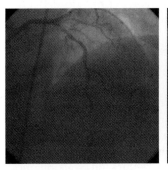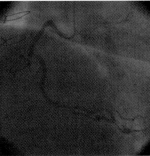

Figure Q36-26

(A) Drug-eluting stent placement
(B) CABG
(C) Balloon angioplasty with bailout stenting
(D) Intense medical therapy and reevaluation in 6 months

36.27 A 58-year-old with a known history of CAD has recurrent angina. He has undergone three prior percutaneous procedures on his middle LAD, including two prior angioplasties and one placement of a drug-eluting stent. During stress testing, his electrocardiogram becomes shows 1.5-mm horizontal ST-segment depression at 3 minutes of exercise with development of chest pain. The radionuclide images show a moderately large area of ischemia in the anterior and anterolateral walls. Repeat angiography shows a 95% lesion of restenosis at the edge of the previously stented segment. Select the BEST management:

(A) Repeat PCI
(B) CABG
(C) Medical therapy alone
(D) Either CABG or PCI

36.28 A 72-year-old-man with a history of myocardial infarction 8 years ago presents with symptoms of stable angina. These symptoms have been present for the past 2 years and occur with moderately severe levels of exertion, such as climbing more than three flights of stairs or after running 2.5 miles. There are no unstable features. Coronary angiography demonstrates a 20-mm-long, calcific total occlusion of the middle right coronary artery with bridging collaterals and Rentrop grade 2 collateralization of the distal vessel from the LAD artery. Select the BEST management:

(A) Rotational atherectomy followed by drug-eluting stenting
(B) Medical therapy
(C) Local infusion of fibrinolytic agents
(D) Controlled antegrade retrograde dissection via septal collaterals

36.29 Select the correct Canadian Cardiovascular Society (CCS) classification of each patient's symptoms:

(A) Class I: Angina occurs on walking uphill or climbing stairs rapidly
(B) Class II: Angina occurs on walking or stair climbing after meals
(C) Class III: Angina occurs on walking more than 2 blocks on the level or climbing more than one flight of stairs
(D) Class IV: Angina occurs on walking 1 to 2 blocks on the level or walking 1 flight of stairs under normal conditions and normal pace

36.30 A 78-year-old woman undergoes coronary angiography for stable angina. She has a history of hypertension, but has no other comorbidities. Her angiogram (Fig. Q36-30) demonstrates a lesion that is treated percutaneously with a 2.75- × 18-mm sirolimus-eluting stent. Which of following are TRUE statements in regard to this patient?

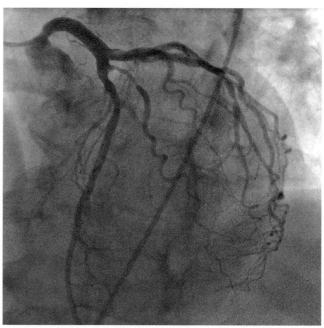

Figure Q36-30

(A) Drug-eluting stent placement and medical therapy achieve comparable relief of symptoms
(B) The rate of target vessel failure for drug-eluting stent placement of such lesions ranges from 5% to 8%
(C) Drug-eluting stent placement results in greater reduction in ischemia than medical therapy alone
(D) Medical therapy alone would have resulted in the same rates of death and nonfatal infarction as that achieved by PCI
(E) B, C, and D

36.31 A 60-year-old woman undergoes placement of a 3.0- × 23-mm everolimus-eluting stent in her middle right coronary artery. She had received 300 mg clopidogrel and aspirin prior to the procedure. There are no postprocedural complications. Which of the following is indicated (more than one answer may be correct)?

(A) Clopidogrel (75 mg daily) and aspirin (81 to 325 mg daily)
(B) Oral hormone replacement therapy
(C) Vitamin E (400 IU daily)
(D) Lipid-lowering therapy with target LDL of <100 mg/dL
(E) A and E

36.32 A 78-year-old woman with stable angina has a discrete 90% lesion in her proximal LAD. PCI with stenting is planned. She has mild chronic renal insufficiency (Cr = 1.4 mg/dL) and drug-treated hyperlipidemia. She takes no medications. There is no history of bleeding or drug allergy. Which of the following antiplatelet therapies are indicated in this patient (more than one answer may be correct)?

(A) Aspirin 325 mg at least 2 hours before PCI

(B) Aspirin 325 mg for 1 month after bare-metal stent placement and then 75 to 162 mg indefinitely

(C) Clopidogrel 600 mg loading dose before PCI

(D) All of the above

36.33 A 62-year-old man returns for follow-up after successful PCI of a chronic total occlusion with placement of a 3.0- × 16-mm paclitaxel-eluting stent in the proximal left circumflex artery. His mildly elevated creatinine is unchanged from baseline (1.4 mg/dL). Current medications are aspirin 162 mg daily, clopidogrel 75 mg daily, metoprolol 25 mg twice daily, and atorvastatin 80 mg daily. The patient is 5'5" and weighs 245 lb. His lipid profile shows a total cholesterol 205 mg/dL, LDL 95 mg/dL, HDL 42 mg/dL, and triglycerides of 501 mg/dL. Which of the following secondary prevention strategies is appropriate?

(A) 30 to 60 minutes of moderate-intensity exercise daily

(B) Reduction in dietary intake of saturated fats to <7% of total calories

(C) Influenza vaccine annually

(D) All of the above

36.34 A 55-year-old male business executive returns for follow-up. He previously was seen for mild symptoms of stable angina, which resolved with medical therapy (metoprolol 25 mg twice daily, atorvastatin 20 mg daily, and aspirin 75 mg daily). His blood pressure is 140/90 mm Hg (heart rate, 80 bpm); the remainder of the physical examination is normal. The resting electrocardiogram is normal. The patient undergoes a treadmill study with Bruce protocol, where he exercises for 5 minutes without electrocardiographic changes or angina. Select the most appropriate next step:

(A) Increase metoprolol dose

(B) Coronary angiography

(C) Echocardiography

(D) Stress nuclear imaging

36.35 Which of the following is an indication for invasive coronary angiography?

(A) A 67-year-old asymptomatic man with a prior history of bypass grafting, mildly positive stress test, and metastatic lung adenocarcinoma

(B) A 42-year-old woman who desires a definitive diagnosis of CAD in the presence of noncardiac chest pain

(C) A 55-year-old man who was successfully resuscitated from ventricular fibrillation

(D) A 74-year-old asymptomatic woman with hypertension, hyperlipidemia, and peripheral vascular disease

36.1 **Answer B.** The patient's symptoms do not meet criteria for typical angina, and thus, non-invasive assessment (e.g., stress echocardiography) may be considered as the next appropriate step in many such patients. However, in this patient's case, the nature of her occupation warrants definitive assessment of the status of her coronary arteries (ACC/AHA Class IIa recommendation).

36.2 **Answer A.** The randomized Bypass vs. Angioplasty Revascularization Investigation (BARI) study demonstrated equivalent long-term survival for angioplasty or bypass grafting among patients with multivessel disease. However, superior survival was observed in diabetic patients who received an internal mammary graft to their left anterior descending (LAD) artery. This finding, which has been corroborated in the Emory Angioplasty vs. Surgery Trial (EAST), supports the ACC/AHA guideline recommendation that CABG is preferred over angioplasty for diabetics with multivessel disease (Class I recommendation). The efficacy of drug-eluting stents vs. bypass grafting in diabetic patients is the subject of ongoing study (the FREEDOM trial). In the BARI 2D study, there was no difference in outcome according to the type of medical therapy for diabetes.

36.3 **Answer C.** The patient is unlikely to derive clinical benefit from revascularization due to the large areas of nonviable myocardium in the absence of ischemia. There are limited studies on the use of viability data in determining appropriateness for revascularization. In the OAT study, where 91% of patients with occluded arteries had mild or no ischemia 3 to 28 hours after infarction, there was no benefit of percutaneous revascularization over medical therapy. In a meta-analysis by Allman and colleagues (*J Am Coll Cardiol* 2002;39:1151–1158), patients with viable myocardium had better clinical outcomes when revascularized, while patients with nonviable myocardium had superior outcomes when not revascularized.

36.4 **Answer A.** Revascularization is not indicated for patients with one- or two-vessel disease without proximal LAD involvement, who have not received an adequate trial of medical therapy and have no demonstrable evidence of ischemia (ACC/AHA Class III recommendation).

36.5 **Answer A.** Equivalent long-term survival has been observed in randomized trials of stenting or CABG in patients with multivessel disease and low-risk anatomy. Patients enrolled in such randomized trials characteristically were relatively young (age 60 years), and most frequently had two-vessel disease, preserved ventricular function, and stable symptoms, although some studies enrolled patients with unstable angina. A cost-effective analysis of the BARI trial demonstrated equivalent costs for either angioplasty or CABG after 12 years, principally due to the need for repeat procedures in the angioplasty group.

36.6 **Answer A.** Although the left main lesion is approachable by PCI because of its distance from the bifurcation of the LAD and circumflex, current guidelines still favor CABG over PCI in patients who are suitable for surgery. In the SYNTAX study, complexity of disease, with or without distal left main involvement, was a major determinant of outcome in comparing CABG to PCI. In 2008, the ACC/AHA guidelines upgraded the recommendation for revascularization of left main disease with PCI from a Class III to Class IIb when anatomy is suitable. Further assessment with intravascular ultrasound or fractional flow reserve would only be indicated in the presence of equivocal angiographic findings.

36.7 **Answer B.** PCI is the most frequent mode of repeat revascularization among patients undergoing CABG with rates of 5% to 6% over follow-up periods of 2 to 3 years.

36.8 **Answer A.** A linear relation between adverse outcomes and all levels of CK rise has been demonstrated, but not for mild elevations of troponin isoforms. However, marked troponin elevations (>5 times normal) are associated with increased mortality. In comparison studies, definitions of periprocedural infarction typically use higher levels of biomarker rise (5 to 10 times normal) for CABG procedures than for PCI.

36.9 **Answer A.** Comparable survival and freedom from infarction has been observed in most of the major trials of stenting vs. CABG (ARTS, ERACI II, SoS, MASS II), including high-risk patients (AWESOME). In SoS, there was a higher mortality in the PCI arm, mainly due to a particularly low surgical mortality and high rate of noncardiac death in the stented patients. Stenting has reduced the need for repeat revascularization by 50% in comparison to rates observed in PTCA trials.

36.10 **Answer A.** The MASS study demonstrated comparable survival for patients with LAD disease, irrespective of whether they received medical therapy, PCI, or CABG. However, revascularization was associated with superior relief of angina and reduced need for antianginal medications. The COURAGE study showed comparable outcomes for PCI vs. intense medical therapy in stable patients. The patient's symptoms are mild. In addition, the Duke treadmill score is +7, which suggests a low annual risk of cardiovascular events (<1% per year) and low likelihood of benefit from any form of revascularization. External extracorporeal counterpulsation is indicated only in patients with severe angina refractory to medical therapy.

36.11 **Answer B.** Few studies have examined the rates of repeat PCI after bare-metal stenting in ≥4.0-mm vessels. In TAXUS V, which compared the paclitaxel-eluting stent with bare-metal stenting in complex coronary artery disease (CAD), 17% of patients were treated with a 4.0-mm stent. The 9-month target lesion revascularization rates were 5% for the bare-metal arm, and 0% in the paclitaxel-eluting stent arm.

36.12 **Answer C.** Although the patient is asymptomatic, there are high-risk features on his nuclear stress study that suggest significant left main or multivessel disease. Few studies have included or focused on asymptomatic patients (e.g. CASS registry, ACIP). The ACC/AHA guidelines recommend coronary angiography for risk stratification with high-risk criteria on noninvasive testing irrespective of anginal severity. As in symptomatic patients, revascularization is indicated for asymptomatic patients when a large ischemic burden is present.

36.13 **Answer D.** While the benefit of aspirin and beta-receptor antagonists in CAD patients is greater in patients with prior infarction, patients with stable angina also likely derive benefit, and

the ACC/AHA guidelines recommend their routine use in patients with CAD irrespective of symptoms. Therapy with ACEIs reduces diabetic complications and cardiovascular events, particularly if hypertension or heart failure is present. In 2008, the ACC/AHA guidelines expanded the Class I indication for ACEIs to all patients with CAD. Although calcium channel blockers are highly effective for the relief of angina, their use in CAD patients has led to higher rates of adverse cardiovascular events in comparison to other therapies, such as ACEIs (e.g., ABCD, FACET studies).

36.14 **Answer E.** Although restenosis may be clinically silent, the prognostic benefit of controlling silent ischemia remains unproven. Thus, stress testing after revascularization should only be performed in patients with a significant change in their angina symptoms (Class I recommendation). For patients with an indication for stress testing, adjunctive imaging is recommended to improve the sensitivity of the test and to help localize the site of ischemia.

36.15 **Answer C.** Angiographic follow-up studies have demonstrated that 6% to 11% of saphenous vein grafts become occluded within the first year after surgery, with greater patency observed in patients treated with platelet inhibition and aggressive lipid-lowering therapy. Use of the internal thoracic artery has greatly improved graft patency with 90% of grafts still functioning >10 years after surgery. Over the same time, saphenous vein grafts have an occlusion rate of 40%, with significant atherosclerosis being present in 50% of those that are still patent.

36.16 **Answer E.** In patients with a normal ECG, no prior myocardial infarction, and no heart failure, routine assessment of left ventricular function is not recommended (Class III recommendation). Of note, several large studies of CAD patients have shown that >90% of patients with a normal ECG have normal left ventricular function.

36.17 **Answer C.** Based on his performance on the treadmill, the patient's prognosis is excellent (Duke score = 6; annual cardiac mortality < 1%) and cannot be improved with revascularization by any means. Revascularization has not been shown to decrease rates of nonfatal infarction.

36.18 **Answer A.** Table A36-18 lists noninvasive findings for prognosis in patients with CAD.

Table A36-18. Noninvasive Risk Stratification

High Risk (>3% annual mortality rate)
1. Severe resting left ventricular dysfunction (LVEF < 35%)
2. High-risk treadmill score (score ≤ −11)
3. Severe exercise left ventricular dysfunction (exercise LVEF < 35%)
4. Stress-induced large perfusion defect (particularly if anterior)
5. Stress-induced multiple perfusion defects of moderate size
6. Large, fixed perfusion defect with left ventricular dilation or increased lung uptake (thallium-201)
7. Stress-induced moderate perfusion defect with left ventricular dilation or increased lung uptake (thallium-201)
8. Echocardiographic wall motion abnormality (involving greater than two segments) developing at low dose of dobutamine (≤10 μg/kg/min) or at a low heart rate (<120 bpm)
9. Stress echocardiographic evidence of extensive ischemia

Intermediate Risk (1%–3% annual mortality rate)
1. Mild/moderate resting left ventricular dysfunction (LVEF = 35%–49%)
2. Intermediate-risk treadmill score (−11 < score < 5)
3. Stress-induced moderate perfusion defect without LV dilation or increased lung intake (thallium-201)
4. Limited stress echocardiographic ischemia with a wall motion abnormality involving less than or equal to two segments only at higher doses of dobutamine

Low Risk (<1% annual mortality rate)
1. Low-risk treadmill score (score ≥5)
2. Normal or small myocardial perfusion defect at rest or with stress[a]
3. Normal stress echocardiographic wall motion or no change of limited resting wall motion abnormalities during stress[a]

[a]Although the published data are limited, patients with these findings will probably not be at low risk in the presence of either a high-risk treadmill score or severe resting left ventricular dysfunction (LVEF < 35%).
LVEF, left ventricular ejection fraction; LV, left ventricular.

36.19 Answer B. For patients with CAD who survive sudden cardiac death, surgical revascularization is recommended over PCI if there is not proximal LAD involvement (ACC/AHA Class I recommendation).

36.20 Answer D. Although there are no strict criteria for defining a significant left main lesion, most studies have supported a minimal lumen area of <7.5 mm². In this patient, revascularization with either CABG or PCI is contraindicated in the absence of demonstrable ischemia on noninvasive testing (ACC/AHA III recommendation).

36.21 Answer A. The majority of enrolled patients in these trials had mild or no symptoms and had preserved left ventricular function. The survival advantage of surgery markedly diminished by 10 years of follow-up, presumably due to graft attrition. Patients who were at high risk of death without surgery were those with left main disease, three-vessel disease and abnormal left ventricular function, two- or three-vessel disease with proximal LAD involvement, a markedly positive exercise test, or an abnormal baseline electrocardiogram.

36.22 Answer A. Even in the absence of symptoms, CABG is recommended for patients with

significant left main disease (Class I recommendation). PCI is contraindicated in patients who are otherwise healthy candidates for CABG (Class IIb recommendation).

36.23 Answer E. Stress testing with adjunctive imaging is recommended over treadmill study alone in patients with prior revascularization who have had a change in clinical status (Class I recommendation). Coronary angiography also may be performed as the initial step in patients with CCS Class III angina despite maximal medical therapy (Class I recommendation).

36.24 Answer A. Coronary angiography, in addition to appropriate medical therapy, is indicated for patients with angina and symptoms and signs of congestive heart failure (Class I recommendation).

36.25 Answer G. All of the above conditions are Class I indications for revascularization.

36.26 Answer B. Both the BARI and the EAST randomized studies demonstrated that diabetics have superior survival with bypass grafting vs. angioplasty, particularly when a left internal mammary graft is placed to the LAD artery.

Thus, in the ACC/AHA guidelines, CABG is preferred over PCI in diabetic patients (Class I recommendation). Nonetheless, the BARI registry data demonstrated that comparable survival for CABG and PCI results when procedural choice is left to the discretion of physicians. In BARI 2D, there was no difference in survival when comparing PCI vs. medical therapy in stable diabetic patients. However, superior survival did occur in the patients randomized to bypass surgery in comparison to medical therapy.

36.27 Answer D. In patients with prior PCI, either CABG or PCI may be performed if a restenosis is associated with a moderate-to-large area of viable myocardium or high-risk criteria on noninvasive testing are present (Class I recommendation).

36.28 Answer B. PCI is not recommended for lesions with mild symptoms and a low likelihood of success (Class III recommendation).

36.29 Answer B. Grading of angina pectoris according to CCS classification is shown in Table A36-29.

Table A36-29.

Class	Description of stage
I	"Ordinary physical activity does not cause angina," such as walking or climbing stairs. Angina occurs with strenuous, rapid, or prolonged exertion at work or recreation.
II	"Slight limitation of ordinary activity." Angina occurs on walking or climbing stairs rapidly; walking uphill; walking or stair climbing after meals; in cold, in wind, or under emotional stress; or only during the few hours after awaking. Angina occurs on walking more than 2 blocks on the level and climbing more than 1 flight or ordinary stairs at a normal pace and under normal conditions.
III	"Marked limitations of ordinary physical activity." Angina occurs on walking 1 to 2 blocks on the level and climbing 1 flight of stairs under normal conditions and at a normal pace.
IV	"Inability to carry on any physical activity without discomfort – anginal symptoms may be present at rest."

36.30 Answer E. Randomized trials of PCI vs. medical therapy consistently have shown superior symptom relief, fewer antianginal medications, and greater functional capacity on objective exercise testing with PCI. No difference in survival or nonfatal infarction has been observed for either PCI or medical therapy in these studies. The rate of target vessel failure for comparable lesions treated with the sirolimus-eluting stent in the SIRIUS study was 5.2% in nondiabetics. In the COURAGE nuclear substudy, PCI was associated with greater reduction in myocardial ischemia than medical therapy alone.

36.31 Answer E. Both dual antiplatelet agents and lipid-lowering strategies are established therapies for patients undergoing to PCI. Despite early promising studies, hormone replacement therapy for postmenopausal women has not been found to be beneficial and may result in harm. In one randomized investigation, hormone replacement therapy resulted in higher rates of myocardial infarction and thromboembolism. Thus, hormone replacement therapy is not recommended in postmenopausal patients for reduction of cardiovascular events (Class IIII recommendation). Vitamin E was examined in a large study (>20,000 patients) and also not found to be beneficial (Class III recommendation).

36.32 Answer D. All of the therapies are Class I recommendations for PCI patients. For patients already taking daily long-term aspirin, a dose of 75 to 325 mg should be administered before PCI (Class I recommendation).

36.33 Answer D. All of the therapies are Class I recommendations, except for B. The blood pressure goal for patients with renal insufficiency or diabetes is <130/80 mm Hg.

36.34 Answer A. Coronary angiography is not indicated in patients with mild symptoms that respond to medical therapy (Class III recommendation). The patient's functional capacity (Duke score = 5) suggests low probability of cardiovascular events (<1% per year), and stress imaging is therefore not indicated. Finally, there are no clinical findings that warrant echocardiography.

36.35 Answer C. Patients with possible or known history of angina and who have survived sudden cardiac death should undergo coronary angiography to establish diagnosis of CAD (Class I recommendation). Coronary angiography would be contraindicated in all of the remaining cases (Class III recommendations).

37

Practice Guidelines in Non–ST-Elevation Acute Coronary Syndromes

Avi Shimony and Mark J. Eisenberg

QUESTIONS

37.1 A 62-year-old woman with diabetes mellitus presents to the emergency room with 3 hours of chest heaviness. Her initial blood work and physical examination are unremarkable. Her electrocardiogram reveals sinus rhythm with anterolateral ST-segment depression. She is diagnosed with a NSTEMI, and coronary angiography is scheduled to be performed within an hour. Her only medication is metformin. What antiplatelet agents should be administered?

(A) Aspirin and abciximab
(B) Aspirin only, and abciximab if a decision is made to proceed to PCI
(C) Aspirin and clopidogrel 600 mg only, and abciximab if a decision is made to proceed to PCI
(C) Aspirin and eptifibatide
(D) Aspirin, clopidogrel 600 mg, and eptifibatide

37.2 A 57-year-old man with diabetes mellitus was diagnosed with NSTEMI at an outside facility and is now being transferred to undergo urgent coronary angiography and possible PCI. He arrives in the catheterization laboratory with no signs of heart failure and no ongoing chest pain. The onset of chest pain was 9 hours ago, and the cardiac enzymes from the outside facility are positive. He received aspirin 325 mg and enoxaparin 1 mg/kg SQ at the outside hospital 8 hours ago. Serum creatinine is normal. Coronary angiography reveals a mid-LAD culprit lesion with a large amount of thrombus. Which of the following anticoagulants would be LEAST recommended at this point?

(A) Unfractionated intravenous heparin
(B) No further heparin
(C) Enoxaparin 0.3 mg/kg IV
(D) Fondaparinux
(E) Bivalirudin

37.3 A 45-year-old man with a history of dyslipidemia and asthma presents to the emergency room with chest discomfort that began 12 hours ago. His physical examination is unremarkable. He is diagnosed with NSTEMI. He is scheduled to have an angiography within 72 to 96 hours. Which of the following should NOT be recommended as an initial treatment?

(A) Aspirin
(B) Upstream eptifibatide
(C) Upstream abciximab
(D) Upstream tirofiban

37.4 A 75-year-old woman with a history of remote coronary artery bypass graft (CABG) surgery presents to the emergency department with 4 hours of chest pain and dyspnea. Her blood pressure is 96/56 mm Hg, and heart rate is 112 bpm. Her ECG reveals sinus tachycardia with anterolateral T-wave inversions. Pulse oximetry is 86% on room air. The patient is diaphoretic. She has a cough productive of pink sputum. She has elevated jugular venous pulsations and bilateral wet crackles midway up the lung fields. Outpatient medications are aspirin and simvastatin. She is diagnosed with an acute coronary syndrome (ACS). Which feature of the patient's presentation is associated with the HIGHEST short-term risk of death or myocardial infarction (MI)?

(A) Prior CABG surgery

(B) T-wave inversions on the electrocardiogram

(C) Pulmonary edema most likely due to ischemia

(D) History of aspirin use

(E) Age of ≥70 years

37.5 Of the following anti-ischemic medications, which does NOT have an ACC/AHA Class I indication for NSTEMI ACS patients?

(A) ACE inhibitor

(B) Beta-adrenergic antagonist.

(C) Dihydropyridine calcium channel blocker

(D) Morphine sulfate

(E) Nitroglycerin

37.6 Of the following antiplatelet or anticoagulant medications, which does NOT have an ACC/AHA Class I indication for NSTEMI ACS patients?

(A) Aspirin

(B) Clopidogrel for patients who have a documented allergy to aspirin

(C) Ticagrelor

(D) Low-molecular-weight heparin subcutaneously

(E) Unfractionated heparin intravenously

37.7 A 66-year-old woman with no prior history of bleeding sustains a NSTEMI. She undergoes coronary angiography, and a recanalized right coronary artery (RCA) culprit lesion with only mild residual stenosis is identified. No PCI is performed. Echocardiography reveals normal ventricular function. Her blood pressure is 107/69 mm Hg, and her lipid profile shows a total cholesterol = 212 mg/dL, HDL = 51 mg/dL, LDL = 141 mg/dL, and triglycerides = 125 mg/dL. She is prescribed aspirin and atorvastatin. Should she also be prescribed clopidogrel on discharge?

(A) Yes, for 1 month

(B) Yes, for 9 to 12 months

(C) Yes, for 2 years

(D) Yes, indefinitely

(E) No

37.8 A 74-year-old man with severe dementia and a history of prior CABG surgery is admitted to the hospital with unstable angina. His HR is 63 bpm and his BP is 111/54 mm Hg. His troponin T level is 0.06 ng/mL. His ECG reveals sinus rhythm and dynamic ECG changes. He and his family refuse cardiac catheterization. He is administered aspirin, enoxaparin, simvastatin, IV nitroglycerin, and IV metoprolol. What is the best way to improve his medical regimen?

(A) Add abciximab

(B) Add clopidogrel

(C) Add eptifibatide

(D) Add tirofiban

(E) Substitute unfractionated heparin for enoxaparin

37.9 A 60-year-old man presents to the emergency department with 10 hours of severe ongoing chest heaviness. The onset began at rest. He has a history of type II diabetes mellitus, hyperlipidemia, hypertension, obesity, obstructive sleep apnea, and renal insufficiency. His CK is 505, CK-MB is 43.7, and TnT is 1.87. His creatinine is 1.7. His ECG reveals sinus rhythm and is otherwise normal. His chest pain is relieved after receiving aspirin, heparin, and nitroglycerin in the emergency department. What is the most appropriate next step in management?

(A) Early invasive strategy

(B) Early conservative strategy, given the absence of chest discomfort and a normal ECG

(C) Resting nuclear sestamibi scan to evaluate for a perfusion abnormality at rest

(D) Continue monitoring his renal function with plans for coronary angiography if renal function improves

(E) Echocardiogram to evaluate the left ventricular function

37.10 A 68-year-old woman presents with unstable angina. She has a history of diabetes and prior CABG surgery (LIMA-LAD, saphenous vein graft [SVG]-OM2, SVG-RPDA). Her ECG reveals 2-mm ST-segment depressions in leads I and aVL during chest discomfort. Troponin is T = 0.07 ng/mL. Coronary and graft angiography reveals severe left main trunk disease, occluded mid LAD, severe proximal circumflex stenosis, and occluded dominant RCA. The LAD and RCA grafts are patent. The midportion of the vein graft to the obtuse marginal branch has a severe ulcerated stenosis with TIMI 2 flow. There is an adequate distal landing zone for an embolic protection device. The best treatment strategy for this patient is:

(A) Medical therapy, because the LAD and RCA grafts are patent

(B) Redo CABG to OM2

(C) PCI to SVG with distal embolic protection

(D) PCI to SVG with adjunctive IIb/IIIa inhibitor

(E) PCI to left main trunk and proximal circumflex

37.11 A 56-year-old woman with hypertension, hyperlipidemia, and obesity presents to the emergency department with chest pain. She is diagnosed with NSTEMI and undergoes a successful PCI with a drug-eluting stent deployed in the LAD. After PCI, her blood pressure is normal. Post-PCI echocardiogram reveals mild mitral regurgitation and normal ventricular function. What should her discharge medications include?

(A) Aspirin 325 mg daily, clopidogrel 75 mg daily, a statin, a beta-adrenergic blocker, and an ACE inhibitor

(B) Aspirin 325 mg daily indefinitely, clopidogrel 75 mg daily, a statin, and a beta-adrenergic blocker

(C) Aspirin 325 mg daily for at least 3 months, clopidogrel 75 mg daily, and a statin

(D) Aspirin 325 mg daily for at least 3 to 6 months, clopidogrel 75 mg daily, a statin, and a beta-adrenergic blocker

(E) Aspirin 81 mg daily, clopidogrel 75 mg daily, a statin, and an ACE inhibitor

37.12 A 53-year-old man with diabetes and obesity is diagnosed with NSTEMI at an outside hospital. He is transferred and undergoes PCI with implantation of 2 drug-eluting stents to the RCA. His ECG reveals sinus rhythm. His bleeding risk is normal. He is prescribed low-dose aspirin. What is the appropriate clopidogrel regimen for this patient?

(A) 150 mg daily for at least 12 months

(B) 150 mg daily for 2 years

(C) 150 mg daily for 9 to 12 months

(D) 75 mg daily for at least 12 months

(E) 75 mg daily for 2 years

37.13 A 63-year-old woman has been having crescendo angina over the last 8 weeks. She is obese but not a diabetic. She had a drug-eluting stent previously placed in the mid LAD. She has been taking atorvastatin, aspirin, clopidogrel, and long-acting niacin. She presents to the emergency department after a severe episode of exertional angina. Her discomfort was relieved after she received two sprays of sublingual nitroglycerin. Cardiac biomarkers are normal, and her ECG shows sinus rhythm with a normal tracing. She is diagnosed with unstable angina and undergoes coronary angiography. The mid-LAD stent is patent with no evidence of in-stent restenosis. A large OM2 branch has a severe stenosis with a Type A lesion. She is sent to undergo PCI with stenting. The optimal adjunctive medical therapy for this patient is:

(A) Bivalirudin only

(B) Heparin only

(C) Heparin and abciximab

(D) Heparin and eptifibatide

(E) Heparin and tirofiban

37.14 A 59-year-old man undergoes PCI to the LAD and D1 with drug-eluting stenting. He is diabetic and overweight. His hemoglobin A1c is 7.6%. His blood pressure is 137/89 mm Hg. His lipid profile shows total cholesterol = 157 mg/dL, HDL = 37 mg/dL, LDL = 95 mg/dL, triglycerides = 135 mg/dL. He has moderate LV dysfunction with LVEF 30%. His inpatient medical regimen consists of aspirin, clopidogrel, atorvastatin, metoprolol, and a multivitamin. Which of the following adjustments to his discharge medications is NOT recommended?

(A) Add an ACE inhibitor to lower his blood pressure and to afford benefits given his diabetes and depressed LVEF

(B) Add a fibrate or niacin to increase HDL

(C) Add metformin to lower HbA1c

(D) Add short-acting nifedipine to lower his blood pressure

(E) Increase atorvastatin dose to lower LDL

37.15 A 45-year-old man presents to the emergency room with episodic rest angina. ECG shows normal sinus rhythm. An ECG obtained during an episode of chest discomfort reveals dynamic ST-segment elevation in leads V3 and V4. The discomfort resolves spontaneously. The cardiac markers are within normal limits. His echocardiogram is normal except for mild posterior mitral valve leaflet prolapse (MVP) with no evidence of mitral regurgitation. Coronary angiography reveals mild coronary disease without flow-limiting lesions. What is the most appropriate next step?

(A) Exercise stress test to evaluate for ischemia

(B) Provocative testing during left heart catheterization with intracoronary methylergonovine, followed by therapy with nitrates and calcium antagonists if the challenge is positive

(C) Provocative testing during left heart catheterization with IV methylergonovine, followed by therapy with nitrates and calcium antagonists if the challenge is positive

(D) Patient education regarding MVP-associated chest pain and instructions for antibiotic prophylaxis with dental procedures

(E) No further therapy for heart disease

37.16 A 43-year-old woman with a remote history of a drug-eluting stent implantation now presents to the emergency department with new-onset atypical chest discomfort at rest. She has severe degenerative lumbar disc disease with debilitating symptoms and is scheduled to undergo an L4/L5 discectomy in 3 weeks. Coronary angiography demonstrates a patent RCA stent and mild LCA disease. Her cardiac medications are aspirin and clopidogrel. Her ventricular function is normal. The patient's back symptoms are severe, and the surgery cannot be delayed. Recommendations include perioperative beta-blockade and minimization of the discontinuation period of aspirin and clopidogrel. What other perioperative recommendations are appropriate?

(A) Continuous ST-segment monitoring following the operation
(B) Pharmacologic stress test with either echocardiographic or nuclear imaging
(C) In-hospital IIb/IIIa therapy during the period of aspirin and clopidogrel discontinuation
(D) Intraoperative monitoring with Swan-Ganz catheter
(E) None

37.17 A 37-year-old obese woman with a history of substance abuse presents to the emergency department with 2 hours of acute-onset chest discomfort at rest. The pain started about 8 hours after snorting cocaine. Cardiac biomarkers are negative. Her ECG reveals sinus tachycardia with upsloping 2-mm ST-segment depression inferolaterally. Her blood pressure is 180/90 mm Hg (equal in both arms), and her lungs are clear. Her chest x-ray is normal. What is the most appropriate management?

(A) IV esmolol
(B) IV labetalol
(C) IV metoprolol
(D) IV morphine
(E) IV nitrates and calcium antagonists, followed by coronary angiography if discomfort persists

37.18 A 37-year-old woman who is 29 weeks pregnant presents to the emergency room with 10 hours of chest pain. Her past medical history is unremarkable. T-wave inversions are observed in leads II, III, and aVF. Her blood pressure is 105/55 with HR of 99. Her initial troponin is 10. She proceeds to the cardiac catheterization laboratory for an emergent angiogram. She is diagnosed with coronary artery dissection. Known risk factors for developing coronary artery dissection include:

(A) Advanced maternal age
(B) Third trimester of pregnancy
(C) Multigravida
(D) All of the above
(E) None of the above

37.19 A 46-year-old obese man is hospitalized with a diagnosis of unstable angina. He recently underwent a resection for colorectal cancer, and he is scheduled for an ileostomy reversal. His left heart catheterization reveals a 90% stenosis in a large diagonal branch. The reference vessel diameter is estimated at 3.0 mm. His other coronary arteries have only mild disease. What is the most appropriate strategy for this patient?

(A) PCI with balloon angioplasty with no stenting
(B) PCI with bare-metal stenting
(C) PCI with paclitaxel-eluting stent
(D) PCI with sirolimus-eluting stent
(E) Single-vessel CABG surgery

37.20 A 76-year-old woman presents to an outside free-standing emergency department with chest pain for 6 hours. She has a previous history of inferior MI. Her ECG shows inferior Q waves and 3-mm ST-segment depressions in V3-V6. She is treated with aspirin, clopidogrel, enoxaparin, tirofiban, and 5 units of reteplase. Her chest discomfort and ST-segment depressions resolve. She is transferred to the ICU and reports no discomfort. Echocardiogram reveals inferior wall hypokinesis. There is no evidence of heart failure. The most appropriate next step is:

(A) Immediate coronary angiography
(B) Immediate stress testing to evaluate for inferior wall ischemia
(C) Continued aspirin, clopidogrel, enoxaparin, and tirofiban, followed by stress testing in 4 to 6 days
(D) Discontinuation of clopidogrel given the high likelihood of urgent CABG
(E) Discontinuation of tirofiban, followed by coronary angiography the next day once the fibrinolytic effect has dissipated

37.21 An 84-year-old man is admitted at midnight with a NSTEMI. He is pain free and hemodynamically stable. He is planned for coronary angiography in the morning. He has long-standing diabetic nephropathy, and his creatinine is 1.9 mg/dL. In addition to minimizing the amount of contrast dye used during the procedure, which of the following is the optimal way to minimize the extent of contrast dye-induced renal injury?

(A) Hydration with normal saline and mucomyst 600 mg

(B) Bicarbonate infusion

(C) The use of iodixanol dye along with biplane imaging system

(D) Mucomyst and bicarbonate infusion

(E) Hydration with normal saline and the use of iodixanol dye

37.22 A 54-year-old obese woman with a history of chronic renal insufficiency presents with new-onset exertional chest heaviness. She is diagnosed with unstable angina and is admitted to the hospital. CK, CK-MB, and troponin T are within normal limits. Her ECG reveals sinus rhythm and a normal tracing. At rest, she is asymptomatic. Her HR is 75 bpm, her BP is 130/90 mm Hg, and her cardiac examination is normal. Prior to the hospitalization, she was not taking any medications. Her creatinine is elevated at 2.5 mg/dL. The best plan for risk stratification is:

(A) Pharmacologic stress test 4 to 6 days after admission

(B) Submaximal exercise stress test 2 to 3 days after admission

(C) Symptom-limited exercise stress test (without echocardiogram or nuclear imaging) 2 to 3 days after admission

(D) Symptom-limited exercise stress test (without echocardiogram or nuclear imaging) 7 to 10 days after admission

(E) Symptom-limited exercise stress test with echocardiogram or nuclear imaging 4 to 6 days after admission

37.23 A 56-year-old man with a history of diabetes, hypertension, and a minor stroke 3 years ago presents to the emergency room with chest pain radiating to both arms and lower jaw for the past 45 minutes. Initial blood pressure is 185/90 mm Hg. His clinical exam is otherwise normal. Recommendations that should be followed or strongly considered (ACC/AHA Class I or IIa) for early risk stratification for this patient include all of the following, EXCEPT:

(A) 12-lead ECG within 10 minutes of emergency department arrival

(B) Cardiac biomarkers

(C) Continuous 12-lead ECG monitoring

(D) Assessment of myoglobin, for patients who present within 6 hours of symptom onset

(E) Repeat measure of initially positive biomarkers

37.24 Which of the following is INCORRECT?

(A) Creatine kinase (CK)-MB is more sensitive, but less specific, for MI than the cardiac troponins

(B) Elevated levels of CK-MB can be found with damage to skeletal muscle

(C) CK-MB has a shorter half-life than troponin

(D) Troponin T and troponin I are derived from heart-specific genes

(E) The timing of elevation for troponin is similar to that of CK-MB, but persists up to 14 days

37.25 A 77-year-old woman with a history of hypertension and diabetes presents to the emergency room. Twenty-four hours prior to her arrival, she experienced 2 hours of chest pain radiating to her left arm and jaw. Her ECG reveals sinus rhythm with 3-mm ST-segment depression in leads V1 to V4 and an elevated troponin I. Her physical examination is unremarkable. Blood oxygen saturation is 98%. Her heart rate is 75 per minute. Currently, she is asymptomatic. Estimated LV ejection fraction by echocardiography is 45%. Which of the following steps are NOT recommended (ACC/AHA Class I/IIa) for her initial therapy?

(A) Oral beta-blocker within the first 24 hours

(B) Oral ACE inhibitor within the first 24 hours

(C) Supplemental oxygen during the first 6 hours

(D) Sublingual nitroglycerin

(E) Bed or chair rest with continuing ECG monitoring in the emergency room

37.26 A 19-year-old man who frequently uses cocaine presents to emergency room with 6 hours of chest pain. His blood pressure is 130/75. The rest of the physical examination is normal. The ER doctor would like your advice about the potential harmful cardiovascular effects of cocaine. All of the statements below are true, EXCEPT:

(A) Cocaine promotes thrombus formation

(B) Cocaine increases myocardial contractility

(C) Cocaine increases platelet activation and decreases plasminogen activator inhibitor

(D) Cocaine increases the production of endothelin

(E) Cocaine accelerates atherosclerosis

37.27 Which of the following can be used for secondary prevention in NSTEMI patients?

(A) Plant sterols

(B) Folic acid

(C) Vitamin E

(D) Vitamin B_6

(E) Vitamin C

37.28 A 67-year-old patient presents to the emergency room with severe shortness of breath and diaphoresis. The patient is producing pink frothy sputum. His blood pressure is 78/45 mm Hg and oxygen saturation on room air is 84%. An intraaortic balloon pump is planned. The risk of limb ischemia is heightened by all the following risk factors, EXCEPT:

(A) Diabetes mellitus
(B) Female sex
(C) Peripheral vascular disease
(D) Smaller catheters (8.0 to 9.5 F)
(E) Postinsertion ankle-brachial index of 0.85

37.29 Which of the following statements is FALSE?

(A) Nitroglycerin is contraindicated in patients who have received sildenafil within the past 48 hours
(B) Abciximab is contraindicated in patients in whom PCI is not planned
(C) Nitrates are contraindicated in patients with a heart rate of 45/min and systolic blood pressure of 120 mm Hg
(D) Intravenous beta-blockers are contraindicated in patients with a low-output state
(E) Angiotensin receptor blockers are contraindicated in pregnant women

37.30 Which of the following is useful to provoke coronary artery spasm in variant angina?

(A) Adenosine with Valsalva
(B) Dipyridamole with histamine
(C) Adenosine with acetylcholine
(D) Dipyridamole with Valsalva
(E) Acetylcholine with hyperventilation

37.31 Which of the following agents should be withdrawn before provocative testing for variant angina?

(A) ACE inhibitors
(B) Beta-blockers
(C) Calcium channel blockers
(D) Diuretics
(E) Digoxin

37.32 The TIMI risk score indicators for UA/NSTEMI patients include all, EXCEPT:

(A) CK-MB elevation
(B) Aspirin used within the last month
(C) Known coronary artery disease >50% stenosis in a major epicardial artery
(D) Age ≥65
(E) ST changes ≥0.5 mm

37.33 The GRACE score for MI includes all, EXCEPT:

(A) Heart rate
(B) Systolic blood pressure
(C) Creatinine
(D) More than three cardiovascular risk factors
(E) ST-segment deviation

37.34 A 49-year-old woman with a family history of coronary artery disease presents to the emergency room with 12 hours of chest heaviness. Her initial blood work and physical examination are unremarkable. Her electrocardiogram reveals sinus rhythm with deep lateral ST-segment depression. She is diagnosed with NSTEMI, and coronary angiography is scheduled to be performed within the next few hours. Her weight is 65 kg. What antiplatelet agents should be administered?

(A) Clopidogrel 150 mg
(B) Prasugrel 10 mg
(C) Prasugrel 60 mg
(D) Aspirin 100 mg

37.35 A 71-year-old homeless woman is admitted to the cardiac care unit with NSTEMI after having 7 days of severe chest pain. Her blood pressure is 90/60 mm Hg. A 4/6 systolic murmur is heard over a large area of the precordium. An echocardiogram confirms the diagnosis of ventricular septal rupture. Which of the following statements concerning ventricular septal rupture is TRUE?

(A) Usually occurs in patients with a previous history of MI
(B) More often associated with atrial fibrillation
(C) Better prognosis when the rupture is in the apical region
(D) More often occurs in younger patients
(E) More often occurs in normotensive patients

37.1 Answer C. Except for patients known to be intolerant of aspirin, all patients with an ACS should be treated with non–enteric-coated aspirin 162 to 325 mg. Patients should also receive an oral loading dose of clopidogrel 300 to 600 mg (the ISAR REACT 2 trial used a loading dose of 600 mg). Platelet glycoprotein (GP) IIb/IIIa receptor antagonists have a further beneficial effect for patients with an ACS undergoing PCI. Of these antagonists, abciximab is supported by the strongest data. Abciximab should be administered only if a firm plan is made to perform PCI; it is contraindicated in patients for whom only medical management is planned.

37.2 Answer D. Currently, unfractionated intravenous heparin remains the recommended anticoagulation regimen during PCI. The SYNERGY trial compared enoxaparin to unfractionated heparin among patients with NSTEMI undergoing PCI. Although there was no significant difference in the ischemic efficacy end points, more bleeding was noted in the enoxaparin group. A post hoc analysis suggested that this increase in bleeding may be attributed to the higher rate of bleeding among patients who were switched from enoxaparin to heparin during the PCI. However, this finding must be prospectively validated before it can be applied in clinical practice. Interestingly, the ACUITY trial also demonstrated that bivalirudin may be safer than, but equally efficacious to, heparin for patients undergoing PCI for non–ST-elevation ACS. Also of note, case reports have documented equipment thrombosis in ACS patients undergoing PCI with only a single preceding dose of subcutaneous enoxaparin. (*Can J Cardiol* 2006;22:511–515.)

37.3 Answer C. Upstream abciximab as the choice for upstream IIb/IIIa therapy is indicated only if there is no appreciable delay to angiography and PCI is likely to be performed (Page e45, 2007 ACC/AHA guidelines for the management of patients with UA/NSTEMI).

37.4 Answer C. In an ACS patient, pulmonary edema is associated with a high short-term risk of death or MI. The other features listed are each associated with intermediate risk. Examples of low-risk features include normal levels of cardiac biomarkers and a normal ECG during chest discomfort.

37.5 Answer C. According to the current ACC/AHA guidelines, long-acting dihydropyridine calcium channel blockers have a Class IIa indication, and immediate release blockers have a Class IIb indication.

37.6 Answer C. Ticagrelor does not have a Class indication as yet.

37.7 Answer B. In the CURE and CREDO studies, the benefit of dual antiplatelet therapy with aspirin and clopidogrel for patients with ACS was seen with 9 to 12 months of clopidogrel use. In terms of recommended duration of clopidogrel treatment, the current ACC/AHA guidelines do not distinguish between medically managed patients and those who undergo revascularization. Although many physicians maintain long-term clopidogrel therapy after implantation of a drug-eluting stent, this is not applicable to the patient in this vignette. Importantly, for patients with stable cardiovascular disease, the CHARISMA trial found no benefit in adding clopidogrel to aspirin.

37.8 Answer B. The CURE trial demonstrated that, compared to aspirin alone in patients with ACS, the addition of clopidogrel was associated with a lower incidence of adverse ischemic events. In this case, clopidogrel should be started and continued for 9 to 12 months. The GUSTO IV trial demonstrated harm with the strategy of administering abciximab to patients without planned PCI. Tirofiban and eptifibatide should not be administered as they are not likely to provide a benefit to medically treated ACS patients. Enoxaparin is superior to unfractionated heparin among medically treated ACS patients.

37.9 Answer A. Multiple clinical trials, including TACTICS TIMI 18, demonstrated that an early invasive strategy is associated with a lower incidence of major adverse cardiac events among NSTEMI patients. An invasive strategy is also favored in a patient with ongoing ischemic symptoms, ischemic ECG changes or electrical instability, or evidence of hemodynamic

Table A37-9. Selection of Initial Treatment Strategy: Invasive Versus Conservative Strategy

Strategy	Status	Patient Characteristic
Invasive	Generally preferred	Recurrent angina or ischemia at rest or with low-level activities despite intensive medical therapy
		Elevated cardiac biomarkers (TnT or TnI)
		New or presumably new ST-segment depression
		Signs or symptoms of HF or new or worsening mitral regurgitation
		High-risk findings from noninvasive testing
		Hemodynamic instability
		Sustained ventricular tachycardia
		PCI within 6 mo
		Prior CABG
		High-risk score (e.g., TIMI, GRACE)
		Mild to moderate renal dysfunction
		Diabetes mellitus
		Reduced left ventricular function (LVEF < 40%)
Conservative	Generally preferred	Low-risk score (e.g., TIMI, GRACE)
		Patient or physician preference in the absence of high-risk features

CABG, coronary artery bypass graft; GRACE, Global Registry of Acute Coronary Events; HF, heart failure; LVEF, left ventricular ejection fraction; PCI, percutaneous coronary intervention; TIMI, thrombolysis in myocardial infarction; TnI, troponin I; TnT, troponin T.
Reprinted from Anderson et al. ACC/AHA UA/NSTEMI Guideline Revision. *Circulation* 2007;116;e148–e304.

instability or heart failure (Table A37.9, Wright RS et al. *Circulation* published online March 28, 2011; doi: 10.1161/CIR.0b013e31820f2f3e). It is also important to continue monitoring renal function and evaluate ventricular function, but as secondary measures to coronary angiography.

37.10 Answer C. Since the graft is on the verge of closing, it is reasonable to expect PCI to provide superior preservation of myocardial function. The risk/benefit ratio for reoperation for a single circumflex territory target is unfavorable. PCI to native coronaries would be more difficult than PCI of the SVG and should be held in reserve as an option for the future. Distal embolic protection devices have been shown to offer benefits in vein graft angioplasty in ACS patients. The benefit of adjunctive IIb/IIIa inhibitors in this patient is modest. Given that the use of a distal embolic protection device has been shown to reduce ischemic complications, and that there is a large amount of thrombotic debris in this case, its use is recommended.

37.11 Answer D. After PCI with implantation of a drug-eluting stent, aspirin and clopidogrel are required medications. For NSTEMI patients treated with DES, aspirin 162 to 325 mg per day should be given for at least 3 months after sirolimus-eluting stent implantation and 6 months after paclitaxel-eluting stent and then continued indefinitely at a daily dose of 75 to 162 mg. In the future, point-of-care testing for aspirin and clopidogrel resistance may yield personalized dosing recommendations for patients. Because this patient has hyperlipidemia, it is important to discharge her on a statin with a goal LDL level <70 mg/dl. Following MI, all patients should be treated with a beta-adrenergic blocker, unless contraindicated. This patient does not require an ACE inhibitor, which is appropriate for patients with ventricular systolic dysfunction, hypertension, or diabetes mellitus.

37.12 Answer D. As drug-eluting stents impede stent endothelialization, many physicians continue clopidogrel for at least 12 months. Case reports have documented stent thrombosis years after implantation of drug-eluting stents, primarily when oral antiplatelet therapy is interrupted. It is currently unknown whether there is a safe time to discontinue clopidogrel. Although the appropriate maintenance dose is also unknown, most physicians use the standard dose of 75 mg daily.

37.13 Answer A. In a patient with unstable angina and a nonthrombotic culprit lesion, the optimal adjunctive pharmacotherapy is bivalirudin. The ACUITY trial demonstrated that, for patients with non–ST-elevation ACS undergoing PCI, bivalirudin is as beneficial as heparin plus IIb/

IIIa inhibitor in terms of ischemic end points, but is safer with respect to bleeding complications. Bivalirudin was especially beneficial in the context of clopidogrel pretreatment. The ISAR REACT 2 trial demonstrated that, in a similar patient population receiving aspirin, clopidogrel loading, and heparin, the addition of a GP IIb/IIIa inhibitor was beneficial among troponin-positive patients. However, in this patient with a negative troponin and a nonthrombotic lesion, bivalirudin is the optimal adjunctive pharmacotherapy.

37.14   **Answer D.** Short-acting nifedipine is not recommended, as it is associated with adverse outcomes among patients with coronary disease. The medications intended to raise HDL and further lower LDL are reasonable given that lipid management is clearly important for this patient. Adding metformin is likely to help him achieve his target Hb A1c of <7%. Adding an ACE inhibitor is also recommended as they are particularly beneficial for diabetics, especially in the context of elevated blood pressure or depressed left ventricular systolic function.

37.15   **Answer C.** Given the patient's coronary anatomy, a stress test would be not be informative. Antibiotic prophylaxis is not required for isolated MVP. The most appropriate step is provocative testing with IV methylergonovine, which is safe and likely to yield a diagnosis of Prinzmetal's angina. Methylergonovine should never be administered via the intracoronary route, as this may cause electric instability and coronary irreversible spasm. Coronary vasospasm may be readily treated with nitrates and calcium channel blockers.

37.16   **Answer E.** No other recommendations need to be implemented. The patient's discomfort does not indicate myocardial ischemia due to coronary disease. The patient is at risk for stent thrombosis due to the upcoming interruption of antiplatelet therapy and the prothrombotic storm that accompanies surgery. However, it is not clear that more intensive monitoring will reduce risk. As there are no flow-limiting coronary stenoses, stress testing is not appropriate. Treatment with IIb/IIIa inhibitors has also not been demonstrated to reduce risk. If clopidogrel must be discontinued for surgery, the duration of cessation should be minimized. If at all possible, low-dose aspirin should be maintained perioperatively. If aspirin must be discontinued, the duration of interruption should also be minimized.

37.17   **Answer E.** Cocaine use is associated with several cardiac conditions including accelerated atherosclerosis, coronary vasospasm, elevated blood pressure, and an increased incidence of aortic dissection and/or MI. For this patient, cautious lowering of blood pressure is the most important next step. Beta-adrenergic blockers should be used with caution as unopposed alpha action may result. Labetalol may be preferable due to its concomitant α-blocking action. However, in this case the concern is less for aortic dissection and more for myocardial ischemia, especially vasospasm. Thus, nitrates and calcium channel blockers are more likely to be effective. Coronary angiography is also advisable if discomfort persists after optimization of the blood pressure.

37.18   **Answer D.** Risk factors for coronary artery dissection include advanced maternal age, multigravida, and being near term or <3 months postpartum.

37.19   **Answer B.** The patient will require an interruption in clopidogrel therapy with his upcoming surgery. Thus, drug-eluting stenting is not recommended for this large-diameter diagonal branch. The most appropriate strategy is bare-metal stenting followed by 1 month of clopidogrel, with surgery scheduled for a later time. The stent will lessen the risk of acute closure and restenosis compared to balloon angioplasty only. Single-vessel surgery is not indicated.

37.20   **Answer E.** It appears the ACS was successfully treated with medical therapy. Of note, reteplase was administered in this patient without appropriate indication (ST elevation or equivalent). This patient is elderly and received 3 antiplatelet medications, heparin, and a fibrinolytic agent. Thus, the risk of bleeding complications is high, and the GP IIb/IIIa inhibitor should be discontinued. Coronary angiography should be delayed until the fibrinolytic effect has dissipated. Routine angiography following successful fibrinolysis may reduce ischemia, although there are no definitive data to guide this. However, in this case, the patient's severe ECG abnormality favors angiography (vs. stress testing). Clopidogrel should be continued because of the low likelihood of urgent CABG.

37.21   **Answer E.** The two most important measures in limiting the injury to kidney are preprocedural hydration with saline and the use of iodixanol (or similar) dye. *N*-acetylcysteine (mucomyst) and bicarbonate infusion may also provide incremental protection, but this is less well established. Biplane imaging often allows for fewer injections, thus affording further nephroprotection.

37.22 **Answer C.** In a patient who is able to exercise, the stress test that provides the most prognostic information is the symptom-limited exercise test. Although echocardiographic or nuclear imaging might provide useful additional information, it is not required in this case because the patient's baseline ECG is normal and would be less cost-effective. The stress test may be safely performed 2 to 3 days after admission, provided that there is no recurrent ischemia during that time.

37.23 **Answer D.** The patient presents to the emergency room with symptoms consistent with an ACS. Rapid assessment and monitoring are needed. Myoglobin is a heme-protein found in cardiac and skeletal muscle. It typically rises early (1 to 4 hours) after onset of MI and returns to normal levels within 24 to 36 hours. It lacks specificity, and its negative and positive predictive values are not high enough to "rule out" or "rule in" an acute MI. The other recommendations are either Class I or Class IIa for early risk stratification for the patient (2007 ACC/AHA guidelines for the management of patients with UA/NSTEMI, p. e18).

37.24 **Answer A.** CK-MB is LESS sensitive and LESS specific for MI than the cardiac troponins. CK-MB appears 4 to 6 hours after onset of symptoms, peaks at 18 to 24 hours, and returns to normal values after 48 to 72 hours (Fig. A37-24). (2007 ACC/AHA guidelines for the management of patients with UA/NSTEMI, p. e25). All the other statements are correct (2007 ACC/AHA guidelines for the management of patients with UA/NSTEMI, p. e25–e26).

defined as the 99th percentile from a normal reference population without myocardial necrosis; the coefficient of variation of the assay should be 10% or less). The earliest rising biomarkers are myoglobin and CK isoforms (*leftmost curve*). CKMB (*dashed curve*) rises to a peak of 2 to 5 times the ULN and typically returns to the normal range within 2 to 3 days after AMI. The cardiac-specific troponins show small elevations above the ULN in small infarctions (e.g., as is often the case with NSTEMI) but rise to 20 to 50 times the ULN in the setting of large infarctions (e.g., as is typically the case in STEMI). The troponin levels may stay elevated above the ULN for 7 days or more after AMI. CK, creatine kinase; CKMB, MB fraction of creatine kinase; CV, coefficient of variation; MI, myocardial infraction; NSTEMI, non–ST-elevation myocardial infarction; UA/NSTEMI, unstable angina/non–ST-elevation myocardial infarction. (Modified from Shapiro BP, Jaffe AS. Cardiac biomarkers. In: Murphy JG, Lioyd MA, eds. Mayo *clinic cardiology: Concise textbook.* 3rd ed. Rochester, MN: Mayo Clinic Scientific Press, New York: Informa Healthcare USA, 2007:773–780. Used with permission of Mayo Foundation for Medical Education and Research).

37.25 **Answer D.** Sublingual nitroglycerin is indicated for ongoing ischemic symptoms; however, the above patient is asymptomatic (2007 ACC/AHA guidelines for the management of patients with UA/NSTEMI, p. e35–e36).

37.26 **Answer C.** Cocaine use is associated with a number of cardiovascular conditions including MI, heart failure, aortic dissection, and arrhythmias. It does so through two main pathways: increased sympathetic output and a local anesthetic effect. Cocaine use is associated with platelet activation, as well as an increased concentration of plasminogen activator inhibitor (*Circulation* 2010;122:2558–2569).

37.27 **Answer A.** Sterols/stanol esters are found naturally in plant foods. An amount of 2 to 3 g/day decreases total and LDL cholesterol by as much as 15% (Table A37-27). Certain food products, such as cereals, margarine, and milk, are enriched with plant sterols/stanol esters (*Nutr Metab Cardiovasc Dis* 2010;20:459–466). Answers B to E were shown to have no beneficial effect on cardiovascular outcomes and in some cases may be harmful (i.e., class III) (2007 ACC/AHA guidelines for the management of patients with UA/NSTEMI, p. e93).

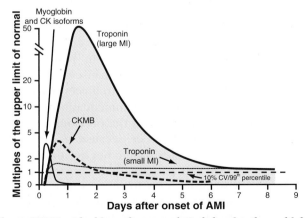

Figure A37-24. The biomarkers are plotted showing the multiples of the cutoff for acute myocardial infarction (AMI) over time. The dashed horizontal line shows the upper limit or normal (ULN;

Table A37-27.   Medications Used for Stabilized UA/NSTEMI Patients

Anti-ischemic and Anti-thrombotic/Antiplatelet Agents	Drug Action	Class/Level of Evidence
Aspirin	Antiplatelet	I/A
Clopidogrel* or ticlopidine	Antiplatelet when aspirin is contraindicated	I/A
Beta-blockers	Anti-ischemic	I/B
ACEI	EF < 0.40 or HF EF > 0.40	I/A IIa/A
Nitrates	Antianginal	I/C for ischemic symptoms
Calcium channel blockers (short-acting dihydropyridine antagonists should be avoided)	Antianginal	I for ischemic symptoms; when beta-blockers are not successful (B) or contraindicated, or cause unacceptable side effects (C)
Dipyridamole	Antiplatelet	III/A

Agents for Secondary Prevention and other Indications	Risk Factor	Class/Level of Evidence
HMG-CoA reductase inhibitors	LDL cholesterol > 70 mg/ dL	Ia
Fibrates	HDL cholesterol < 40 mg/ dL	IIa/B
Niacin	HDL cholesterol < 40 mg/ dL	IIa/B
Niacin or fibrate	Triglycerides 200 mg/dL	IIa/B
Antidepressant	Treatment of depression	IIb/B
Treatment of hypertension	Blood pressure > 140/90 mm Hg or > 130/80 mm Hg if kidney disease or diabetes present	I/A
Hormone therapy (initiation)†	Postmenopausal state	III/A
Treatment of diabetes	HbA$_{1c}$ > 7%	I/B
Hormone therapy (continuation)†	Postmenopausal state	III/B
COX-2 inhibitor or NSAID	Chronic pain	IIa/C, IIb/C or III/C
Vitamins C, E, beta-carotene; folic acid, B$_6$, B$_{12}$	Antioxidant effect; homocysteine lowering	III/A

*Preferred to ticlopidine.
†For risk reduction of coronary artery disease.
ACEI, angiotensin-converting enzyme inhibitor; CHF, congestive heart failure; COX-2, cyclooxygenase 2; EF, ejection fraction; HDL, high-density lipoprotein; HMG-CoA, hydroxymethyl glutaryl coenzyme A; INR, international normalized ratio; LDL, low-density lipoprotein; NSAID, nonsteroidal anti-inflammatory drug; NSTEMI, non–ST-segment elevation myocardial infarction; UA, unstable angina.

37.28 **Answer D.** Large IABP catheters may cause limb ischemia due to reduced blood flow and the promotion of thrombus formation. It is mandatory to monitor for limb ischemia following the insertion of an IABP. Smaller IABP catheters reduce the risk of limb ischemia (Libby, *Braunwald's heart disease: A textbook of cardiovascular medicine*, 8th ed. Chapter 19).

37.29 **Answer A.** The vasodilator effect of sildenafil and nitroglycerin is mediated by the release of nitric oxide. The combination can cause severe hazardous hypotension and is thus contraindicated—especially in patients with coronary artery disease. Because of sildenafil's half-life of 3 to 4 hours, nitroglycerin is contraindicated (Class III recommendation) after the use of sildenafil within the previous 24 hours. Answer C is incorrect because, according to guidelines, nitrates should not be administered to UA/NSTEMI patients with severe bradycardia (<50 beats/min) in the absence of symptomatic HF, or right ventricular infarction (Class III, level of Evidence C). (2007 ACC/AHA guidelines for the management of patients with UA/NSTEMI, p. e36).

37.30 **Answer E.** Variant angina (Prinzmetal's angina) is a form of unstable angina that typically occurs spontaneously at rest and is associated with transient ST elevation. It often occurs in clusters with long periods of no attacks. Variant angina is caused by coronary spasm that occurs in either normal or diseased vessels. Coronary spasm leads to myocardial ischemia and chest pain. Variant angina can usually be reversed by nitroglycerin or calcium channel blockers. Diagnostic tests for variant angina are based on the documentation of transient ST-segment elevation during an episode of chest pain. Acetylcholine and hyperventilation can be useful to provoke coronary artery spasm. (2007 ACC/AHA guidelines for the management of patients with UA/NSTEMI, p. e116).

37.31 **Answer C.** Coronary spasm in variant angina is often responsive to nitrates and calcium channel blockers. The clinical effect of beta-blockers is controversial. A number of provocative tests can be used to precipitate coronary spasm. Nitrates and calcium channel blockers should be withdrawn well before provocative testing to prevent false-negative results (2007 ACC/AHA guidelines for the management of patients with UA/NSTEMI, p. e116).

37.32 **Answer B.** The TIMI risk score developed for UA/NSTEMI patients is a simple tool composed of seven risk indicators that help predict the risk of cardiac events (Table A37-32). The rates of all-cause mortality, MI, and severe recurrent ischemia prompting urgent revascularization through 14 days increase as TIMI risk score increases.

Answer B is incorrect because aspirin used within the last 7 *days* is one of the risk indicators (*JAMA* 2000;284:835–842).

Table A37-32. TIMI Risk Score for Unstable Angina/Non–ST-Elevation MI

TIMI Risk Score	All-Cause Mortality, New or Recurrent MI, or Severe Recurrent Ischemia Requiring Urgent Revascularization Through 14 d After Randomization,%
0–1	4.7
2	8.3
3	13.2
4	19.9
5	26.2
6–7	40.9

The TIMI risk score is determined by the sum of the presence of 7 variables at admission; 1 point is given for each of the following variables: age 65 y or older; at least 3 risk factors for CAD; prior coronary stenosis of 50% or more; ST-segment deviation on ECG presentation; at least 2 anginal events in prior 24 h; use of aspirin in prior 7 d; elevated serum cardiac biomarkers. Prior coronary stenosis of 50% or more remained relatively insensitive to missing information and remained a significant predictor of events.

CAD, coronary artery disease; ECG, electrocardiogram; MI, myocardial infarction; y, year.

Reprinted from Antman EM, Cohen M, Bernink PJ. et al. TIMI risk score for unstable angina/ non-ST elevation MI: a method for prognostication and therapeutic decision making. *JAMA* 2000;284:835–842, with permission. Copyright © 2000 American Medical Association.

37.33 **Answer D.** Criterion D is taken from the TIMI risk score. The GRACE score for ACS patients (UA/NSTEMI and STEMI) was developed on the basis of over 11,000 patients in the GRACE registry. The 8 variables used in the GRACE risk model are age, Killip class, systolic blood pressure, serum creatinine level, heart rate (defined as continuous outcomes), ST-segment deviation, cardiac arrest at admission, and positive cardiac biomarkers level (defined as binary outcomes) (*Arch Intern Med* 2003;163:2345–2353) A patient's GRACE risk score is calculated by adding points corresponding to all these variables.

37.34 **Answer C.** For patients with NSTEMI in whom PCI is planned, Prasugrel 60 mg should be given and no later than 1 hour after PCI. This new recommendation is based on the pivotal trial for prasugrel, TRITON-TIMI 38. Prasugrel 10 mg is the daily maintenance dose. Clopidogrel loading dose is 300 to 600 mg. Based on the CURRENT-OASIS-7 trial, the use of a loading dose of 600 mg clopidogrel, followed by a higher maintenance dose of 150 mg daily for 6 days, then 75 mg daily in patients with low risk for bleeding may be considered (Class IIb indication).

37.35 **Answer C.** Ventricular septal rupture is a rare mechanical and potentially lethal complication of MI. It occurs in about 0.2% of patients in the era of reperfusion therapy. Known risk factors include older age, female gender, hypertension, absence of smoking history, and Killip class 3–4. The prognosis is worse when the rupture is in the basal septum commonly associated with right ventricular infarction (Libby, *Braunwald's heart disease: A textbook of cardiovascular medicine*, 8th ed. Chapter 51).

38 Percutaneous Coronary Interventions: ACC/AHA/SCAI Guidelines

Leslie Cho

QUESTIONS

38.1 A 54-year-old female with a history of radical mastectomy, chemotherapy, and radiation therapy for left breast cancer presents for a second opinion regarding her coronary artery disease. She has been having difficulty breathing with exertional chest pain and underwent stress testing that showed LV dilatation during stress. She then underwent catheterization at an outside hospital. This showed 40% to 50% ostial left main trunk (LMT) by angiography and normal left anterior descending (LAD) and circumflex coronary artery (LCX) and ostial 80% right coronary artery (RCA) lesion. She underwent drug-eluting stent (DES) implantation to her ostial RCA. Her symptoms never improved. She underwent repeat catheterization by the same interventionalist and was told that she is fine. You reviewed her catheterization and elect to repeat it with intravascular ultrasound (IVUS) of her LMT. Figure Q38-1 is the finding of her LMT IVUS. Based on the finding, what would you recommend?

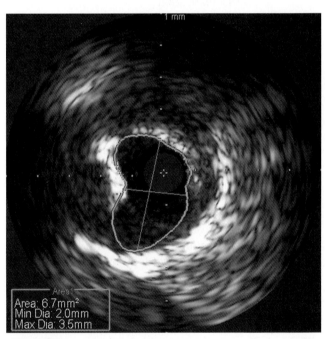

Figure Q38-1

    (A) Medical management
    (B) Percutaneous coronary intervention (PCI) of LMT
    (C) Coronary artery bypass graft (CABG)
    (D) Exercise stress testing

38.2 A 67-year-old woman with history of hypertension and hyperlipidemia who underwent LAD stenting 2 years ago for angina presents to your office for a second opinion. She has been on atenolol, amlodipine, atorvastatin, aspirin, and nitrates with minimal angina. She underwent her annual stress test where she exercised for

10 minutes on a modified Bruce protocol and achieved 10 Mets. Her ejection fraction at rest was 60%. There was no evidence of ischemia with stress. She underwent cardiac CT at her own request and was found to have significant stenosis in her LCX artery. She then underwent catheterization that showed 30% mid LAD stenosis, a large dominant RCA with 40% distal RCA stenosis, and 80% proximal stenosis in moderate-size LCX artery. On exam, her blood pressure is 104/68 with a heart rate of 58 without any evidence of heart failure. She wants your opinion regarding revascularization. You would advise:

(A) Continue current medication regimen but no revascularization
(B) Fractional flow reserve (FFR) of LCX artery, and if <0.80 proceed to PCI
(C) PCI of LCX artery
(D) Add clopidogrel therapy but no revascularization

38.3   She is not satisfied with your answer and goes to another cardiologist. She undergoes FFR of the LCX artery that was 0.86, and IVUS of the lesion showed 70% area stenosis. She is still asymptomatic and returns to your office wanting your opinion regarding revascularization.

(A) There are data to support IVUS over FFR; therefore, PCI to LCX should be performed
(B) Clinical outcome among patients with a significant lesion based on IVUS is poor; therefore, FFR result should be ignored and PCI to LCX should be planned
(C) Clinical outcome when deferring coronary intervention for stenosis with normal physiology (FFR) is very good. There is no need for PCI
(D) Single-vessel bypass is warranted given the uncertainty

38.4   A 76-year-old male with hypertension, diabetes, coronary artery disease, hyperlipidemia, and history of congestive heart failure presents to the emergency room (ER) with increasing shortness of breath and chest pain. His past medical history is notable for CABG 5 years ago. He had been doing well until a few weeks ago when he experienced mild chest pain while mowing his lawn. Since then he has noticed increasing chest pain with exertion. On the day of admission, he had chest pain at rest with increasing shortness of breath. In the ER, his ECG showed ST elevation in leads II, III, and aVF. His blood pressure was 126/90 with a heart rate of 100, and his cardiac exam revealed regular rhythm and rate,

normal S1, S2 with S3, and elevated JVP. He is taken to the catheterization laboratory. His catheterization reveals normal LMT, 100% mid LAD, 60% proximal LCX stenosis, 100% RCA, patent LIMA to LAD with minimal distal LAD stenosis, 95% stenosis in the saphenous vein graft (SVG) posterior descending artery (PDA) with TIMI I flow, and 90% SVG-to-D1 lesion. His EF is 55% with 2–3+ MR. SVG to PDA is thought to be the culprit lesion, and successful PCI is performed using emboli filter device and stent. His general cardiologist would like you to fix his SVG to D1 lesion as well. Do you agree?

(A) Yes, in light of his heart failure symptoms, it is best to open all significant lesions based on the SHOCK trial
(B) No, elective PCI should not be performed in a non–infarct-related artery at the time of primary PCI of the infarct-related artery in patients without hemodynamic compromise
(C) Yes, elective PCI should be performed in a non–infarct-related artery at the time of primary PCI of the infarct-related artery in patients without hemodynamic compromise
(D) No, the patient is over the age of 75. In the SHOCK trial, multivessel revascularization was only beneficial in patients younger than 75 years of age

38.5   A 46-year-old male with a history of hyperlipidemia and tobacco use presents with chest pain for 3 months. He undergoes a stress thallium test where he exercised to 11 METS and at stress showed a large anterior wall ischemic defect. His EF is 70%. The patient undergoes cardiac catheterization, which shows 75% mid LAD, noncalcified, and nontortuous stenosis. The lesion appears to be low risk. He is scheduled for PCI at the same hospital. While you are explaining the risks and benefits of PCI, he becomes concerned about the risk of possible urgent CABG. What is the exact percentage of this risk?

(A) ≤1%
(B) 2% to 3%
(C) 4% to 5%
(D) ≥5%

38.6   The same patient undergoes successful PCI to LAD with sirolimus-eluting stent and is now ready for discharge. Your nurse practitioner asks about discharge medications. The patient and his wife are extremely worried about bleeding complications after reading about clopidogrel. They want a minimal duration on antiplatelet therapy. Based on current recommendations, what should his oral antiplatelet regimen be?

(A) Aspirin 325 mg daily for 1 month and then aspirin 81 mg daily for life and clopidogrel 75 mg a day for at least 3 months

(B) Aspirin 81 mg daily for life and clopidogrel 75 mg daily for 3 months

(C) Aspirin 325 mg daily for 1 month and then aspirin 81 mg daily for life and clopidogrel 75 mg daily for at least 9 months

(D) Aspirin 81 mg daily for life and clopidogrel 75 mg daily for 12 months

38.7 A 54-year-old woman presents to the ER with chest pain and is found to have nonspecific ST-segment changes in leads II, III, and aVF and a troponin I level of 2.3 ng/mL. Her medical history is notable for morbid obesity, diabetes, hypertension, history of TIA, and active smoking. She is given aspirin 325 mg and 5,000 units of IV heparin in the ER. She is taken immediately to the catheterization laboratory. Her diagnostic catheterization reveals a 99% mid RCA stenosis with a 60% proximal LCX lesion, and a 60% mid LAD lesion. You proceed with PCI of the RCA. The best antiplatelet and antithrombotic regimen for this patient prior to PCI based on the current body of evidence would be:

(A) Prasugrel 60 mg and bivalirudin

(B) Heparin, clopidogrel 600 mg load, and GP IIb/IIIa inhibitor

(C) LMWH, prasugrel 60 mg loading, and GP IIb/IIIa inhibitor

(D) Bivalirudin only

38.8 A 78-year-old retired cardiologist with a history of CABG in 1990 and 1999 presents to your office with increasing chest pain with exertion. He undergoes a cardiac catheterization and is found to have severe ostial SVG-to-LCX disease, patent LIMA to LAD, patent SVG to PDA but with a significant distal SVG lesion. Other grafts are patent without significant disease including SVG to D1 and SVG to LCX. His SVG to LCX is from his 1990 surgery and SVG to PDA is from his 1999 surgery. You proceed to intervene upon SVG to LCX and SVG to PDA. He wants to talk about his chances of final patency. In both lesions, there is diffuse disease, but the lesions are not friable or degenerative. You state:

(A) Patency rates are the same for both grafts

(B) The older graft has less likelihood of patency

(C) Patency rates are equivalent since emboli protection devices will be used for both grafts

(D) The lesion location is a predictor of final patency with ostial lesions having a lower likelihood of patency

(E) The lesion location is a predictor of final patency with distal lesions having a lower likelihood of patency

38.9 You are called to evaluate a 69-year-old woman with ST-segment elevation in the anterior leads. She underwent CABG 3 days ago including LIMA to LAD, SVG to OM2, SVG to PDA, and SVG to posterior lateral branch (PLB). She was doing well until 3 hours ago when she started complaining of chest pain. In the catheterization laboratory, she is found to have a 90% stenosis at the anastomosis of the LIMA to LAD graft. You should:

(A) Proceed to balloon dilatation

(B) Proceed to balloon dilatation and stent placement

(C) Proceed to open native LAD

(D) Do not perform PCI since it is not safe to proceed with PCI so soon after CABG

38.10 A 74-year-old female presents to an outside ER with respiratory failure. She was found in severe respiratory distress by the paramedics and was intubated in the field. According to her husband, she started experiencing chest pain 2 hours ago. She has a history of hypertension and hyperlipidemia and has been healthy until 2 hours ago. According to the ER physician, her blood pressure is 80/60 on IV norepinephrine, and her heart rate is 110. Her ECG shows 5-mm ST elevation in the anterior leads. The emergency room, located 3 hours from your hospital, has a catheterization laboratory. The ER physician is certified to place an intra-aortic balloon pump (IABP). What should be done next?

(A) Fibrinolytic therapy if there are no contraindications and emergency transfer

(B) No fibrinolytic therapy and emergency transfer

(C) Intraaortic balloon pump and emergency transfer

(D) Fibrinolytic therapy, IABP, and emergency transfer

38.11 The patient in Question 10 is transferred to your hospital. You are waiting for her in the catheterization laboratory. She still has ST elevation, and she is still on IV norepinephrine with blood pressure of 80/60 and heart rate of 120. She undergoes emergent catheterization and is found to have multivessel disease with chronically occluded long RCA stenosis, 80% lesion type A lesion in a moderate size LCX artery, and a 100% LAD lesion. The proximal LAD is filled with thrombus but is a PCI-approachable lesion. What should be done next?

(A) Proceed with multivessel PCI, and plan on PCI to LAD and LCX
(B) Proceed with infarct-related artery PCI only
(C) Refer to CABG
(D) Proceed with LAD PCI and if there is no improvement then PCI to LCX

38.12 A 79-year-old male presented to an outside hospital 3 days ago with chest pain for 10 hours. At that time, he had ST-segment elevation in the inferior leads and received fibrinolytic therapy because he did not want to be transferred to another hospital. At that time his BP was 130/80 with HR of 94, and he did not have a physical exam consistent with heart failure. With fibrinolytic therapy, there was no ST resolution, and he continued to have chest pain, which is resolved in 6 hours. His peak troponin was 6.5 ng/mL. Currently, he is doing well without chest pain, and there has been no ST depression on his monitor. His children want him to undergo catheterization. His general cardiologist performed an angiogram that showed 100% PDA lesion, moderate diffuse 50% lesion in LAD, and LCX and inferior hypokinesis on LV gram. They would like you to intervene on his RCA. The patient's daughter, a nurse, wants to know if PCI will improve his prognosis. What do you think?

(A) Extrapolating from NSTEMI data, there is reason to believe that invasive therapy will decrease major adverse cardiac events in these patients
(B) There are no convincing data to support the routine use of late adjuvant PCI days after failed fibrinolysis in patients who are hemodynamically and electrically stable without any evidence of ischemia
(C) On the basis of observational and experimental data, infarct artery patency favorably influences LV remodeling and electrical stability; therefore, PCI to RCA is recommended
(D) Based on the recent DANAMI trial, PCI of an infarct-related artery resulted in fewer major adverse cardiac events

38.13 You are called to see a patient in the catheterization laboratory. Your partner is doing a catheterization on a 69-year-old male with hypertension and hyperlipidemia who presented with STEMI. The patient received 600 mg of clopidogrel and aspirin and was transferred immediately from the ER. He underwent catheterization and has a lesion in LAD (Fig. Q38-13). He wants to talk about DES vs. bare-metal stent (BMS) in this patient. What is the latest guideline recommendation regarding DES in STEMI patients?

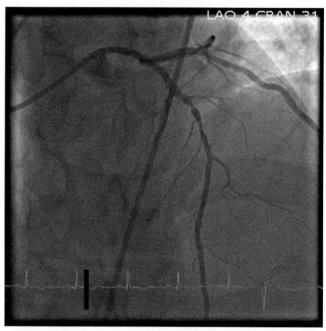

Figure Q38-13

(A) Guideline gives no recommendation on DES vs. BMS in STEMI patients
(B) Guideline gives preference to BMS due to high stent thrombosis rates in STEMI receiving DES
(C) Guideline gives preference to DES due to high repeat revascularization rates in BMS
(D) Guideline recommends that is it reasonable to use DES as an alternative to BMS for primary PCI.

38.14 You are contacted by a lawyer for the plaintiff of a case involving a 57-year-old female catheterization laboratory nurse with acute MI. She presented to the ER within 3 hours of chest pain and was found to have ST-segment elevation anteriorly with reciprocal changes. She was given aspirin 325 mg, 300 mg of clopidogrel, eptifibatide bolus and infusion, and 5,000 U of heparin in the ER. Her blood pressure was 110/70 with HR of 110. She was taken to the catheterization laboratory and found to have 100% occlusion of a large LAD. Her door-to-balloon time was 90 minutes. She underwent successful PCI to LAD with sirolimus-eluting stent. However, subsequently her post-PCI course was complicated by retroperitoneal bleeding that required 2-U blood transfusion and 3 additional days of hospitalization. Also, her EF following PCI was 30%. She is suing because she feels that abciximab should have been used rather than eptifibatide. What is your response?

(A) You agree that based on literature abciximab should have been used because abciximab is superior to other IIb/IIIa inhibitors in STEMI

(B) You think the regimen should be bivalirudin alone since it has the best data

(C) Based on the available literature, IIb/IIIa inhibitors are equivalent in primary PCI

38.15 The same patient is also stating that she should have received fibrinolytic therapy instead of primary PCI. She wants to know what evidence supports PCI vs. fibrinolytic therapy in STEMI?

(A) Primary PCI patients have lower mortality, fewer reinfarctions, and less bleeding

(B) Primary PCI patients have lower mortality, fewer reinfarctions, and more bleeding

(C) Primary PCI patients have similar mortality, fewer reinfarctions, and less bleeding

(D) Primary PCI patients have similar mortality, fewer reinfarctions, and more bleeding.

38.16 The same patient referred to in Question 38.15 also asks for clinical evidence regarding primary PCI with stent vs. balloon angioplasty.

(A) Primary PCIs with stent patients have lower death and reinfarction rates compared to the balloon angioplasty group

(B) Primary PCIs with stent patients have similar death rate as primary balloon angioplasty group but less reinfarction rates

(C) Primary PCIs with stent patients vs. primary balloon angioplasty groups have similar death and reinfarction rates

(D) Primary balloon angioplasty group have lower bleeding rates

38.17 A 75-year-old male smoker presents to the ER with STEMI. He has ECG changes consistent with an inferior wall MI. He is brought to your catheterization laboratory. He has received 325 mg of aspirin, 600 mg of clopidogrel, and heparin in the ER. He undergoes catheterization, and there is an occlusion of the RCA (Fig. Q38-17). He undergoes PCI with bivalirudin. He receives a BMS and does well. During your weekly interventional conference, a question is brought up by your partner that the patient should have received IIb/IIIa based on recent ACC/AHA STEMI guidelines. What is your opinion?

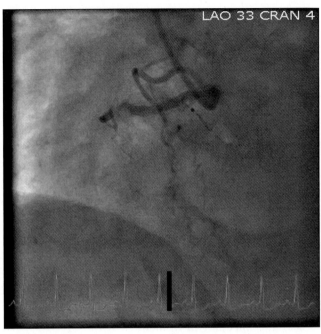

LAO 33 CRAN 4

Figure Q38-17

(A) Based on the guideline, routine IIb/IIIa should be used during STEMI PCI

(B) Based on the guideline, routine IIb/IIIa is not necessarily recommended during STEMI PCI

(C) Based on the guideline, routine IIb/IIIa use is recommended only if the patient received 300 mg of clopidogrel loading

38.18 You have recently been elected to the quality review board of your hospital. They are reviewing a protocol of cardiac biomarker (CK-MB, troponin I or T) blood draws after every PCI. They are being pressured by insurance companies to stop this procedure. Based on current data, what are the recommendations?

(A) Biomarkers should not be drawn since they add little value to prognosis or diagnosis of the patient

(B) All patients who have signs or symptoms suggestive of MI during or after PCI and those with complicated procedures should have biomarkers measured after the procedure only. Routine measurement is not recommended

(C) Only in patients who are admitted with STEMI, NSTEMI, or unstable angina

(D) In addition to patients who have signs or symptoms suggestive of MI during or after PCI and those with complicated procedures, routine measurement in all patients undergoing PCI is reasonable 8 to 12 hours after the procedure

38.19 A 71-year-old woman with a history of CABG in 2003 undergoes SVG-to-D1 intervention due to unstable angina. The intervention was performed with an emboli filter device, abciximab, and bare-metal 5.0/18 mm stent. PCI was uneventful; however, 3 hours after the case she complains of abdominal pain, and her BP is 70/50 with HR of 110. Her Hgb that was 12 g/dL at the start of PCI is now 8.8 g/dL. Due to her profound hypotension, she requires 2 U of blood transfusion. She stabilizes and is discharged home 3 days later. She does well; however, she is angry about her complication. She states that she bled from abciximab administration and that you should have never used abciximab because it is known to cause more major bleeding in women. Which of the following statements is CORRECT?

(A) Abciximab causes more major and minor bleeding in women

(B) Abciximab causes more major bleeding but similar rates of minor bleeding in women

(C) Abciximab causes similar major bleeding but more minor bleeding in women

(D) Abciximab does not cause more major or minor bleeding in women

38.20 A 63-year-old diabetic hospital administrator presents to your office for a second opinion. She has been experiencing increasing dyspnea on exertion and had a stress echocardiogram that showed a left ventricular ejection fraction (LVEF) of 55% and lateral ischemia. She exercised for only 6 minutes. She underwent catheterization and was found to have three-vessel disease with a 90% focal proximal LAD bifurcation lesion that involves a large-sized diagonal artery, an LCX with mild disease but extremely (110 degrees) angulated, a 90% moderately tortuous OM2 lesion, a 95% distal diffuse RCA lesion that measures 15 mm, and a 100% chronically occluded PDA and PL branch with bridging collaterals. She was offered CABG; however, she is adamant that she does not want CABG unless her lesions are high risk. Which of these lesions is high risk?

(A) All of them
(B) All except the OM2 lesion
(D) All except the distal RCA lesion
(D) All except the proximal LAD lesion

38.21 A 49-year-old trial lawyer presents to your office for a consultation. He has a family history of heart disease and has been on simvastatin for several years. He is not a diabetic and has no history of congestive heart failure. After recently experiencing chest pain at work, a stress test showed inferior and lateral ischemia at peak stress. He underwent catheterization and was found to have three-vessel disease with normal LV function. He has 80% mid LAD, and 90% LCX and 95% RCA lesions. The lesions are amenable to PCI, but he has heard about minimally invasive CABG and is interested. He has been emotionally debilitated since his catheterization and feels that he needs to proceed with whatever mode of revascularization is going to make him live longer and have fewer heart attacks. What do you recommend?

(A) CABG. Mortality and morbidity are lower with CABG in three-vessel disease

(B) CABG. There is no difference in mortality between CABG and PCI; however, the PCI group has more myocardial infarctions later

(C) Either one. There is no difference in mortality or myocardial infarction rate between the two

(D) CABG due to LAD disease. Only if LAD is involved is CABG superior to PCI in terms of lower mortality and morbidity

38.22 A 76-year-old retired acupuncturist presents to your office with increasing shortness of breath. The patient's history is only remarkable for hyperlipidemia for which he uses red rice yeast. He undergoes a stress test and is found to have anterior ischemia, and his catheterization shows a 90% mid LAD lesion with no significant disease in other arteries and a normal ejection fraction. He states that he is willing to take "western medicine" but does not want PCI or CABG. His wife is very concerned about his risk and wants to know which modality is best for long-term survival?

(A) Medical therapy since it is not a proximal LAD lesion

(B) CABG for symptom relief as well as mortality benefit

(C) Either revascularization therapy since either one provides similar mortality benefit over medicine

(D) There is no mortality difference between medical therapy, PCI, or CABG

38.23 A 71-year-old retired executive presents to your office for a second opinion. She underwent a routine stress test at the urging of her primary care provider even though she had no symptoms and was found to have inferior and posterior ischemia. She also underwent ambulatory

ECG monitoring, which also showed ST-segment depression in the inferior and lateral leads. She then underwent cardiac catheterization and was found to have a nondominant RCA with minimal disease, hyperdominant LCX with a severe 95% proximal stenosis, and minimal disease in her LAD. She was offered PCI and now wants your opinion regarding the matter. What would you tell her?

(A) Angina-guided drug therapy is equivalent to PCI in major adverse cardiac event rates

(B) Angina plus ischemia-guided drug therapy is equivalent to PCI in major adverse cardiac event rates

(C) Revascularization with PCI lowers major adverse cardiac events

(D) There is no difference between either medical therapy or revascularization in terms of major adverse cardiac event rates

38.24 You are asked to provide your opinion regarding on-site PCI privileges for a colleague. He is an experienced, board-certified interventional cardiologist who performed 130 PCIs and 600 diagnostic angiograms last year. He has recently fought with his partners and is opening his own practice at a local community hospital. The community hospital does not have on-site cardiac surgery and is located 40 minutes from the nearest high-volume hospital with on-site cardiac surgery. He wants to start doing diagnostic angiograms and elective PCIs. Based on current literature, what is the recommendation for performing elective PCI in a hospital without surgery backup?

(A) Elective, low-risk PCI may be performed in a hospital without on-site cardiac surgery if it is done by high-volume operators

(B) Elective low- or high-risk PCI may be performed in a hospital without on-site cardiac surgery if it is done by a high-volume operator in a high-volume center

(C) It is not recommended that elective PCI be performed at an institution that does not provide on-site cardiac surgery

(D) Elective PCI may be performed if there is a cardiac surgery program within 90 minutes from the hospital.

38.25 A colleague of yours has been called by the state medical board for violation. He performed primary PCI at a community hospital without on-site cardiac surgery in a 64-year-old female with acute lateral MI. She presented to the hospital with 2 hours of chest pain and was hemodynamically stable. Her catheterization showed 60% LMT, 50% mid LAD, large LCX with proximal 100% occlusion, and nondominant RCA with minimal disease. During her LCX PCI, she went into ventricular fibrillation and died. The patient's family has filed a complaint to the state medical board. They have requested your opinion. What is the current recommendation regarding performing primary PCI without on-site cardiac surgery?

(A) Primary PCI in selected cases by an experienced operator in a well-equipped lab with trained staff is acceptable

(B) Primary PCI should never be performed without on-site cardiac surgery

(C) Primary PCI should be performed by any trained interventionalist on all acute MI patients regardless of whether the hospital has on-site cardiac surgery

38.26 A 46-year-old female physician presents to your office for a second opinion. She underwent a stress test for chest pain and was found to have lateral ischemia. She then underwent catheterization and was found to have diffuse proximal LCX 90% stenosis. Her only risk factors are family history, early menopause, and hyperlipidemia. She is not diabetic. She underwent successful PCI to LCX with 3.5/23 mm Xience DES about 18 months ago. She has been taking clopidogrel and aspirin and has been doing well. She would like to know when she can discontinue clopidogrel. What is the guideline recommendation?

(A) Clopidogrel for ≥ 3 months after DES

(B) Clopidogrel for ≥ 12 months after DES

(C) Clopidogrel for 24 months after DES

(D) Clopidogrel lifelong

38.27 A 68-year-old male nurse presents to your office for a fourth opinion. He underwent RCA PCI a year ago for exertional chest pain, which was complicated by coronary artery dissection. He had a 3.5/18-mm paclitaxel stent placed for mid CA lesion, which was postdilated with a 4.5/15-mm noncompliant balloon since the reference diameter of the RCA was 4.4 mm. After the balloon dilatation, there was a long spiral dissection that required 3 subsequent stents and a loss of PL branch as well as increase in his troponin. Since then he has done well and only has occasional chest pain with heavy exertion. He does not have ischemia on his most recent stress thallium. Nevertheless, he is very upset and feels that they should have never placed a DES. In the trials of bare-metal vs. DESs (such as RAVEL, TAXUS, SIRIUS), what size of vessel required intervention?

(A) 2.0 to 3.5 mm

(B) 2.5 to 4.0 mm

(C) 2.75 to 4.0 mm

(D) 2.75 to 3.75 mm

38.28 A 68-year-old male from Asia presents to your office to establish care. He comes with his son who is his interpreter. He has diabetes, hyperlipidemia, and hypertension. He is on aspirin 325 mg, clopidogrel 75 mg, simvastatin 80 mg, metoprolol 75 mg twice daily, and enalapril 10 mg twice daily. He underwent a catheterization last month where they found 70% proximal LMT disease with minimal disease in LAD, LCX, and RCA. His EF was 65%. He underwent PCI to unprotected LMT with IVUS guidance and a 5.0/12-mm BMS. He denies any chest pain or shortness of breath and feels well. He was told by his physician that he should undergo another cardiac angiogram in 6 months. He does not want to do this since he has no symptoms and is feeling well. He seeks your opinion.

(A) In light of no symptoms and a good medical regimen, he does not need angiogram; he can follow up in 6 months

(B) It is not reasonable to perform catheterization; obtain a stress test and if it is positive, then perform catheterization

(C) It is not reasonable to perform catheterization; obtain an echocardiogram if his ejection fraction is changed, then perform catheterization

(D) It is reasonable to perform catheterization in 6 months

38.29 The same gentleman has been told by his outside physician to get a platelet aggregation study. He had this done at another hospital in your city and was told that there was less than 50% inhibition of platelet aggregation. What should you do next?

(A) Change aspirin 325 mg to twice daily

(B) Switch to ticlopidine

(C) Switch to prasugrel

(D) Add cilostazol to the current regime

38.30 A 63-year-old male presents for preoperative evaluation for back pain. His risk factors include hyperlipidemia, anemia, and hypertension. He undergoes a stress test and has RCA-territory ischemia with LVEF of 50%. He then undergoes catheterization, which shows a severe, diffuse RCA lesion, which is amenable to PCI. This is a type C lesion. He is a Jehovah's witness and does not want any blood products. His baseline

hemoglobin is 9. He had an aspirin load the day prior to catheterization and was given 60 U/kg of heparin and no GP IIb/IIIa inhibitor due to his anemia. His procedural ACT after heparin is 260 using the Hemochron device. Based on literature, what is the optimal ACT for patients not on GP IIb/IIIa inhibitor?

(A) Hemochron 300 to 350 seconds

(B) Hemochron 200 to 250 seconds

(C) Hemochron 250 to 300 seconds

(D) Optimal ACT studies have not been done with Hemochron, only HemoTec device

38.31 A 59-year-old cardiothoracic surgeon with hypertension, hyperlipidemia, and a 20-year smoking history presents to the ER with chest pain for 5 hours. He is found to have nonspecific ST-segment changes and is admitted. He is placed on enoxaparin, aspirin, clopidogrel, atorvastatin, and metoprolol. He no longer has chest pain. He refuses to have a stress test and just wants to have an angiogram. His catheterization shows a severe proximal LAD stenosis. It is amenable to PCI and the decision is made to proceed. You ask for an abciximab bolus and IV, and the nurse wants to know if you would like additional unfractionated heparin since the patient received his enoxaparin 7 hours ago. His ACT is 180 seconds.

(A) Yes, he needs additional 50 U/kg of unfractionated heparin

(B) Yes, he needs to receive his enoxaparin IV now

(C) No, he is within 8 hours of his last enoxaparin dose

(D) No, he is within 12 hours of his last enoxaparin dose

38.32 A 49-year-old diabetic, HIV-positive patient is undergoing PCI to LAD for exertional chest pain. He is on aspirin, pravastatin, ezetimibe, protease inhibitors, and metoprolol and received 300 mg clopidogrel load yesterday. He had his diagnostic catheterization a week ago by a general cardiologist and presents to you now for PCI. He has a chronically occluded large LCX that is being fed by a diffusely diseased LAD. The mid LAD lesion is tortuous and diffusely calcified and diseased. He is adamantly refusing CABG and wants you to be aggressive and fix his disease. You decide to use bivalirudin and GP IIb/IIIa infusion during PCI due to the large myocardium at risk. You are able to cross the lesion after multiple attempts. The case is very time-consuming. During the case, the nurse tells you his ACT is 450. You would:

(A) Hold bivalirudin infusion and recheck in 5 to 10 minutes

(B) Continue bivalirudin infusion but stop tirofiban infusion

(C) Stop both bivalirudin and GP IIb/IIIa infusion

(D) Continue both bivalirudin and tirofiban infusion

38.33 You are asked to be an expert witness in a case involving the death of a 56-year-old male diabetic with hypertension, hyperlipidemia, and CKD. He presented to another hospital with 2 hours of chest pain on a Friday night. His ECG at time of presentation showed ST depression and T wave flattening. He was given aspirin, loaded on 600 mg of clopidogrel and NTG with prompt resolution of his chest pain. His first set of enzymes was negative and his second set of troponin T 0.02 ng/mL. He was admitted to the hospital and started on IV heparin. His third set of troponin T was 1.26 ng/mL. CKMB was not done. His echocardiogram during the weekend shows EF of 30%. He was taken to the catheterization laboratory on Monday morning and found to have severe three-vessel disease. He underwent CABG, and during CABG he expired. The case centers around when the patient should have been taken to the catheterization laboratory.

(A) There is no difference in mortality between patients who underwent catheterization early (<24 hours) vs. late (>36 hours)

(B) Patients taken to the catheterization laboratory early (<24 hours) had improvement in death or MI

(C) Patients taken to the catheterization laboratory early (<24 hours) had less death, MI, or refractory ischemia

(D) Patients taken to the catheterization laboratory early had less troponin elevation based on ABOARD study

38.34 You are reviewing a case for your hospital intervention program. You notice that a particular colleague of yours is doing FFR with every case. You are asked to assess a case of a 79-year-old patient who is hypertensive by the hospital review board. She underwent stress testing that showed large lateral wall ischemia in setting of increasing shortness of breath and chest pain. She underwent catheterization with the following angiogram (Fig. Q38-34). The patient then underwent FFR, which showed 0.61. She then had DES to the artery. The review board wants to know the evidence of using FFR in this setting. Based on your reading of the guideline, what would you say?

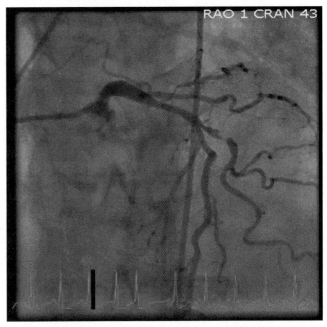

Figure Q38-34

(A) Based on the guidelines, FFR is indicated even with positive stress test, given the high false-positive rate of the stress test

(B) Based on the guideline, there is no role for routine FFR in the setting of angiographic disease in the same vascular distribution as a positive unequivocal stress test

(C) The guidelines make no mention of FFR and stress test. Thus, no recommendation can be made

38.1 **Answer C.** The IVUS of the LMT shows area of 6.7 mm². Therefore, since it is <7.5 mm², she should undergo CABG.

38.2 **Answer A.** There are no data to support PCI in an asymptomatic patient with Class I angina. This patient has no evidence of ischemia in the moderate LCX artery distribution and already had an exercise stress test that showed no evidence of ischemia. Although adding clopidogrel therapy might seem reasonable, there is no evidence to support its routine use in an asymptomatic patient. This is a Class III indication for PCI.

38.3 **Answer C.** There are no data on IVUS and clinical event rates with normal FFR. There is evidence of low clinical event rates at 2 years with normal FFR. Therefore, there is no need for PCI. This is a Class III indication.

38.4 **Answer B.** This patient is not in cardiogenic shock, does have frank heart failure, and does not have hemodynamic compromise. Therefore, elective PCI should not be performed in a non–infarct-related artery at the time of primary PCI. This is a Class III indication for PCI in the 2005 ACC/AHA guidelines.

38.5 **Answer A.** Multiple large-scale registries and prospective studies show the need for emergent CABG to be <1%.

38.6 **Answer D.** Based on the new guideline, patients with DES should be on aspirin 81 mg indefinitely and 75 mg of clopidogrel for at least 12 months. The aspirin dose was based on the CURRENT-OASIS 7 trial.

38.7 **Answer B.** History of CVA or TIA is a contraindication to prasugrel use. The guideline gives a broad range of clopidogrel loading, 300 mg or 600 mg, as being acceptable. One dose over another is not specified.

38.8 **Answer D.** Final patency after PCI is greater for distal SVG lesion than for ostial or mid SVG lesions. Stenosis location appears to be a better determinant of final patency than graft age or the type of interventional device used.

38.9 **Answer A.** Based on case reports, balloon dilatation across suture lines has been accomplished safely within days of surgery. Recurrent ischemia early postoperatively reflects graft failure and may occur in both saphenous vein and arterial graft conduits. Urgent coronary angiography is indicated to define the anatomic cause of ischemia and to determine the best course of therapy. Emergency PCI of a focal graft stenosis may successfully relieve ischemia is the majority of patients. This is a Class I indication.

38.10 **Answer D.** Fibrinolytic therapy is recommended if there is a more than 90-minute delay to PCI, 3 hours prior to onset of STEMI symptoms, and no contraindication to fibrinolytic therapy. IABP is recommended when shock is not quickly reversed with pharmacologic therapy, as a stabilizing measure for patients who are candidates for further invasive care.

38.11 **Answer C.** Early mechanical revascularization with PCI/CABG is a Class I recommendation for candidates younger than 75 years of age with ST elevation who develop shock less than 36 hours from STEMI and in whom revascularization can be performed within 18 hours of shock. In the SHOCK trial, the average patient underwent 2.3-vessel revascularization. A more thorough revascularization should be attempted in patients who have shock. Therefore, in light of chronic total occlusion of RCA, CABG would provide more complete revascularization (Fig. A38-11).

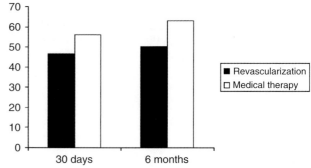

Figure A38-11. Mortality rate (%) in SHOCK trial at 30-days (46.7% vs. 56.0%) and 6 months (50.3% vs. 63.1%).

38.12 **Answer B.** This is a Class III indication for PCI. There are no data to date that support routine use of PCI days after failed fibrinolysis in patients who are hemodynamically and electrically stable and who do not have ischemia. DANAMI tested the hypothesis of PCI in patients who have spontaneous or inducible angina after STEMI. Our patient does not fit the criteria. Also, the OATS study shows no benefit of opening CTO.

38.13 **Answer D.** The 2009 Guideline for ST elevation MI states that DES is a reasonable alternative to BMS for primary PCI. There appears to be no difference between BMS and DES in mortality or MI rates and no difference in stent thrombosis risk. The major advantage of DES over BMS was reduction of TVR rates.

38.14 **Answer C.** Two meta-analyses of randomized trials were published that compared abciximab with small molecule IIb/IIIa inhibitors in primary PCI patients. In both studies, there was no statistical difference in 30-day mortality and reinfarction between the two groups.

38.15 **Answer B.** Primary PCI patients have lower mortality, fewer reinfarctions, and fewer hemorrhagic strokes. They do have higher overall bleeding rates (Fig. A38-15).

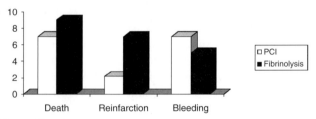

Figure A38-15

38.16 **Answer C.** Primary PCI with stent patients vs. primary balloon angioplasty groups have similar death and reinfarction rates. Restenosis rates are lower with stents.

38.17 **Answer B.** Based on a recent 2009 STEMI guideline, use of IIb/IIIa is given a Class IIa recommendation, meaning it is a reasonable therapeutic consideration.

38.18 **Answer D.** All patients who have signs or symptoms suggestive of MI during or after PCI and those with complicated procedures should have biomarkers measured after the procedure. This is a Class I indication. Routine measurement is a Class IIa indication.

38.19 **Answer C.** The patient had a major bleeding episode in the hospital. Major bleeding in many protocols is defined as intracranial, intraocular, or retroperitoneal hemorrhage or any hemorrhage requiring a transfusion or surgical intervention or that results in a hematocrit decrease of >15% or hemoglobin decrease of >5 g/dL. Abciximab is not associated with an increased risk of major bleeding in women but does increase the rate of minor bleeding.

38.20 **Answer C.** See Table A38-20.

Table A38-20.

Anatomic criteria for high-risk lesion

Diffuse disease—length >2 cm
Excessive tortuosity of proximal segment
Extremely angulated segments, >90 degrees
Total occlusion for longer than 3 mo and/or bridging collateral
Inability to protect major side branches
Degenerated vein grafts with friable lesions

38.21 **Answer C.** ERACI, ARTS, SoS, and BARI have all addressed the question of PCI vs. CABG in patients. This patient is nondiabetic and has three-vessel disease without proximal LAD involvement. Therefore, the totality of data suggests that PCI or CABG would offer similar mortality and myocardial infarction rates. PCI has a higher revascularization rate. The data on DES vs. CABG for multivessel disease again show similar findings of increased revascularization in DES patients compared to CABG.

38.22 **Answer D.** MASS study tested medical therapy, PCI, or CABG in patients with isolated LAD disease. They found similar mortality rates in all groups. Proximal LAD lesion appears to benefit from revascularization; however, mid LAD lesions, such as with this patient, generally have good prognosis. Other trials, such as ACME and RITA-2, have tested medical therapy vs. PCI. They also found no difference in mortality.

38.23 **Answer C.** This scenario was tested in ACIP study. Patients who underwent revascularization had a lower death or MI rate. ACIP suggests that outcomes of revascularization with CABG surgery or PCI are very favorable compared with medical therapy in patients with asymptomatic ischemia with or without mild angina.

38.24 **Answer C.** This is a Class III indication. It is not recommended that elective PCI be performed by either low- or high-volume operators at low- or high-volume centers without on-site cardiac surgery.

38.25 **Answer A.** The guideline recommends that primary PCI for patients with STEMI might be considered in hospitals without on-site cardiac surgery provided that it is done by a high-volume operator with an experienced catheterization team in a well-equipped catheterization laboratory and provided that there is a proven plan for rapid transport to a cardiac surgery operating room in a nearby hospital with hemodynamic support capability for transfer. Also, they recommend avoiding intervention in STEMI hemodynamically stable patients with significant unprotected left main stenosis upstream from an acute occlusion in the left coronary system, extremely long or angulated infarct-related lesions with TIMI 3 flow, infract-related lesion with TIMI 3 flow in stable patients with three-vessel disease, and infarct-related lesions of small or secondary vessels or hemodynamically significant lesions in other than infarct artery.

38.26 **Answer B.** The recommendation is that patients be on aspirin 81 mg indefinitely and clopidogrel for 12 months. The ideal duration is unknown at this time but based on consensus documents, clopidogrel is recommended for ≥12 months. She had a single stent and has no other significant risk factors for stent thrombosis; thus, the answer for this question is ≥12 months.

38.27 **Answer D.** In RAVEL, Taxus, and SIRIUS, patients with 2.75- to 3.75-mm reference diameter were intervened upon. A DES may be considered for use in anatomic settings in which the usefulness, effectiveness, and safety have not been fully documented in published trials. The use of smaller DES postdilated with a much larger-sized balloon for a large-vessel PCI have not been studied. It is a Class IIb indication.

38.28 **Answer D.** The new recommendation from the guideline does not recommend routine angiography to assess LMT stent patency. The prior recommendation for routine angiographic follow-up was deleted.

38.29 **Answer C.** In patients in whom stent thrombosis may be catastrophic or lethal, such as those

with unprotected left main stent, bifurcating left main, or last patent coronary vessel stent, platelet aggregation studies may be considered. Since he does not have contraindication to prasugrel, it is reasonable to switch him. Another reasonable option might be to increase clopidogrel to 150 mg/day and recheck his platelet aggregation study. There are no clinical trials evidencing an optimal approach for such cases.

38.30 **Answer A.** In patients who do not receive GP IIb/IIIa inhibitor, the recommendation based on literature is ACT of 250 to 300 with the HemoTec device and 300 to 350 with the Hemochron device. With GP IIb/IIIa inhibitor, it should be ACT of 200s with either the HemoTec or Hemochron device. The currently recommended target ACT for eptifibatide and tirofiban is <300 seconds during PCI.

38.31 **Answer C.** In patients who received the last subcutaneously administered dose of enoxaparin within 8 hours, no additional anticoagulant therapy is needed before PCI. In patients who received the last subcutaneously administered dose of enoxaparin between 8 and 12 hours before PCI, an additional 0.3 mg/kg dose of enoxaparin should be administered intravenously before PCI.

38.32 **Answer D.** Ecarin clotting time provides a more accurate assessment of bivalirudin-mediated anticoagulation and bivalirudin concentration during PCI than the ACT. The lack of strong correlation between ACT and bivalirudin levels may explain why previous studies have failed to show a relation between bleeding complications and the relatively high ACT values observed in the setting of direct thrombin inhibitors.

38.33 **Answer C.** Based on the TIMAC study, patients with NSTEMI who were taken to the catheterization laboratory early (<24 hours, median time was 14 hours) had less death, MI, or refractory ischemia. However, mortality benefit was not seen. In the ABOARD study, there was no difference in troponin rates between patients taken immediately to the catheterization laboratory vs. delayed therapy.

38.34 **Answer B.** Based on guidelines, this is a Class III indication for FFR. In patients with angina, unequivocal stress test in the same vascular distribution as severe angiographic coronary artery lesion, there is no need for routine FFR.

References

1. ACC/AHA/SCAI 2005 Guideline Update for Percutaneous Coronary Intervention—Summary article: A report of ACC/AHA Task Force on Practice Guideline. *Circulation* 2006;113:156-175.

2. 2009 focused updates: ACC/AHA guidelines for the management of patients with ST elevation MI (updating 2004 guideline and 2007 focused updates) and ACC/AHA/SCAI guideline on percutaneous coronary intervention (updating 2005 guideline and 2007 focused update): A report of the ACC/AHA task force on practice guideline. *J Am Coll Cardiol* 2009;54:2205-2241.

39 ST-Elevation Myocardial Infarction: ACC/AHA Guidelines

Brion M. Winston and David P. Faxon

QUESTIONS

39.1 You are called by the emergency department about a 54-year-old woman with interscapular pain radiating to the left shoulder that began 6 hours ago. She has history of diabetes, hypertension, hyperlipidemia, and tobacco smoking. Per report, her physical exam reveals: blood pressure (BP) 155/70 mm Hg, pulse 71, respiratory rate 18, 98% oxygen saturation on 2-L nasal cannula, normal jugular venous pressure, clear lungs, and normal first and second heart sounds. Her ECG is shown in Figure Q39-1. Which of the following treatment goals is optimal in this patient?

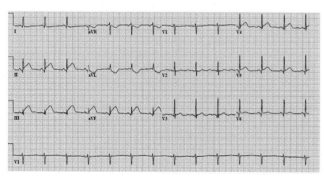

Figure Q39-1

   (A) ED arrival-to-femoral arterial puncture time of <60 minutes
   (B) Total ischemic time of <150 minutes
   (C) Total ischemic time of <180 minutes
   (D) Less than 60 minutes from ED arrival to intravenous bolus of alteplase
   (E) Less than 90 minutes from ED arrival to manual aspiration thrombectomy

39.2 A 57-year-old man with hypertension, who is a current tobacco user, presented to the emergency

department with substernal chest pain. The chest pain started 90 minutes ago and is associated with nausea and diaphoresis. A prior electrocardiogram (ECG) from 1 year ago and his current ECG on presentation are shown in Figure Q39-2A-B. On physical examination his BP is 146/84 mm Hg, with a pulse of 84 bpm. His lungs are clear to auscultation. His neck veins are flat. He has a regular rate and rhythm with no murmurs, rubs, or gallops. He has 2+ pulses in his distal extremities. He is placed on telemetry and is given aspirin 325 mg PO, nitroglycerin 0.4 mg SL, metoprolol 5 mg IV Q5min times three, and started on an IV unfractionated heparin (UFH) drip. He has some relief in his chest pain. The most appropriate next step in this patient's management should include:

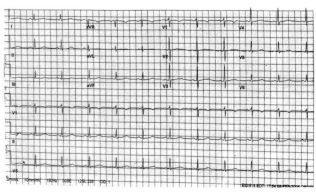

Figure Q39-2A

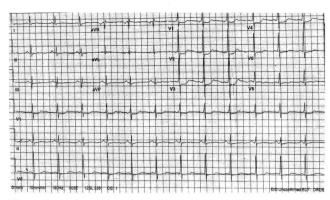

Figure Q39-2B

(A) Initiation of eptifibatide: 180 µg/kg IV bolus, followed by an infusion at 2 µg/kg/min IV and admit to the cardiac care unit

(B) Admission to the cardiac care unit for further monitoring while awaiting results of serial cardiac biomarkers

(C) Order a single photon emission computerized tomography (SPECT) radionuclide imaging stress test

(D) Activate the catheterization laboratory for possible primary angioplasty

39.3 A 49-year-old man with hypertension began experiencing chest "tightness" and shortness of breath while at work as a construction contractor. The patient's father died of a "massive heart attack" at age 52. His coworkers called 911, and the Emergency Medical Services (EMS) arrived on the scene within 10 minutes. Upon arrival, EMS gave the patient a chewable aspirin (325 mg), nitroglycerin SL (0.4 mg), and IV morphine (2 mg). He was started on oxygen 2 L through nasal cannula. Which of these prehospital therapies has been shown to have the most benefit on mortality?

(A) Chewable aspirin (325 mg)

(B) Nitroglycerin SL (0.4 mg)

(C) IV morphine (2 mg)

(D) Oxygen 2 L through nasal cannula

39.4 A 62-year-old male with history of tobacco smoking and hypertension develops sudden onset chest heaviness radiating to both arms while shoveling snow associated with nausea and diaphoresis. His spouse promptly drives him to the emergency department of a hospital with PCI capability. His ECG, obtained 5 minutes after arrival in the ED and approximately 30 minutes after the onset of symptoms, reveals anterolateral ST elevations consistent with myocardial injury. He has no contraindications to PCI or thrombolysis. You are the sole interventionalist available that day and are contacted by the ED physician about this patient

in the middle of a complicated case of elective bifurcation PCI involving rotational atherectomy. You estimate that your ongoing case will require another 50 minutes. In addition to aspirin and clopidogrel, which of the following is the most appropriate advice for the ED physician based on ACC/AHA guidelines for management of STEMI?

(A) Abciximab and heparin with PCI upon completion of your ongoing case

(B) Heparin with PCI upon completion of your ongoing case

(C) Heparin and half-dose alteplase with PCI upon completion of your ongoing case

(D) Heparin and alteplase 15 mg IV bolus followed by a weight-based infusion

39.5 You are called by the emergency department physician about a 76-year-old man who presents with epigastric pain and shortness of breath for the past 10 hours. He has history of right MCA stroke at age 73 with minimal residual deficits, hypertension, hyperlipidemia, tobacco smoking, and family history of premature CAD. He has history of peptic ulcer disease with upper GI bleeding episodes 1 year ago. His examination reveals: 165/85 mm Hg, pulse 82, respiratory rate 22, 98% oxygen saturation on 3-L nasal cannula; his lungs are clear with normal first and second heart sounds and warm extremities. His medications include aspirin 81 mg daily, amlodopine 5 mg daily, and hydrochlorothiazide 12.5 mg daily. His ECG is shown in Figure Q39-5. His telemetry shows paroxysms of wide complex tachycardia. His epigastric pain, shortness of breath, and wide complex tachycardia have improved with aspirin, metoprolol, and morphine. The ED physician states that the patient has expressed a strong preference for coronary artery bypass grafting should he have any blocked arteries because "his brother did very well with surgery." In addition to starting heparin, which of the following strategies in the emergency room is most supported by the ACC/AHA guidelines for STEMI management as you prepare for emergency coronary angiography?

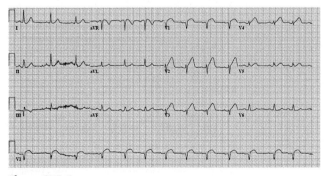

Figure Q39-5

(A) Clopidogrel 600 mg PO × 1

(B) Prasugrel 60 mg PO × 1

(C) Clopidogrel 600 mg PO × 1 and double bolus eptifibatide

(D) Double bolus eptifibatide

39.6 After primary PCI, which of the following findings is associated with the worst mortality?

(A) Thrombolysis in myocardial infarction (TIMI) 2 flow grade

(B) Transient no-reflow

(C) Persistent ST-segment elevation

(D) TIMI 1 myocardial perfusion grade

39.7 Immediate β-blockers should NOT be used in which of the following situations?

(A) Non–ST-segment elevation myocardial infarction

(B) Heart rate (HR) < 70 bpm

(C) Systolic blood pressure (SBP) < 100 mm Hg

(D) Patients undergoing primary PCI

39.8 Which of the following strategies has NOT been shown to reduce door-to-balloon time in management of STEMI?

(A) catheterization laboratory activation by emergency department physician

(B) In-house interventional cardiologist on call

(C) Cath team arrival in <20 minutes from alert

(D) Biannual feedback between catheterization laboratory and emergency department

(E) Emergency department makes a single contact to all members of the cath team

39.9 You receive a call from an intensive care unit physician at a community hospital without PCI capability (but catheterization laboratory is available 20 minutes away) where a 53-year-old woman with family history of premature CAD was admitted with 6 hours of chest pain. Her initial ECG revealed anterolateral ST elevations. She received intravenous alteplase, heparin, nitroglycerine and fentanyl, as well as clopidogrel, aspirin, and metoprolol. Her initial troponin I was 20 times the upper limit of normal. Her chest pain subsided in the first hour after thrombolysis and her ST-segment elevations resolved. Thereafter, her chest pain returns despite increasing doses of nitrates, and she has 0.5-mm re-elevations of the anterolateral ST segments on ECG. BP is 100/60 mm Hg and pulse is 110 bpm. She appears cold and clammy. Which of the following should be done next?

(A) Repeat bolus and infusion of alteplase

(B) Metoprolol 5 mg IV

(C) Immediate transfer to a catheterization laboratory for emergency cardiac catheterization

(D) Intravenous dobutamine 5 µg/kg/h

39.10 A 51-year-old male with history of HIV on antiretroviral therapy and family history of premature CAD is admitted from an outside hospital with an episode of crushing substernal chest pain while walking in his home, which resolved with aspirin, heparin, nitrates, and metoprolol. His initial troponin I is twice the upper limit of normal. His initial ECG revealed small anterolateral T wave inversions. He has another episode of chest pain overnight after transfer to your hospital, while walking to the bathroom, which quickly resolves with rest and his vital signs remain stable. During 6 AM phlebotomy, approximately 18 hours after his initial presentation, he again develops crushing substernal chest pain, shortness of breath, and hypotension. The two ECGs in Figure Q39-10A,B are obtained, and the patient is taken for emergent cardiac catheterization. What is the most likely finding on angiography?

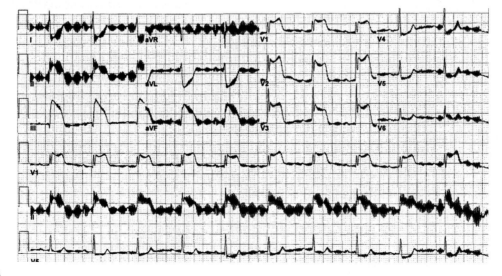

Figure Q39-10A

Right Sided Precordial Leads

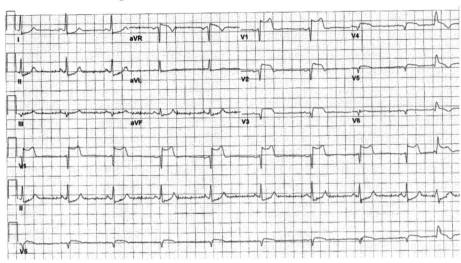

Figure Q39-10B

(A) Total proximal occlusion of a dominant RCA
(B) Coronary spasm of the proximal LAD
(C) Thrombotic lesions of both the LAD and RCA
(D) High grade stenosis of a "wrap-around" LAD
(E) Spontaneous dissection of the left main

39.11 Angiography of the patient mentioned in Question 39.10 is shown in Figure Q39-11A-B. The patient requires dopamine and norepinephrine for hypotension, which persists despite TIMI 3 flow. What is the likely cause of the hypotension?

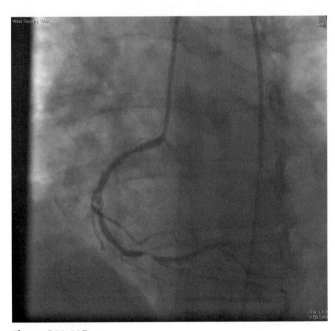

Figure Q39-11B

(A) Retroperitoneal bleed
(B) Multiple culprit lesions requiring treatment
(C) Myocardial stunning
(D) Allergic reaction to contrast

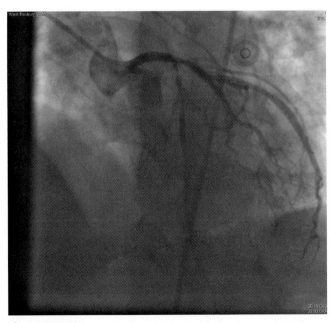

Figure Q39-11A

39.12 Which of the following statements is TRUE regarding facilitated PCI compared to primary PCI?

(A) TIMI flow grade is worse
(B) Major bleeding risk is higher
(C) Mortality risk is lower
(D) Urgent target vessel revascularization rates are lower
(E) Stroke risk is equal

39.13 Which of the following statements about heparin plus a glycoprotein IIb/IIIa inhibitor vs. bivalirudin in STEMI is supported by findings from HORIZONS-AMI?

(A) Stroke risk was lower
(B) Major adverse cardiac event rates are similar
(C) Major bleeding risk is similar
(D) Thrombocytopenia is less common
(E) Revascularization rates were significantly lower for bivalirudin

39.14 Which of the following statements is TRUE regarding patients with STEMI managed with the device depicted in Figure Q39-14 followed by PCI as compared to primary PCI alone?

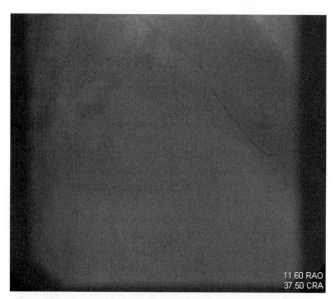

Figure Q39-14

(A) Major bleeding risk is lower
(B) Myocardial blush grade is equal
(C) ST segment resolution occurs over a similar period
(D) Mortality at 1 year is reduced

39.15 A 61-year-old man with history of hypertension, obesity, and tobacco smoking presents to an emergency department of a community hospital without PCI capability with jaw and bilateral arm pain, shortness of breath, and diaphoresis of 5 hours duration. An ECG obtained within 5 minutes of arrival reveals 2-mm anterior ST-segment elevations. On physical examination he is diaphoretic, 105/85, pulse 104, 91% on room air, respiratory rate 21. He has jugular venous distension to 8 cm, bibasilar rales, a normal first and second heart sound, a third heart sound heard best at the apex, no murmurs or rubs, and diminished pedal pulses. He receives aspirin 325 mg,

clopidogrel 600 mg, heparin, and tenecteplase. Which of the following outcomes is more likely if the patient is transferred immediately for PCI at a PCI-capable hospital?

(A) A higher risk of death
(B) A lower risk of cardiogenic shock
(C) A lower risk of reinfarction
(D) A lower risk of new congestive heart failure

39.16 Which of the following patients should be transferred urgently to a PCI capable hospital after thrombolysis based upon the ACC/AHA STEMI guidelines?

(A) All patients
(B) Only high risk patients
(C) Patients at high risk of reinfarction
(D) Patients with new right bundle branch block and left anterior hemiblock

39.17 Which of the following contrast agents is recommended for patients with chronic renal insufficiency undergoing coronary angiography?

(A) Iodixanol
(B) Iohexol
(C) Ioxaglate
(D) All of the above

39.18 A 60-year-old man with hyperlipidemia, hypertension, and diabetes presents with substernal chest pain for 1 hour and the ECG is shown in Figure Q39-18A. On exam his BP is 130/70, pulse 105, and he is breathing at 24/minute, oxygen saturation 98% on 2 L. He is anxious, his lungs are clear, he has a normal first and second heart sound with no rubs, murmurs, or gallops, his jugular venous pressure is not elevated, and his extremities are warm. Coronary angiography is shown in Figure Q39-18B. Which of the following interventions would you recommend for this patient?

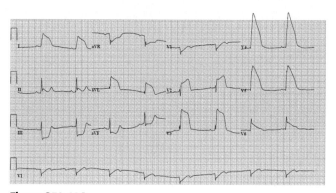

Figure Q39-18A

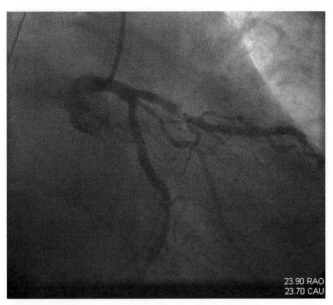

23.90 RAO
23.70 CAU

Figure Q39-18B

(A) A bare-metal stent
(B) A drug-eluting stent
(C) Either a drug-eluting stent or bare-metal stent
(D) Balloon angioplasty only

39.19 Which of the following outcomes occurred in the HORIZONS AMI Trial?

(A) The 1-year stent thrombosis rate was higher for paclitaxel stents
(B) The 1-year major adverse cardiac event (death/MI/Stroke) rate was similar for bare-metal and paclitaxel stents
(C) The rate of ischemic target vessel revascularization was higher in the bare-metal stent group
(D) All of the above
(E) B and C

39.20 A 61-year-old male with hypertension and hyperlipidemia presents to the emergency department with 2 hours of substernal chest pain radiating to his jaw that began during an argument with his wife. His ECG reveals 3-mm ST-segment elevations in leads II, III, and aVF and V5 to V6. On exam he is diaphoretic and anxious, pulse 61 bpm, 105/70 mm Hg in the left arm 118/76 in the right arm, breathing at 16/minute, 98% on 3-L nasal cannula. He has jugular venous distension to 6 mm above the sternal angle. His lungs are clear to auscultation. His point of maximal impulse is nondisplaced; he has a normal S1 and S2 with no rubs, murmurs, or gallops. His distal pulses are 2+ and his extremities are warm

without cyanosis, clubbing, or edema. In the emergency department he is loaded with prasugrel 60 mg before primary PCI. The findings of TRITON TIMI 38 suggest which of the following relative risks for patients such as this one treated with prasugrel instead of clopidogrel?

(A) Stent thrombosis is lower
(B) Death from a cardiovascular cause is similar
(C) Urgent target vessel revascularization is lower
(D) All of the above

39.21 Which of the following statements regarding arterial access in patients undergoing primary PCI for STEMI is supported by the ACC/AHA guidelines?

(A) Transfemoral access is preferred for primary PCI
(B) Transradial access is reasonable for primary PCI
(C) Either is acceptable

39.22 You are called to the emergency department to evaluate a 71-year-old man with history of a pacemaker, hypertension, diabetes, and 6 hours of upper back and nck pain. An ECG obtained within five minutes of ED arrival reveals an ectopic atrial rhythm at 86 BPM with left bundle branch block. You confirm this by placing a magnet over the implanted device. He has received aspirin 162 mg and morphine 2 mg IV. His daughter has stated that the patient has a slow heart rate, but she is unaware of the LBBB through his primary care physician, and that for 2 weeks his father has been complaining of increasing fatigue. On exam he appears uncomfortable, 100/85 mm Hg on the right, 95/80 on the left, pulse 105 and regular, respiratory rate 20 on 3-L nasal cannula, 97% oxygen saturation. His neck veins are distended to 6 cm above the sternal angle. Auscultation reveals trace bibasilar rales, and his cardiac exam reveals a laterally displaced point of maximal impulse, a paradoxically split second heart sound, and II/VI holosystolic murmur loudest at the apex. His feet are cool with 2+ edema to his ankles. Chest x-ray is shown in Figure Q39-22A,B. Which of the following should be done next?

(A) Chest CT with contrast
(B) Coronary angiography
(C) Thrombolysis
(D) Myocardial perfusion imaging
(E) Medical therapy with serial cardiac enzymes

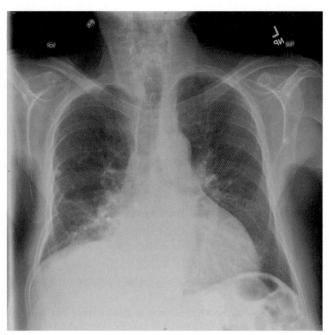

Figure Q39-22A

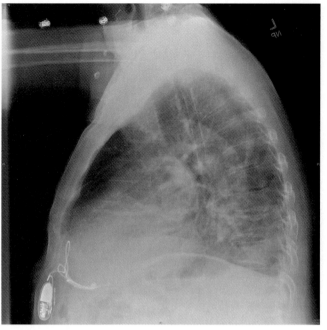

Figure Q39-22B

39.23 A 62-year-old woman with coronary artery disease presents with anterior STEMI and is taken for primary PCI. She has the angiogram shown in Figure Q39-23. At the conclusion of diagnostic catheterization, the patient is dyspneic and restless, her central aortic pressure has fallen to 80/65, and her heart rate has increased to 130 despite initiation of dopamine infusion. She requires emergent endotracheal intubation for hypoxic respiratory failure. Which of the following cardiac assist devices would you recommend based upon the ACC/AHA guidelines?

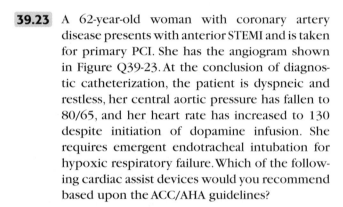

(A) Extracorporeal membrane oxygenation
(B) Percutaneous ventricular assist device
(C) Surgically placed ventricular assist device
(D) Intra-aortic balloon pump

39.24 Which of the following time delays in primary PCI is associated with the highest mortality?

(A) Door-to-balloon time
(B) Door-to-balloon time minus door-to-needle time
(C) Symptoms-to-balloon time
(D) Symptoms-to-door time

39.25 Which of the following interventions to reduce reperfusion injury have been shown to reduce infarct size in humans?

(A) Superoxide dismutase
(B) Glucose–insulin–potassium (GIK) infusion
(C) Pexelixumab (complement inhibitor)
(D) Ischemic preconditioning

39.26 Which of the following patients is most likely to have acute shortness of breath with no chest pain as their presenting symptoms of a STEMI?

(A) A 75-year-old white woman
(B) A 49-year-old white man
(C) A 49-year-old white woman
(D) A 75-year-old African American man

39.27 A 49-year-old man with hypertension presents to the emergency department with 16 hours of severe substernal chest pain. The initial ECG

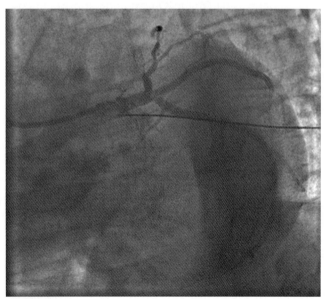

Figure Q39-23

shows Q waves and 1-mm ST-segment elevation in leads V1 to V4. He continues to have 3/10 chest discomfort despite nitroglycerine (NTG) and morphine. On physical examination, his BP is 110/60 with a pulse of 95 bpm. An S3 is present with rales halfway up both lung fields. The monitor shows two 10-beat runs of nonsustained VT at 160 beats/minute. The patient is started on lidocaine. What would be the next step in the management of this patient?

(A) Immediate catheterization and possible PCI
(B) IV β-blocker and IV lasix with medical management
(C) IABP insertion with medical management
(D) PA catheter insertion with medical management

39.28 A 67-year-old woman presents to the emergency department with 4 hours of substernal chest pain and shortness of breath. ECG shows 4-mm ST-segment elevation in II, III, and aVF. Physical examination shows a BP of 140/70 with a pulse of 80 bpm. An S4 is audible. The patient is given aspirin, heparin, SL NTG, and clopidogrel, and is taken to the catheterization laboratory. She is found to have a 99% lesion of the proximal RCA with large clot burden and TIMI 2 flow. The LAD has a 50% midlesion, and first obtuse marginal branch has an ostial 70% lesion. The patient had ventricular ectopy during the contrast injections. The patient is started on abciximab. What additional therapy is indicated prior to primary angioplasty?

(A) IV β-blocker
(B) IV lidocaine
(C) IC tissue plasminogen activator t-PA
(D) IC adenosine

39.29 A 65-year-old man presented to the emergency department with a 2-hour history of "indigestion" and shortness of breath. His ECG showed 2-mm ST-segment elevation in leads II, III, and aVF. He received prompt reperfusion therapy with fibrinolytic agents in addition to aspirin, heparin, and β-blockers. Ninety minutes after the initiation of fibrinolytic agents, his chest pain has resolved and he has minimal residual ST-segment elevation on the repeat ECG. His vital signs have remained stable: BP 126/64 and pulse of 59 bpm. The rhythm in Figure Q39-29 (below) is observed on the telemetry monitor. What medical treatment should be added at this point?

(A) IV amiodarone
(B) IV lidocaine
(C) IV procainamide
(D) Continue to observe

39.30 Primary angioplasty with stenting compared with primary angioplasty with balloon angioplasty alone has been shown to:

(A) Reduce restenosis and target vessel revascularization (TVR)
(B) Reduce restenosis and reinfarction
(C) Reduce restenosis and mortality
(D) Reduce restenosis, mortality and congestive heart failure (CHF)

39.31 A 59-year-old previously healthy woman presented with fatigue and a 4-hour history of chest discomfort. Her ECG demonstrated ST-segment elevations in V3 to V6. She was started on aspirin, heparin, NTG, and metoprolol. Primary PCI was chosen as the strategy for reperfusion. En route to the catheterization laboratory, she became unresponsive. The monitor showed ventricular fibrillation (VF). She was successfully

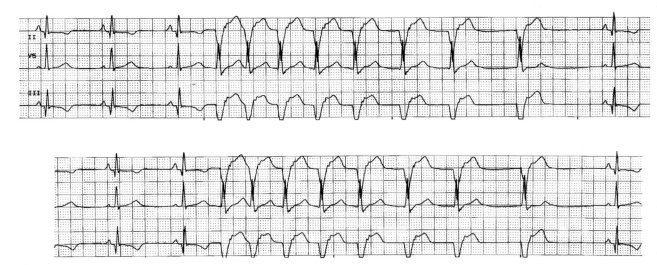

Figure Q39-29

defibrillated with 150 J of biphasic energy. At catheterization, she had a total occlusion of the proximal to mid-LAD. The lesion was stented with an excellent angiographic result with restoration of TIMI 3 flow. A transthoracic echo done 1 day after presentation showed an EF of 30% with hypokinesis of the anterior and lateral walls and apical akinesis. She has had no evidence of recurrent ischemia and no further ventricular arrhythmias. She has no evidence of congestive heart failure. Her medical regimen now includes aspirin, clopidogrel, metoprolol, lisinopril, and atorvastatin. What additional step should be taken in regard to the patient's episode of VF?

(A) Implantable cardioverter defibrillator (ICD) placement before discharge
(B) Electrophysiologic (EP) study before discharge
(C) ICD placement 1 month post discharge
(D) Reassessment of left ventricular (LV) function 40 days post infarct

39.32 According to the ACCF/ASNC/ACR/AHA/ASE/SCCT/SCMR/SNM appropriateness criteria for nuclear imaging, for patients with STEMI who do not undergo primary PCI or angiography, and who remain hemodynamically stable without angina or congestive heart failure, the use of nuclear imaging within 3 months of the infarct is:

(A) Appropriate
(B) Inappropriate
(C) Uncertain

39.33 A 67-year-old woman presents with confusion and shortness of breath that started 8 hours ago. Her ECG shows 3-mm ST-segment elevation and Q waves in II, III, aVF, and V4 to V6. On physical examination, she has no focal neurologic signs. Her BP is 120/80 and pulse 90 bpm. She has minimal crackles at the base of the lung fields. She is given aspirin, IV heparin, SL nitroglycerin, and IV reteplase. Within 30 minutes, the ST elevations have decreased. At 60 minutes, she becomes unresponsive. Her BP is 130/90 and pulse 100 bpm. What should you do now?

(A) Obtain transesophageal echocardiogram (TEE)
(B) Obtain head CT

(C) Take the patient to the catheterization laboratory emergently
(D) Stop heparin and obtain head CT

39.34 Each of the following should be part of the clinical performance measurement of STEMI care as outlined by the ACC/AHA, EXCEPT:

(A) Aspirin at arrival
(B) Beta blocker at arrival
(C) Fasting lipid panel within 24 hours
(D) Adult smoking cessation advice/counseling

39.35 A 41-year-old obese man with no known past medical history presents with chest pain while shoveling snow. ECG obtained on EMS arrival reveals inferolateral STEMI. He remains hemodynamically stable and primary PCI is planned. A point of care glucose measurement obtained in the ambulance was "out of range high," and repeat serum glucose available to you during post dilation of the stent placed to a large first obtuse marginal artery is reported to you as 620 mg/dL (normal 70 to 100 mg/dL). Which of the following statements is supported by the ACC/AHA guidelines?

(A) Insulin should be given to all STEMI patients with glucose > 200 mg/dL to achieve a serum glucose of 70 to 140 mg/dL
(B) An insulin infusion to normalize blood glucose is recommended for patients with STEMI and complicated courses
(C) It is reasonable to use an insulin-based regimen to achieve and maintain glucose levels <180 mg/dL while avoiding hypoglycemia for patients with STEMI with either a complicated or uncomplicated course

39.36 Which of the following agents is recommended as first line therapy for management of chronic musculoskeletal pain in patients post-STEMI?

(A) Acetaminophen
(B) Ibuprofen
(C) Ketorolac
(D) All of the above

39.1 **Answer E.** When thrombolysis is the strategy for management of STEMI, the "door-to-needle" time should be <30 minutes. When primary PCI is the revascularization strategy, the door-to-primary device time should be <90 minutes. This period is commonly referred to as "door-to-balloon" time but would also include first deployment of a manual or mechanical thrombectomy device or direct deployment of a stent. Total ischemic time of <2 hours, and ideally <1 hour, is the overall goal of systems based management of STEMI care and is defined as the onset of symptoms to needle or balloon time (ACC/AHA 2007).

39.2 **Answer D.** The ECG demonstrates a true posterior MI with tall R waves and ST depressions in the right precordial leads (V1 to V2). In addition to standard medical treatment for acute STEMI (aspirin, β-blocker, etc.), a strategy for early reperfusion should be implemented in a timely fashion. The pertinent American College of Cardiology/ American Heart Association (ACC/AHA) guidelines (ACC/AHA 2004 guideline update 2004) are:

- Class I: All STEMI patients should undergo rapid evaluation for reperfusion therapy and have a reperfusion strategy implemented promptly after contact with the medical system (*Level of Evidence: B*).
- Class I: If immediately available, primary PCI should be performed in patients with STEMI (including true posterior MI) or MI with new or presumably new LBBB who can undergo PCI of the infarct artery within 12 hours of symptom onset (*Level of Evidence: A*).
- Class IIa: In the absence of contraindications, it is reasonable to administer fibrinolytic therapy to STEMI patients with symptom onset within the prior 12 hours and 12-lead ECG findings consistent with a true posterior MI (*Level of Evidence: C*).

39.3 **Answer A.** The use of prehospital aspirin is strongly encouraged in patients suspected of having a STEMI as its potential benefits outweigh the risks (*Arch Intern Med* 1996;156:1506–1510). Although empiric treatment of patients with suspected STEMI with morphine, oxygen, nitroglycerin, and aspirin (MONA) is part of the recommended prehospital protocol, aspirin is the only therapy shown to decrease mortality. The sooner aspirin is administered, the greater impact on outcomes. The pertinent ACC/AHA guidelines are:

- Class I: Prehospital EMS providers should administer 162 to 325 mg of aspirin (chewed) to patients with chest pain suspected of having STEMI unless contraindicated or already taken by the patient. Although some trials have used enteric-coated aspirin for initial dosing, more rapid buccal absorption occurs with non–enteric-coated formulations (*Level of Evidence: C*).

39.4 **Answer D.** This patient presents with anterior STEMI shortly after the onset of symptoms (within the "Golden Hour"), during which time the overall benefit for thrombolysis and PCI is greatest and similar. If door to balloon time is expected to exceed 30 minutes in a PCI capable hospital, thrombolysis with concomitant aspirin, clopidogrel, and unfractionated heparin reduces major adverse cardiac events compared to delayed PCI (ACC/AHA class I). A large meta-analysis showed that for every 30 minute delay in primary PCI compared to thrombolysis, mortality increased by 10% (*Circulation* 2006;114:2019–2025). See Figure A39-4. The facilitated PCI strategy of half dose alteplase with planned PCI within 90 minutes has uncertain benefit (ACC/AHA class IIb).

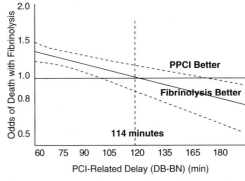

PCI-related Delay and Mortality
NRMI 2-4 (N=192,509, 645 hospitals)

Figure A39-4. Pinto Ds, Kirtane AJ, Nallamothu BK, et al. Hospital delays in reperfusion for ST-elevation...a reperfusion strategy. *Circulation* 2006;114:2019–2025.

39.5 **Answer A.** Loading with clopidogrel or prasugrel as early as possible is recommended for all STEMI patients. If angiography and clinical factors favor a surgical revascularization strategy the thienopyridine should be held for 5 to 7 days before surgery to minimize perioperative bleeding. If a patient for whom surgical bypass is planned develops hemodynamic or electrical instability before the 5 to 7 days "washout" period, the guidelines support earlier operative intervention. Prasugrel is contraindicated in patients with prior stroke or TIA, as the risk of intracranial hemorrhage is higher in these patients (*N Engl J Med* 2007;357:2001–2015). The role for glycoprotein IIb/IIIa inhibitors before coronary angiography in STEMI where PCI is planned is uncertain (ACC/AHA Class IIb), and would pose an additional risk for major bleeding in this patient with prior upper GI hemorrhage.

39.6 **Answer D.** Despite TIMI 3 flow in an epicardial vessel after reperfusion, impaired myocardial perfusion may still be present and is associated with worse outcomes. The TIMI myocardial perfusion grading system (TMPG) or myocardial blush grade is a marker of myocardial perfusion and corresponds to higher mortality rates independent of epicardial flow (*Circulation* 2000;101:125–130). TMPG grade 0 is defined as no apparent tissue-level perfusion (no ground-glass appearance of blush or opacification of the myocardium) in the distribution of the culprit artery. TMPG grade 1 indicates presence of myocardial blush but no clearance from the microvasculature (blush or a stain is present on the next injection). TMPG grade 2 blush clears slowly (blush is strongly persistent and diminishes minimally or not at all during three cardiac cycles of the washout phase). TMPG grade 3 indicates that blush begins to clear during washout (blush is minimally persistent after three cardiac cycles of washout). No-reflow is defined as a profound reduction in antegrade coronary blood flow despite vessel patency and the absence of dissection, spasm, or distal macroembolus. It is presumed to reflect microvascular dysfunction and appears to be more common in diabetic patients. TIMI myocardial perfusion grade is a stronger independent predictor of mortality outcomes in STEMI patients after reperfusion therapy than persistent ST-segment elevations, TIMI flow grade, or the presence of no-reflow. Patients with TIMI grade 2 flow may have a normal TMPG grade secondary to collateral circulation. Patients with both normal epicardial flow (TIMI grade 3 flow) and normal tissue-level perfusion (TMPG grade 3) have an extremely low risk of mortality (*Circulation* 2002;105:1909–1913).

39.7 **Answer C.** SBP < 100 mm Hg. The current ACC/AHA guidelines in regard to immediate administration of β-blockers are:

- Class I: Oral β-blocker therapy should be administered promptly to those patients without a contraindication (*Level of Evidence: B*).
- Class I: Patients with contra-indications to β-blockers in the first 24 hours of STEMI should be re-evaluated for their use (*Level of Evidence: C*).
- Class I: Patients with moderate or severe LV dysfunction should receive β-blockers for secondary prevention, gradually titrated (*Level of Evidence: B*).
- Class IIa: It is reasonable to administer IV β-blockers promptly to STEMI patients without contraindications who are hypertensive (*Level of Evidence: B*).

The following are relative contraindications to β-blocker therapy: HR < 60 bpm, systolic arterial pressure < 100 mm Hg, moderate or severe LV failure, signs of peripheral hypoperfusion, shock, PR interval > 0.24 second, second- or third-degree atrioventricular (AV) block, active asthma, or reactive airway disease. The Clopidogrel and Metoprolol in Myocardial Infarction Trial/Second Chinese Cardiac Study (COMMIT/CCS-2) enrolled 45,852 patients at 1,250 centers (*Lancet* 2005;366:1622–1632). COMMIT/CCS-2 was a randomized, parallel-controlled trial that used a 2 × 2 factorial design to assess the effects of adding 75 mg of clopidogrel (vs. placebo) and the effects of adding the β-blocker metoprolol (vs. placebo) in patients with acute MI on aspirin therapy (162 mg daily). The study enrolled patients with suspected acute MI (ST change or new LBBB) within 24 hours of symptom onset. Patients with shock, SBP < 100 mm Hg, HR < 50 bpm, or second- or third-degree AV block were excluded. The findings on metoprolol showed that giving three intravenous doses of 5 mg metoprolol followed by daily oral doses of 200 mg reduced the relative risks of reinfarction and vascular events by 15% to 20%, but increased the relative risk of cardiac shock by 30%, especially during the first day of treatment. This finding emphasizes that the β-blocker therapy in the setting of acute STEMI should be tailored to the individual patient. In patients at high risk of cardiogenic shock (borderline BP or those presenting in Killip class III), β-blockers should either be delayed until such patients are hemodynamically stable or they should be slowly up-titrated.

39.8 **Answer D.** Feedback between the emergency department and catheterization laboratory regarding efficiency of STEMI care and door-to-balloon times should happen on a real-time basis, within hours or days of the event so that swift system improvements to PCI management are possible. In a multicenter study of 365 acute care hospitals with PCI capability who performed 25 or more PCIs for STEMI annually the following six factors were associated with reduced door-to-balloon times: real time feedback, single call to the cath team, emergency department activation of the cath team, an in-house interventionalist, arrival of the cath team in <20 minutes from the STEMI alert, and having the emergency department physician activate the catheterization laboratory while the patient is enroute (*N Engl J Med* 2006;355:2308–2320).

39.9 **Answer C.** This patient is unstable after thrombolysis for STEMI. Transfer directly to a catheterization laboratory with acute care capability for PCI is indicated for persistent ST elevations 90 minutes after thrombolysis or with clinical instability (*N Engl J Med* 2005; ACC/AHA class I). Based on the SHOCK registry, approximately 5% of patients with STEMI develop cardiogenic shock (*N Engl J Med* 1999;340:1162–1168). STEMI patients with cardiogenic shock should be managed with a primary PCI strategy (ACC/AHA class I). Oral beta blockers are preferred to IV beta blockers due to a higher risk of worsening congestive heart failure and precipitating cardiogenic shock with IV agents (ACC/AHA class I).

39.10 **Answer C.** This patient presents with hyperacute myocardial injury in two major epicardial vascular distributions. The ECG evolves from a current of injury in both the left and right ventricle to a current of injury only in the LAD territory as seen on the second ECG with right precordial leads. With resolution of the ST elevations in II, III, and aVF, the evolution of ST elevations and Q waves in right sided V1 to V6 most likely reflects ongoing left ventricular injury "seen" even from the right precordial leads, and reperfusion of the right ventricle, as opposed to worsening right ventricular injury. Spontaneous left main dissection is more common among pregnant women and young men after vigorous exercise.

39.11 **Answer B.** In a three vessel intravascular ultrasound study of patients presenting with acute coronary syndromes, 79% of patients had plaque rupture apart from the culprit lesion, and 70% of these ruptured lesions were in a non-infarct artery (*Circulation* 2002;106:804–808). The significance of these non-infarct-related laque

ruptures requires further study. Given the persistence of hypotension despite revascularization of the LAD and requirement for vasopressors in this patient, revascularization of the RCA is indicated in this patient as it is a true second, contemporaneous infarct artery. Revascularization of a non-infarct-related artery in the same catheterization laboratory visit as primary PCI for STEMI is associated with a twofold higher 1-year mortality compared to revascularization during a second visit within 60 days of STEMI (*JACC Cardiovasc Interv* 2010;3:22–31). PCI should not be performed in a noninfarct artery at the time of primary PCI in the absence of hemodynamic compromise (ACC/AHA class III).

39.12 **Answer B.** Facilitated PCI is the use of pharmacologic agents, alone or in combination, such as glycoprotein IIb/IIIa inhibitors, high dose heparin, half-dose thrombolysis, or full dose thrombolysis, before PCI in the management of STEMI. Half-dose reteplase with or without abciximab before PCI was associated with more major bleeding than abciximab at the time of PCI, and no improvement in major adverse cardiac event rate (*N Engl J Med* 2008;358:2205–2217). A large meta-analysis showed that facilitated PCI was associated with higher rates of death, stroke, urgent revascularization, reinfarction, and major bleeding, although TIMI flow grade on initial angiography was better in the pharmacologically pretreated patients (*Lancet* 2006;367:579-588). Facilitated PCI has an ACC/AHA class IIb recommendation.

39.13 **Answer B.** The results of HORIZONS-AMI suggest that bivalirudin vs. heparin plus a IIb/IIIa inhibitor in STEMI show no significant difference for major adverse cardiac events or stroke (*N Engl J Med* 2008;358:2218–2230). While thrombocytopenia was significantly more common in the IIb/IIIa inhibitor group, bleeding risk was significantly lower in the bivalirudin group. There was a numerically higher rate of target vessel revascularization in the bivalirudin group which did not reach statistical significance. Supportive use of either heparin with or without a IIb/IIIa inhibitor or bivalirudin at the time of PCI is an ACC/AHA class I recommendation (*Circulation* 2009;120;2271–2306).

39.14 **Answer D.** Manual aspiration thrombectomy with the Export Aspiration Catheter (Medtronic, Minneapolis, MN) has shown superiority to PCI alone with shorter time to ST segment resolution, better myocardial blush grade, and lower 1-year mortality (*N Engl J Med* 2008;358:557–567;

Lancet 2008;371:1915–1920). These benefits were seen despite the angiographic appearance of thrombus, and the majority of aspirates showed platelet rich material. Aspiration thrombectomy in STEMI is supported by an ACC/AHA class IIa recommendation.

39.15   **Answer C.** TRANSFER AMI was a multicenter randomized trial of high risk STEMI patients undergoing thrombolysis at hospitals without PCI capability (*N Engl J Med* 2009;360:2705–2718). After the initiation of tenecteplase, patients were randomized to transfer for PCI as follows: (1) immediate transfer for PCI within 6 hours of thrombolysis; (2) delayed transfer in patients with persistent ST elevations, hemodynamic instability or chest pain; (3) delayed transfer for angiography > 24 hours after thrombolysis in patients with successful reperfusion. This study showed that the immediate and delayed transfer strategies were equivalent with respect to mortality, but reinfarction and recurrent ischemia were significantly less common in the immediate transfer group (Fig. A39-15). Immediate transfer post thrombolysis is an ACC/AHA class IIa recommendation for high risk STEMI patients with marked ST elevations or reciprocal ST depressions, evidence of extensive myocardial injury such as new LBBB or RV infarction, or features of heart failure or cardiogenic shock (*Circulation* 2009;120;2271–2306).

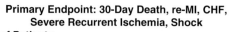

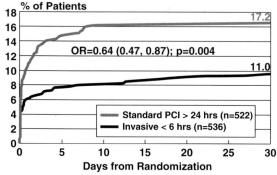

Figure A39-15

39.16   **Answer B.** It is reasonable to transfer high risk patients post-thrombolysis (class IIa). Transfer of non–high-risk patients may be considered (class IIb). The decision to transfer post-thrombolysis must be made on a case-by-case basis where success of pharmacologic reperfusion, patient comorbidities, and patient preferences are weighed.

39.17   **Answer A.** Isosmolar and lower-molecular-weight contrast agents have a class I recommendation for angiography in patients with chronic kidney disease not undergoing dialysis. Iodixanol is a low-molecular-weight agent associated with less contrast-induced nephropathy than iohexol and ioxaglate (*Circulation* 2007;115:3189–3196; *J Am Coll Cardiol* 2006;48:924–930).

39.18   **Answer C.** This ECG reveals a marked anterolateral current of injury with reciprocal inferior ST depressions consistent with evolving acute anterolateral MI. This patient's angiogram reveals a thrombotic 90% lesion in the proximal LAD. A bare-metal stent for STEMI is preferred in patients with bleeding conditions, poor medication compliance, or difficulty with medication access due to the requirement for long term dual antiplatelet therapy. A drug-eluting stent is a reasonable alternative to a bare-metal stent in STEMI patients (class Ia). For patients with diabetes, long lesions, or small vessels a drug-eluting stent should be considered. Either a bare-metal or drug-eluting stent would be reasonable in this patient based on his ability to comply with prolonged dual antiplatelet therapy.

39.19   **Answer E.** HORIZONS AMI, in addition to comparing bivalirudin with heparin and a glycoprotein IIb/IIIa inhibitor for STEMI, also compared paclitaxel-eluting stents with bare-metal stents in a 3:1 randomization (*N Engl J Med* 2009;360:1946–1959). The paclitaxel stent arm had less target vessel revascularization and a similar rate of death or recurrent MI compared to the bare-metal stent arm. Stent thrombosis was similar (Fig. A39-19).

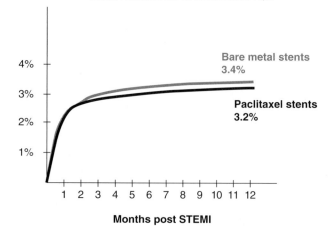

Figure A39-19.   Adapted from Stone GW, Lansky AJ, Pocock SJ, et al. Paclitaxel-eluting stents versus bare-metal stents in acute myocardial infarction. *N Engl J Med* 2009;360:1946–1959

39.20 **Answer D.** Use of prasugrel vs. clopidogrel in STEMI is associated with lower risk of the combined primary end point of death from cardiovascular causes, nonfatal MI, or nonfatal stroke (*N Engl J Med* 2007;357:2001–2015). Prasugrel is also associated with a lower risk of stent thrombosis and urgent target vessel revascularization. There is a higher rate of major non–CABG-associated bleeding with prasugrel. The number needed to treat for benefit over clopidogrel was 46. The number needed to harm was 167 (Fig. A39-20). Prasugrel 60 mg should be given as early as possible for STEMI patients (ACC/AHA 2009 class Ib).

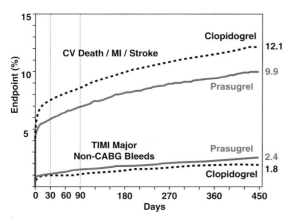

Figure A39-20. Adapted from Wiviott SD, Braunwald E, McCabe CH, et al. Prasugrel versus clopidogrel in patients with acute coronary syndromes. *N Engl J Med* 2007;357:2001–2015

39.21 **Answer C.** The ACC/AHA guidelines do not make specific recommendations for arterial access in primary PCI. While transfemoral access is most commonly used for primary PCI, there are multiple randomized studies showing similarity with transradial access for procedural time and procedural success, and a lower incidence of bleeding complications (*Heart* 2010;96:1341–1344). The impact on major adverse cardiac events of transradial access is not clear, but appears to be no worse than for transfemoral access (Fig. A39.21).

39.22 **Answer B.** Given his advanced age and risk factors for coronary artery disease the pre-test likelihood of obstructive coronary artery disease in this man is high. A new LBBB is a STEMI equivalent and an ACC/AHA class I indication for primary PCI or thrombolysis. PCI is preferred over thrombolysis except where this would require delay, where vascular access is difficult, and where PCI staff is not skilled for acute MI care (ACC/AHA guidelines, 2004). This chest x-ray reveals cardiomegaly and increased pulmonary vascularity as well as a subxiphoid permanent pacemaker. The chronicity of the LBBB in this case is in doubt so immediate thrombolysis would be inappropriate. Further testing with emergent diagnostic angiography is the best answer.

Transradial vs. transfemoral access in primary PCI

Study name	N	Minutes (TRA vs TFA)	Success (%) (TRA vs TFA)	Bleeding (%) (TRA vs TFA)	30 day MACE (%) (TRA vs TFA)
TEMPURA	149	44 vs 51	96 vs 97	0 vs 2.8	17.8 vs 24.2
FARMI	114	45 vs 39	91 vs 96	5.3 vs 7.1	–
Vazquez-Rodriguez et al	439	21 vs 18	91 vs 93	0.5 vs 2.2	5.9 vs 6.4
RADIAL AMI	50	49 vs 47	96 vs 100	4 vs 16	0 vs 4.1
Li et al	370	56 vs 55	95 vs 94	1 vs 3.8	–
RADIAMI	100	58 vs 55	100 vs 98	6 vs 14	–
Yan et al	103	44 vs 41	97 vs 96	1.8 vs 13.1	5.3 vs 6.5

Figure A39-21. Reproduced from Amoroso G, Kiemeneij F. Transradial access for primary percutaneous coronary intervention: the next standard of care? *Heart* 2010;96:1341–1344, with permission from BMJ Publishing Group Ltd.

39.23 **Answer D.** This angiogram reveals stent thrombosis of the LAD. The 2004 ACC/AHA guidelines acknowledge the potential utility of all the devices listed for the management of STEMI complicated by cardiogenic shock. However, only the intra-aortic balloon pump is specifically recommended (class Ib) and is also widely available.

39.24 **Answer C.** Symptoms-to-balloon time. Symptom onset to balloon inflation represents the true ischemic time in patients undergoing primary PCI. De Luca et al. demonstrated that for every 30-minute delay from the onset of symptoms to balloon inflation, the risk of 1-year mortality is increased by 7.5% (*Circulation* 2004;109:1223–1225). Figure A39-24 depicts this relationship between ischemic time and 1-year mortality (the dotted line represents 95% confidence intervals of predicted mortality).

Ischemic Time and Mortality in 1° PCI

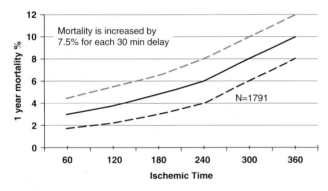

Figure A39-24. **DeLuca et al.** *Circulation* **2004;109:1223–1225**

39.25 **Answer D.** Ischemic preconditioning is the phenomenon in which brief nonlethal episodes of ischemia protect the myocardium before a subsequent prolonged ischemic event through a variety of adaptive physiologic measures. This concept was initially described in animal models, but it has subsequently been described in humans and shown to decrease infarct size. It likely accounts for some of the cardiovascular benefit seen in individuals who exercise. Superoxide dismutase is an endogenous free radical scavenger that has been studied in a variety of animal models of reperfusion injury. To date, no human studies have shown a reduction in infarct size. The effects of GIK therapy were studied in the CREATE-ECLA trial (*JAMA* 2005;293:437–446). Patients presenting with STEMI within 12

hours of symptom onset were randomized to GIK infusion or placebo. There was no difference in all-cause mortality, cardiac arrest, cardiogenic shock, or reinfarction. Pexelizumab is a monoclonal antibody against C5 complement and functions to inhibit the activation of the complement system. Complement activation is a mediator of inflammatory damage seen with reperfusion injury. In the COMMA trial (*Circulation* 2003;108:1184–1190), pexelizumab was administered (bolus alone or bolus plus infusion) to patients with STEMI undergoing mechanical reperfusion. Administration of this monoclonal antibody failed to show a reduction in infarct size, but patients receiving the bolus plus infusion showed a significant reduction in 90-day mortality. Other agents have also been unsuccessful in clinical trials. This includes monoclonal antibodies against white cell CD11/18 integrin receptors, calcium channel blockers, the Na/H exchange inhibitor, cariporide, the K_ATP channel opener, nicorandil, and adenosine. Whereas adenosine showed benefit following thrombolysis in initial trials, subsequent trials in patients undergoing primary PCI have been negative.

39.26 **Answer A.** McSweeney et al. (*Circulation* 2003;108:2619–2623) retrospectively surveyed a group of women diagnosed with acute MI to determine the symptoms at presentation. In this cohort of predominantly white women, the most frequent presenting symptoms were shortness of breath (58%), weakness (55%), and fatigue (43%). Acute chest pain was absent in 43% of patients. In general, women and the elderly present with more atypical symptoms leading to delays in presentation and diagnosis.

39.27 **Answer A.** This patient is presenting >12 hours after his initial symptoms. However, he has evidence of heart failure, electric instability, and persistent symptoms. An emergent cardiac catheterization should be performed. The pertinent ACC/AHA guidelines are:

- Class IIa: It is reasonable to perform primary PCI for patients with onset of symptoms within the previous 12 to 24 hours and one or more of the following:
- Severe CHF (*Level of Evidence: C*)
- Hemodynamic or electrical instability (*Level of Evidence: C*)
- Persistent ischemic symptoms (*Level of Evidence: C*).

39.28 **Answer A.** Administration of β-blockers in the acute phase of a STEMI diminishes myocardial oxygen demand, reduces systemic arterial pressure, and reduces myocardial contractility. β-Blockers are part of the standard of care for STEMI management except for scenarios reviewed in Question 39.7. Through a reduction in HR and prolongation of diastole, β-blockers are thought to augment myocardial perfusion. β-Blockers have been shown to decrease the size of infarction, decrease the rate of reinfarction, and decrease the frequency of life-threatening ventricular arrhythmias regardless of the reperfusion strategy. Several nonrandomized trials (e.g., PAMI and CADILLAC) have shown improved short- and long-term mortality with pretreatment with β-blockers in patients undergoing primary PCI.

39.29 **Answer D.** The rhythm is an accelerated idioventricular rhythm. This rhythm is frequently seen in the first 12 hours of infarction, but it is not a risk factor for the development of ventricular fibrillation. Accelerated idioventricular rhythms are thought to be related to reperfusion. They should be managed with observation rather than with antiarrhythmic agents. Prophylactic use of antiarrhythmics for treatment of isolated PVCs or nonsustained VT or suppression of accelerated idioventricular rhythm should not be a part of STEMI management (ACC/AHA class III).

39.30 **Answer A.** Compared with PTCA, several studies show that intracoronary stents achieve better immediate angiographic results with a larger arterial lumen. No significant differences in mortality or reinfarction have been observed, but with primary stenting, there is less vessel reocclusion and restenosis, leading to less target vessel revascularization (*J Am Coll Cardiol* 1998;31:1234–1239).

39.31 **Answer D.** This patient has ventricular fibrillation in the setting of acute myocardial infarction. With prompt reperfusion therapy for STEMI and medical optimization in the ensuing weeks, it is likely that her left ventricular function will improve and that her risk of a recurrent lethal arrhythmia is very low. The relevant guidelines come from the ACC/AHA/HRS consensus document (*Circulation* 2008;117:2820–2840).

- Class I: ICD therapy is indicated in patients who are survivors of cardiac arrest due to ventricular fibrillation or hemodynamically unstable sustained VT after evaluation to define the cause of the event and to exclude any completely reversible causes. (*Level of Evidence:A*)
- Class I: ICD therapy is indicated in patients with LVEF ≤ 35% due to prior myocardial infarction who are at least 40 days post–myocardial infarction and are in NYHA functional class II or III. (*Level of Evidence:A*)
- Class I: ICD therapy is indicated in patients with LV dysfunction due to prior myocardial infarction who are at least 40 days post–myocardial infarction, have an LVEF ≤ 30%, and are in NYHA functional class I. (*Level of Evidence:A*)

39.32 **Answer A.** The relevant appropriateness criteria from the ACCF/ASNC/ACR/AHA/ASE/SCCT/SCMR/SNM 2009. Appropriate use criteria for cardiac radionuclide imaging Cardiac Radionuclide Imaging Writing Group et al. *Circulation* 2009;119:e561.

Risk Assessment: Within 3 Months of STEMI:

- Hemodynamically stable, no recurrent chest pain symptoms or no signs of HF
- To evaluate for inducible ischemia
- No prior coronary angiography

39.33 **Answer D.** An abrupt decline in consciousness or other new central nervous system deficit in a patient undergoing thrombolysis is an immediate indication to stop further fibrinolysis, anticoagulation, and antiplatelet agents. PT, aPTT, platelets and fibrinogen should be drawn. STAT brain imaging and consultation with neurology should be obtained. Protamine, cryoprecipitate, fresh frozen plasma, or platelets should be given where clinically indicated. This is based on the algorithm for evaluation of intracranial hemorrhage complicating fibrinolytic therapy for STEMI (ACC/AHA, 2004).

39.34 **Answer B.** ACC/AHA (*Circulation* 2006;113:732–761) inpatient measures are aspirin at arrival, aspirin prescribed at discharge, β-blocker prescribed at discharge, LDL-cholesterol assessment, lipid lowering therapy at discharge, ACEi or ARB for LV systolic dysfunction at discharge, time to fibrinolytic therapy, time to PCI, reperfusion therapy, and adult smoking cessation advice/counseling. Based on new studies, as of November 10, 2008, the ACC/AHA Task Force on Performance Measures has removed the measure "AMI-6" (β-blocker received within 24 hours after hospital arrival) from their list of supported performance measures.

39.35 **Answer C.** Level IIa: It is reasonable to use an insulin-based regimen to achieve and maintain glucose levels < 180 mg/dL while avoiding hypoglycemia for patients with STEMI with either a complicated or uncomplicated course. (*Level of Evidence: B*) (ACC/AHA guidelines, 2009)

39.36 **Answer A.** The pertinent guideline (ACC/AHA 2007 class I) is:

• At the time of preparation for hospital discharge, the patient's need for treatment of chronic musculoskeletal discomfort should be assessed and a stepped-care approach to pain management should be used for selection of treatments. Pain relief should begin with acetaminophen or aspirin, small doses of narcotics, or nonacetylated salicylates. (*Level of Evidence: C*)

40

Ethical Issues and Risks Associated with Catheterization and Interventional Procedures

David C. Booth and Christopher Walters

QUESTIONS

40.1 A 65-year-old man presents to the local emergency department with 2 hours of severe substernal chest pain. The initial 12-lead electrocardiogram (ECG) (Fig. Q40-1) reveals an acute injury pattern with a 2 mm ST-segment elevations in leads II, III, aVF, as well as V_5 and V_6. His blood pressure is 125/75 mm Hg and his heart rate is 90 beats/min and regular. The chest examination reveals rales throughout the lung fields. His pain is mostly relieved by ianntravenous nitroglycerin infusion. There is no on-site cardiac surgery capability at this facility, but a board-eligible interventional cardiologist has recently been added to the medical staff, and an acute interventional program has been initiated at the hospital. The nearest facility with on-site surgery is approximately 30 minutes away by ambulance. What is the appropriate management of this patient?

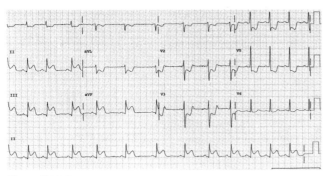

Figure Q40-1

(A) Treat the patient with IV thrombolytic therapy along with routine medical therapy and observe for evidence of reperfusion

(B) Because the patient's discomfort has been largely relieved by intravenous nitroglycerin,

admit the patient to the coronary care unit (CCU) for observation

(C) Proceed with urgent cardiac catheterization for possible coronary intervention

(D) Give thrombolytic therapy and immediately transfer to the nearest facility with both interventional and surgical backup

(E) Transfer immediately to the nearest facility with both interventional capability and surgical backup without initiating thrombolysis

40.2 Your catheterization laboratory is reviewing policy concerning which personnel are qualified to perform coronary interventions. Which of the following statements is FALSE?

(A) A physician must be a full member of the hospital staff to be granted privileges to perform percutaneous coronary intervention (PCI) in the cardiac catheterization laboratory

(B) A primary operator must have completed an accredited fellowship in interventional cardiology and therefore be board-eligible, or must have earned an American Board of Internal Medicine (ABIM) Certificate of Added Qualification in Interventional Cardiology

(C) The primary operator for PCI must have performed >250 coronary interventions in training and must perform >75 PCI per year as primary operator

(D) An invasive cardiologist who has watched or participated in a total of 100 interventional procedures at a neighboring tertiary referral hospital, where the cardiologist drove once weekly to participate in cases, may be granted privileges to carry out interventional cardiology procedures

481

40.3 A 45-year-old man with a history of hypertension and cigarette smoking presents to the office of a board-certified interventional cardiologist with coronary and peripheral artery expertise, with recent-onset exertional chest discomfort as well as pain in the right calf with walking. The cardiac exam and resting ECG are normal. Exercise echocardiography results are consistent with inferior ischemia. Coronary arteriography is subsequently performed and demonstrates important two-vessel involvement amenable to PCI, with a 90% unstable-appearing proximal right coronary artery stenosis and a 75% left anterior descending stenosis, but no significant left main or circumflex disease. There is difficulty noted in guidewire passage into the central aorta from the right iliac. Left ventriculography demonstrates normal wall motion. After completion of the diagnostic portion of the procedure, the patient reports he has been experiencing chest discomfort and discomfort in the right thigh that has worsened as the procedure has progressed. Right iliac and femoral angiography demonstrates a 90% right common iliac stenosis. On the basis of these findings, how best should the interventional cardiologist proceed?

(A) End the procedure and schedule the patient for left anterior descending and right coronary PCIs and right iliac intervention at three separate procedures

(B) Carry out PCI only for right iliac stenosis and have the patient return for coronary intervention at a later date

(C) Perform PCI for both coronary lesions and have the patient return at a later date for iliac intervention

(D) Carry out right coronary and right common iliac interventions and have the patient return for left anterior descending intervention

40.4 An 80-year-old woman with a history of chronic obstructive pulmonary disease who is 2 days status post total arthroplasty following right hip fracture develops respiratory distress that responds to continuous positive airway pressure with a mask, but from which the patient subsequently cannot be weaned. Cardiac markers include a troponin I of 6.25. Coronary arteriography demonstrates serial severe left anterior descending lesions. The circumflex is dominant and free of hemodynamically significant-appearing disease. The patient is restive from

the beginning of the procedure, then becomes agitated and combative—twice contaminating the catheterization fields. The interventional cardiologist does not have privileges for deep conscious sedation, defined at the institution as bolus or brief continuous administration of general anesthetic agents such as propofol, but feels that deeper sedation is the optimum means of managing the patient's combativeness. Which of the following is the optimal approach for managing the patient's sedation and airway during the procedure?

(A) Stop the procedure and refer the patient for emergency surgical revascularization

(B) Administer increasing doses of fentanyl and midazolam in an effort to sedate the patient

(C) Contact Anesthesiology for stat administration of propofol

(D) Use forcible restraints to prevent the patient from contaminating the field

(E) The interventional cardiologist should break scrub and administer a propofol 50 mg intravenous bolus and initiate 0.1 to 0.2 mg/kg/min continuous infusion, and then rescrub and perform PCI for the left anterior descending

40.5 An interventional cardiologist in a highly competitive environment is considering strategies to increase market share. Of the following options, which would constitute an ethical way of garnering more patient referrals?

(A) Contract with an advertising firm for an Internet and billboard campaign that describes the physician as "the Heavy Hitter in Interventional Cardiology in Our Area," and "the Sheriff Who'll Put Those Outlaw Stenoses Behind Bars for Good," and also encourages "Go to PlaqueBlaster.com"

(B) Have in practice a seasonal gift-giving plan in which physicians who refer five or more patients are sent a minimum of $1,000 for professional development purposes, and monies for these payments are derived from the collections from the respective patients

(C) Initiate a system whereby in return for patient referrals, the interventional cardiologist will send the patient back to the referring physician for nonindicated procedures such as surveillance radionuclide stress testing

(D) Have in place a system whereby in return for referring friends and acquaintances, patients will be charged "Insurance Only"

40.6 An 80-year-old woman with a history of age-related cognitive decline, who resides in an assisted living facility, has been admitted to hospital with a non–ST-segment elevation myocardial infarction. The patient's husband is deceased. There are five children, all of whom frequently visit the patient. The eldest daughter has power of attorney. There is a valid Living Will. An interventional cardiologist has been following the patient and discusses treatment options with the siblings, who agree on an initial course of conservative management, with aspirin, clopidogrel, β-blockade, and statin therapy, and reiterate the patient's request in the Living Will to not be resuscitated. The patient had been admitted to the CCU and has now been transferred to a nontelemetry floor bed. On the floor, the patient has experienced two episodes of prolonged chest discomfort associated with ST-segment depression on the ECG. The children have met, and four out of the five, including the daughter with power of attorney, wish to continue conservative management. The youngest son has demanded that the patient be taken for coronary arteriography and percutaneous coronary revascularization and that the patient be resuscitated in the event of an arrest. What is the CORRECT approach in this situation?

(A) The interventional cardiologist is supremely confident in his ability to see patients safely through complex, high-risk interventional procedures. The youngest son tells the physician that he has spoken with the rest of the family, and that they now agree with him. Using an informed consent signed by the youngest son, the interventional cardiologist takes the patient to the cardiac catheterization laboratory

(B) The interventional cardiologist realizes the legal significance of power of attorney and recommends a joint meeting with all five siblings. The youngest son resists this suggestion and initially threatens to leave the hospital. Ultimately, with the intervention of an experienced palliative care nurse, he agrees to join his brothers and sisters in a meeting

(C) Discuss the situation with the telemetry floor nursing staff, who have dealt with many such situations

(D) Because of the family strife, the interventional cardiologist notifies the family of his withdrawal from management of the patient

40.7 What, if any, federal regulation exists concerning self-referral?

(A) The Belmont Statute

(B) The Stark Law

(C) The Medicare-Medicaid Anti-Kickback Statute

(D) The Proxmire Designated Health Services Law, also referred to as the Golden Fleece Law

(E) There is no federal regulation regarding self-referral in medicine

40.8 You are actively enrolling patients at your institution in an ongoing clinical trial and have provided scientific, privacy-protected information to the study sponsor, while at the same time ensuring that patient care is not negatively impacted by your financial relationship to the study. In addition to the study, you have begun to do continuing medical education (CME) presentations that are underwritten by the study. To date, you have received approximately $7,500 in compensation for your participation in the CME activities. What level of compensation is considered significant?

(A) Any compensation is considered significant for CME activities

(B) Any compensation >$500

(C) Any compensation ≤$10,000

(D) Any compensation >$10,000

40.9 You are the medical director of a catheterization laboratory, which has just hired a female radiology technologist to assist with the increasing volume of cases. She is well-trained and eager to help. The catheterization laboratory nurse manager reports to you that a catheterization laboratory employee has recounted overhearing another male employee speak in overt sexual contexts both around and directly to the new female technician. The new female staff member confirms that these conversations took place, but she assures you that she is not affected by this environment. However, you feel that she is simply trying to protect her new job, and that such coworker behavior is inappropriate and unprofessional. What is the most appropriate way to handle this situation?

(A) Refer to the policy of your institution regarding sexual harassment in the workplace, then instruct the catheterization laboratory nurse or technical manager to address this issue directly with the coworker at the earliest opportunity, enforcing the principles of professionalism and the consequences (both legal and professional) of sexual harassment either real or perceived

(B) Reassure the employee that this conduct is likely due to the predominance of men in the workplace and that this behavior is a benign part of male-dominated workplaces

(C) Because the female technician stated that such conduct did not bother her, take no further action at this point

(D) See that the particular offending male staff members and physicians avoid working with the new female technician

40.10 You are carrying out a coronary interventional procedure in a live-demonstration course and will be using an investigational device as part of the procedure. An informed consent for the procedure includes consent for participation in the live demonstration that was electronically signed and is in the electronic record. The intervention is complex but proceeds smoothly and successfully until near the conclusion of the procedure, when the patient acutely develops diaphoresis and asks for the live demonstration to be terminated. A guidewire perforation is noted on arteriography. Despite efforts, a covered stent cannot be delivered to remedy the perforation. Attempts at coil embolization of the artery at the perforation are successful, and the patient stabilizes. Which of the answers best summarizes the conduct of the case?

(A) Rather than agreeing to the patient's request to terminate the live demonstration, efforts should be directed at identification of the problem and stabilization of the patient

(B) The informed process for the live demonstration and use of an investigational device were appropriate

(C) The informed consent process was appropriate, but the live demonstration should have been terminated at the instant of the patient's request

(D) There are ethical problems with the informed consent process, and the patient may terminate the live demonstration at any time

40.11 A 75-year-old man is known to have a history of diabetes mellitus, hypertension, dyslipidemia, and >50 pack-years of smoking, and the patient is referred by the primary care provider for stress testing. The stress test is abnormal, with high-risk features, and the patient subsequently undergoes uncomplicated drug-eluting stent placement to the mid-left anterior descending. One hour after the catheterization, the patient complains of severe pain at the femoral access site, and a 4-cm hematoma is noted. Of the clinical and/or procedural factors listed in the following text, which is most closely associated with the development of femoral catheterization site injury?

(A) Age > 70 years
(B) Male gender
(C) Sheath size > 6 French
(D) Use of a coronary stent during the procedure
(E) Use of mechanical clamp device for hemostasis

40.12 At a case conference with your colleagues, you discuss a 50-year-old patient who presented overnight with a non–ST-elevation acute coronary syndrome and was stabilized on medical therapy with class I indications. The next morning the patient underwent uncomplicated primary stent placement in the circumflex, and 4 hours later developed ventricular fibrillation on the telemetry ward, could not be resuscitated, and died. What is the unadjusted in-hospital mortality from PCI?

(A) Less than 0.5%
(B) 0.5% to 1.5%
(C) 1.5% to 3.0%
(D) Greater than 3.0%

40.13 A 78-year-old woman undergoes elective PCI with a drug-eluting stent to the mid-left anterior descending via femoral access with no immediate complications. Intravenous heparin and a glycoprotein IIb/IIIa inhibitor are used, and the patient received a loading dose of a thienopyridine at the completion of the case. In the catheterization recovery area 30 minutes following the procedure, the patient develops back pain and becomes diaphoretic. A 12-lead ECG is normal. Acute retroperitoneal hemorrhage is suspected. What is the best clinical predictor of retroperitoneal hematoma (RPH) formation after PCI?

(A) Preexisting poorly controlled hypertension
(B) Arterial sheath size > 7 French
(C) Female gender
(D) Glycoprotein IIb/IIIa use
(E) Body surface area (BSA) < 1.73 m²

40.14 It was your anniversary, you were not on call, and you had already left the hospital when you were notified about your patient, a 78-year-old woman now 45 minutes status post percutaneous circumflex coronary intervention, with flank pain, diaphoresis, and suspected retroperitoneal hemorrhage. The patient has a BSA of 1.6 m² and a history of systolic hypertension, and in spite of 2,000 mL of crystalloid administered, the systolic blood pressure in the catheterization laboratory recovery area remains 90 to 100 mm Hg. The IIb/IIIa glycoprotein inhibitor was stopped. The ECG remains normal. The physician now responsible has seen the patient and is moving her to the CT scanner for imaging. On the way to the scanner, the systolic blood pressure falls to 70 mm Hg, necessitating return of the patient post haste to the catheterization laboratory recovery area for further resuscitation. What of the options below is NOT part of the optimal treatment approach in this case?

(A) Sufficient volume expansion to stabilize the blood pressure before imaging to confirm retroperitoneal hemorrhage
(B) Type and cross-match for blood transfusion
(C) Rather than return to the recovery area, continue on to the radiology suite for CT scanning to confirm the diagnosis of retroperitoneal hemorrhage
(D) Obtain immediate consultation from vascular surgery and/or peripheral interventional cardiologist, in order to prepare for possible catheter-based closure of a retroperitoneal leak
(E) Ascertain the availability in the catheterization laboratory inventory of embolization coils and covered stents of sufficient size to repair an iliac perforation

40.15 A 72-year-old woman with a history of hypertension, insulin-dependent diabetes mellitus, and chronic renal insufficiency (serum creatinine 2.2 mg/dL) is scheduled to undergo diagnostic coronary angiography and possible PCI, after presenting with a history consistent with Canadian Cardiovascular Society Class III angina. An exercise echocardiogram demonstrated a large reversible anteroseptal wall motion abnormality. Should the patient develop acute kidney injury (AKI) after a PCI procedure, what is the effect on her mortality?

(A) In-hospital mortality has been shown to increase dramatically in patients who develop AKI after PCI, and increases even more in patients who require hemodialysis (acute renal failure requiring dialysis [ARFD])
(B) In-hospital mortality is not impacted, but survival at 1 year is significantly decreased
(C) In-hospital mortality is only affected by development of ARFD, but not just development of AKI
(D) There are no data to suggest that development of ARFD after PCI affects overall mortality

40.16 A 73-year-old man with known coronary artery disease, severe left ventricular systolic dysfunction, and NYHA Class III heart failure symptoms presents by emergency medical transport to the emergency department with an unequivocal anterior ST-segment elevation myocardial infarction (STEMI). The patient has altered mental status, a blood pressure of 90 mm Hg palpable systolic, a heart rate of 100 beats/min, and is unable to give informed consent. He is well known to you from follow-up in your clinic and has no living relatives. Recently, although in a better state of health, the patient told you that it is his desire to have no further cardiac interventions in the future, and he indicated that he had completed appropriate "Do Not Resuscitate (DNR) Orders" with his primary care provider. What option in the following text offers the most optimal and appropriate cardiovascular care for this patient?

(A) In addition to standard medical therapy, begin dopamine infusion due to hypotension, providing only bag-mask ventilation to see if he stabilizes
(B) Quickly confer with other medical professionals in the emergency room and proceed to the catheterization laboratory under an emergency informed consent signed by you
(C) Tell the patient that you feel he needs to go directly to the catheterization laboratory or he will likely die
(D) Consider thrombolytic therapy along with aspirin, oxygen, nitroglycerin, and heparin, and pressor support, if necessary, and move the patient to the CCU for further management and observation

40.17 A colleague consults you regarding a patient who has undergone diagnostic coronary angiography. Your colleague has identified a single lesion that he feels would benefit from PCI. Informed consent for possible PCI had been obtained before the procedure, and the patient is aware that you would be performing the procedure. You initially agree to perform the procedure, but as the equipment for the intervention is being pulled from electronic cabinets, your earlier doubt that the procedure is indicated intensifies because you, in fact, believe the stenosis is not hemodynamically significant. How do you proceed?

(A) Tell the patient you are uncertain of the potential benefit of the planned procedure, and ask if he chooses to proceed

(B) Tell the patient that your assessment is that the procedure is not indicated and should be canceled and that you will review his records further and discuss your findings with him

(C) Advise the patient that although you are unsure of the ultimate outcome, the potential risks of the procedure are low and proceed

(D) Proceed without expressing your opinion to the patient in deference to both your colleague's opinion and the catheterization laboratory schedule

40.18 Before proceeding with a planned percutaneous mitral valvotomy, you explain the procedure to the patient, along with the risks, benefits, and alternatives. The patient is 75 years of age and has a history of "a touch of Alzheimer disease," according to a daughter who accompanies him. He is otherwise independent, and no separate provision such as a health care power of attorney has been established. What is the proper way to proceed with ensuring that informed consent is obtained?

(A) Ask your nurse to spend extra time assessing the patient's understanding of the procedure and let you know if the patient seems to understand the plan

(B) Ask the daughter if she understands the procedure and if she is agreeable to proceeding

(C) Have the daughter convince the patient to proceed and sign the consent form despite his reluctance

(D) Ensure that the patient displays competence, understanding, and autonomy in providing consent free of undue influence or coercion

40.19 You are carrying out a coronary intervention that has immediately followed the diagnostic procedure. The patient is a 68-year-old woman with no history of drug allergies who underwent an uncomplicated renal arteriogram several years ago, and since that procedure has been taking lisinopril for control of hypertension. Within the past week, a lung nodule was found on chest x-ray, and coincidentally, the patient has experienced several episodes of chest discomfort radiating to the left arm lasting for 10 to 15 minutes. Because her son was in town for the procedure, they went out for soft-shell crabs at the local French restaurant the night before the procedure. The precatheterization ECG is normal. For the procedure, the patient has received aspirin, clopidogrel, intravenous β-blocker, heparin, small doses of fentanyl and midazolam, and 150 mL of low-osmolality nonionic contrast material. The procedure has been going smoothly, but you have just encountered difficulty advancing a drug-eluting stent across a target lesion that was predilated with an appropriately sized balloon, when the patient first says, "I feel funny," and then a minute later complains of intense itching, queasy stomach, and a feeling of being unable to clear her throat, and the blood pressure has dropped to 80 mm Hg systolic. On examination the patient is found to have diffuse raised urticaria, including a 10-cm diameter right neck lesion extending from dorsal of the right ear lobe to the sternal notch. What is the most likely explanation for the patient's findings?

(A) The patient is having an immune-mediated reaction to contrast material

(B) The patient is having a delayed hypersensitivity reaction to the soft-shell crab she had for dinner the night before the procedure

(C) The patient is experiencing an anaphylactoid reaction to iodinated contrast material

(D) The episode constitutes evidence that the patient has a paraneoplastic syndrome in which a tumor is producing histamine

(E) The cutaneous findings are angioedema due to lisinopril

40.20 Several months after an acute coronary event, you are seeing a 40-year-old man in follow-up in the clinic. In the course of left leg trauma from a motor vehicular accident, the patient sustained an inferior myocardial infarction (MI), for which you performed PCI of the right coronary artery, including placement of a stent. You noted during the catheterization that the coronary arteries appeared smooth and normal, with the exception of the right coronary occlusion, which had the appearance of a meniscus convex in the direction of vessel origin (retrograde), suggesting an embolic coronary occlusion, which could have occurred as a result of the leg trauma, rather than a primary plaque rupture. Following the interventional procedure, you had ordered an echocardiogram including contrast study, which was performed in the catheterization laboratory holding area, but it was a busy day in the laboratory, and the patient passed to the care of trauma surgery without disposition on the echocardiographic findings. In fact, the echocardiographic contrast study had demonstrated passage of contrast from the right atrium into the left atrium, consistent with a patent foramen ovale (PFO). As a result of the leg trauma, the patient underwent left below-the-knee amputation, and now will require reconstructive knee surgery. In the clinic, now several weeks later, your adept midlevel associate has uncovered the echocardiographic contrast result. What is the best approach to convey this overlooked result to the patient?

(A) The echocardiographic contrast result should be conveyed to the patient as having been an incidental finding on the echocardiogram during the hospitalization

(B) A personal policy of full disclosure should be held by the physician, and in this case, the physician should explicitly relate to the patient that the echocardiographic contrast result was overlooked, followed by a discussion of the test's potential significance

(C) The echocardiographic result need not be discussed with the patient, because the findings are not germane to the present illness

(D) The interventional cardiologist should disclose the echocardiographic findings to the patient and tell him that it was the responsibility of the trauma surgeon to notify the patient of the echocardiographic findings

40.1 **Answer C.** The ECG is diagnostic for an acute inferolateral STEMI. The results of the ISIS-4 trial (*Lancet* 1995;345:669–685) demonstrated no survival benefit of nitrates in STEMI; and, therefore, B is incorrect. Option C is the most rapid option for reperfusion. The issue of coronary intervention for STEMI at sites without surgical backup is less clear. Aversano et al. (*JAMA* 2002;287:1943–1951) have reported superior outcome in the 6-month composite end point of death, recurrent MI, and stroke in patients with STEMI randomly assigned to PCI at 11 community hospitals without surgery backup, compared with patients assigned to thrombolytic therapy. The 2005 revision of the American College of Cardiology Foundation (ACCF)/American Heart Association (AHA)/Society of Cardiac Angiography and Interventions (SCAI) remains the latest guideline statement regarding PCI without on-site cardiac surgery and states that emergency PCI without surgical backup has class IIb indication, and should only be done at facilities with a proven plan for rapid access (within 1 hour) to a cardiac surgery operating room. This indication assumes that the hospital without a cardiac surgery program performs high-quality acute interventional procedures. At a practical level, there should be virtually no "practice-makes-perfect interval" series of cases for the operator and the catheterization laboratory team that performs acute percutaneous intervention without immediate access to surgery backup. If a hospital with no heart surgery backup is incapable of offering acute intervention 24 hours, 7 days a week, the program should be considered suboptimal. In acute PCI, the current standard for door-to-balloon (D2B) time remains 90 minutes, but every effort should be made to achieve shorter D2B times. To be considered qualified to perform such acute cases, the operator must perform >75 PCIs per year, 11 of which are for acute MI, and the facility >36 primary PCIs per year. A program of performance assessment and continuous improvement should be in place, as is afforded by a database such as the National Cardiovascular Data Registry of the American College of Cardiology. In the event the operator at the facility with no backup does not meet these criteria, for the physician who first encounters the patient with acute STEMI there can be no constraint with regard to transfer of the patient to a larger cardiac center, particularly a patient with Killip Class 3 or 4, as described in this scenario. Regarding the issue of thrombolytic therapy vs. transfer for acute coronary intervention, based on the DANAMI-2 trial (*Am Heart J* 2003;146:234–241) and earlier smaller studies, a consensus began to emerge that PCI has superior efficacy to thrombolytic therapy even when the patient with STEMI is transferred from a non-catheterization- capable hospital. The results of the CARESS-in-AMI trial (*Lancet* 2008;371:559–568) and the TRANSFER-AMI trial (*N Engl J Med* 2009;360:2705–2718) have allowed for coalescence of a specific guideline pathway in the latest guideline update for those patients presenting to a PCI-capable facility and those presenting to a non–PCI-capable facility (*American College of Cardiology Foundation/American Heart Association Focused Updates* 2007 and 2009). For those presenting to a PCI facility, the patient should be moved "expeditiously" to the catheterization laboratory, with appropriate antithrombotic therapy for catheterization and PCI. Those patients presenting to non-PCI facilities should be triaged to either immediate transfer for PCI or to thrombolytic therapy plus probable transfer, as the preponderance of data from the transfer studies demonstrate a benefit of rescue PCI. The decision will depend on the mortality of risk of the MI, the risk of fibrinolytic therapy, the duration of the symptoms when first seen, and the time required for transport to a PCI-capable facility.

40.2 **Answer D.** The 2008 ACCF Training Statement endorsed by the SCAI for diagnostic and interventional cardiac catheterization (*J Am Coll Cardiol* 2008;51:355–361) and the 2007 ACCF/AHA/SCAI guideline update on clinical competence in cardiac interventional procedures (*J Am Col Cardiol* 2007;50:82–108) address the requirements to achieve and maintain proficiency in performing PCI. Formal training in interventional cardiology in an accredited program is a requirement. Level III training proficiency, that is, trainees who will perform diagnostic and interventional cardiac catheterization procedures, must be completed during the 4th year of cardiology fellowship dedicated to coronary interventional training, with performance of at least 250 coronary interventions as the primary operator, each patient counting as one intervention regardless of the number of vessels that are treated. Maintaining proficiency requires >75 PCI cases per year. It is recommended that a physician who is not a full member of the hospital staff should not be given privileges in the cardiac catheterization laboratory. Regarding professional certification to perform coronary interventions, eligibility for the interventional cardiology board examination through the "practice pathway," that is, without having completed an Accredited Council for Graduate Medical Education (ACGME)-accredited interventional training program, ended in 2002; and, therefore, physicians should not be privileged to perform coronary interventions unless board-certified or board-eligible.

40.3 **Answer D.** The ethical choice for managing the patient is to ameliorate the unstable coronary lesion, and as long as the coronary intervention is uncomplicated, to carry out right iliac intervention as well because the patient has experienced leg pain at rest during the procedure, and schedule the patient to return at a later date for left anterior descending intervention. Had not the right iliac lesion been present and produced symptoms during the procedure, consideration of two-vessel coronary intervention at the same setting would have been reasonable. Detailing options for treatment is part of the informed consent process; and, therefore, it is appropriate before catheterization to discuss surgical revascularization as an option for managing selected subsets of coronary anatomy. In some instances, reimbursement may be influenced by whether multiple coronary interventions are carried out at the same or in different settings. In these cases, it is essential for the well-being of the patient that the interventional cardiologist's efforts be directed solely toward what is most right for the patient. In the absence of the peripheral artery situation described in this case, a reasonable approach in multivessel cases is to take into account the complexity of the lesions to be intervened and endeavor to complete all the interventions in no more than two separate procedures; however, the approach should be guided by lesion complexity.

40.4 **Answer C.** Further narcotics and benzodiazepines in this patient may not result in the desired level of sedation, and apnea could result. The lack of deep conscious sedation privileges presents the interventional with an ethical dilemma. Lacking these, the interventional cardiologist does not have the authority to administer propofol, although this is the most medically optimal approach. Forcible restraints may keep the patient from contaminating the field, but they will not stop the patient's movement. A valid Advanced Cardiac Life Support (ACLS) card may not constitute sufficient expertise in airway management to afford the interventional cardiologist deep conscious sedation privileges. Although deep sedation during interventional procedures is rarely necessary, in our experience most such patients can safely be administered propofol without resorting to elective intubation of the patient, utilizing the deep conscious sedation monitoring protocol of the catheterization laboratory; however, it is incumbent upon the interventional cardiologist to have the appropriate hospital privilege, as otherwise, to administer a drug that has the potential to result in apnea would be unethical. If the cardiac catheterization laboratory is staffed by a full-time certified nurse anesthetist, this individual may administer drugs such as propofol, but under current nurse professional guidelines, as well as Joint Accreditation of Hospital Organization assessments, nurses with critical care qualifications are not authorized to administer deep sedation unless the patient is already intubated. Therefore, if he or she had the appropriate privilege in the present case, the interventional cardiologist could break scrub and personally administer therapy of deep sedation.

40.5 **Answer A.** Although the Internet-Billboard scheme may be unappealing, there would be nothing unethical about such an advertising campaign. The remaining options are either unethical, illegal, or both. Option B constitutes payola, a kickback to the primary physician in return for the referral of a patient and is a prosecutable offense under the Medicare-Medicaid Anti-Kickback provision in Chapter 42 of the United States Code. Similarly, charging "insurance only" is considered Medicare fraud and is a practice that is prohibited by the Commission for Medicare and Medicaid Services. Any such *quid pro quo* arrangements are unethical. Similarly, the practice of referring patients for any procedure that is not indicated is to be decried. For a Medicare patient, it would constitute fraud.

40.6 **Answer B.** Continued communication with the youngest son is essential to the well-being of this grief-stricken individual and the well-being of the family unit. Regarding clinical decisions, the physician is legally obligated to follow the instructions of the power of attorney, and the law is clear in this situation that only the power of attorney's signature constitutes valid informed consent. Therefore, whether the procedure was successful, Option A would result in legal action by the family. Option D is unsavory and comes close to an abdication of the physician's covenant to care for the patient, who should never be abandoned in time of medical need. Open, inclusive, and compassionate communication by engaged care providers virtually never fails to aid bereaved relatives, such as the youngest son, and an approach by the physician in concert with other providers such as the patient's nurse can gently move the process forward. Palliative care services are now available in many inpatient health facilities and can provide significant benefit in the management of bereavement and comfort to the patient (*J Am Coll Cardiol* 1999;58:386–396; *Chest* 2009;135:1360–1369).

40.7 **Answer B.** The Federal Physician Self-Referral Law, also known as the Stark Law, United States Code Section 1395nn) prohibits referrals by a physician for "designated health services" covered by Medicare or Medicaid to entities in which the physician has a financial relationship (broadly defined as an ownership interest or compensation agreement). As the following figure demonstrates, there has been dramatic growth in the volume of both invasive and noninvasive procedures over the past decade. The impact of this law in cardiology practice is ACCF/AHA Consensus Conference Report on Professionalism and Ethics (*J Am Coll Cardiol* 2004;44:1740–1746). The Stark Law was conceived to curtail unnecessary usage of limited resources. The Medicare-Medicaid Anti-Kickback Statute (Chapter 42, United States Code Section 1320a–7b[b]) prohibits individuals or entities from knowingly and willfully offering, paying, soliciting, or receiving remuneration to induce referrals of items or services covered by Medicare or Medicaid. The Stark legislation is complex, but in essence is an attempt to control self-referrals motivated by personal or financial gain, hence creating overutilization of resources. The Stark Laws are distinct from the Anti-Kickback Statute in that Stark focuses on the financial aspects of referral relationships, and is a civil rather than criminal statute. Regarding Answer D, there is no such statute as the Proxmire Designated Health Services Law. The late Senator William Proxmire, Wisconsin, was a force against overcharging of

the federal government by private industry, and for many years recognized egregious examples of bilking with the Golden Fleece Award. He is perhaps better known as the Senate sponsor of legislation in 1987 ratifying the International Convention on the Prevention and Punishment of the Crime of Genocide approved by the United Nations General Assembly in 1948.

40.8 **Answer D.** Transparency is the key to ensuring that the public and individual patients feel confident that we as cardiovascular clinician-researchers are keeping the public's best interests at the forefront of our activities. Beginning in January 2009 the pharmaceutical industry agreed to a voluntary moratorium on gifts to physicians, from pens and coffee mugs to more expensive goods and services such as tickets to concerts and junkets to resorts. The plan was prepared by Pharmaceutical Research and Manufacturers of America, an industry group in Washington, DC. In addition to the banishment of gifts, the moratorium asks companies to refrain from interfering with the selection content of continuing medical courses, which they may finance. When activities such as the CME in the example create conflicts of interest, it is incumbent upon the physician to understand what the patient and fellow professionals expect regarding disclosure. The professional community has not been silent on these issues, and guidelines for conduct and disclosure are available. The 2004 ACCF/AHA Consensus Conference Report on Professionalism and Ethics (*J Am Coll Cardiol* 2004;44:1722–1723) states that disclosure of financial arrangements should be mandatory for educational activities and scientific publications. The American College of Cardiology Foundation Statement on Relationships with Industry, revised in May 2010 and available at the ACC website, states that relevant financial relationships between the clinical researcher and industry should be defined in terms of levels of compensation and support: None, Modest (≤$10,000), and Significant (>$10,000). These levels are in keeping with previous guidelines offered by the NIH (The National Institutes of Health 2004) and FDA (The Food and Drug Administration 2000). In this case, the $7,500 the physician has been compensated, although considered "modest" under the guidelines, is clearly more than none and should be disclosed by the physician when delivering talks, as well as when asking for patients' participation in the trial. There is impetus, for example, at the NIH, to lower the Modest-Significant cut-off to $5,000, and many consumer watchdog entities consider any remuneration to be significant. Disclosure of financial interest is required to ensure transparency of potential financial conflicts of interest to the trial participants and to the institutional review boards, whenever human subjects are being enrolled and a financial relationship exists between the sponsor and the investigator.

40.9 **Answer A.** Given your concerns regarding this conduct, you should personally review your established policies regarding sexual harassment and promptly address the issue with the employee who is making the inappropriate comments, and review the Sexual Harassment policy with the entire catheterization laboratory staff. Stated succinctly, there should be zero tolerance for sexual harassment in the workplace. As the laboratory director, you have the obligation to ensure that all policies are current, available, and in practice on a daily basis in the catheterization laboratory. It is the supervisor's responsibility to provide a professional atmosphere and a safe, nonhostile working environment (*J Am Coll Cardiol* 2001;37:2170–2214). Employees should participate in regular sexual harassment training and understand that harassment is a violation of federal, state, and local laws. The first federal guidelines regarding sexual harassment in the workplace were published by the Equal Employment Opportunity Commission (EEOC) in 1980. The EEOC is the federal organization that is responsible for enforcing and interpreting federal discrimination laws. The EEOC defines sexual harassment as:

- Unwelcome sexual advances, requests for sexual favors, and other verbal or physical conduct of a sexual nature, where,
  - Submission to such conduct is made either implicitly or explicitly a term or condition of employment; or
  - Submission to or rejection of such conduct by an individual is used as a basis for employment decisions affecting the individual
- Unwelcome sexual advances, requests for sexual favors, and other verbal or physical conduct of a sexual nature, where such conduct has the purpose or effect of unreasonably interfering with the individual's work performance or creating an intimidating, hostile, or offensive working environment. (*United States Equal Employment Opportunity Commission* 2001:186–192).

In this case, it is reasonable to conclude that the explicit and suggestive behavior of the male colleague could interfere substantially with the ability of the female technician to carry out her work because the environment is offensive, hostile, and intimidating. Therefore, such behavior must be considered inappropriate and a potential violation of federal antiharassment laws. If a "zero tolerance" policy is to be effective, there must be strict enforcement of the antiharassment policies and bylaws that are in place. While the female technician suggests that such explicit language and behavior does not excessively bother her, it is incumbent upon you as laboratory director to take the necessary actions to ensure that all staff members are free to work in a nonoffensive, nonhostile environment free of harassment.

40.10 **Answer D.** A work group of the SCAI, ACCF, the Heart Rhythm Society, the European Society of Cardiology, the Sociedad Latinoamericana de Cardiología Intervencionista, and the Asian Pacific Society of Interventional Cardiology has recently published a consensus document on the use of live case demonstrations at cardiology meetings (*J Am Coll Cardiol* 2010;56:1267–128). It is worthwhile to keep in mind the Belmont principles, beneficence, respect for persons, and justice. These guiding tenets can serve not only as the ethical basis for Best Clinical Practice in the conduct of human research, but also as the model for activities involving patients such as live demonstrations, even the basis for how to provide care to patients. The consensus document notes that a potential conflict of interest will exist when using investigational devices in a live demonstration, and the well-being of the patient takes precedence. In the case presented, there of course should have been a signed informed consent approved by the human investigations and studies committee (IRB) to participate in an IRB-approved study involving an investigational device. In addition, the writers of the consensus document recommend an IRB-approved informed consent be utilized for live demonstration participation. As with consent to participate in a human investigation, so, too, the patient may withdraw consent to participate in a live demonstration at any time and the request should be honored. Beneficence, respect for persons, justice should prevail.

40.11 **Answer D.** The risks of coronary interventional procedures vary on a case-by-case basis according to a mix of clinical and procedural characteristics, which can be predicted with relative accuracy before the procedure, and explanation of these risks is part of the informed consent process for each patient. Peripheral vascular complications are the most common morbidity encountered in the setting of PCI and, arguably, although still relatively uncommon, have become more frequent in an era of potent antiplatelet and anticoagulant drugs. Serious vascular access complications include hematomas with significant blood loss, arterial pseudoaneurysm, and arteriovenous fistulas, and to this list, RPH should probably be added as an access complication. Data from trials such as CAVEAT-1 (*J Am Coll Cardiol* 1995;26:922–930) indicate that the frequency of such complications ranges from 3% to 5% in noncomplex PCI. Results from the Evaluation of c7E3 for the Prevention of Ischemic Complications (EPIC) trial (*Am J Cardiol* 1998;81:36–40) demonstrate that more potent anticoagulant and antiplatelet regimens do increase risk of minor and major bleeding. Konstance et al. (*J Interv Cardiol* 2004;17:65–70) examined independent clinical and procedural risk factors for major vascular complications and determined that *stent usage* is the strongest independent predictor of a vascular access complication in univariate and multivariate analysis. Age > 65 and female gender are both independent risk predictors for vascular access complications as well. Sheath size has been shown to be associated with vascular complications, with studies showing up to fivefold increases in vascular access complication rates when upgrading from a 6-French to an 8-French sheath. Use of anticoagulants and procedure duration may play a role. The use of a mechanical clamp for hemostasis increases the risk of complication, but is not as strongly associated as is the use of stents, female sex, or sheath size. Compelling data such as the PRESTO-ACS substudy (*Am J Cardiol* 2009;103:796–800) and the MORTAL study (*Heart* 2008;94:1019–1025) demonstrate that radial artery access for coronary interventional procedures is associated with less bleeding complications and possibly, better long-term outcome.

40.12   Answer B. A review of the literature shows that unadjusted in-hospital mortality following PCI is approximately 0.5% to 1.5%. Abrupt coronary artery occlusion with associated left ventricular failure is noted as the primary cause of PCI-associated mortality. The clinical and angiographic variables associated with increased mortality include advanced age, female gender, diabetes, prior MI, multivessel disease, left main

or equivalent coronary disease, a large area of myocardium at risk, preexisting impairment of left ventricular dysfunction or abnormal renal function, and collateral vessels supplying significant areas of myocardium that originate distal to the segment to be dilated. Unadjusted mortality rates do not take into account the different settings in which PCI is performed or certain patient characteristics that may influence outcome. Multivariate models have been published that can be utilized to estimate the mortality risk of PCI (*Circulation* 1997;95:2479–2484; *JAMA* 1997;277:892–898; *Circulation* 2003;107:1871–1876; *J Am Coll Cardiol* 1999;34:674–680; *Circulation* 2001;104:263–268; *J Am Coll Cardiol* 2002;39:1104–1112). Findings from the American College of Cardiology National Cardiovascular Data Registry indicate a univariate mortality rate of 0.5% for patients undergoing elective PCI, a mortality rate of 5.1% for patients undergoing primary PCI within 6 hours of the onset of STEMI, and a mortality rate of 28% for patients undergoing PCI for cardiogenic shock (*J Am Coll Cardiol* 2002;39:1104–1112). Therefore, stratification by clinical setting of PCI is helpful in estimating individual patient mortality risk. Finally, as is well described in the ACCF/AHA/SCAI 2007 cardiac interventional procedure update (*J Am Coll Cardiol* 2007;50:82–108), procedural complication rate declines while procedural success rate increases with numbers of cases, leveling off at approximately 200 cases per operator-year and 600 cases per institution-year.

40.13   Answer E. Farouque et al. reviewed the incidence, features, and risk factors for the formation of RPH in 3,508 patients undergoing PCI in which current techniques including glycoprotein IIb/IIIa receptor antagonists were utilized (*J Am Coll Cardiol* 2005;45:363–368). Approximately one-third of these patients had presented with an acute coronary syndrome. The authors demonstrated that BSA < 1.73 m^2 conferred the highest multivariable risk for RPH, odds ratio 7.1, $p = 0.008$. Female gender was a significant factor, odds ratio of 5.4, $p = 0.005$. The only other predictor with independent significance in high femoral puncture site, defined as above the middle third of the femoral head on fluoroscopy, odds ratio 5.3, $p = 0.013$. Body surface area and femoral artery size correlated in a linear regression analysis, thus, it is possible that small arterial size may have a role. The incidence of RPH was 0.74%, and mortality associated with RPH 4%, similar to previous studies. Again, it is worth noting that retroperitoneal would be a vanishingly rare complication when PCI is performed via the radial approach (*Am J Cardiol* 2009;103:796–800).

40.14 **Answer C.** The management of acute hypotension in patients postcatheterization is fundamentally the same as in any other setting. At times we in cardiology may err in overthinking cardiac etiologies for hypotension. A 12-lead ECG is appropriate. The presence of bradycardia and vagal symptoms should alert the clinician to the possibility of vasovagal (autonomic) hypotension, as well as anaphylactoid reaction, the latter especially if there is stridor, wheezing, or dyspnea. For postintervention patients with hypotension, in whom heparin, low-molecular-weight heparin, IIb/IIIa glycoprotein inhibitors, or a direct thrombin inhibitor will have been used, retroperitoneal hemorrhage or abdominal rectus hematoma should be given high priority in the differential. It is to be emphasized that key management is like a trauma alert, with all the effort directed at normalization and stabilization of the blood pressure (*J Am Coll Cardiol Cardiovasc Interv* 2010;3:845–850) *before* considering diagnostic testing. The need for intravenous pressors for blood pressure support is an indication for consideration of catheter or surgical intervention. Combined covered stent placement and coil embolization are emerging as an effective strategy in the management of retroperitoneal hemorrhage with hemodynamic instability (*Ann Vasc Surg* 2010;25:352–358).

40.15 **Answer A.** The development of AKI after PCI is a marker for poor outcomes. Multiple studies have now shown that both in-hospital and long-term mortality increase significantly in patients developing AKI, and higher still in patients who require dialysis. The incidence of AKI after PCI is approximately 3%. Studies have demonstrated that preexisting renal insufficiency confers the highest risk for developing acute renal failure after PCI. The incidence increases linearly with increasing baseline creatinine levels. A history of diabetes, congestive heart failure, and acute MI are among other risk factors that significantly increase the chance of developing AKI (*Circulation* 2002;105:2259–2264). AKI is usually defined as a >25% rise in serum creatinine over baseline levels. In a retrospective analysis of the Mayo Clinic PCI registry, Rihal et al. evaluated the incidence and prognostic importance of AKI following PCI. Of the 7,586 patients

included, there was a 22% in-hospital mortality rate in patients developing AKI compared with a mortality of 1.4% in patients who did not. The trend toward higher mortality was also noted at 1 and 5 years of follow-up (*Circulation* 2002;105:2259–2264). Regarding preexisting renal insufficiency, Gruberg et al. evaluated 439 consecutive patients undergoing PCI in a tertiary facility who were not on dialysis but with a baseline serum creatinine > 1.8 mg/dL. Patients developing a >25% increase over baseline creatinine had an in-hospital mortality of 14.9%, vs. 4.9% in those with no such increase in creatinine. In patients requiring dialysis, the in-hospital mortality was 22.6%. The cumulative 1-year mortality was 45.2% for those who required dialysis, 35.4% for those who did not require dialysis, and 19.4% for patients with no creatinine increase ($p = 0.001$) (*J Am Coll Cardiol* 2000;36:1542–1548). The development of AKI or the need for dialysis following PCI portends poorer outcomes both in-hospital and over time. Other than periprocedural shock, the strongest predictor of in-hospital death following PCI is the development of AKI (*Circulation* 2002;105:2259–2264; *Am J Med* 1997;103:368–375). Recent PCI data indicate an increasing risk of contrast-induced nephropathy (CIN), defined as a >25% increase in creatinine within 72 hours of the PCI procedure, with increasing doses of contrast (*Ann Int Med* 2009;150:170–177), with the lowest risk in patients receiving 30 to 175 mL of contrast material (about 30% of the patients in this study had creatinine clearance < 60 mL/min). Prevention of volume contraction appears as effective as any other strategy in prevention of CIN, as convincing data to support a beneficial effect of *N*-acetylcysteine, isosmolar contrast material, sodium bicarbonate are lacking. For every promising small-scale study, a larger randomized clinical trial has demonstrated no benefit (see ACT study, *AHA Scientific Sessions* 2010). However, a sufficiently large factorial design trial patients with Stage 2 to 3 chronic kidney disease, who receive a sufficiently large contrast dose (i.e., a diagnostic + PCI dose), comparing crystalloid alone, *N*-acetylcysteine, sodium bicarbonate, and iloprost has not been carried out. It would not be sinful to address CIN with such a study.

40.16 **Answer D.** Advanced directive dilemmas are relatively common for the interventional cardiologist. The issue of advance directives (ADs), advanced care plans (ACPs), Living Wills, and

DNR orders will become increasingly prominent in cardiovascular medicine practice as the patient population continues to age and with the presentation of patients who have higher morbidity. Individuals have the right to forgo potentially life-sustaining treatment based on the principle of patient autonomy, which is the ethical centerpiece of the doctor–patient relationship. In this case, a competent patient has expressed directly and in writing that he desires to have no further invasive procedures, even in an emergency. In patients who cannot make competent decisions, the issue of substitute decision making arises. The "substitute" decision maker must approximate the patient's wishes. Who can legally assume the role of substitute decision maker and act as a proxy for the patient, as well as manage legal aspects of ADs, ACPs, Living Wills, and DNR orders, varies by jurisdiction. However, the underlying ethical principles that guide therapy in this situation should not vary, and it is paramount to respect patient autonomy and decision making, recognizing that patients do have the right to refuse potentially life-saving therapies. The surrogate decision maker must consider in decreasing order of priority the patient's wishes, the patient's values and beliefs, and then patient's best interests (*J Am Coll Cardiol* 1998;31:917–925). In the case presented the patient's wishes are clear: no further invasive procedures, and he does not wish to be resuscitated in the event of an emergency. A key responsibility in the physician's job description is to inform, counsel, and guide patients and families through this process. The choice of starting pressor drugs and using bag-mask ventilation is not appealing, because these treatments are often precluded in the setting of a DNR order. Physicians should familiarize themselves with state law and advance directive policies in their practice settings. In the present scenario, there is ample information about the patient's prior wishes to proceed with palliative therapy, though one may feel that PCI is the best option. This approach respects the patient's autonomy and protects his trust.

40.17 **Answer B.** In this scenario, in which the first interaction with the patient is in the catheterization laboratory itself, the interventional cardiologist has a duty to advise the patient of his/her assessment of the findings and either evaluate the hemodynamic significance of the stenosis or cancel the procedure. It is unethical for the interventional cardiologist to perform a procedure that he/she in fact judges to not be indicated, and in the present scenario would amount to a failure to take part in the clinical decision-making process, and would violate all three Belmont principles. It would be better that the interventional physician does what he or she judges to be the right thing for the patient than to later have to reconcile a complication during a nonindicated procedure. In our experience, a true colleague will virtually always understand such a change in management when the physician's best judgment is the basis for taking the alternate approach. Like all physicians, the interventional cardiologist's first responsibility is to be an advocate for the patient, be free of avoidable conflicts of interest in decision making, and use ethical judgment in providing patient care. The interventional physician is responsible for determining the appropriateness and timing of a procedure and ensuring that the patient is informed of the various options, risks, and benefits of any planned procedures. (*Catheter Cardiovasc Interv* 2004;61:157–162). In many historians' opinion, Henry Clay, the senator from Kentucky known as the Great Compromiser, staved off the Civil War for 30 years by appealing to the gentler sensibilities of statespersons like Daniel Webster and John C. Calhoun. A way out of the present case that both protects the patient's interests and addresses the physiologic significance of the lesion in question, of course, is Fractional Flow Reserve (FFR), the invention of the redoubtable Niko Pijls, most recently showcased in the FAME study (*N Engl J Med* 2009;360:213–224).

40.18 **Answer D.** Neglect of ensuring proper informed consent can occur. The concept of informed consent is integral to the good clinical practice of any physician. Appropriate informed consent procedures must be maintained and constitute the main method of demonstrating respect for patient autonomy and protecting the patient's trust in the physician. In the present scenario, the interventional cardiologist must spend adequate time to ensure that the patient possesses competence to understand the risks, benefits, and alternatives to the procedure, and does so with autonomy, that is, free of undue influence or coercion. Generally accepted essential elements of informed consent include:

- Documentation of full disclosure of the risks and benefits of the planned procedure;
- Demonstration that the patient possesses the proper understanding of the planned procedure;

- Demonstration of patient competence to understand the procedure as well as the risks and benefits it entails;
- Demonstration of autonomy to make decisions regarding care without undo influence or coercion;
- Documentation that the patient, after having displayed competence, understanding, and autonomy, has authorized the operator to proceed with the planned procedure (*Nurs Crit Care* 1996;1:127–133).

The patient was mentally capable of presenting a cogent history of exertional dyspnea, which signifies a level competency sufficient to consent to a procedure intended to relieve symptoms. As a general rule, the patient should be considered competent to provide informed consent unless there is a legally authorized health care power of attorney. However, in the course of the informed consent process, if the physician performing the anticipated procedure and an independent health provider such as a catheterization laboratory holding area nurse agree an informed consent problem exists, the process should continue until such time as acceptable informed consent is obtained, if necessary involving next-of-kin in the consent, and documenting the process in the progress notes. Proceeding when there is a lack of agreement about the quality of consent among providers is a recipe for problems for the patient and practitioners.

40.19 **Answer C.** When a patient undergoing a catheterization procedure says, "I feel funny," in the next minute the patient may be incommunicative (procedural stroke) or, as in the case presented, have an anaphylactoid reaction, unless the patient received intravenous lidocaine instead of heparin (labeling containers on the table is worthwhile). Although an anaphylactic reaction, an IgE-mediated immune response such as to a bee sting, is possible, the incidence of immunoglobulin E (IgE) antibodies in patients who have sustained immediate hypersensitivity reactions in the catheterization laboratory is vanishingly low, and the likelihood is that the patient is experiencing an anaphylactoid reaction, most probably to iodinated contrast material. Angioedema due to lisinopril would be in the differential, but is unlikely because the patient has been taking this drug for several years. So-called anaphylactoid reactions to contrast material are uncommon, especially in the era of the newer contrast agents, but such reactions do occur and have manifestations similar to the classic

anaphylactic reaction. Anaphylactoid reactions, as can be judged by the name, resemble anaphylactic reactions, but are nonimmune mediated. These reactions are characterized by the release of vasoactive substances such as histamine and serotonin, presumably through a cytokine mechanism that is triggered by contrast administration, leading to the development of urticaria, indigestion, and hypotension, and respiratory distress that are usually manageable by appropriate medical interventions. Iodine contained in the contrast material is not necessarily the only anaphylactoid trigger. The "queasy stomach" is a clinical sign of endogenous histamine release giving rise to secretion of stomach acid. If the patient in fact had IgE antibody to contrast material, an anaphylactic reaction would have been likely to occur immediately upon the initial administration of contrast, and would have been associated with laryngeal edema and stridor, which in this patient did not occur. There is some delay in the development of a contrast reaction, as described in the scenario. Treatment consists of volume expansion, intravenous diphenhydramine and H2 receptor blocker, and intravenous glucocorticoid, and if necessary, administration of a pressor such phenylephrine. Epinephrine 0.1 to 0.3 mL should be administered intramuscularly (1:1,000 dilution) for moderate reactions (*J Invasive Cardiol* 2009;21:548–551). In the event of a severe reaction, such as severe bronchospasm, laryngeal edema or cardiopulmonary arrest, intravenous epinephrine may be given in a diluted form (1:10,000) at a dose of 1 to 3 mL, recognizing that nearly all adverse outcomes caused by epinephrine result when given intravenously. Completion of the patient's interventional procedure should be delayed until the patient has been stabilized. Rarely, the hypotension of an anaphylactoid event can be sustained and sluggishly responsive to volume expansion and phenylephrine, and it is in these cases that postponement of the process becomes an option. An ounce of prevention: for patients who give any history of contrast reaction, pretreatment with the preventive agents above beginning 24 hours before and again at the time of the procedure is the best practice. It is possible that the patient is experiencing a delayed hypersensitivity reaction to the soft-shell crab, but such a reaction would most probably have awakened the patient in the middle of the night before the procedure.

40.20 **Answer B.** Honesty, coupled with full disclosure, is always the best policy when disclosing medical errors. The physician has only to fully disclose the echocardiographic contrast findings to the patient, explicitly take responsibility that the oversight was his/her error alone, and the patient, although perhaps briefly dismayed about this health history development, will see that the physician has the patient's best interest as the first priority. Any approach other than full disclosure constitutes dissembling, and there could be no other conclusion by the patient in that event other than the physician wishes to hide something. In the present scenario, nothing untoward has occurred as a result of the patient's PFO, but the possibility of paradoxic embolism as a cause of MI must be introduced to the patient. For errors of commission or omission, an approach of full disclosure allows the patient and physician to proceed without emotional encumbrances, and for the physician precludes feelings of guilt for not having been forthcoming to the patient. In the present case allows the

physician to proceed with a positive discussion regarding management of the PFO, including the odds that the patient's left leg trauma resulted in either a thromboembolism or fat embolism that could have passed paradoxically to the right coronary artery. Lack of full disclosure leads down the path to repeated dissembling, after dissembling, loss of the patient's trust, dissolution of the physician–patient relationship, and litigation. Litigation risk is not the reason to be honest. Quality patient trust and care are. Breach of the physician–patient relationship as result of dishonesty will likely result in litigation (*Arch Intern Med* 2005;165:1819-1824; *Ann Intern Med* 1999;131:963-967; *Acta Anaesthesiol Scand* 2005;49:728-734). Full disclosure is not just owed to the patient, it is part of the physician–patient covenant, and as ably demonstrated by Kraman and colleagues, it works (*Brit Med J* 2007;334:490; *Ann Int Med* 1999;131:963-967).

41

Statistics Related to Interventional Cardiology Procedures

Eric Reyes, Karen Pieper, and Robert A. Harrington

QUESTIONS

41.1 A recent journal article reported the results of a randomized clinical trial (RCT) comparing two medical therapies used in conjunction with transcatheter aortic valve implantation. The primary end point was 30-day mortality. In addition to the results for the overall study population, results of a subgroup analysis by gender were also reported by the investigators (Fig. Q41-1). Based upon these results, you conclude the following:

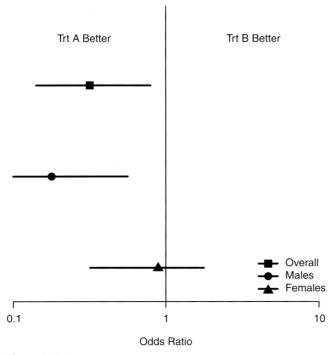

Figure Q41-1

(A) Females can be treated with either treatment
(B) Females should be treated with treatment B
(C) Neither treatment is effective at reducing 30-day mortality
(D) The results for the overall study population contain the most information

41.2 A catheterization laboratory colleague practicing at a hospital in North Carolina is preparing to treat a patient who has a very long lesion (>25 mm) in the right coronary artery. She is considering two approaches: overlapping two drug-eluting stents (DES-DES) or overlapping a drug-eluting and bare-metal stent (DES-BMS). She brings you two articles to review and asks your advice on how to proceed. The first reports the results of a large, well-powered, RCT in South African patients. The trial found DES-DES to be a safer and more effective means of treatment than the alternative approach. The second article reports the results of a large observational study in the United States, which found no significant advantage to either treatment over the other. What do you recommend?

(A) She should proceed with DES-DES, because randomized trials are more reliable than observational studies
(B) She can treat with either, because observational studies are more reliable than randomized clinical studies
(C) She should broaden her literature review to include RCTs conducted in the United States before making her decision
(D) She should broaden her literature review to include observational studies conducted in South Africa before making her decision

41.3 You are given access to data collected from a large randomized trial designed to compare the effectiveness of a new intracoronary stent (Stent A) in reducing mortality compared with Stent B. While the primary end point of the original study was mortality, patients were also followed to determine if repeat revascularization was required following the index procedure. Demographic data, such as a patient's diabetic status, age, race, etc., were also recorded. You would like to use this dataset to determine if Stent A is effective in diabetic patients. After removing nondiabetic patients, 1,000 patients remain, 500 randomized to Stent A, and 500 to Stent B. You are considering the composite end point of mortality or revascularization. The statistician on the project summarizes the data in Figure Q41-3. Based on the figure, the composite end point is a reasonable end point to consider since there will be so many more events with the inclusion of revascularization, which will in turn increase statistical power.

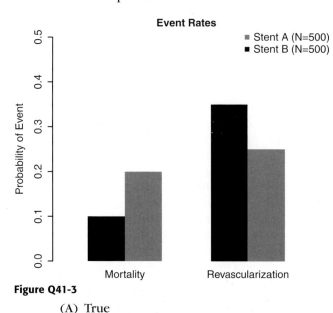

Figure Q41-3

(A) True
(B) False

41.4 The Framingham Heart Study can best be described as what type of clinical study?

(A) Cohort study
(B) Randomized clinical trial
(C) Case–control study
(D) Community intervention study

41.5 Table Q41-5 reports the baseline characteristics of patients with de novo left main disease from two different studies. Both studies compared the efficacy of percutaneous coronary intervention (PCI) using paclitaxel-eluting stents and coronary artery bypass graft treatment. Based on these characteristics, which study most likely corresponds to the randomized Synergy Between PCI with TAXUS and Cardiac Surgery (SYNTAX) trial and which belongs to an observational study?

Table Q41-5.

	Study A		Study B	
	CABG	**PCI**	**CABG**	**PCI**
Age, years	65.6	65.4	61.3	58.6
Men, %	75.6	72.0	73.9	70.1
Left main only	14.1	11.8	10.0	41.8
Diabetes mellitus, %	25.6	23.8	31.0	23.9
Prior myocardial infarction (MI), %	24.0	17.9	12.7	8.2

All continuous covariates are presented as the mean value, and categorical measures presented as percents.

(A) Study A most likely corresponds to the SYN-TAX trial
(B) Study B most likely corresponds to the SYN-TAX trial
(C) Not enough information to decide

41.6 You have been approached to help in the planning of a multicenter study that will examine a potential difference in the restenosis rates of two commonly used DESs. The plan is to conduct a randomized controlled trial. As you begin discussions with your colleagues and the study sponsor, the first question that might arise is how many subjects will be needed for an adequate experiment. Which factor is NOT relevant to the ensuing scientific discussions?

(A) Anticipated event rate in the control group
(B) Estimated difference between the groups
(C) Amount of time required to complete enrollment
(D) Composition of the primary end point

41.7 A pharmaceutical sales representative is presenting his company's literature on the use of a medical treatment for coronary artery disease (CAD). The medical treatment, if beneficial, would reduce the need for PCI when treating CAD. He describes a large randomized trial investigating the superiority of the medical treatment when compared with PCI. The primary end point of the study was periprocedural or spontaneous MI. The sales representative presents the Kaplan–Meier estimates of the survival curves over the first 48 hours following treatment for both treatment groups (Fig. Q41-7). Which of the following is a possible explanation for the results seen in the figure?

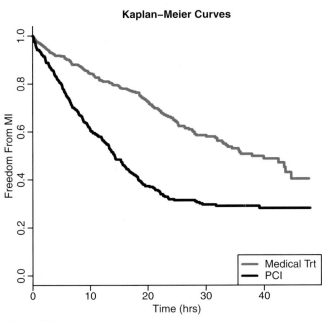

Kaplan–Meier Curves

Figure Q41-7

(A) Medical treatment is superior to PCI
(B) The inclusion of periprocedural MI in the end point definition is biasing the results in favor of medical treatment
(C) Both A and B
(D) Neither A nor B

41.8 You are part of a proposed study's steering committee, which has been charged with designing a clinical trial to test whether new stent A is better than old stent B. The new stent has many attractive design features and your research group would like to be sure that the study is large enough to definitively conclude that stent A is truly superior to stent B if the rates hypothesized are seen. Which component of sample size calculation does this refer to?

(A) Type I error
(B) Type II error
(C) Number needed to treat (NNT)
(D) Study *p*-value

41.9 In Figure Q41-9, which study demonstrates non-inferiority of Treatment A to Treatment B (MID: Minimally important difference)?

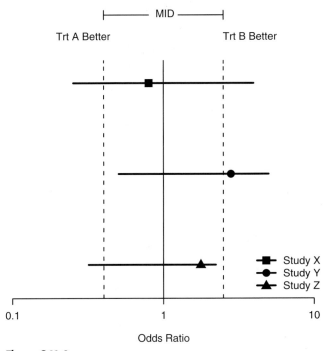

Figure Q41-9

(A) Study X
(B) Study Y
(C) Study Z
(D) None of the above

41.10 Two years ago, a new DES was introduced into a practice within a community-based catheterization laboratory that performs approximately 500 PCIs per year. It quickly became popular and was used in 45% of procedures. The laboratory collects information at the time of procedure and over the first year following discharge. You have noticed that there have been several recent cases of subacute stent thrombosis and wonder if these events are related to the new stent. You are preparing a proposal to investigate this relationship for the director of the laboratory. What is the most appropriate study design to get information quickly in this setting that might be useful in addressing your concerns?

(A) Case–control study
(B) Nonrandomized observational registry
(C) Cohort study
(D) Randomized clinical trial

41.11 Regardless of your answer to Question Q41.10, suppose you decide to perform a cohort study. You divide patients into two groups: those whose interventions included the new DESs and those whose interventions did not, and you follow them for the next year. You calculate the rate of subacute stent thrombosis in each group and determine the odds ratio (OR) (Fig. Q41-11). You conduct your study at a 0.05 nominal level. What do you conclude?

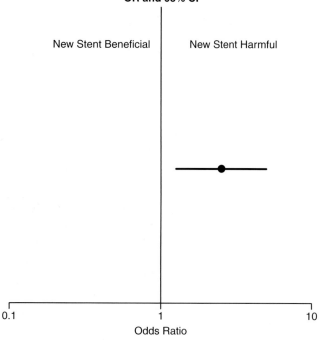

Figure Q41-11

(A) Due to the randomization in a cohort study, you can easily conclude that the stent is harmful

(B) Due to the lack of randomization in a cohort study, you cannot conclude the stent is harmful without first adjusting for other possible confounders

(C) Regardless of the randomization, the stent is harmful

(D) Regardless of the randomization, the stent is beneficial

41.12 For which of the following reason(s) is blinding (or "masking") in a clinical trial important?

(A) It helps prevent introduction of treatment-specific biases

(B) It helps maintain objectivity in assessment of clinical events

(C) It preserves Type I error rate

(D) A and B

41.13 A new treatment is being considered as a low-cost alternative to the current standard of care. As the primary benefit of this new treatment will be the lower cost, a large noninferiority trial was conducted to investigate the performance of the new treatment; see Figure Q41-13 for a summary of the findings. Some patients randomized to receive the new low-cost treatment were inadvertently given the old treatment. The decision was made to analyze the data with an intention-to-treat protocol (ITT). The study reported the findings to be inconclusive. Which of the following statements is a possible explanation of the results?

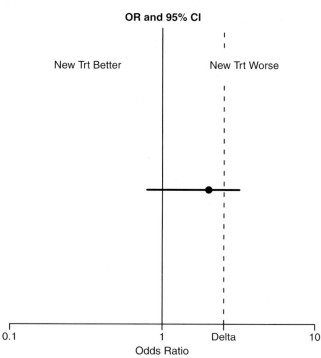

Figure Q41-13

(A) The study was underpowered to correctly determine noninferiority, resulting in a wide confidence interval

(B) The ITT analysis favored the inferiority hypothesis, resulting in a wide confidence interval

(C) Both A and B

(D) Neither A nor B

41.14 You are interpreting the results of a clinical trial that compared fibrinolysis with primary angioplasty for ST-segment elevation acute myocardial infarction. There were 6,600 patients randomly assigned to one of two treatments, with 3,300 patients in each group. If there were 300 deaths in the fibrinolysis group and 200 deaths in the PCI group, what is the OR that most appropriately compares the two groups?

(A) 0.065
(B) 0.10
(C) 0.65
(D) 9.1%

41.15 The results of a clinical study are provided in Table Q41-15. Your local formulary committee asks you to put this into clinical context and provide them the NNT with the new drug to prevent one myocardial infarction. The NNT is:

Table Q41-15.

	Placebo	Treatment	Total
MI	10	8	18
No MI	90	92	182
Total	100	100	200

(A) 0.02
(B) 0.50
(C) 42
(D) 50

41.16 Some of the ways to describe continuous data include:

(A) Medians
(B) Standard deviation
(C) Interquartile ranges
(D) None of the above
(E) All of the above

41.17 You are conducting a case–control study to compare the long-term efficacy of BMS and DES in your local catheterization laboratory. Looking through the database available, you find that patients are categorized based on the type of stent implanted. All patients had a follow-up exam 12 months following their index procedure, and the amount of restenosis in the artery was recorded. In conducting this case–control study, you use propensity scores to match each DES patient with a similar BMS patient. The matching is done to account for possible confounders, such as age, gender, BMI, etc.; see Figure Q41-17. Is this figure an appropriate way to visually compare these data?

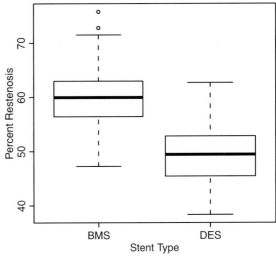

Figure Q41-17

(A) Yes
(B) No

41.18 A recently completed, randomized, active control clinical trial comparing new Drug A with old Drug B enrolled 10,000 patients. The sample size was chosen to maintain a Type I error rate of 0.05 and detect a meaningful difference with 80% power. The trial reported a 15% improvement with the new drug, $p = 0.06$. What is the most appropriate interpretation of these results?

(A) Drug A is statistically superior to Drug B
(B) Drug A is comparable to Drug B
(C) Drug A is definitely inferior to Drug B
(D) Drug A is not statistically superior to Drug B

41.19 Your colleague hypothesizes that the amount of restenosis 10 years following the implantation of a stent is associated with the BMI of the patient at the time of the PCI. Using a preexisting database from a clinical trial comparing two stents that measured a patient's BMI and other risk factors, he divides patients into two groups: those with a BMI >20 at the time of PCI and those with a BMI no more than 20 at the time of PCI. His analysis, summarized in Figure Q41-19, found little relationship between BMI and the amount of restenosis 10 years following PCI. He submits the article for publication. Which of the following is a possible response from a reviewer?

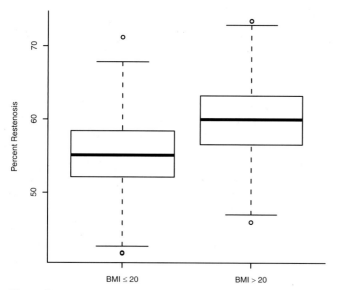

Figure Q41-19

(A) BMI should not be broken up into two arbitrarily defined categories, as this might mask the effect of BMI on restenosis

(B) The amount of restenosis is a categorical variable and therefore a boxplot is not an appropriate method of displaying the data

(C) When considering various groups based on a variable, you should consider at least 10 groups

(D) None of the above

41.20 As you read the medical literature, you note that p-values are variously reported as being significant at very different levels, including ones listed as <0.05 and others listed as <0.01. Which of the following is most helpful in interpreting the reported clinical data?

(A) "Lower is better"

(B) "Higher is better"

(C) Any p-value <0.05 is considered significant

(D) The pretest nominal p-value

41.1 **Answer D.** Clinical trials are typically designed and powered to answer one question, represented by the primary end point. Subgroups of patients, defined by patient characteristics (such as gender or age) or disease characteristics (such as the presence or absence of diabetes or other risk factors), are best viewed for consistency. If there is a positive treatment effect in favor of one therapy over another, there may well be *quantitative* differences (differences in the absolute treatment effect) in the magnitude of the observed treatment effect that favor certain subgroups, but it is unlikely that there will be important *qualitative* differences (treatment effect that is truly directionally different from the main result) among subgroups. The most appropriate way to view RCT results is from the perspective of the overall trial results.

41.2 **Answer C.** While RCTs are generally preferred to observational studies, the results of the trial should be generalizable to the patient of interest before making treatment decisions. In this case, the randomized trial was conducted solely in South Africa while the patient of interest is from the United States. Because of differences in patient characteristics, the result seen in the trial may not generalize to the patient of interest. If randomized trials including U.S. patients are available, these results should be considered prior to making a treatment decision. If such trials are not available, the results of the South African trial are likely more useful and reliable than the US-based observational study.

41.3 **Answer B.** The figure illustrates that Stent A appears to be associated with a lower revascularization rate, but it also appears to be associated with an increased mortality rate. Since Stent A has a different effect on each of the components of the composite, considering a composite end point with these two events would be inappropriate.

41.4 **Answer A.** The Framingham Heart Study is an example of a cohort study (*Am J Public Health* 1951;41:279–281). Patients are identified in a community and are followed for a long time, with periodic assessments to observe outcomes. Patients are examined as having some characteristic habits (e.g., smoking) and are defined as an "exposed" group. They may be compared with a "nonexposed" group to allow insight into the effects of exposure over time. There are no attempts to introduce an intervention in this study, either randomized or nonrandomized.

41.5 **Answer A.** The primary benefit of randomizing patients into treatment groups is that the groups are then "balanced" across other covariate information. This ensures that any associations we observe are due to the treatment under study and not to extraneous covariate differences (confounding). In the table, the data related to Study A appear to be balanced (similar between the two treatment groups), while in Study B, the characteristics differ between the groups. Notice that without knowing if the sample sizes are similar for the two studies, the balance only refers to the additional covariate information. Since the SYNTAX trial is a randomized study, it most likely corresponds to Study A.

41.6 **Answer C.** While the length of time required to enroll patients into the study is an important part of feasibility discussions and considerations, it does not affect the total number of patients required to adequately answer the question of interest. Calculation of sample size depends on multiple factors, including the Type I error rate, the Type II error rate, the end point to be analyzed, the estimated value for the end point occurring in the control arm, the estimated improvement in the treatment arm, the amount of variation in the end point measured, and the statistical method to be used in analyzing the end point. Sample size is also influenced by the decision to undertake a superiority, noninferiority, or equivalence trial.

41.7 **Answer C.** The survival curve for medically treated patients is shifted upward from that corresponding to patients undergoing PCI. Therefore, it is possible that the medical treatment is indeed reducing the risk of myocardial infarction. However, the inclusion of periprocedural MI in the end point definition will bias the results in favor of medical treatment. That is, since those patients undergoing medical treatment do not undergo a procedure, by definition, they cannot experience a periprocedural MI, and the survival probability for the PCI group will look worse at first (carry an early hazard). If periprocedural MI is not included in the end point, PCI might actually appear similar or even superior to the medical treatment. It is important to carefully consider the definition of an end point and the definition of the treatment under study when examining study results.

41.8 Answer B. The Type II error (β) occurs when no effect is seen between the studied treatments when in fact a treatment effect truly exists. One minus the Type II error ($1 - \beta$) is also known as the *trial's power*. By understanding the risk of a Type II error, or conversely, the importance of power in examining clinical trial results, one can appreciate whether a study actually had adequate power or was truly large enough in size to answer the desired question. Many studies that fail to show a statistical difference between therapies suffer from a lack of power; that is, the study design accepted a large potential Type II error (*Prog Cardiovasc Disc* 1985;27:335–371). By convention, a well-powered clinical trial accepts a potential β error of <10% to no more than 20%. In the example given, one would want to be sure that the planned trial had a minimum of 80% power (but preferably ≥90%) to definitively conclude that stent A was truly superior to stent B.

41.9 Answer C. We are interested in whether the CI falls below the bound (the minimally important difference or MID) for Drug A being no worse than Drug B. As therapies for acute cardiovascular disease proliferate, equivalence and noninferiority trials are becoming critical in assessing the therapeutic value of new drugs and devices. Noninferiority and equivalence trials are most useful when the experimental therapy is unlikely to prove superior to established therapy, but may provide incremental benefit. These benefits may include a reduction in adverse events, easier administration of the therapeutic agent, or reduced cost. For both noninferiority and equivalence studies, establishing the MID boundary is of primary importance, and the criteria for its establishment should be well described in the trial's methods.

41.10 Answer A. The case-control study is well suited for providing preliminary information on a question using previously collected data (*Circulation* 1996;93:667–671). Since you can identify patients who have experienced stent thrombosis and a matched group who have not, you should be able to get some preliminary information regarding the factors that are associated with the outcome. There are problems with the case-control study, most notably bias that arises from the data already collected before occurrence of the event. Randomized trials prove the overall best method of evaluating and comparing treatments, but such studies are much larger and take longer than is practical to provide some preliminary insight into your concerns.

41.11 Answer B. Observational studies do not randomize patients. As no attempts were made to account for the effect of possible confounders, we cannot make a strong causal interpretation of the results. It is possible that the difference observed is due to differences in the age of the patients receiving the different types of stent. For example, suppose all patients who received the new stent are older than those patients who did not; then, it is not possible to determine if the observed effect is due to the stent or the age of the patient. This is a limitation of observational studies. The use of analytical methods such as propensity scores to match patients is an example of how one might attempt to overcome this drawback by accounting for the effects of other confounders, such as age. This example demonstrates why RCTs are seen as the gold standard in the evaluation of new therapies. The randomization allows us to make causal links based on the results as the treatment groups are balanced (i.e., the same) except for the randomly assigned treatment.

41.12 Answer D. Blinding in a clinical trial can reduce the likelihood of biased behavior on the part of investigators, patients, or other study personnel. For example, knowledge of the treatment assignment might cause an investigator to look harder for certain drug effects, both expected and unexpected. For trials that include an independent assessment of the study's end point events, such as review by a clinical events committee, blinding is essential to maintain the integrity of a process that relies on a completely objective determination of suspected end point events (*Curr Control Trials CardiovascMed* 2001;2:180–186).

41.13 Answer C. When a study is underpowered, the resulting confidence intervals for an estimate are very wide. That is, it is difficult to detect whether a treatment is noninferior (or superior, depending on the context). In addition, ITT analyses are conservative in a superiority trial, but are not so in a noninferiority trial. Suppose that the new treatment is superior, the patients who incorrectly took the standard treatment will bias the estimated treatment effect in favor of the standard treatment. This will result in a wider confidence interval and can lead to inconclusive or even incorrect conclusions. In most trials that are testing first for superiority, the ITT analysis is the appropriate one; in a noninferiority test, it is frequently preferred to use a treatment received or even an on-treatment comparison for the most informative assessment.

41.14 **Answer C.** ORs and risk ratios are two of the more common ways to display comparative data in the medical literature. To calculate the odds of having an event in any one group, we divide the number of events in that group by the number of patients in that group who did not have an event. The OR is the ratio of those two odds. Risk is calculated by dividing the number of events by the total number of patients in a group. Risk ratios are then calculated by dividing the risks of the individual groups. In the example given, the odds of dying in the fibrinolysis group are 0.10 (300/3,000) and in the PCI group are 0.065 (200/3,100). This provides an OR of 0.65 (0.065/0.10).

41.15 **Answer D.** The NNT is defined as 1/(risk difference). The risk under placebo is 10% (10/100), and the risk under the treatment is 8% (8/100), giving a risk difference of 2%. To calculate NNT, we take 1/0.02 = 50.

41.16 **Answer E.** To describe continuous data (such as age or body weight), we can calculate measures of the center of the distribution. For example, the mean is the average of the measures and the median is the middle value, or 50th percentile, of the distribution. Measures of the variability around the center might be described as the range of the data (maximum value–minimum value), the standard deviation or variance, or the difference in the 25th and 75th percentiles (interquartile range or IQR).

41.17 **Answer B.** No, we cannot use the boxplots to compare the data. The existence of confounders has been accounted for by matching each DES patient to a similar BMS patient. However, this creates a correlation structure in the data.

That is, each matched pair is more similar to one another than to other patients in the sample. For example, suppose we recorded blood pressure on 10 individuals before and after a stress test. The two measurements taken on patient 1 will be more similar to one another than the measurements of patient 1 and patient 2. So, the data are not independent. When the data are correlated, other visual and statistical methods must be considered that account for this correlation.

41.18 **Answer D.** Trials that compare therapeutic strategies frequently are designed to test whether the new or experimental therapy is better than (superior to) a control therapy. The control therapy might be a placebo, or it might be an established therapy, often referred to as an active control. Sample size calculation for clinical trials requires that the investigator consider the acceptable Type I error. A Type I error is when an effect is observed when in truth no effect exists. This trial, as is convention (*Ann Epidemiol* 1998;8:351–357), set the Type I error rate at 5% (0.05). For example, if the same trial were conducted 1,000 times, then by chance alone, 50 studies would demonstrate the new treatment superior to the old treatment even if there were no true difference between the therapies. Nominal statistical significance requires the testing procedure to have a significance level less than or equal to the prospectively declared nominal level (0.05 in this case). However, *p*-values greater than this nominal level do not allow us to conclude that the new treatment is *definitely* worse than the old treatment. We can only conclude that the new drug is not statistically superior to the old drug. Despite how close the *p*-value is to the nominal level, we cannot conclude comparability without more information, such as a formal test for noninferiority based upon a predefined boundary of the MID.

41.19 **Answer A.** Continuous variables, such as age, BMI, and creatinine clearance, typically should not be broken into categories (called discretizing). This process discards potentially valuable information and can actually mask the effect. For example, suppose the relationship between BMI and the amount of restenosis was curved; then, by grouping patients based on an arbitrary cut point of BMI, it is possible to miss the underlying effect in the analysis.

41.20 **Answer D.** A *p*-value is the probability of obtaining the results (or even more extreme results) observed if the effect is really due to random chance alone. For example, a p-value of ≤ 0.05 indicates that a difference of at least the amount observed in the experiment would occur in ≤ 50 out of 1,000 similar experiments if the treatment studied had no effect on the measured outcome. Before conducting a clinical study, one must prospectively state the hypothesis being tested, the statistical test that will be used on this hypothesis (to reject the null hypothesis, meaning the rejection of the statement that there is no difference between the treatment groups), and the critical (or nominal) value for declaring significance (the Type I error rate). By convention, the nominal value for declaring significance in much medical research is set at 0.05. However, it is appropriate for certain types of studies to set a different level of nominal significance, for example at 0.025 or 0.001. The key concept is that the level of significance is determined by the pretest establishment of the Type I error (*Ann Epidemiol* 1998;8:351–357).

42 Approach to Interventional Boards and Test-Taking Strategies

Joseph D. Babb and Steven R. Daugherty

QUESTIONS

42.1 You have just finished reading through all of your study materials for the Board exam and you have some additional time before the date at which you are scheduled to take the exam. To make the best use of this remaining preparation time you should:

(A) Do as many practice questions as possible in the time you have left
(B) Do some practice questions and let the ones you get wrong tell you what to go back and study again
(C) Find and review new study material to give you an alternative perspective on the core concepts for the exam
(D) Read over your study materials again
(E) Take a break from study so you will be fresh for the exam itself

42.2 Once you gather the material you need to study for the Board exam, you are ready to start your preparation. After acquiring your study material for the Board exam you should organize your study plan to:

(A) Begin with the subject matter you know best to build your confidence
(B) Focus on doing practice questions
(C) Focus on the content you have heard is most important for the exam
(D) Map out how many pages of material you will cover each day
(E) Start by focusing on the content area where you are least confident

42.3 There is a lot of information to commit to memory for the Board exam. The most efficient way to commit critical study material to memory is to:

(A) Copy the details from your study material into a personal study notebook
(B) Do a lot of practice questions
(C) Organize the material into clusters
(D) Read over it repeatedly
(E) Talk it over with a friend or colleague

42.4 There is a lot of material to study for the Board exam, and many people feel some frustration at some point in the study process. When you feel frustrated in the middle of your study process, the best thing to do is:

(A) Find a different source to study from
(B) Shift to a different topic area
(C) Stop studying for the day and come back to look at the material the next day
(D) Take a 10-minute break from study
(E) Take a deep breath and focus your attention on the material before you

42.5 When answering questions during the Board exam, if you are able to eliminate all but two of the presented options, but cannot come up with a reason to select one or the other, the best strategy is to:

(A) Go back and re-read the questions to check for important details you might have missed
(B) Make an argument to yourself about why one, then the other, option must be right
(C) Read each option again and think about what it reminds you of
(D) Read each option again and think carefully about the exact wording
(E) Take a guess

507

42.6 Taking time to do practice questions is an important part of preparation for the Board exam. The best strategy for getting the most benefit out of practice questions is to:

(A) Do as many practice questions as you can from as many different sources as you can

(B) Focus on a particular set of questions and do them repeatedly until you get them all correct

(C) Save your practice questions until you have completed your study of content material

(D) Take your time when doing practice questions to give yourself a chance to think clearly about each one

(E) Use questions you get wrong to guide you as to what to go back and review again

42.7 In medical practice, experts often disagree as to the proper course of action in a given circumstance. When confronting a presented situation in an exam question where you know there may be some difference of opinion among practitioners in the field, the best way to decide on an answer is:

(A) Become familiar with clinical findings and research published in the last year

(B) Consider what you think most of the colleagues you know would do in a similar situation

(C) Select an answer based on existing practice guidelines

(D) Think about how you would handle the situation in your own practice

(E) Think back to the direction you received in handling similar situations when you were in residency and fellowship training

42.8 People have a lot of different advice as to how to best prepare for the Board exam. Some of this advice is good and some is not. Most people find that the best way to understand and remember important information for the Board exam is to:

(A) Focus on linking the material you study to real life patients you have encountered

(B) Rearrange study materials to focus on differences among concepts

(C) Re-read the details to reinforce their importance

(D) Try hard to remember the material exactly as it was presented

(E) Write everything out longhand in parallel with your study material

42.9 Preparation for the exam usually does not occur all at once, but in a series of study sessions across several weeks or months. The best thing to do at the end of each of these study session is to:

(A) Chart your progress in covering the material you will need to master for the exam

(B) Look ahead at the study material you have left for the specific topic you are studying

(C) Map out what you will study next

(D) Summarize for yourself the key concepts covered during your study session

(E) Think about something besides the study material to give yourself as mental break

42.10 To do well on the Board exam you have to apply the knowledge you have learned to the questions presented. During the actual exam, after first reading through the clinical information presented in the stem of a question, the next thing you should do is:

(A) Focus on the question at the end of the clinical case

(B) Go back over the presented content and check on relevant details

(C) Read down over the presented options to see what comes to mind

(D) Take a moment and think about the issues that the presentation brings to mind

(E) Try to connect what you have read to a real-life patient you have encountered

42.11 Practice questions are usually a part of everyone's preparation for the Board exam. The best way to integrate practice questions into the weeks and months of your study is to:

(A) Begin doing a few questions early and increase the number as the exam gets closer

(B) Don't limit practice questions to study time, but do them whenever you have a spare moment in your day

(C) Hold off doing practice questions until you have completed your content study

(D) Spend most of your study time on practice questions and reading the annotated answers

(E) Start your study by doing a lot of questions to guide you as to what to study

42.12 Different people need to take different amounts of time to prepare for the Board exam depending on their general familiarity with the material. The best way to decide how much time you need to take to prepare for your Board exam is to:

(A) Assume that you will need about 2 weeks of preparation for every year that you are out of my fellowship

(B) Begin preparation early to get a sense of what is familiar and your comfort with the material

(C) Check with people who took the exam in the past few years and see how long they took

(D) Decide how many pages of study material you can cover in a week and project the time needed to complete the material

(E) Take a practice exam and see how well you do

42.13 The way we learn should be different for different types of material and different kinds of tests. The best way to get ready for a multiple choice exam is to:

(A) Focus on memorizing important details just as they are presented in study materials

(B) Organize material in modules, and modules in clusters that emphasize differentiation

(C) Read your study material aloud to make sure you cover it all and to help with memorization

(D) Talk to colleagues who have taken the exam in the past and focus your study on the things that were featured prominently on their exam

(E) Write or type out explanations of important concepts in sentence form to get familiar with the essential details

42.14 Some of the material you have to learn for the Board exam will be relatively easy and simple memorization will suffice. Other material is more complex and will require more sophisticated techniques to master. When trying to master difficult or complex material for the Board exam, the best strategy is to:

(A) Block out time and sit studying the material until you have mastered it

(B) Focus on practice questions so you will know how it will appear on the exam

(C) Gather all the reference material you can on the subject and work your way through all of it

(D) Look at it for a little bit of time every day until you feel comfortable with it

(E) Skip it completely and hope that it will not account for much of the exam

42.15 For people who have recently completed a relevant fellowship prior to taking the Interventional Boards, the best suggestions for planning how to spend study time would be:

(A) Feel confident that your fellowship has given you exposure to the best and most recent information and work on maintaining confidence and getting well rested

(B) Organize a study group of colleagues who you know from your fellowship program

(C) Plan an extensive review based on notes and materials collected from the recently completed fellowship

(D) Select study material independent of your fellowship and organize your time for a complete review of all of it

(E) Wait to study until right before the exam so that your knowledge will be as fresh as possible

42.16 The best motto for helping yourself remember and understand the material at the level you will need for the Board exam is:

(A) Be consistent: Doing the same study procedures every day is the key to success

(B) Follow your nose: Trust your instincts as to what is important and what you need to learn

(C) Nose to the grindstone: Keep at it and do not stop until you have completed the task

(D) Repetition is best: Reading over material again is always a good use of time

(E) Variety is the spice of life: Doing different things with the material will give better results than getting stuck on one approach

42.17 In the week immediately leading up to the exam, the best strategy to maximize by performance on the exam would be to:

(A) Maintain my clinical schedule, but do as many practice questions as possible in the evening

(B) Maintain my clinical schedule, but meet with colleagues in the evening to have them grill me on essential concepts

(C) Stick with my regular professional routine to maintain the appropriate clinical perspective

(D) Take time off from clinical work and spend all the time possible in intensive reading and study

(E) Take time off from clinical work and spend the day alternating between doing practice questions and reviewing material as you decide you need to

42.18 Because the Board exam is a timed test, it is important to have a developed strategy for managing time over the course of the exam. For this exam, the best strategy to manage your time would be:

(A) Answer easy questions and very hard questions quickly so you will have the time to think about questions when you need it

(B) Go slow and concentrate in the beginning of the exam and pick up the pace if you find you run short of time

(C) Practice allocating time evenly and spending the same amount of time on each question

(D) Relax and proceed at a measured pace without focusing on the time issue

(E) Work as quickly as possible from the very beginning to be sure that there is enough time

42.19 When you feel short of time during the Board exam, the best strategy to pick up speed would be to read:

(A) The first line and the last line of the question stem and then move to the options

(B) The last line of the stem, the actual question, and take your best guess at an answer after looking at the options

(C) The presented options first so you will know what the key issues are as you read though the question stem

(D) Through the question stem carefully and spend just enough time on the presented options to make a decision

(E) Through the question stem quickly so you will have time to think about the answer options

42.20 Some people are concerned that the makeup of the board examination is unknown and obscure and this makes it difficult for them to study for the examination correctly. This concern is often heightened as they discover that few of their colleagues who have previously taken the examination have been helpful in telling them what questions were asked and what types of material was covered other than to say "everything." In the face of this uncertainty, the best strategy for getting a clear sense of what is tested on the Board exam is to:

(A) Buy a couple of large textbooks on interventional cardiology and read each one cover to cover, focusing on memorizing as much as possible

(B) Contact the College of Education at a local university for insight and advice on how to prepare for these examinations

(C) Hire an educational/testing consultant to assist you in preparation

(D) Rely on your developed clinical instincts as to what is most important and most likely to be tested

(E) Visit the ABIM Web site for guidance

42.21 The ABIM Web site states that "the examination will assess the candidate's knowledge and clinical judgment in aspects of interventional cardiology required to perform at a high level of competence." Since performing at a high level of competence demands current knowledge and good clinical judgment demands that you be aware of the latest thinking and trends, your best sources of information for studying will be:

(A) Controversies and debates at the most recent appropriate annual professional meetings

(B) Materials for a board review course run last year

(C) Recent ACCEL and other media releases

(D) Recent issues of major cardiovascular journals dealing with interventional cardiology

(E) Textbooks and practice guideline documents published at least 6 months before the exam

42.22 As you prepare for your exam, you run into a subject or issue that you are having a hard time understanding. The best way to deal with this would be:

(A) Stick with it until you get it no matter how long it takes

(B) Put the topic aside and come back to it after you have finished everything else

(C) Move on to another topic and come back to review the first topic the next time you study

(D) Skip it completely and move on to something else

(E) Seek different review materials that can make the topic clear to you

42.23 Sometimes what physicians do in practice and what the research suggests is best may be different. On the ABIM exam, the CORRECT answer will most likely be defined by:

(A) The consensus of actual practice by the physicians in the specialty

(B) What the leading physicians in the specialty are doing

(C) Standards set by the Institute of Health

(D) Historical standards for practice in the specialty

(E) The most recent peer-reviewed publications

42.24 When taking your exam, you read the question and are about to select an answer choice. At that moment, you remember something from your recent studies that suggests that the answer is different than that you are about to select. At this point, your best course of action would be to:

(A) Reread the question again to gain a fresh perspective
(B) Mark the answer you had selected first
(C) Move on to the next question and come back to sort it out later
(D) Mark the second answer as suggested by your studies
(E) Make a random choice between the two options you are considering

42.25 As you are studying for your exam, you find that you have a hard time remembering the names of some newer pharmacology options. The best way to help you remember these new options would be to:

(A) Think about the drug as one of set of options along with other similar drugs and focus on what sets it apart from the others
(B) Read the details about the drug over and over and over again until you can remember it
(C) Associate the drug with a patient you can remember from your own practice
(D) Associate the drug with the representative from the company who markets the drug
(E) Look up the fact sheet provided by the company that makes the drug and spend time reading over the provided material

42.26 Finding time to study for your exam in the middle of a busy professional practice and personal life can be difficult. The best way to organize your study time would be to:

(A) Block out one full day a week to study until you take the exam
(B) Keep study material with you and study any moment that you get
(C) Set aside the same time each day and commit yourself to using it for study
(D) Just focus on doing questions whenever you have a chance
(E) Focus on your practice and take a week off before the exam to do whatever study you need

42.27 On previous exams, you sometimes have felt yourself to be nervous, jumpy, and to have a hard time concentrating. For this exam, the best way to deal with these feelings would be to:

(A) Tell yourself that these reactions are not helpful and they need to stop
(B) Consider taking a 1-week course of bupropion just before the exam
(C) Stop thinking about what might happen during the exam and focus on your study and preparation
(D) Do several practice exams before the actual exam to become more accustomed to the exam situation
(E) Consider psychotherapy to address you exam reactions

42.28 Of all the material that you have to review for your exam, there is one topic that you just cannot stand. You do not deal with it during your clinical practice and really do not feel comfortable with the material. The best way to deal with this topic as you prepare for your exam would be to:

(A) Begin your studies with the topic
(B) Ignore the topic completely and study what makes more sense
(C) Find a colleague who can explain the details of the topic to you
(D) Focus on the topic right before the exam so it will be fresh in your mind
(E) Find as many questions as you can on the topic and do them all

42.29 You have been unhappy with one of the partners in your medical practice for some time. The week before you are scheduled to take your exam he/she does something that really annoys you. Your best course of action would be to:

(A) Sit down with the partner and talk about the most recent event that annoyed you
(B) Just ignore it for the time being
(C) Complain to a colleague, but avoid talking with the partner who annoys you
(D) Write down some things that you want to say to the partner, and then put them away until after the exam
(E) Sit down with the partner and talk about all of the things that you have found annoying over the years

42.1 **Answer B.** Do some practice questions and let the ones you get wrong tell you what to go back and study again. Questions benefit you in two ways. First, they give you experience in the behaviors and thought processes you need for the exam. Second, they can uncover weaknesses in your knowledge and understanding before the real exam. Your task is to take the information provided by questions you miss and do something about it. If you find you do not understand a concept, go back and look at it again. And do not just look at the exact issue you missed. If you missed one issue in a subject area, the odds are you have other weaknesses there are well. Just doing a lot of questions provided no real benefit. All you are doing is retesting yourself, but doing nothing to improve and increase your chances of success. Looking at brand new study material will simply expand the amount of material you have to master and likely result in you feeling confused or overloaded. Rereading repetitiously increases boredom, but does little to give you a better grasp or increased understanding of material. Replowing the same field over and over again does not give you a better crop. You have time to prepare more. The issue now is to move from simple repetition to something that will help direct your study efforts. Question guided study will do that.

42.2 **Answer E.** Start by focusing on the content area where you are least confident. Most people when they sit down to study like to spend the most time on the things that they already know fairly well. Although this might make you feel good, it does little to identify and correct deficits that should be the main goal of your exam preparation. Starting with the weakest subject assures that you will give it the time and attention it deserves. It is simply easier to bring your worst subject area to average than to try to make your best subject areas even better. Starting with what you know may make you feel good, but will not resolve essential difficulties you have. Doing practice questions too early is like hunting without ammunition. You have to have a good sense of the material already before practice questions can really guide your further review. Focusing on what others have told you can be dangerous. First, memory of exam takers is selective and

what people remember is often not a good representation of what was really on the exam. In addition, what was on the exam last year may not be your best guide as to what will be on the exam that you take. Trying to cover a set number of pages each day misses the fact that some content will be easy and some will be hard for you. You need to spend enough on a subject until you get it, but not waste on content you already know fairly well. Covering a set number of pages per day means you are not tailoring your study time to your specific needs.

42.3 **Answer C.** Organize the material into clusters. Our minds are not wired to learn lists, but classes of things. You must organize study to take advantage of this fact. Group like content together. What are key differentials? How will you decide when to choose among a select set of procedures or techniques? These are the questions you will be called upon to address on the exam. Organize your study to anticipate this. Copying details from your study material takes quite a bit of time and does not provide much return. Keeping things in the format of your study material does not render it in a form that has the most resonance with you and focusing on all the details risks having you overwhelmed by the weight of the particulars. Questions test what you know, but do not help you with the process of memorization. Rereading gets boring and eventually results in diminishing returns. Mechanically rereading means that you must cover a lot of material you already know just to uncover a few nuggets of new insight. Talking with a friend can really help you sort out and learn to articulate your understanding of difficult concepts, but memorization is an individual process done in private.

42.4 **Answer D.** Take a break from study. Nothing fuels frustration as much as to keep pushing on the thing that is frustrating you. You need to walk away briefly and take a mental break. When you return to the material you will find you have a different perspective and what was obscure before now makes sense. Changing to a different source risks increasing the volume of material you have to study and can result in overload. There is no reason that our break should be 24 hours. A short time way from the content is usually all it takes. Shifting topics can make your study schedule choppy, make it hard to track what you have and have not studied, and often means that you never do return to the point of frustration to clarify it and achieve resolution.

42.5 **Answer E.** If you are able to eliminate all but two options and you do not know which one to select, you have taken the questions as far as you can. You now have a 50% shot. Take it and run. It is time to guess and move on to the next question. Most people get <½ of these questions correct because they do one of several bad strategies. They reread the questions, which takes time and usually does not clarify. Making an argument usually means inventing a different question and losing track of exactly what it is you are supposed to answer. Reading each option again and reflecting usually causes you to think about things not anticipated by the questions writer. And looking carefully at the wording of options often causes you to over interpret simple wording and talk yourself out of a right answer. When you get to two and you are through, it is time to guess.

42.6 **Answer E.** Use questions you get wrong to guide you as to what to go back and review again. Questions test you, but do not teach you. The learning occurs when you respond to the deficit uncovered by the questions by fixing it. Usually this means returning to your primary study materials and reexamining the sections relevant to the question you just got incorrect. Doing a lot of questions from a lot of different sources will have you spend your time getting comfortable doing questions, but will not help you improve your score. Doing more questions without additional review simply gives a more reliable assessment of your current level of expertise. Doing the same questions over and over will help you to memorize those questions, but will not help you to learn the material in a way you will need for the new questions you will face on the board exam. Saving practice questions until the end of studying means you will not have the benefit of a reminder of what it is you are preparing for. You needed to be reminded of the task at hand to help you focus on what is essential rather than what is simply interesting. And because the exam is timed, you should do your practice questions under timed conditions to get used to the pressures of the exam. Doing well on the exam means not just being able to answer the questions, but being able to answer them within the given timeframe.

42.7 **Answer C.** Select an answer based on existing practice guidelines. Established practice guidelines represent the consensus of the best minds in the field. When question writers are constructing questions, they are very likely to use existing guidelines as templates for writing questions and as arbiters for what makes the best answer. The most recently published clinical work is likely to be too new and was not available when the questions for your exam were written. What everyone thinks is right is not always what objective research tells us is correct. Consider that questions writers are especially likely to write a question about a topic where what many practitioners actually do is not supported by the empirical research. When everyone knows the right thing to do, it simply does not make a very good question. And keep in mind that the field is constantly undergoing changes. What was state-of-the-art several years ago may not be so today. In residency, the right answer is whatever your current attending physician says it is. On the Board exam, the right answer is what the committee of experts relying on empirical research says that it is.

42.8 **Answer B.** Rearrange study materials to focus on differences among concepts. This is one of the most important issues for efficient study. Your task on a multiple choice exam is to select among presented options. To do your best, you need to study the same way. Focus on learning sets options and then how to choose among those options. Learning all the details of something will not be nearly as useful as knowing what clinical detail makes one option better than another. Differential diagnosis should be your template. You need to be able to do more than recognize a patient with a certain condition. You need to be able to tell yourself why it is that condition and not something similar. The same logic holds for choosing among procedures, techniques, and patient management options. Real life cases may not offer the type of choices you will be given on the actual exam. Rereading and remembering something exactly as they are presented helps memorize the text but does not give you an understanding of the material in your own words and on your own terms. Material memorized does not help you decide. Material you have organized in your head for that purpose does. And writing everything out longhand just takes too much time given the amount of material you have to master for your exam.

42.9 **Answer D.** Summarize for yourself the key concepts covered during your study session. A quick mental review of what you have covered is the best way to get closure for your study session, to facilitate remembering key concepts, and forcing you to think about things in your own terms rather than just mimicking the words you have studied. Focusing on where you are in your progress tends to make the task seem longer. Each time you focus on looking ahead you risk your inner child asking, "Are we there yet?" Before you look ahead, be sure of what you have just covered. Looking ahead to the next topic can make it hard to concentrate on and retain the current issues under study. And at the end of your study session, you will have a mental break as you move on to other things in your life. Just be sure to summarize and reinforce what you have just done before moving on.

42.10 **Answer A.** Focus on the question at the end of the clinical case. One of the most common, and avoidable, mistakes on a multiple choice exam is to answer the questions you wanted or expected rather than the one you were actually asked. This error costs otherwise well prepared people valuable points they deserve to have. After reading the case, you must pay careful attention to what it is that has been asked about the case. Learn this when you are doing your practice questions and you will not make the mistake during the real exam when it counts. Going back over the case takes time you do not have. You must get key information on the first reading. Looking at options before you focus on the question is really putting the "cart before the horse." Without the guidance of the questions, options tend to only confuse you. And thinking in general or about a real life patient takes you away from that matter at hand. Focus on the questions asked and let your thinking be about that!

42.11 **Answer A.** Begin doing a few questions early and increase the number as the exam gets closer. Questions are the target that you are in training to hit. You need to be reminded of why you are studying. Start doing practice questions, just a few, early in you study. As you progress through the material, day by day you can increase the number of questions you do and the time you spend reviewing them. Do not do questions haphazardly in spare moments, but keep your practice as close as you can to the real exam situation. This means questions should be done in cluster and with a clock. Do a set of questions before looking up the answer to any

one question. But also remember that questions themselves will not get you where you need to be. The hard work of study is how you learn what you need to learn. Questions just help you refine your knowledge and gain perspective on how an issue might be approached on an exam question. Study is first. Questions are second. Just do not leave them until the end.

42.12 **Answer B.** Begin preparation early to get a sense of what is familiar and your comfort with the material. One size does not fit all. There is no magic number of days, weeks, or months required to prepare for the exam. You simply need to make sure that you have the time that *you* need, which may be different than that of other people. By starting early you will ensure that you have the time if you need it, and will be able to get a real concrete sense of how familiar or unfamiliar the material might be. The key is not to adopt some formula like a set number of weeks or a certain number of pages per day, but to select a solution and study schedule that meets your particular needs. A practice exam is always a nice idea, if possible, and can pinpoint areas of weakness, but it cannot tell you how long you, personally, need to prepare. When are you ready to take the exam? When you get it! You should be at the level of being able to argue and explain the material to others. Most people have pretty good gut instinct as to when they have reached this level.

42.13 **Answer B.** Organize material in modules and modules in clusters that emphasize differentiation. The two most important issues for study are to organize the material in a way that makes sense to you, and make sure you focus on being able to make choices among presented options. If you can lay out everything that is known about a procedure or a technique, this will not help you. You will not be asked to lay out everything you know. Instead, you will have to be able to say why "this" and not "that." Details that help you make these kinds of decisions are essential. Details that do not are mere knowledge ornamentation with no value for improving your exam performance. Not all the details matter. Everything in your study material is not important. Make choices and focus on what matters. Review courses help you with this, but you can also give yourself guidance by remembering the type of decisions the exam will ask you to make. Reading aloud is a good way to reinforce memory regarding difficult concepts, but simply takes too long given the body of material you have to master, nor does reading someone else's words help to get concepts framed in the way that makes the most sense to you. Studying what was on the exam last year can be a recipe for disaster. Board exams tend to shift content year to year. Study for *this* exam, not for the one last year. Outlines and tales showing similarities and difference among concepts are much better choices than writing out content in full sentences.

42.14 **Answer D.** Look at it for a little bit of time every day until you feel comfortable with it. Sequential study sessions over a period of days are by far the most effective and efficient way to master complex materials. Learning theory tells us that "Spaced practice is better than massed practice," which means that sitting and trying to grasp content all at once is not nearly as effective as looking at it repeatedly over time. Trying to get it all in one day is a residual of the days when you had to cram for an exam in only a day or two. Preparing for the Board exam is different. You will be studying over weeks and months and have the time to take the time when you need it. Practice questions are an excellent vehicle to get you to think about the exam and to break you from the monotony of rote rereading of material, but they will likely not show you the material just as you will encounter it on the exam. Most people walk out of the exam surprised that although practice questions do cover much of the same information as on the exam, they do so in a different, and sometimes, surprising way. You cannot anticipate all the questions, but you can arm yourself with the information you need and train yourself to be able to think with it and solve whatever problem you are presented with. Gathering all the reference material available is a sure way to end up overloaded and overwhelmed. Do not skip over complex material. Complex material is more likely than easier material to be the source of questions. Take the time you need, look at it repeatedly, and you will find you are able to master what you could not master before.

42.15 **Answer D.** No matter how well known and structured the program and how compulsive the fellow, it is unlikely that any program will impart all of the possible testable knowledge in an ABIM examination. In each program or curriculum, there is an intended curriculum (objectives, examination blueprint, etc.) and an informal curriculum (content emphasized during lectures and small group discussions, etc.) (McLaughlin K, Codere S, Woloschuk W, et al., *BMC Education* 2005;5:69). Frequently it is the informal curriculum that flavors a trainee's data retention and clinical practice patterns. The examiners for the ABIM-sponsored examinations are focused on assessing core knowledge of generally accepted practice standards, however. Therefore, it is important to recognize that the examiners' perception of core knowledge may not be consonant with the exam takers experience with an informal curriculum. All programs have strengths and weaknesses, and it is the latter components in which it is particularly important to study and increase one's knowledge. A casual attitude of preparation is likely to lead to disappointing results in testing.

42.16 **Answer E.** Variety is the spice of life: Doing different things with the material will give better results than getting stuck on one approach. Effective study requires a series of steps in which you do different things with the material as your familiarity with it changes. Step 1 is to decide what you will study. Step 2 requires repetition and reading over the essential material. Step 3 requires fostering recall by doing something active with the material such as making outlines, drawing pictures, talking to yourself about it, or talking with others. Step 4 moves on to practice using the material as you focus on practice questions. Doing the exact same things every day does not makes sense as your understanding changes and improves. Following your instincts will likely have you study what you like, but avoid what you hate. You need guidance as to what to study beyond your personal preferences. Pushing on for weeks at a time without a break is emotionally damaging and cognitively ineffective. Schedule some pauses in your study. You will come back to it fresher, with more insight, and more motivation. Re-reading helps to get content into your head, but does not help you get it out when you need it. At some point, you need to change from repetition to active processes that promote recall.

42.17 **Answer E.** Take time off from clinical work and spend the day alternating between doing practice questions and reviewing material as you decide you need to. The Board exam will require different mental processes and a different perspective than daily clinical work. Taking a break from your clinical duties will aid you in making this transition. It will also help to ensure that you do not walk into the exam sleep deprived by giving up sleep in order to try to do your usual work and your exam preparation at the same time. When you take time off, do not spend every waking moment in preparation. Instead, set up each day like a job, put in the time you planned, and then stop and allow yourself some down time to relax.

42.18 **Answer A.** Answer easy questions and very hard questions quickly so you will have the time to think about questions when you need it. The essential notion here is to have the time when you need it by not wasting it on difficult questions you do not know or lingering over easy questions when the answer is obvious to you. Going slow and focusing on concentration will result in you having too little time at the end. Not all questions take the same amount of time. Spend just what is needed on each one and then move on. If you do not think about time at all, you will be ambushed by a shortage of time at the end of the exam period. The trick is to track the time without being panicked by the ticking of the clock. Working as quickly as possible makes most people feel rushed and unable to have that moment of reflection that makes the difference. Questions will require you to think. You need to move efficiently through the exam. But not at the expense of giving up applying your intelligence and thinking through to the best answer.

42.19 **Answer D.** Read though the question stem carefully and spend just enough time on the presented options to make a decision. The question stem is your friend. It must, by the rules, give you everything that you need to analyze the question and come up with the best answer. The options are the enemy. Their task is to confuse you and con you into picking the wrong answer. Time spent reading the question is time well spent. Focus on reading what is presented and thinking about the issues involved. Spend as little time on the options as possible. Make a choice and move on! Skipping over parts of the question stem is a high-risk strategy. It may work for you sometimes, but usually, you will miss some key detail or some essential clue, and therefore, not converge on the keyed answer. We all tend to like the options because options are the way out of the question. But be careful. Getting to the options before reading and processing the clues given in the question is essentially hunting in the dark. You will pick an option and get out

of the questions all right. But, you are unlikely to get the right option that gives you the point and improves your chances of passing.

42.20 **Answer E.** To get specific information about the exam you are preparing for, go right to the source. An educational consultant or the local College of Education at the university will provide useful information about the broad field of study techniques, improving data retention, and the like. They will not be knowledgeable about the structure of the ABIM CAQ in Interventional Cardiology, however. Knowing that structure can help you target your preparation better. It is available at the ABIM Web site (www.abim.org) and currently has a Web address of www.abim.org/cert/aqic.shtm. The primary content areas and their relative proportions on the examination as of April 2006 are:

Table A42-20.

Content Area	Relative Proportion (%)
Case selection and management	25
Procedural technique	25
Basic science	15
Pharmacology	15
Imaging	15
Miscellaneous	5

The Web site provides additional information as to what the specific contents are within each of these broad areas. Merging this information with your own awareness of strengths and weaknesses in your own knowledge base allows you to tailor your study, spending more time on relatively weaker areas of knowledge and slightly less in areas of greater proficiency.

42.21 **Answer E.** Board questions are focused on core knowledge required to support excellent clinical judgment. As such, the boards do not examine on the latest and greatest theories, ideas, and personal opinions of interventional thought leaders. Guidelines documents are a rich source of information as they are robust, amply referenced, and based on levels of evidence. Since they are evidence based, they provide a rich source of potential examination material with "single best answers." Textbooks are also excellent sources of information but this information is often a bit more dated. Nonetheless, such information is often highly relevant and "testable". Remember that the board questions are written, vetted, and "put to bed" several months before the actual examination. The ABIM has never given an exact cut-off date for inclusion of information in the examination, but a general time frame of 6 to 9 months pre-examination has been suggested as reasonable. Data more recent than that is not felt to be widely enough known, disseminated, and incorporated to provide valid test material. Also, the controversies or debates at large annual meeting, recent reports and opinions for interventional cardiology leaders, and other such opinion-based material is not the core information used for ABIM testing. Board review courses are rich sources of information for preparation as they are focused on core knowledge and not the latest, hottest new topics.

42.22 Answer C. Moving on and then coming back helps to avoid frustration and helps to guarantee that you will not neglect the topic. Content that many people find difficult is especially likely to be on your test. Neglecting the topic means you are taking a risk with your score. On the other hand, staying with the topic while frustration builds is unlikely to be productive. When you come back to a topic, you do so with fresh eyes, and that which made no sense before is very likely to be clearer the second or third time. Seeking new sources for study can be productive if your basic study material is inadequate. But seeking an alternative on a regular basis simply multiples your study material and increases the burden of preparation. When you want to understand a topic and have good recall, multiple exposures, over time, maximizes what you will gain for your effort.

42.23 Answer E. One of the aims of this certification exam is to be sure you are abreast of current medical knowledge. Medicine and the standards for good practice do not stand still. What might have been the best practice yesterday may not be today. The best physicians change what they do as medical knowledge changes. It takes a while for physicians to change their habits, so what everyone around you is doing may not actually be the best practice, and therefore, not the best answer on your exam. The Institutes of Medicine or medical specialty societies may set forth practice guidelines from time to time. You may even be asked to participate in this process. But, these guidelines are based on the best knowledge available, which means concrete evidence as presented in publication that were able to stand the test of peer review. The best answer on your exam is not what everyone does, but what everyone ought to do, based on the most current knowledge.

42.24 Answer D. In spite of what has become common wisdom, your first impulse is not necessarily your best answer. Research has shown us that changing your mind when new information occurs increases your score when compared to always sticking to the first answer that occurs to you. This is different from second guessing yourself or simply having doubts. In those instances, your first instinct is likely your best. But when you are thinking about a problem and new information occurs to you, that new information is likely useful and your response should change accordingly. Note that moving away from the question and coming back later interrupts the thought process in which you were engaged. When you come back, you must reengage the question and repeat the thought process all over again.

42.25 Answer A. Comparing the drugs with other options creates an anchor for the new information and fosters retention. Remember that our brains are basically lazy and retain information only if we are going to use it or if it connected to other information of value. By thinking about how these new drugs are similar to and different than the pharmacology you already know, you have placed the drugs in a content from which they are easier to recall. Reading about the drugs over and over again is an exercise in brute memory. This type of memory is short term and the information is easily forgotten when you move on to something else. Linking the drug to a patient is only useful if the exam presents to you the same type of patient and you have some actual experience using the drug. Thinking about the pharmacy representative removes you from the clinical thought process the exam question will require of you when thinking about the drug on an exam question.

42.26 Answer C. Learning is most efficient when it occurs regularly over time. Having study time as a part of your routine makes it less likely that you will forget to put the time in or be distracted by something else. Blocking out one day a week can be difficult in the face of clinical practice demands and can create as feeling that too much has to be accomplished on this day. Trying to study every spare moment can be fatiguing and can distract you from clinical and personal life demands. Questions are a great way to self-evaluate and get guidance for future study, but do not by themselves give you the overview and content you need to make sense of material. Waiting until the last week before the exam to study may mean that you do not have enough time to really prepare and is unlikely to allow you to reflect on and think about the material as you study.

42.27 **Answer D.** Familiarity tends to lessen anxiety. Spending time in practice situations will help you have more emotional control during the exam when it matters. This process has the added benefit of providing the questions which you get wrong to give you guidance as to what you should study as your exam preparation moves forward. Telling yourself to not have your emotional reactions is rarely effective. Our cognitive processes can influence, but often have little control over our emotional reactions. Self-medication is never a good idea and when the trigger for anxiety is situational rather than systemic, general antianxiety medications are not the answer. Trying not to think about something that is a worry for you often enhances, rather than suppresses, our emotional reaction. The reaction you have is real and cannot simply be ignored. Finally, having some nervousness during exams is relatively normal and does not suggest the need for psychotherapy. Remember that getting nervous during exams is normal. The issue is to get used to the situation so anxiety does not rise to the level of becoming a problem.

42.28 **Answer A.** We all have material we do not like and do not want to study. The best way to tackle this material is to get it out of the way early. If you put it off, you will likely find that you never really have time to get to it and your score will suffer correspondingly. If you are going to run the race, tackle the big hill at the start of the race; do not wait and let it defeat you at the end of the process. Getting a colleague to talk to you about the topic may prove difficult. If you do not deal with these issues in your own practice, you may not know who to approach. Even if you do find someone, just because they can explain it to you does not mean that you will gain the understanding you need. You need to make the content yours, which means getting an understanding in ways that make sense to you. Doing questions will confirm that you do not know the topic, but will not teach it to you. Start with the hardest stuff first in your study. This will give you the time you need to master it. And once you have mastered the hard stuff, the rest is (literally!) easy.

42.29 **Answer D.** This partner has been annoying for a long time. Talking to them about what you find annoying is likely to require more than one conversation and may well involve some level of emotional exchange. All of this is a distraction as you are trying to focus on your coming exam. On the other hand, just ignoring it is often ineffective. Interpersonal annoyances tend to grab our attention and make it hard to focus on something else. Complaining to a colleague may help you vent your frustration, but also risks setting of a chain of events that will call for your attention over the next few days. Writing down what you have to say lets you vent some of your feelings and help you move beyond the annoyance for the moment. This technique also has the benefit of helping you think through what you really want to say to your partner after you sit for your exam.